THE WRIST

THE WRIST

Julio Taleisnik, M.D.

Assistant Clinical Professor of Orthopaedic Surgery
University of California, Irvine
California College of Medicine
Irvine, California

CHURCHILL LIVINGSTONE
NEW YORK, EDINBURGH, LONDON, AND MELBOURNE 1985

Acquisitions editor: *Toni M. Tracy*
Copy editor: *Ann Ruzycka*
Production designer: *Karen Goldsmith Montanez*
Production supervisor: *Sharon Tuder*
Compositor: *Progressive Typographers, Inc.*
Printer/Binder: *Halliday Lithograph*

Distributed in the United Kingdom by Churchill Livingstone, Robert Stevenson House, 1-3 Baxter's Place, Leith Walk, Edinburgh EH1 3AF and by associated companies, branches and representatives throughout the world.

First published 1985

Printed in USA

ISBN 0-443-08134-4

9 8 7 6 5 4 3 2 1

Library of Congress Cataloging in Publication Data

Taleisnik, Julio
  The wrist.

  Includes bibliographies and index.
    1. Wrist — Wounds and injuries.   2. Wrist — Surgery.
  3. Rheumatoid arthritis — Surgery.   I. Title.
  [DNLM: 1. Arthritis, Rheumatoid.   2. Joint Instability.
  3. Wrist.   4. Wrist Injuries.   WE 830 T123w]
  RD559.T35   1985   617′.574   85-13264
  ISBN 0-443-08134-4

Manufactured in the United States of America

To Chela

Foreword

To surgeons dealing with impaired function of the hand the key joint in controlling digital motion has always been the wrist. For this reason maintenance of a good range of motion and avoidance of ankylosing procedures were taught as basic principles in reconstructive surgery of the hand. In the past, when disease or injury to the wrist components themselves resulted in pain or restricted motion and the whole hand suffered, our knowledge of anatomy and function and the means available for relief were much limited. Now, with the aid of studies such as those reported here, we can utilize better methods of diagnosis and treatment of this most important joint.

Because of the complex nature, the multiple parts, and the almost infinite number of motions possible in this intercalary joint, locating the causes of impairment is difficult. One needs a detailed knowledge of the static and the dynamic anatomy of this region and an understanding of the response of its tissues to normal use, to the forces of trauma, and to the results of disease in order to interpret the results of arthrographic, cineradiographic, and scanning techniques. Although x-rays have been used since Roentgen's discovery, it is only in recent years that newer techniques have given us a better understanding of wrist function.

Many of the relevant findings contributing to our current views have been published in less widely read journals and are thus lost to those who chauvinistically refer to the "literature" as those works written only in their mother tongue. Fortunately in this volume we can find the substance of such studies given the rightful place in the development of our present knowledge. These thorough reviews are combined with the results of the author's own studies and those of colleagues to allow the logical development of a consistent system of treatment.

Bringing together all this information makes it now possible for many to understand the pathomechanics of this most important joint. Dr. Taleisnik's skill in anatomy and orthopedics, his concentration on surgery of the upper extremity, particularly the wrist, and his multilingual capability have resulted in a book that will be regarded as a classic in its field.

Joseph H. Boyes, M.D., F.A.C.S., F.R.C.S.Ed., F.R.A.C.S.

Preface

In the year 1900 Lewis A. Stimson, in the third edition of his treatise on fractures and dislocations, devoted less than one page to the wrist. His opening statement proclaimed that "simple fractures of the carpal bones appear to be rare. Only a few cases have been reported in which the nature of the injury was shown by direct examination." This was 5 years after the discovery of x-rays by Wilhelm Roentgen and four years after Etienne Destot began a radiographic study of the wrist, which was first published in 1923. Destot's treatise, "Traumatismes du Poignet et Rayon X," is a classic and the culmination of an era of brilliant clinical and experimental studies of the wrist, also represented by the works of Fick, Navarro, Jeanne, Mouchet, Bryce, Tavernier, Testut, Poirier, Johnston, von Mayersbach, and a few others whose names will become familiar to the readers of this book. Much was learned from these investigators, although the painful wrist, particularly when accompanied by few, if any, clinical or radiographic findings, remained an enigma. Even today, many wrist problems are still labeled as sprains, in spite of Punch's admonition, quoted by Todd in 1921: "to those about to diagnose sprained wrist — don't."

The past 15 years have witnessed a resurgence of interest in wrist anatomy, biomechanics, diagnosis, and treatment. During its first 5 years of existence, the *Journal of Hand Surgery* published 52 articles and letters dealing with the wrist. During the following 3 years, from 1980 to 1983, 77 additional papers were published. Articles dealing with the wrist were second in frequency only to those on finger and tendon injuries. It is this surge of interest that justifies the publication of this book. Dr. Joseph H. Boyes greatly influenced my decision to make this a single-author text. I am indebted to Dr. Boyes for this, as well as for his encouragement in continuing my studies of the wrist, and for his help in proofreading and correcting the manuscripts.

I did not intend this book to be a definitive study of the wrist. It simply provides information that has served me well in understanding and treating wrist problems. I hope that this text will be useful as an introduction to the subject and as a foundation for future work. It is intended for the general orthopedist and the orthopedic resident. A thorough review of the literature is included for each subject. In deference to historical accuracy, recognition is given to the work of early investigators which was often not appreciated, or was quickly forgotten.

There are many repetitions of concepts and techniques throughout the text. This was done so that each chapter represents the complete source of information for the treatment of a specific problem. The first five chapters review the basic concepts of anatomy, biomechanics, and radiography that have been so helpful in the interpretation of wrist injuries and disease. Chapters 6 through 9 deal with carpal fractures, including Kienböck's disease, and with carpal and radiocarpal dislocations and fracture-dislocations. Chapters 10 through 13 are entirely devoted to a relative newcomer to the field of wrist injuries, carpal instability. The final chapters include a review of rheumatoid arthritis and of the soft tissue, joint, and bone procedures commonly utilized in its treatment.

When I first decided to take on this project, I did not envision the tremendous investment in time that it would represent. This time had to be carved out of a busy schedule, and of the time that was previously shared with family, friends, and associates. Without their understanding, support, and cooperation this book would not have been possible.

Julio Taleisnik

Contents

1. The Bones of the Wrist   **1**

2. The Ligaments of the Wrist   **13**

3. Carpal Kinematics   **39**

4. The Vascular Anatomy of the Wrist   **51**

5. Radiographic Examination of the Wrist   **79**

6. Fractures of the Scaphoid   **105**

7. Isolated Injuries to Carpal Bones Other Than Scaphoid and Lunate   **149**

8. Kienböck's Disease   **169**

9. Dislocations and Fracture-Dislocations of the Carpus   **195**

10. Classification of Carpal Instability   **229**

11. Scapholunate Dissociation   **239**

12. Medial Carpal Instability   **281**

13. Proximal Carpal Instability   **305**

14. Rheumatoid Arthritis of the Wrist   **327**

15. Surgery for the Rheumatoid Wrist: Indications and Timing   **329**

16. Evaluation of the Rheumatoid Wrist   **335**

17. Mechanism of Wrist Deformity in Rheumatoid Arthritis   **357**

18. Treatment: Soft Tissue Procedures   **365**

19. Treatment: Bone and Joint Procedures   **387**

20. The Distal Ulna in the Wrist with Rheumatoid Arthritis   **421**

Index   **437**

1 The Bones of the Wrist

Wrist, from the old teutonic "wraestan": to twist.[7]

Wrist, from the Old English and German "rist": back of hand.[27]

Carpus, from the Greek "karpos": wrist. Found in the writings of Galen.[30]

The wrist is a complex joint; it includes the multiple bones and articulations of the carpus, the distal radius, and the structures contained within the ulnocarpal space (Figs.1-1 and 1-2). The inferior radioulnar joint should probably be excluded,[5] since it is a part of the forearm functional complex. Jeanne and Mouchet[11] defined the wrist as a unit composed of the carpus and the distal radius, from where the radius "starts to enlarge in order to supply an articular plateau and where the origin of the anterior border of the styloid process appears." In practice, it corresponds to a line passing 3 cm proximal to the radiocarpal space. Essentially the same approach was adopted by Destot,[6] placing the proximal limit of the wrist at "about 33 mm above the radiocarpal space" based on the frequency of fractures of the distal radius within this boundary. This proximal limit need not be precisely defined. It should be determined on functional rather than on anatomic or radiologic grounds. Injuries to the distal radius, even if extraarticular, are considered wrist injuries when they directly interfere with wrist function. Distally, the wrist ends at the carpometacarpal joint level.[11] The proximal surface of the carpus is an oblong condyle articulating with the composite surface of the radius and triangular fibrocartilage. The palmar surface is concave, and constitutes the floor and walls of the carpal canal (Fig. 1-3).

THE CARPAL BONES

The initial recognition of the carpus as an anatomic entity has been attributed to Andreas Vesalius.[33] In the first edition of his monumental work *De Humani Corporis Fabrica* (1543) Vesalius identified all the carpal bones and numbered each, beginning with the scaphoid and ending with the hamate. More than a century later, Michael Lyser first proposed proper names for each carpal bone, but these terms were not used until Alexander Monro published his *Anatomy of the Humane Bones* in 1726.[13,23] The present official nomenclature for the human carpus was established in 1955, a revised version of the Birmingham Revision (1933) of the *Basle Nomina Anatomica* (1895).[2]

Most modern reptiles and mammals have eight carpal bones. Napier points out that in certain orders reductions and fusions have taken place, and he specifically mentions a single scapholunate bone in carnivores.[24] The human carpus is not, however, a mere relic of an earlier ancestral configuration[5]; this arrangement of several multifaceted bones is a superb solution to the need for mobility and stability in the human being. From a purely descriptive standpoint carpal bones are arranged in two rows of four bones each. With the exception of humans and some African apes, the proximal carpal

1

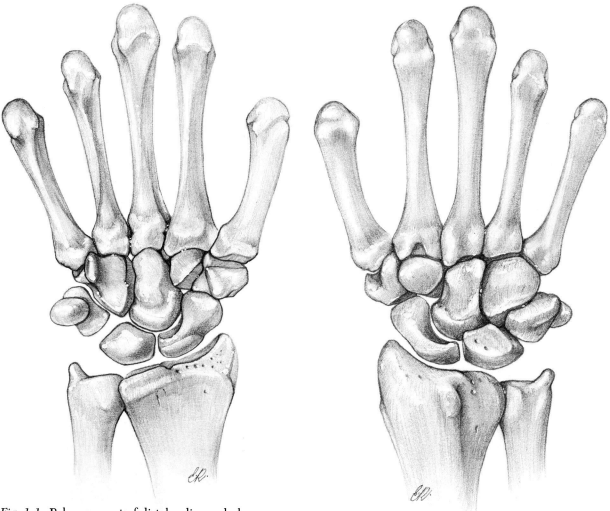

Fig. 1-1. Palmar aspect of distal radius and ulna, carpus and metacarpals.

Fig. 1-2. Dorsal aspect of distal radius and ulna, carpus and metacarpals.

row in primates includes one extra bone, the os centrale. In the human embryo the os centrale appears in the sixth week of gestation and fuses with the scaphoid in the eighth, remaining only as a small irregular prominence[4] (Fig. 1-4). Bogart[3] and Jones[13] have reported that in some wrists the os centrale degenerates into a fibrous structure represented in the adult carpus by an "inconsiderable ligament" present between scaphoid and capitate. When this occurs, radiographs may demonstrate an open space between capitate and hamate (Fig. 1-5). Painful clicking of the wrist during motion has been attributed to the persistence of a mobile cartilaginous os centrale in a patient with such

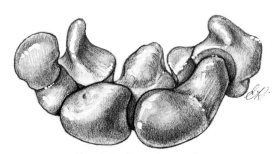

Fig. 1-3. Carpal tunnel.

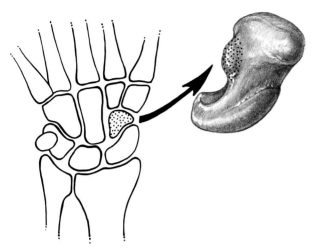

Fig. 1-4. Os centrale: appears in the 6th week of gestation, fuses with the scaphoid in the 8th. It remains as a small irregular prominence in the adult scaphoid.

a wide scaphocapitate space.[28] The scaphoid, lunate, triquetrum, and pisiform form the proximal carpal row, and the trapezium, trapezoid, capitate, and hamate form the distal carpal row.

The Scaphoid

The *scaphoid* is a bridge or rod across the lunocapitate (midcarpal) joint (Figs. 1-1, 1-2). Most of its surface is covered by hyaline cartilage for articulation with the radius, the trapezium and trapezoid, and the lunate and capitate. The facet for the radius is the largest, occupying the entire proximal pole. The articular surface of the distal pole is divided by a superficial ridge into two facets, one for the trapezium and the other for the trapezoid. The direction of this ridge, from dorsal and radial to volar and ulnar, coincides with the maximum plane of wrist motion and corresponds to the joint space between the trapezium and the trapezoid. The medial facet is actually composed of two surfaces, one distally for the head of the capitate and the other a more proximal, very small, semilunar facet for articulation with the lunate. The extreme volar portion of the facet for the lunate contains a shallow fossa for the insertion of the radioscapholunate ligament. The nonarticular surface is narrow, and is commonly referred to as the waist of the scaphoid (Fig. 1-6). It twists around the bone, mostly on the lateral aspect, directly opposite the facet for the capitate. It ends at a large distal pole, the tubercle of the scaphoid, onto which the transverse carpal ligament and the palmar intrinsic and radiocarpal ligaments are inserted.[31] In the narrow waist or groove are numerous foramina for blood vessels. It is also the site of attachment for important ligaments and capsules.

The Lunate

On the lateral aspect of the lunate is an articular surface containing a small shallow fossa for the insertion of the radioscapholunate ligament.[15,31,32] The medial facet of the lunate for articulation with the triquetrum is much larger than the scaphoid facet and more rectangular in shape. Antuña Zapico,[1] in an exhaustive morphologic study of 100 lunate specimens, observed that, when viewed from their volar aspect, some lunates were largely rectangular, whereas in other cases proximal (radial) and medial (triquetral) surfaces joined into a peak or apex, giving the lunate a conical shape. He proposed an "angle of inclination" as an expression of these morphologic changes. The angle is drawn between lateral (scaphoid) and proximal (radial) surfaces (Fig. 1-7). Based on the values of the angle, Antuña Zapico classified lunates into three types. In type I, the angle of inclination was 130 degrees or more; this was found in 30 percent of his specimens. Type II presented an angle of inclination of approximately 100 degrees, and was the most common variety; it was seen in 50 percent of the specimens. Type III occurred least frequently, with a proximal articular surface of the lunate with two distinct facets, one for the radius and the other opposite the triangular fibrocartilage; this was present in 18 percent of his specimens. The larger the angle of inclination, the shorter the lunate facet for the scaphoid. Antuña Zapico further observed that in both volar and dorsal surfaces the perforations or vascular foramina concentrated predominantly in proximal triangular areas. These anatomic characteristics may be important in the pathogenesis of Kienböck's disease (see Chapter 8). In sagittal sections the lunate is wedge-shaped, the height of its volar pole greater than that of the dorsal pole.[11,17] It is this wedge shape that explains the tendency of the lunate to rotate into dorsiflexion, a

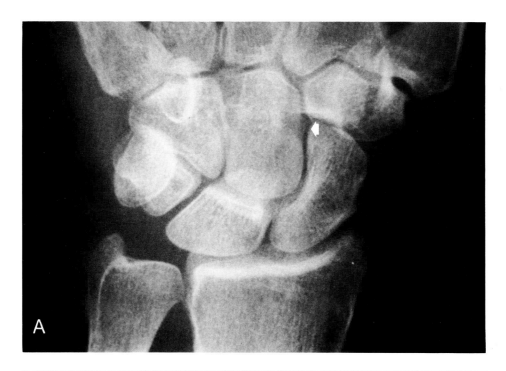

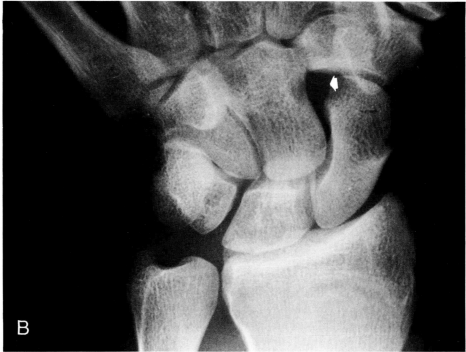

Fig. 1-5. Radiographs of normal adult carpus. *A:* Congruent scaphocapitate relationship (arrow). *B:* Wide scaphocapitate space (arrow) suggests presence of a ligamentous structure, remnant of os centrale.

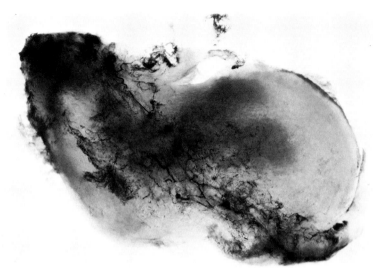

Fig. 1-6. Cleared adult scaphoid specimen (Spalteholz technique) injected with India ink. Palmar aspect of the scaphoid is at the top of the photograph, distal facet to the left. The waist of the bone extends from the proximal end of the dorsal surface to the base of the tubercle in a helicoidal fashion. (From Taleisnik J, Kelly PJ: The extraosseous and intraosseous blood supply of the scaphoid bone. J Bone Joint Surg [Am] 48:1125, 1966.)

tendency independent of the relative position of the capitate to the radius. Kauer[16,17] points out that, for an intercalated bone such as the lunate, this nonconcentric wedge shape and the consequent tendency to rotate in one direction are advantages because only a single force applied in an opposite direction is required to realign the lunate in a neutral position.[21] This palmarflexing force is provided by the scaphoid (Fig. 1-8). The distal articular surface of the lunate is traditionally described as a biconcave facet for articulation with the central, biconvex facet on the head of the capitate. Both the radiocarpal and midcarpal joints, on account of this configuration, have been classified as condylar.[11] In 1921 Navarro[25] pointed out that this central portion of the radiocarpal joint is actually a double trochlea, between the radius, the triangular fibrocartilage, and the lunate proximally, and between the lunate, the capitate, and the hamate distally (Fig. 1-9). In such a type III lunate the proximal articular surface may have a distinct crease,[29] separating a lateral facet for articulation with the radius from a medial facet opposite the triangular fibrocartilage.[1] Shepherd[29] had also observed that this medial facet of the lunate varied in size in different subjects, and in direct proportion to the size of the proximal articular surface of the neighboring triquetrum: the larger the triquetrum, the smaller the lunate surface opposing the triangular fibrocartilage, and vice versa. The distal trochlea is composed of the lunate proximally and the capitate, hamate, and triquetrum distally (Fig. 1-9). Navarro compared this joint to that between the humerus and the ulna, and he observed that, unlike a condylar joint, a trochlear system allows only flexion and extension and a variable degree of lateral displacement and angulation, but does not allow any rotation at all.

The Triquetrum

The triquetrum, on the surface toward the hamate, has an inferior (distal), shallow, saddle-shaped facet. At approximately 90 degrees to this facet is the flat, large articular surface for the lunate (Figs. 1-1, 1-2, 1-9). The relationship between the two facets is such that during ulnar deviation the triquetrum glides distally on the hamate, as if descending a spiral staircase. Its distal facet rotates from facing laterally to facing dorsally, causing the

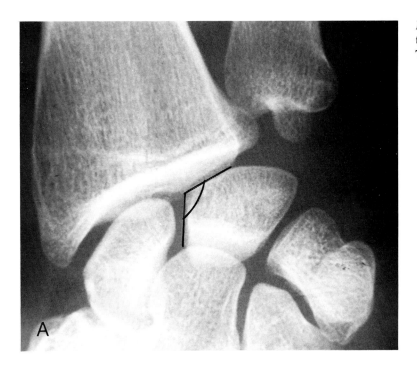

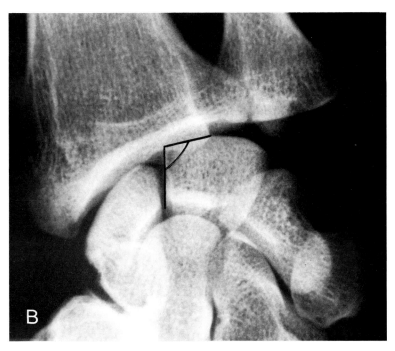

Fig. 1-7. "Angle of inclination" (Antuña Zapico, Ref. 1) of the lunate. *A:* Type I. *B:* Type II.

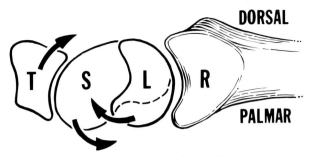

Fig. 1-8. Wedge-shaped lunate (L) tends to rotate into dorsiflexion (palmar pole larger than dorsal pole), scaphoid (S) counteracts this tendency, providing a palmar-flexing force induced by the trapezium and trapezoid (T). R, radius.

proximal facet for the lunate to dorsiflex (Fig. 1-10). Thus a relatively small, piston-type motion of the distal facet, articulating with the hamate, results in an effective force to dorsiflex the lunate. The plane of the triquetrolunate joint is oblique distally and radially. Virchow (quoted by Fick[9]) in-

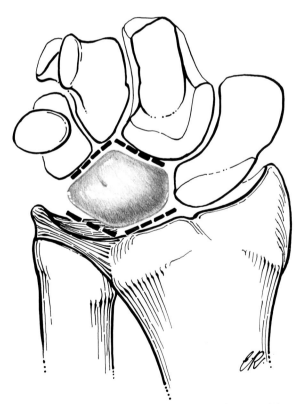

Fig. 1-9. Navarro's concept of the double trochlear articulation of the wrist (see text).

dicated that this obliquity allowed a proximal to distal displacement of the triquetrum on the lunate when the wrist is taken from radial to ulnar deviation. The proximal-medial facet is in contact with the ulnocarpal complex. There are two main nonarticular areas: one dorsal and one volar. Unlike most other carpal bones, where palmar ligament attachments are all-important, the triquetrum is the site of insertion of equally strong dorsal and palmar fascicles, the dorsal radiocarpal and intercarpal, and the palmar lunotriquetral ligament[31] (see Chapter 2). When the radiotriquetral fascicle of the *dorsal* radiocarpal ligament, and the *volar* lunotriquetral ligament itself (taken as just the distal half of a radiolunotriquetral fascicle) are considered together, they form the posterior and anterior pillars of a harness from the radius to the triquetrum, described by Kuhlmann[19] as the "frondiform ligament."

The Pisiform

The pisiform is the only carpal bone to have a tendon insertion from a forearm muscle.[10] Part of the transverse carpal ligament also attaches to it. According to Kadasne and Bansal,[14] the pisiform develops within the substance of the flexor carpi ulnaris tendon, not as a sesamoid, but independently. Distally, the tendon of the flexor carpi ulnaris continues as the pisohamate and pisometacarpal ligaments.[34] Navarro[25,26] stressed the importance of what he called a "triquetropisiform system." He stated that "the pisiform, anatomically and physiologically, is a part of the triquetrum" and from the functional standpoint both, together, are the equal, on the ulnar side of the carpus, to the scaphoid on the lateral side. Morphologically, the lunotriquetropisiform unit resembles a scaphoid (Figs. 1-11 and 1-12). The synovial cavity of the pisotriquetral joint is continuous with that of the wrist joint.[34] Although seemingly tethered in all directions by tendons and ligaments, the pisiform is very mobile, pulled distally during radial deviation and dorsiflexion by pisohamate and pisometacarpal ligaments and proximally during ulnar deviation and palmar flexion by the action of the flexor carpi ulnaris tendon (Fig. 1-13).

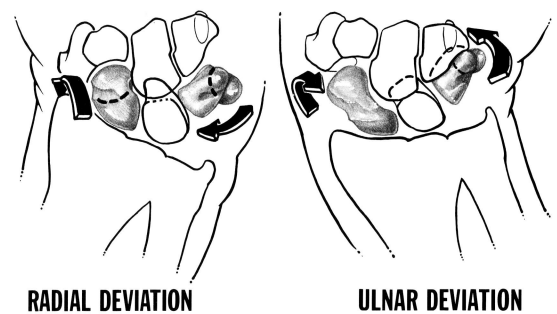

RADIAL DEVIATION   ULNAR DEVIATION

Fig. 1-10 In radial deviation the proximal row is palmar flexed. Scaphoid appears foreshortened, lunate triangular in shape, and triquetrum proximal in relation to the hamate. In ulnar deviation proximal row is dorsiflexed. Scaphoid appears elongated, lunate shape is trapezoidal, triquetrum is distal in relation to the hamate.

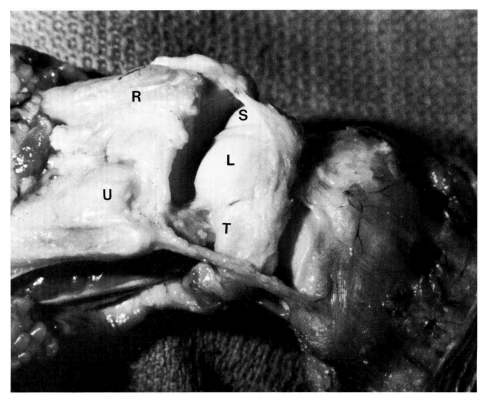

Fig. 1-11. Lunotriquetral unit resembles a scaphoid. L, lunate; T, triquetrum; S, scaphoid; R, radius; U, ulnar head.

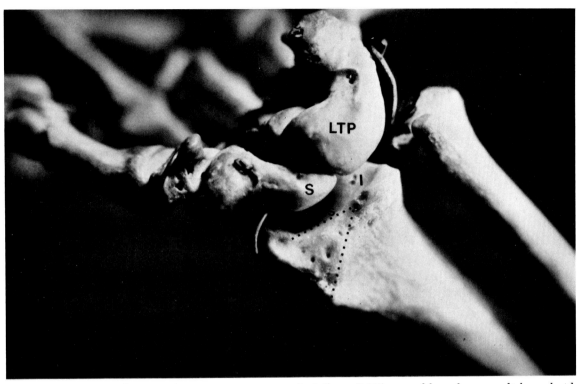

Fig. 1-12. Synostoses between lunate, triquetrum, and pisiform (LTP) resembles a large medial scaphoid. Triangular area on palmar-distal surface of radius, is for the origin of the deep palmar radiocarpal ligaments. Radial articular facets for the scaphoid (s) and lunate (l) are also shown.

The Hamate

The hamate is pyramidal in shape, with a base for articulation with the fourth and fifth metacarpals, and a blunt proximal apex, shaped as a rounded anteroposterior border, articulating with the lunate (Figs. 1-1, 1-2). This border results from the proximal confluence of a flat lateral surface facing the capitate and a helicoidal medial facet facing ulnarward and proximally. The medial facet is actually two surfaces in different alignment. The distal half is almost horizontal and has been compared[25] to the surface created by the trapezium and trapezoid for the acceptance and support of the distal pole of the scaphoid. This, in effect, completes Navarro's analogy of the scaphoid laterally and the triquetropisiform system medially. The difference in magnitude and amplitude of motion between the scaphoid and the triquetropisiform system has been attributed to the need to provide specialized support to the thumb in humans because of its particular function as an opposable digit. The entire facet of the hamate winds along the medial side "as if the bone had been caught at its apex and twisted"[12] (Fig. 1-14). It is on this facet that triquetrohamate displacements take place. The hook or hamulus arises from the palmar surface of the body of the hamate to constitute the medial wall of the carpal tunnel, as well as the distal and lateral wall of the canal of Guyon (Fig. 1-3). It lies between the flexor tendons in the carpal tunnel and the ulnar neurovascular bundle, particularly the motor branch of the ulnar nerve, which winds around its base before entering the deep palmar compartment. The hamulus is the major medial bony attachment for the flexor retinaculum.[18]

The Capitate

The capitate occupies the center of the carpus (Figs. 1-1, 1-2). It articulates with the second, third, and fourth metacarpals distally, with the trapezoid radially, and with the hamate medially. The head of the capitate is large and contains three

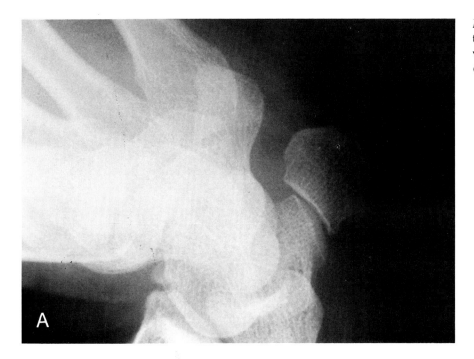

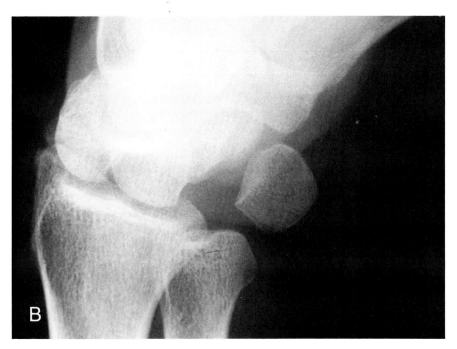

Fig. 1-13. Normal mobility of the pisiform from radial deviation *(A)* to ulnar deviation *(B)*.

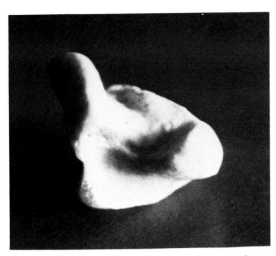

Fig. 1-14. Articular facet of hamate for articulation with triquetrum is helicoidal in shape. (Reproduced by permission from Taleisnik J: Wrist: Anatomy, function, and injury. Am Acad Orthop Surgeons Instruct Course Lect 27:61. St Louis, 1978, The C. V. Mosby Co.)

facets of different degrees of curvature for articulation with the scaphoid, lunate, and hamate.[20] The palmar surface is nonarticular. The area immediately distal to the articular surface of the head is particularly rough, and gives attachment to the "V" or deltoid intrinsic palmar carpal ligament[31] (see Chapter 2 and Fig. 1-2).

The Trapezoid

The trapezoid articulates with the scaphoid proximally, the capitate medially, the trapezium on its lateral aspect, and the second metacarpal distally. It is the only bone in the distal carpal row that articulates with a single metacarpal.[8]

The Trapezium

The trapezium is most important as the link between the carpus and the very mobile thumb metacarpal. The articular surface facing the metacarpal is traditionally described as "saddle-shaped." The proximal articular surface of the trapezium, together with that of the trapezoid, constitute a broad facet for the distal pole of the scaphoid. Medially, the trapezium articulates with the trapezoid. It has a prominent tubercle on the palmar

surface, making up a portion of the lateral wall of the carpal canal where the tendon of the flexor carpi radialis lies (Fig. 1-3). All four bones in the distal carpal row fit tightly against each other and are held together by stout, unyielding interosseous ligaments.

THE DISTAL RADIUS

The carpal articular surface of the radius is grossly triangular in shape, its apex toward the radial styloid, its base next to the articular cavity for the head of the ulna. This surface is divided into two facets by a shallow anteroposterior crest. The lateral facet articulates with the scaphoid, the medial with the lunate (Fig. 2-10). Anteriorly, the dividing crest ends at the volar rim of the radius, creating a small notch or tubercle for the origin of the radioscapholunate ligament.[31] This notch, in turn, represents the apex of a large, triangular, smooth impression,[22] with numerous vascular foramina,[15] situated on the anterior aspect of the styloid process of the radius (Fig. 1-12). The deep volar radiocarpal ligaments originate from this surface.[11,22] Jeanne and Mouchet[11] point out that this surface can be reached by deep palpation, between the tendons of the abductor pollicis longus and flexor carpi radialis, where tenderness may be consistently elicited in the sprained wrist. The distal articular surface faces in a palmar and ulnar direction. The proximal joint surface for the radiocarpal joint is completed by the triangular fibrocartilage (Figs. 1-9, 2-10).

REFERENCES

1. Antuña Zapico JM: Malacia del semilunar. Tesis doctoral, Universidad de Valladolid, Industrias y Editorial Sever-Cuesta, Valladolid, 1966
2. Birmingham Revision of the Basle Nomina Anatomica (Anatomical Society of Great Britain and Ireland). University Press, Glasgow, 1933
3. Bogart FB: Variations of the bones of the wrist. Am J Roentgenol 28:638, 1932
4. Boyes JH: Bunnell's Surgery of the Hand. 5th Ed. Lippincott, Philadelphia, 1970
5. Braus H, Elze C: Anatomie des Menschen; ein Lehr-

buch für Studierende und Ärzte. Vol. 1. Springer Verlag, Berlin, 1954

6. Destot E: Injuries of the Wrist, a Radiological Study. Ernest Denn, London, 1925
7. Dobyns JH, Linscheid RL: Editorial comment, carpal bone injuries. Clin Orthop 149:2, 1980
8. Fahrer M: Introduction to the anatomy of the wrist. In Tubiana R (ed): The Hand. Vol. I. Saunders, Philadelphia, 1981
9. Fick R: Handbuch der Anatomie und Mechanik der Gelenke: III. Spezielle Gelenk- und Muskelmechanik. G. Fischer, Jena, 1911
10. Hollinshead WH: Anatomy for Surgeons. 2nd Ed. Vol. 3. Hoeber, New York, 1969.
11. Jeanne LA and Mouchet A: Les lésions traumatiques fermées du poignet. 28th Congrès Français de Chirurgie, 1919
12. Johnston MB: Varying positions of the carpal bones in the different movements at the wrist. J Anat 41:109, 1907
13. Jones FW: The Principles of Anatomy as seen in the Hand. 2nd Ed Baillière, Tindall and Cox, London, 1949
14. Kadasne DK, Bansal PG: Origin of human pisiform bone. J Anat Soc India 14:23, 1965
15. Kaplan EB: Functional and surgical anatomy of the hand. 2nd Ed. Lippincott, Philadelphia, 1965
16. Kauer JMG: The interdependence of carpal articulation chains. Acta Anat 88:481, 1974
17. Kauer JMG: Functional anatomy of the wrist. Clin Orthop 149:9, 1980
18. Kauer JMG, Landsmeer JMF: Functional anatomy of the wrist. In Tubiana R (ed): The Hand. Vol. I. Saunders, Philadelphia, 1981
19. Kuhlmann N: Anatomía descriptiva y funcional del carpo en relación con la patología traumática del mismo. Rev Esp Cir Mano 5:13, 1977
20. Lamoen in Matricali EAM van: Ontleedkundig-Functioneel Onderzoek van het Polsgewricht. Thesis: Leiden, Holland, 1961
21. Landsmeer JMF: Studies in the anatomy of articulation. I. The equilibrium of the "intercalated" bone. Acta Morphol Neerl Scand 3:287, 1961
22. Lewis OJ, Hamshere RJ, Bucknill TM: The anatomy of the wrist joint. J Anat 106:539, 1970
23. McMurrich JP: The nomenclature of the carpal bones. Anat Rec 8:173, 1914
24. Napier, J: Hands. Pantheon, New York, 1980
25. Navarro A: Luxaciones del carpo. An Fac Med Montevideo, 6:113, 1921
26. Navarro A: Anales del Instituto de Clinica Quirurgica y Cirugia Experimental. Imprenta Artistica de Dornaleche Hnos, Montevideo, 1935
27. Nordby EJ: Editorial comment. Clin Orthop 83:2, 1972
28. Sack SC: Painful clicking wrists associated with os centrale. S Afri Med J 23:766, 1949
29. Shepherd FJ: A note on the radio-carpal articulation. J Anat 25:349, 1890
30. Sobotta J: Atlas of human anatomy. 8th Engl Ed. by Figge FHJ. Hafner, New York, 1968
31. Taleisnik J: The ligaments of the wrist. J Hand Surg 1:110, 1976
32. Testut L, Latarjet A: Tratado de anatomia humana. 9th Ed. Vol. 1. Salvat. Editores, Buenos Aires, 1951
33. Vesalius A: De humani corporis fabrica, Libri septem, Basilae, 1543. Ex. officina I. Oporini, Bruxelles, 1964
34. Weston WJ: Functional anatomy of the pisi-cuneiform joint. Br J Radiol 46:692, 1973

2 The Ligaments of the Wrist

During wrist motions the behavior of individual carpal bones, and of the carpus as a whole, is determined to a considerable degree by interacting contact pressures from all bone surfaces, controlled by a highly developed, complex ligamentous system. In most joints the function of ligaments is limited to restriction and support; Ghia[10] called them "ligaments of arrest." In the wrist, ligaments constitute a sophisticated net of fibers, capable of inducing bony displacements and of transmitting very precise tension loads at a distance. The volar ligaments are thick and strong. Their strength and disposition correlates with the primitive palmigrade position of the limbs in primates.[27] The dorsal ligaments are much thinner, fewer in number, and functionally and structurally reinforced by the floor and septi of the fibrous tunnels through which the extensor tendons pass on the dorsum of the wrist.

The ligaments of the wrist are divided into two major groups[37,38]: *extrinsic ligaments*, which course between the carpal bones and the radius or the metacarpals, and *intrinsic ligaments*, which originate and insert on the carpal bones (Fig. 2-1).

EXTRINSIC LIGAMENTS

The extrinsic ligaments are located between the radius and the carpus (proximal extrinsic ligaments) (Fig. 2-2) and between the carpals and metacarpals (distal extrinsic ligaments). The proximal extrinsic ligaments occupy all four quadrants of the wrist joint: radial, volar, ulnar, and dorsal.

The Radial Collateral Ligament

The radial collateral ligament (Figs. 2-3 and 2-4) is actually more volar than lateral.[37] It originates from the volar margin of the radial styloid, courses volar to the transverse axis of wrist motion, and attaches on the tuberosity of the scaphoid and the walls of the osteofibrous tunnel for the flexor carpi radialis tendon. Rather than a collateral ligament, it should be viewed as the most lateral of all volar radiocarpal fascicles (Fig. 2-2).[37] The function of a true collateral structure, as seen in hinge or ginglymal joints, is not possible in a joint like the wrist, with the anatomic appearance of a condylar or trochlear articulation but the actual function of a multiaxial enarthrosis. Collateral ligaments would be justified only if radiocarpal motions were limited to flexion and extension. When ulnar and radial deviation are added, however, any static collateral ligament system would in effect restrain lateral and medial angulatory displacements. Jeanne and Mouchet,[13] in their extensive presentation on carpal injuries to the 28th French Congress of Surgery, had suggested that some of the tendons "may be considered as true ligaments." In 1979 Kauer[18] stated that the unique range of wrist motion "excludes collateral ligaments as components of the ligamentous apparatus of the wrist." He proposed an "adjustable collateral system" of muscles acting as true collateral support, the extensor carpi ulnaris for the ulnar side of the wrist (Fig. 2-5), and the extensor pollicis brevis and abductor pollicis long for the radial side (Fig. 2-4). Lateral wrist stability,

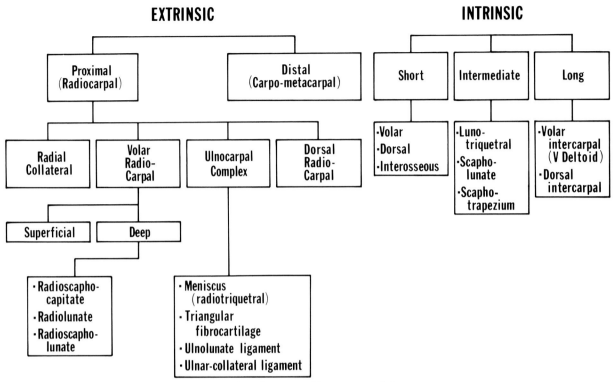

EXTRINSIC

- Proximal (Radiocarpal)
  - Radial Collateral
  - Volar Radio-Carpal
    - Superficial
    - Deep
      - · Radioscapho-capitate
      - · Radiolunate
      - · Radioscapho-lunate
  - Ulnocarpal Complex
    - · Meniscus (radiotriquetral)
    - · Triangular fibrocartilage
    - · Ulnolunate ligament
    - · Ulnar-collateral ligament
  - Dorsal Radio-Carpal
- Distal (Carpo-metacarpal)

INTRINSIC

- Short
  - · Volar
  - · Dorsal
  - · Interosseous
- Intermediate
  - · Luno-triquetral
  - · Scapho-lunate
  - · Scapho-trapezium
- Long
  - · Volar intercarpal (V Deltoid)
  - · Dorsal intercarpal

Fig. 2-1. Classification of ligaments of the wrist.

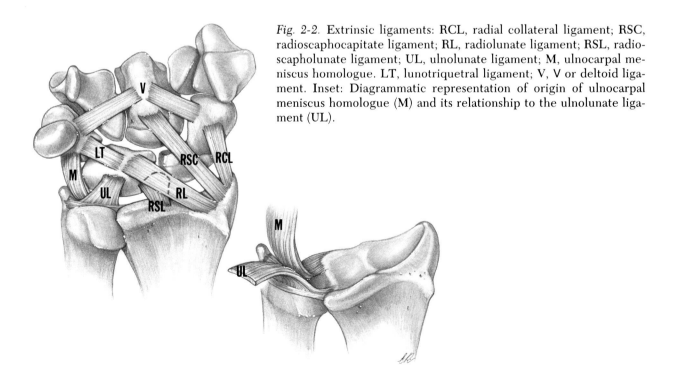

Fig. 2-2. Extrinsic ligaments: RCL, radial collateral ligament; RSC, radioscaphocapitate ligament; RL, radiolunate ligament; RSL, radioscapholunate ligament; UL, ulnolunate ligament; M, ulnocarpal meniscus homologue. LT, lunotriquetral ligament; V, V or deltoid ligament. Inset: Diagrammatic representation of origin of ulnocarpal meniscus homologue (M) and its relationship to the ulnolunate ligament (UL).

Fig. 2-3. Radial collateral ligament is palmar to axis of rotation of the wrist. (From Taleisnik J: The ligaments of the wrist. J Hand Surg 1:110, 1976.)

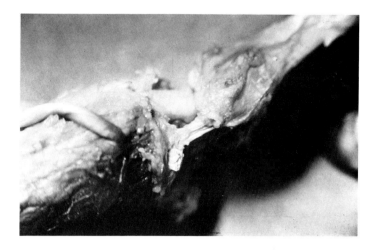

therefore, does not depend on the presence of collateral ligaments, but rather is based on a precise fitting of multiple radiocarpal surfaces and on this adjustable adaptable collateral system.

The Volar Radiocarpal Ligaments

The volar radiocarpal ligaments are superficial and deep (Fig. 2-6). In the superficial layer most fibers assume a V shape, the apex attached to capitate and lunate, the two arms diverging proximally, toward radius and ulna. Their radial attachment is on an osseous crest at the base of the anterior surface of the radial styloid (Fig. 1-12). The deep volar radiocarpal ligaments are three strong fascicles, best seen from within the joint.[27] These ligaments are named according to their points of origin and insertion (Figs. 2-7, 2-8).

The most lateral is the *radiocapitate* (or radioscaphocapitate) *ligament.* It originates from the triangular surface on the anterior aspect of the radial styloid (Fig. 1-12) and attaches on the capitate. On the way, it courses across the volar concave aspect of the scaphoid, onto which it gains a rather weak attachment.[37] Because of its direction, Weitbrecht named this ligament "obliquum" (quoted by Poirier[34]). Medial to it is the *radiolunate ligament,* a very massive bundle of almost transverse fibers. For this fascicle Weitbrecht (quoted by Poirier[34]) reserved the name "rectum." Still more medial, and deeper, is the *radioscapholunate ligament,*[40] or

"ligament of Kuenz and Testut" (Figs. 2-8, 2-9). It originates from the small tubercle or notch at the intersection of the volar rim and the articular crest separating scaphoid and lunate facets in the distal articular surface of the radius. This ligament inserts primarily into the small fossae in the articular surfaces between lunate and scaphoid. It also covers the scaphoid-lunate interspace (Fig. 2-7). The lunate insertion is strong.[13,40] In full volar flexion of the scaphoid the radioscapholunate ligament, along with the radioscaphocapitate fascicle, tethers the proximal pole of the scaphoid to the volar margin of the radius. In maximum dorsiflexion of the scaphoid, it provides an anterior restraint against excessive volar displacement of the proximal pole.

In a biomechanical study of the human carpal ligaments,[30] the tensile properties of the radiocapitate, radiolunate, and lunotriquetral ligaments were investigated. The radioscaphoid fibers were considerably more elastic and showed elastic fibers within the compact collagenous portion of this ligament in preliminary histologic studies. The amount of ligament elongation before failure was higher in the radiocapitate ligament (74%), compared with the radiolunotriquetral ligament (57%). The latter was the strongest of all palmar intracapsular radiocarpal ligaments. The weakest were on the radial side, the radioscaphoid portion of the deep radioscapholunate and the radiocapitate ligaments, suggesting that failure is more likely to occur on the radial than on the ulnar carpus.

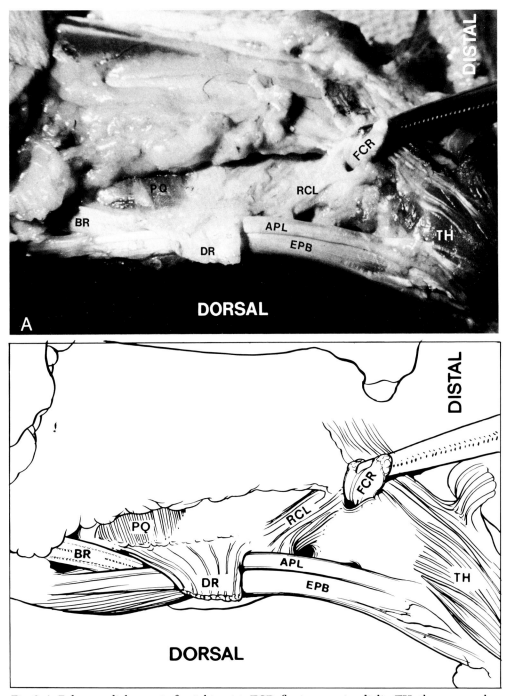

Fig. 2-4. Palmar radial aspect of a right wrist. FCR, flexion carpi radialis; TH, thenar muscles; RCL, radial collateral ligament; PQ, pronator quadratus; BR, brachioradialis; EPB, extensor pollicis brevis; APL, abductor pollicis longus; DR, radial origin of dorsal extensor retinaculum. (From Taleisnik J: Current concepts of the anatomy of the wrist. In Spinner M: Kaplan's Functional and Surgical Anatomy of the Hand. 3rd Ed. Lippincott, Philadelphia, 1984.)

Fig. 2-5. Supratendinous and infratendinous layers of retinaculum. *A*: extensor carpiulnaris; *B*: infratendinous retinaculum joining *C*: supratendinous retinaculum at insertion into triquetrum (arrow); *D*: pisiform. (From Taleisnik J, Gelberman RH, Miller BW, Szabo RM: The extensor retinaculum of the wrist. J Hand Surg 9A:495, 1984.)

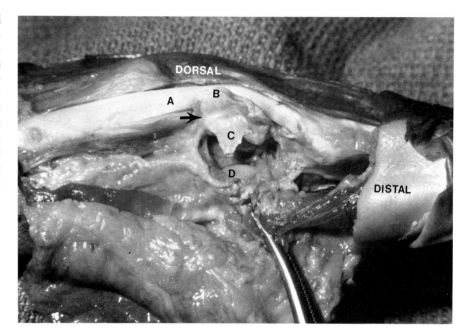

The Ulnocarpal Complex

The ulnocarpal complex occupies the ulnar quadrant of the wrist joint. This is an intricate ligamentous system of considerable functional significance. In the lower primate the ulnar styloid articulates with the triquetrum.[27] Phylogenetic development suggests a tendency of the ulnar styloid to gradually recede from the carpus. In humans this leaves an ulnar styloid of variable length (Fig. 2-10) and a void that is replaced by a cartilaginous filler, the *ulnocarpal meniscus homologue* (Fig. 2-2).[27] Frequently this structure is separate from the *triangular fibrocartilage* (Fig. 2-11),

Fig. 2-6. Proximal aspect of scaphoid (S), lunate (L) and ulnocarpal meniscus (M). Arrow points to superficial (1) and deep (2) palmar radiocarpal ligaments. (From Taleisnik J: The ligaments of the wrist. J Hand Surg 1:110, 1976.)

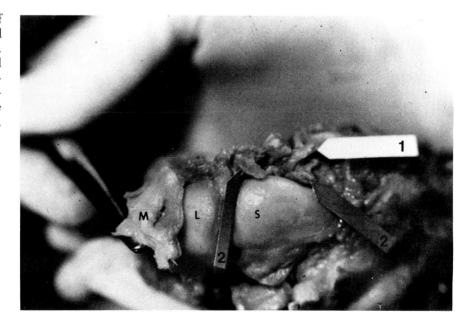

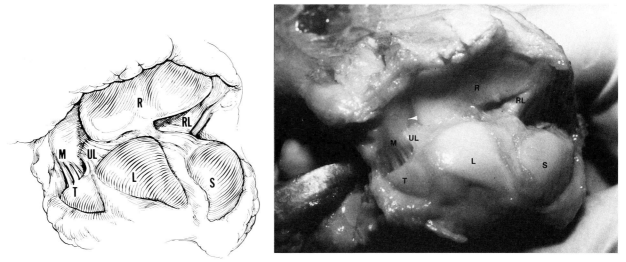

Fig. 2-7. Palmar structures shown from within the joint. S, scaphoid; L, lunate; T, triquetrum; RL, radiolunate ligament; R, radius; UL, ulnolunate ligament shown arising from palmar margin of triangular fibrocartilage (arrow). These and ulnocarpal meniscus homologue (M) form a poorly differentiated structure.

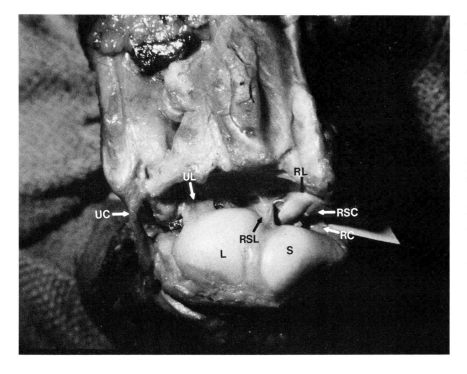

Fig. 2-8. Deep palmar radiocarpal ligaments (right wrist) seen from within the joint. RC, radial collateral ligament; RSC, radioscaphocapitate ligament; RL, radiolunate ligament; UL, ulnolunate ligament; UC, ulnar collateral structure; RSL, radioscapholunate ligament; L, lunate; S, scaphoid. (From Taleisnik J: Current concepts of the anatomy of the wrist. In Spinner M (ed): Kaplan's Functional and Surgical Anatomy of the Hand. 3rd Ed. Lippincott, Philadelphia, 1984.)

Fig. 2-9. Palmar half of coronal section of the wrist. RSL, radioscapholunate ligament. (From Taleisnik J: The ligaments of the wrist. J Hand Surg 1:110, 1976.)

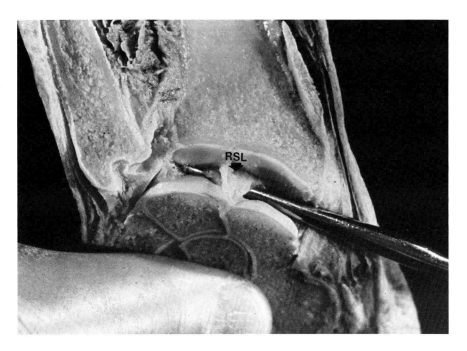

with which it should not be confused. Triangular fibrocartilage and ulnocarpal meniscus homologue share a common proximal and dorsal origin from the dorsoulnar corner of the radius. From here the ulnocarpal meniscus homologue swings around the ulnar border of the wrist to a triquetral insertion (Figs. 2-2 and 2-12), while the triangular fibrocartilage spreads across to reach the head of the ulna (Fig. 2-11). It inserts at the junction of the base of the styloid process and the ulnar head. In those wrists where the ulnocarpal meniscus homologue appears as an identifiable, separate structure, it presents a free border to the joint, and between this border and the overlying triangular fibrocartilage there is an opening that leads to a space surrounding the ulnar styloid, the prestyloid recess

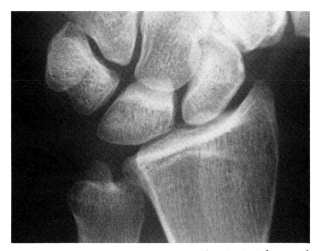

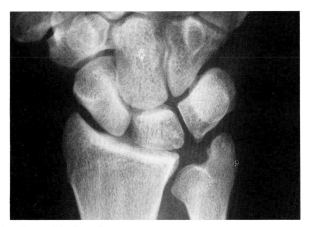

Fig. 2-10. Ulnar styloids of variable lengths.

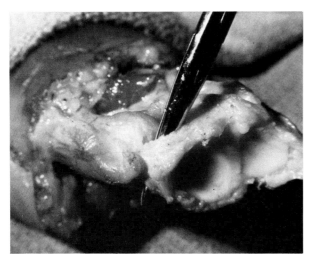

Fig. 2-11. Triangular fibrocartilage, right wrist. (From Spinner M (ed): Kaplan's Functional and Surgical Anatomy of the Hand. 3rd Ed. Lippincott, Philadelphia, 1984.)

(Figs. 2-13, 2-14).[27,37,38,40] This space is filled with synovium, and may assume pathologic significance when synovitis is present, such as in rheumatoid disease.[27] Within this space, long ulnar styloids may be seen, covered with hyaline cartilage and

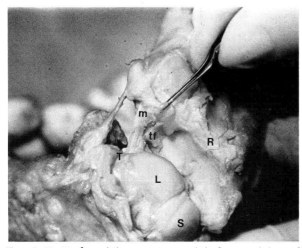

Fig. 2-12. Radius (R), triquetrum (T), lunate (L), and scaphoid (S) shown from within the joint and from the dorsum. Forceps is holding the common origin of ulnocarpal meniscus homologue (M) and of triangular fibrocartilage (tf) from dorsal and ulnar corner of distal radius.

free of ligamentous attachments. Short styloids tend to be covered by capsular and ligamentous fibers.

In many specimens triangular fibrocartilage and ulnocarpal meniscus homologue cannot be clearly differentiated,[17,33] and remain fused throughout their length into a more amorphous cartilaginous mass (Fig. 2-7). This mass extends in part medially to insert in the caput ulna, and in part continues along the ulnar border of the wrist to the volar aspect of the triquetrum. In the dorsum some of its fibers join the extensor carpi ulnaris sheath, and through this the ulnocarpal cartilaginous system may reach as far as the base of the fifth metacarpal.[27,29] The triangular fibrocartilage is thicker at both ends, and also along its anterior and posterior borders, also referred to as the anterior and posterior distal radioulnar ligaments. The center of this fibrocartilaginous formation is thinner,[33,40] at times perforated, allowing the radiocarpal joint to communicate with the synovial pouch of the distal radioulnar joint, the recessus sacciformis.

Palmer and collaborators[33] described three anomalies frequently seen in association with perforation of the triangular fibrocartilages: a kissing area of lunate chondromalacia, an ulna-plus variant, and a tear of the lunotriquetral ligament. The *ulnolunate ligament* (Figs. 2-2, 2-7, 2-8) connects the anterior border of the triangular fibrocartilage to the lunate. The last component of this ulnocarpal complex is the *ulnar collateral ligament.* This ligament has been depicted as arising from the tip of the ulnar styloid,[12] from the fovea at the base of the styloid, next to the insertion of the triangular fibrocartilage,[5] or from the outer, medial contour of the base of the styloid process, together with the wrist capsule.[40]

Although there is some agreement as to the lack of ligamentous attachments on the tip of the ulnar styloid,[5,40] Dameron depicts the tip of the styloid outside the ulnocarpal joint capsule, rather than within it, in relationship with the prestyloid recess.[37,40] The ulnar collateral ligament is not actually a distinct fascicle, but a thickening of the joint capsule, in relationship with the overlying sheath of the extensor carpi ulnaris (Fig. 2-5).[18,19]

Leeuw[26] clarified the structural characteristic of the extensor carpi ulnaris tunnel, dorsal and distal to the ulnar head. In the distal forearm the extensor

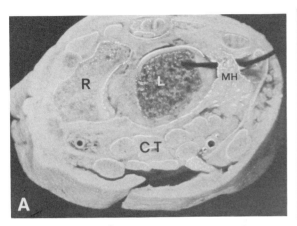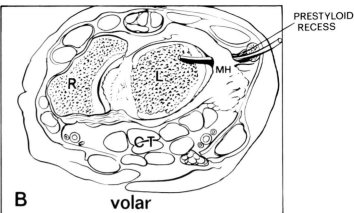

Fig. 2-13. A and B: Transverse section. Specimen shows cut ulnocarpal meniscus homologue, with dark marker placed underneath, from radiocarpal joint to prestyloid recess. R, radial styloid; L, lunate; MH, meniscus homologue; CT, carpal tunnel. (From Taleisnik J: Current concepts of the anatomy of the wrist. In Spinner M (ed): Kaplan's Functional and Surgical Anatomy of the Hand. 3rd Ed. Lippincott, Philadelphia, 1984.)

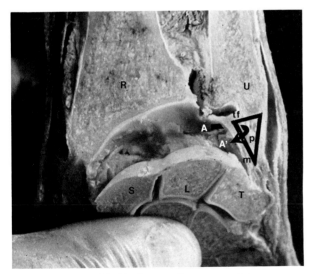

Fig. 2-14. Dorsal half of coronal section of the wrist. R, radius; U, ulna; T, triquetrum; L, lunate; S, scaphoid. Triangular fibrocartilage (tf) and ulnocarpal meniscus (m) share a common origin from the dorsal and ulnar corner of the radius, and delineate a triangular space (p), the prestyloid recess filled with synovial tissue. Arrow (A-A) shows communication between prestyloid recess and radiocarpal joint. (From Taleisnik J: The ligaments of the wrist. J Hand Surg 1:110, 1976.)

carpi ulnaris is held in position under a sheath, an extension of the deep layer of the antebrachial fascia (Fig. 2-15). Distally, this sheath gradually merges into the dorsal retinaculum, which, like the sheath itself, is separated from the ulnar head, on which it does not attach. Were this not the case, the extensor carpi ulnaris would be bound to the ulnar head, interfering with pronation and supination. Instead, this tendon shifts freely over the ulnar head during rotation of the forearm. Therefore, unlike the bony grooves seen in the distal radius for all other extensor tendons, there is no osteofibrous tunnel on the ulnar head for the extensor carpi ulnaris tendon. Distal to the ulnar styloid, however, the extensor carpi ulnaris is encased in a fibrous sheath, which, also unlike the other extensors, has a carpal attachment (on the triquetrum).[25] This strong sheath assures that the approach of the extensor carpi ulnaris to the carpus remains unchanged, regardless of the shifting of the tendon, proximal to the ulnar styloid, during pronation and supination (Fig. 2-15). Leeuw's investigation showed that the ulnar collateral ligament is in fact a part of the dorsal carpal retinaculum, and that a distinct attachment of this ligament to the ulna could not exist.

Anatomic studies[39] show that the ulnar collateral ligament does not act as an actual fascicular constraint, whether independent or in conjunction with the dorsal retinaculum. I believe that when

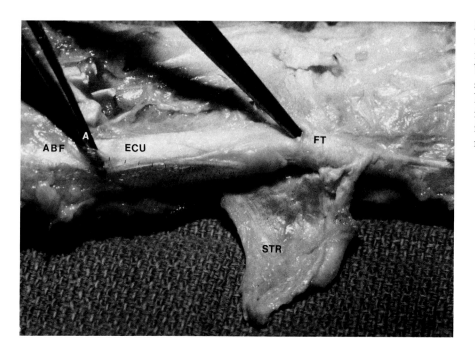

Fig. 2-15. Support mechanism for the extensor carpi ulnaris tendon (ECU). **FT,** fibrous tunnel for the ECU; small markers delineate the linea jugata, also elevated by forceps **A; ABF,** antebrachial fascia; **STR,** supratendinous retinaculum.

dissection techniques that attempt to expose an ulnar collateral ligament are used, thinner areas are excised and thicker fibrous structures are left behind. These fibers from the confluence of the dorsal retinaculum, the floor of the extensor carpi ulnaris, and the joint capsule (Fig. 2-5) artificially create an ulnar collateral system.

In summary, the dorsoulnar and volar-radial corners of the radius are strongly bound to the *volar* carpus through a fibrocartilaginous "sling" (Fig. 2-16).[37,38] The head of the ulna is strictly not a part of the wrist joint.

The Dorsal Radiocarpal Ligament

The dorsal radiocarpal ligament is also very strong, but wider and with a more laminar appearance than the volar radiocarpal ligaments. It originates from the dorsal rim of the radius, and inserts firmly into the lunate, the triquetrum, and the scaphoid. This dorsal radiotriquetral fascicle, and a similar palmar radiotriquetral ligament (radiolunate + lunotriquetral), make up the posterior and anterior pillars of a radiotriquetral harness called "the frondiform ligament" by Kuhlman.[23] There may be a capsular fold arising from the radius and inserting into both lunate and triquetrum. Delbet

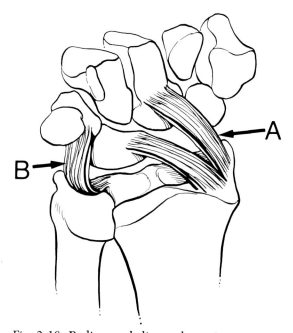

Fig. 2-16. Radiocarpal sling, schematic representation as seen from palmar aspect. *A:* Palmar radiocarpal ligaments. *B:* Ulnocarpal meniscus homologue.

Fig. 2-17. Deep dorsal radio-lunotriquetral ligament (RLT) was detached from dorsal origin (a) and folded distally (a¹). R, radius; U, ulnar head; L, lunate; T, triquetrum; LTI, lunotriquetral intrinsic ligament.

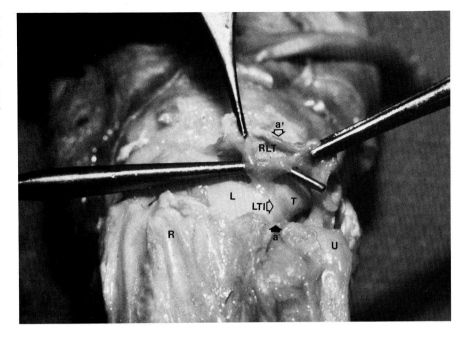

(quoted by Jeanne and Mouchet[13]) called this structure the posterior "frenulum" of the lunate. This formation in the dorsum of the wrist is analogous to the volar radioscapholunate ligament, although certainly not as direct nor as well developed (Fig. 2-17). Because of this similarity, however, this structure has been called the deep radiolunotriquetral ligament.[15]

INTRINSIC LIGAMENTS

Intrinsic ligaments of the wrist originate and insert on the carpal bones. According to their length, and the relative intercarpal motion they allow, these ligaments may be grouped into three categories: short, intermediate, and long.[37]

Short Intrinsic Ligaments

Short intrinsic ligaments are stout and tightly bind adjacent carpal bones to one another (Fig. 2-18). The interosseous ligament between capitate and hamate is particularly large and strong. In effect, all four bones of the distal carpus are converted into one functional unit because of their interconnecting intrinsic fascicles.

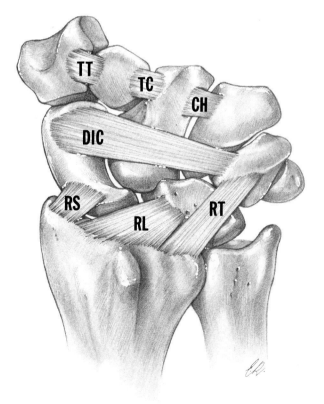

Fig. 2-18. Dorsal ligaments. TT, trapeziotrapezoid; TC, trapeziocapitate; CH, capitohamate; DIC, dorsal intercarpal; RS, RL, RT, radioscaphoid, radiolunate, and radiotriquetral fascicles of the dorsal radiocarpal ligament.

Intermediate Intrinsic Ligaments

Intermediate intrinsic ligaments are disposed between scaphoid and trapezium, lunate and triquetrum, and scaphoid and lunate. There are three main *scaphoid-trapezium ligaments:* volar, dorsal, and lateral (Fig. 2-19). These allow the trapezium and trapezoid to ride dorsal to the distal pole of the scaphoid, a mechanism that forces the scaphoid into volar flexion during radial deviation of the wrist.[14,19]

The *lunotriquetral* fascicle is very strong, contin-

uing the overal direction of the radiolunate ligament past the lunate onto the triquetrum (Fig. 2-19). Both these fascicles may be thought of as a single radiotriquetral ligament.[3,29] There is also a lunotriquetral interosseous ligamentous component (Fig. 2-17), which is not as slack as that between the scaphoid and the lunate, making for a more solid relationship between lunate and triquetrum than that existing between lunate and scaphoid. This ligament arrangement allows a distal-to-proximal lunotriquetral motion in a piston-type manner, as described by Virchow (quoted by Fick[8])

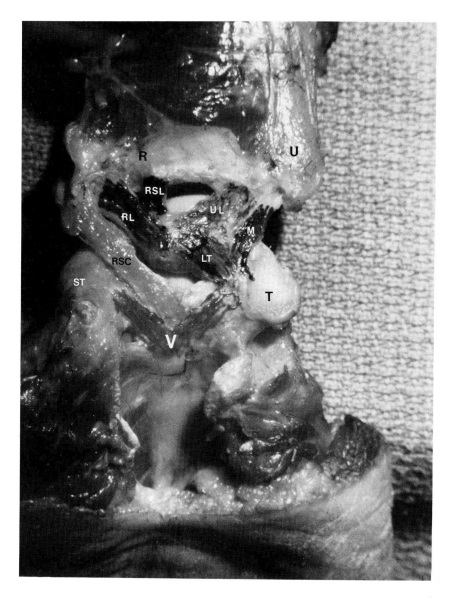

Fig. 2-19. Palmar ligaments. RSC, radioscaphocapitate; RL, radiolunate; RSL, deep radio-scapholunate; UL, ulnolunate, LT, lunotriquetral; M, ulnocarpal meniscus homologue; V, V or deltoid ligament; ST, scaphotrapezium capsule; R, radius; U, ulnar head; T, triquetrum. (From Taleisnik J: Current concepts of the anatomy of the wrist. In Spinner M (ed): Kaplan's Functional and Surgical Anatomy of the Hand. 3rd Ed. Lippincott, Philadelphia, 1984.)

and also the transmission of dorsiflexion torque from the triquetrum to the lunate during ulnar deviation.[14]

The *scapholunate* ligaments are found on both the volar and dorsal surfaces. They course obliquely from lunate to scaphoid, and allow considerable motion between these two bones.[3,13,14,15] From neutral-to-full dorsiflexion, the lunate rotates approximately 28 degrees and the scaphoid 30 degrees.[42] From neutral-to-complete volarflexion, the lunate rotates 30 degrees and the scaphoid 60 degrees. Both ligaments twist as dissimilar scapholunate rotations occur in volar flexion, to unwind as the carpus returns to neutral.[10,37] The dorsal ligament is shorter and more dense than the volar,[16,19] allowing for anterior scapholunate gaping during motion. Kauer[16,19] described a third type of scapholunate displacement, in addition to rotation and "gaping." This displacement occurs because of the difference in the degree of curvature between the proximal pole of the scaphoid and the proximal articular surface of the lunate. The scaphoid curvature is greater; therefore it must shift proximally during volar flexion, in relationship to the lunate, in order to maintain its surface contact with the radius.

Long Intrinsic Ligaments

The long intrinsic ligaments are volar and dorsal. Although the volar ligament appears more formidable, and therefore more important, there is increasing evidence of the functional importance of the dorsal ligament.

The *volar intercarpal ligament* has been called deltoid, radiate, arcuate, or, more simply, V ligament (Fig. 2-19). Some of the discrepancies in descriptive terminology arise from the different appearance of the ligament in different specimens. At times, there is a continuous fan-shaped array of fibers from the capitate to the triquetrum, lunate, and scaphoid, hence the name deltoid or radiate ligament. Frequently, however, the central fibers to the lunate are absent, leaving a more familiar V-shaped structure, with the lunate in its center. The lateral (capitoscaphoid) fascicle of the V ligament contributes to the support of the distal pole of the scaphoid, together with the radial collateral ligament. It may extend to the trapezium, an actual capitoscaphotrapezium ligament.[13] The medial (capitotriquetral) fascicle of the V ligament is the only volar structure, other than the scaphoid, to cross and therefore stabilize the midcarpal joint.[28]

The *dorsal intercarpal ligament* (Fig. 2-18) is a ribbonlike structure that originates from the triquetrum and courses laterally and obliquely to insert on the scaphoid, and on the trapezium.[13,40] It skirts about the neck of the capitate, leaving an area of weakness between the proximal border of this dorsal intercarpal fascicle and the more proximal insertion of the dorsal radiocarpal ligament on the lunate.

WRIST LIGAMENTS: RECAPITULATION

Each individual radiocarpal and intrinsic carpal ligament is integrated into a sophisticated system that assists in the control of the extent of intercarpal displacement, and the gradual smooth movement of carpal bones on each other, through a full range of motion of the wrist. Four bones receive the bulk of the volar ligamentous attachments (Figs. 2-2, 2-19)[37]: capitate, lunate, scaphoid, and triquetrum. The *capitate* is at the apex of a V-shaped complex of fibers that originates proximally and laterally from the radius and scaphoid, and proximally and medially from the triquetrum. Contained within this V is a second V made up of the radiolunate and ulnolunate ligaments[6] converging to a broad and strong insertion on the volar aspect of the *lunate.* Traumatic detachment of this insertion is infrequent. An important source of blood supply reaches the lunate in vessels following these fascicles. There is frequently an area of weakness on the volar wrist capsule, the "space of Poirier" caused by the absence of a volar lunocapitate ligament. Poirier[34] had actually described "small hernias" of synovial membrane protruding between ligaments, two of which were more constant on the palmar aspect: one between the two systems of V-shaped ligaments, and a second between the radius and the proximal V. Poirier also described similar pouches on the dorsal aspect, which he related to the development of dorsal ganglions. As we have seen, when a lunocapitate bundle is present, the volar intercarpal V ligament changes into a radiate or deltoid structure.[12] When absent, however, a potential cause of instability is created. Fisk[9] believed that carpal support depended on the integrity of the volar lunocapitate capsule, and stated that the midcarpal joint did not become unstable until this capsule was divided. Navarro[31] had suggested that the absence of lunocapitate support could be an "explanation of carpal subluxations." In addition to this anatomic characteristic, some normal individuals show a form of systemic articular laxity or hypermobility, which may predispose to wrist instability.[22,36] In these individuals a dorsal force applied to the hand can easily bring the capitate very close to subluxing on the lunate.[6,37,38]

Ulnar and radial deviation are not the result of pure angular displacements of the carpus. For these motions to be completed, some carpal bones move simultaneously around or along three axes. The double V ligament system is well suited to control this type of displacement (Fig. 2-20). Actually, this V shape is apparent only when the wrist is examined in neutral position, but it changes alignment during ulnar and radial deviation. In ulnar deviation, for instance, both the capitate as the representative of the distal carpal row and the lunate representing the proximal row rotate into ulnar deviation. In addition, the lunate will translate radially and rotate into dorsiflexion. Because the anteroposterior axis for this motion passes through the head of the capitate, very close to the articular surface with the lunate, the capitate will by necessity rotate distal to the axis, in the opposite sense to that of the lunate, into volarflexion and ulnar translation. The net result is one of ulnar deviation, since opposing rotations around other axes will cancel each other out.

In ulnar deviation the medial fascicle of the proximal V (ulnolunate ligament) becomes largely transverse, to check radial displacement of the lunate, while the lateral fascicle (radiolunate) aligns more longitudinally to control lunate dorsiflexion. The proximal V has now changed into an L. The distal V undergoes a similar transformation, but in the opposite direction. It is the lateral (capitoscaphoid) fibers that become transverse, to check translation of the body of the capitate in an ulnar direction, while the medial (capitotriquetral) fascicles assume a longitudinal orientation, for the control of capitate volar flexion. The distal V ligament has also changed into a L but facing in a direction opposite to that of the proximal L. A similar but

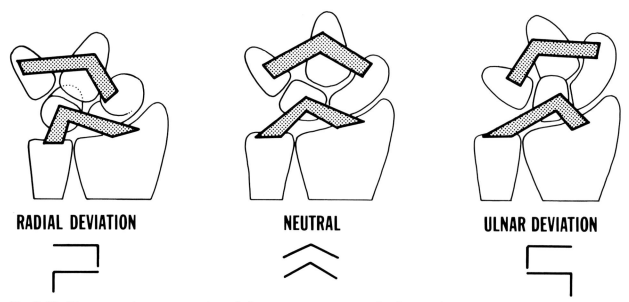

RADIAL DEVIATION   **NEUTRAL**   **ULNAR DEVIATION**

Fig. 2-20. Diagrammatic representation of changes in orientation of palmar radiocarpal ligaments during radial deviation, neutral, and ulnar deviation.

opposite mechanism takes place during radial deviation. Thus, some fibers of each ligament fascicle remain taut throughout ulnar and radial deviation of the wrist.

On the volar aspect of the *scaphoid*, there are three well-defined ligamentous zones: *proximal*, for the control of rotation of the proximal pole on the radius (radioscapholunate ligament) and lunate (intrinsic scapholunate ligament); *distal*, for the distal pole or tuberosity, connected to the radius (radial collateral ligament) and the capitate (volar intercarpal V ligament); and *central*, for the radioscaphocapitate or "sling" ligament. The scaphoid rotates on this ligament as a gymnast balances on a horizontal bar when executing a hip circle (Fig. 2-21).[37] The contact point between the "sling" ligament and the scaphoid coincides with the transverse axis for scaphoid rotation from volarflexion to dorsiflexion. Both the radioscaphocapitate and the radioscapholunate ligaments tether the proximal pole of the scaphoid to the volar radius. The radioscapholunate ligament is particularly important and is tense at both ends of scaphoid rotation. As long as these fascicles are intact, rotatory subluxation of the scaphoid cannot occur even if the scapholunate interosseous ligaments are severed, an anatomic observation[29,38] confirmed by experimental kinematic studies.[2]

The *triquetrum* is the point of convergence of multiple strong volar and dorsal fascicles (Figs. 2-2, 2-19). These originate from the ulnocarpal complex (ulnotriquetral attachment of the ulnocarpal meniscus homologue), the lunate (lunotriquetral ligament), and the capitate (capitotriquetral fascicle of the V ligament) in the volar aspect. In the dorsum, with the wrist in neutral position, the radiotriquetral portion of the dorsal radiocarpal ligament and the dorsal intercarpal ligament attach on the triquetrum at nearly right angles to each other (Fig. 2-18). This overall ligament distribution is

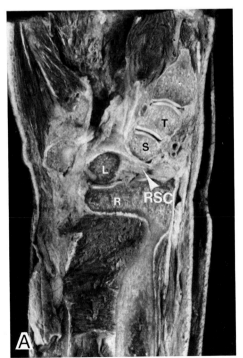

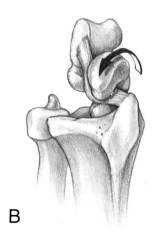

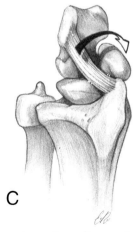

Fig. 2-21. Radioscaphocapitate ligament. *A:* Palmar half, coronal section; RSC, radioscaphocapitate ligament, obliquely across waist of scaphoid (S); R, radius; L, lunate; T, trapezium. The scaphoid rotates on the radioscapholunate ligament from palmar flexion (*B*) to dorsiflexion (*C*).

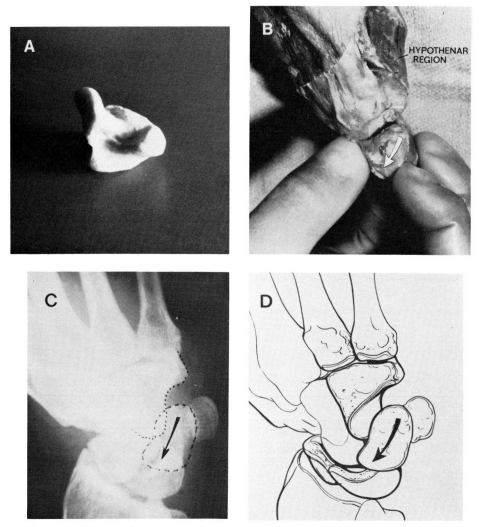

Fig. 2-22. A: Helicoidal surface of hamate for articulation with triquetrum. *B, C, D:* Triquetrum in a proximal ("high") position.

ideal for the control of the smooth pistonlike progression of the triquetrum on the helicoidal surface of the hamate from a high (proximal) position in radial deviation to a low (distal) position in ulnar deviation[41] (Fig. 2-22). Particularly important are the radiotriquetral fascicle of the dorsal radiocarpal ligament and the medial or capitotriquetral fascicle of the deltoid ligament. The latter is the only palmar structure, other than the scaphoid, to cross the midcarpal space and is therefore important in stabilizing the medial half of this joint.[28] Loss of this support may be responsible for the development of medial carpal instability. Poirier[34] had observed that the very oblique direction of the palmar and dorsal ligaments was related to their "carrying" the hand during pronation and supination. He called the "obliquum" ligament of Weitbrecht the "supinator" ligament and the dorsal radiotriquetral ligament the "pronator" ligament.

The importance, indeed the actual existence, of a collateral ligament system for the wrist has been discussed. The presence of anteroposterior and lat-

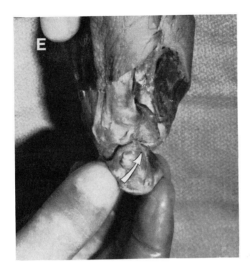

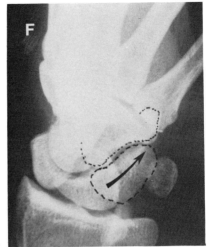

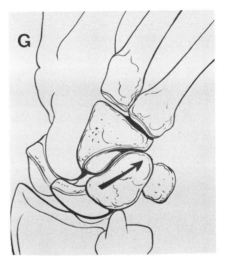

Fig. 2-22 (cont.) E, F, G: Distal ("low") position (From Taleisnik J: Current concepts of the anatomy of the wrist. In Spinner M (ed): Kaplan's Functional and Surgical Anatomy of the Hand. 3rd ed. JB Lippincott, Philadelphia, 1984.)

eral movements, as well as circumduction in this joint argues against a functionally efficient collateral system.[18,26] Kauer[18,20] pointed out that from neutral deviation to full radial or ulnar deviation, true collateral ligaments would need to bridge ever increasing distances. Therefore they would be lax in neutral deviation and consequently useless when needed the most, during dorsiflexion and volarflexion. Lateral stability depends instead on the shapes of the bones, enhanced by an "adaptable collateral system"[18] provided by the extensor carpi ulnaris, the extensor pollicis brevis, and the abductor pollicis longus.

THE DORSAL RETINACULUM OF THE WRIST°

There are two layers of forearm fascia: superficial and deep. Only the latter contributes to the formation of the extensor retinaculum of the wrist.[1] Likewise, the retinaculum itself presents two layers, both extensions of the deep antebrachial

° The author wishes to thank Dr. R. H. Gelberman, Dr. B. Miller, and Dr. R. M. Szabo for their contribution to this study, and for the use of their material.

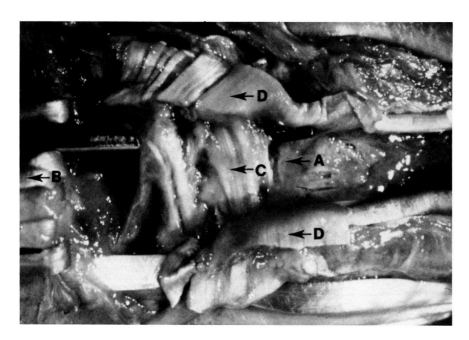

Fig. 2-23. Supratendinous and infratendinous portions of extensor retinaculum: *A*: Distal radius. *B*: Extensor tendons of fourth compartment incised and reflected distally. *C*: Infratendinous retinaculum elevated by probe. *D*: Incised supratendinous retinaculum. (From Taleisnik J, Gelberman RH, Miller BW, Szabo, RM: The extensor retinaculum of the wrist. J Hand Surg 9A:495, 1984.)

fascia, one superficial (supratendinous) and the other deep to the extensor tendons (infratendinous) (Fig. 2-23).

The Supratendinous Extensor Retinaculum

The supratendinous extensor retinaculum[39] first becomes apparent 2 to 3 cm proximal to the radiocarpal joint. Because the radial half is still thin at this same level, the retinaculum resembles an L, with the base of the L along the ulna. The supratendinous retinaculum thickens gradually as it progresses distally. It ends at the level of the carpometacarpal joints. The most proximal retinacular fibers are more transverse, and become more oblique distally (Fig. 2-24). In general, these fibers are parallel except for a small area of crisscrossing, measuring 1 cm × 1 cm, over the first and second extensor compartments.

The retinaculum has three distinct insertions on the radial side of the wrist (Fig. 2-25). Proximally it wraps around the wrist, surrounds the flexor carpi radialis tendon (with more deep than superficial fibers), and blends with the anterior antebrachial fascia (Fig. 2-26). Central fibers insert into the radius (Fig. 2-27), and distal fibers terminate by blending with the thenar fascia.

The medial supratendinous retinaculum extends over the distal ulna, without attaching to the ulna itself. The retinaculum can be followed around the medial aspect of the wrist to three distinct insertions (Fig. 2-28). Proximally the retinaculum surrounds the flexor carpi ulnaris tendon, as it did the flexor carpi radialis tendon laterally, also with more deep than superficial fibers. These fibers also blend with the anterior antebrachial fascia. The central insertion is on the triquetrum and pisiform (Fig. 2-29). Beyond the pisiform, these fibers blend with the volar carpal ligament. The distal attachment is into the hypothenar fascia and, deep to this, into the fifth metacarpal. The total length of the broad ulnar retinaculum averages 32 mm (range 26–41 mm). The lack of attachment of the supratendinous retinaculum on the head of the ulna guarantees free rotation during pronation and supination.[7,15,20,21,25,35,40]

The Infratendinous Retinaculum

The infratendinous retinaculum extends only from the radiocarpal to the carpometacarpal joint (Fig. 2-23). It is distinct only deep to the fourth and fifth dorsal extensor compartments. At this level, it tends to blend with the dorsal capsule of the wrist

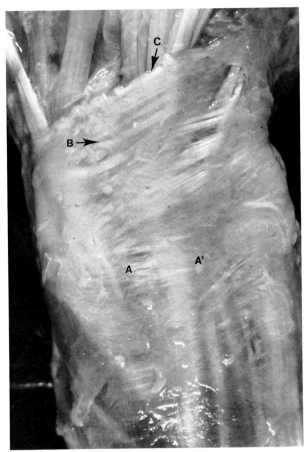

Fig. 2-24. Supratendinous extensor retinaculum. *A.A*¹:
Proximal transverse fibers. *B*: Distal oblique fibers. *C*:
Well-defined, thicker distal margin.

joint from which it can be laboriously dissected.
This feature may be utilized during dorsal surgical
exposures of the wrist: the fourth compartment can
be elevated with all its tendons still within their
tunnel, leaving behind the dorsal capsule for later
reconstruction or repair. There is no infratendinous retinaculum under the lateral three compartments. Medial to the extensor digiti quinti the
infratendinous retinaculum continues deep to the
sixth compartment; it forms a fibrous tunnel for the
extensor carpi ulnaris (Figs. 2-5, 2-15) and continues past the extensor carpi ulnaris to insert into
the triquetrum in common with the wrist capsule
and the central fibers of the supratendinous retinaculum.

Retinacular Septa and Extensor
Compartments

There are six septa separating six dorsal compartments.

The *first septum* is the central insertion of the
supratendinous retinaculum on the radius (Fig.
2-27). It arises from the periosteum of the distal
radius, averages 18 mm in length and terminates
distally at the radiocarpal joint level.

The *second septum*, between the first and second
compartments, is created by the tight adhesions of
the supratendinous retinaculum to a triangular
bony prominence of the distal radius (Fig. 2-30); in
effect, this creates a broad wall with one septum on
each side of the bony prominence, shorter on the
lateral side and longer on the medial side. The second septum terminates at the end of the distal
radius and averages 16 and 22 mm for its two portions.

The *third septum* separates the second from the
third compartments. It also arises from an osseous
eminence, Lister's tubercle, and averages 15 mm
in length.

The *fourth septum*, between the third and fourth
compartments, originates from the periosteum of
the distal radius, and blends distally with the transverse fibers of the infratendinous retinaculum. This
creates a circular tube for the extensor digitorum
communis and the extensor indicis proprius (Fig.
2-23). This tube averages 15 mm in length.

The *fifth septum*, between the fourth and fifth
compartments, constitutes the medial wall of the
fibrous tube for the extensor digitorum communis
and extensor indicis proprius (Fig. 2-23). It originates from the distal radius and terminates over the
proximal carpal row in line with the base of the
fourth metacarpal. It averages 22 mm in length.

The *sixth septum*, between the fifth and sixth
compartments, is entirely fibrous (Fig. 2-31). It
does not originate from the ulna, but from the dorsoulnar corner of the radius, and extends for an
average of 22 mm over the proximal and distal carpal rows. This strong attachment of the sixth septum forms, with the common origin of the ulnocarpal complex and the dorsal distal radioulnar
ligament,[37] a fibrous nucleus similar to the "nucleus of assemblage" described by Zancolli[43] for

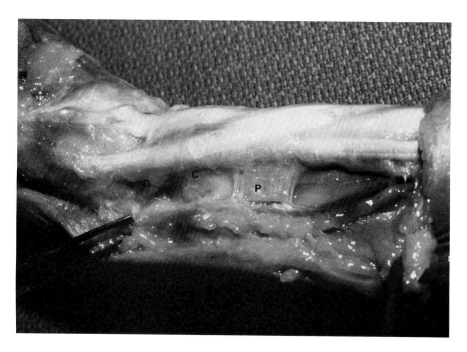

Fig. 2-25. Radial insertion of extensor retinaculum. P, proximal; C, central; D, distal.

the palmar aspect of the proximal joints of the fingers. The insertion of the sixth septum into the radius and not into the ulna assures that the function of the extensor digiti quinti, to extend the little finger, will not be embarrassed during varying degrees of rotation of the forearm.[35]

The six septa described create six tunnels or compartments.

The *first compartment* contains the abductor pollicis longus and extensor pollicis brevis. A small fibrous wall may exist separating these two tendons (Fig. 2-32). Giles[11] noted this septum in 20 percent

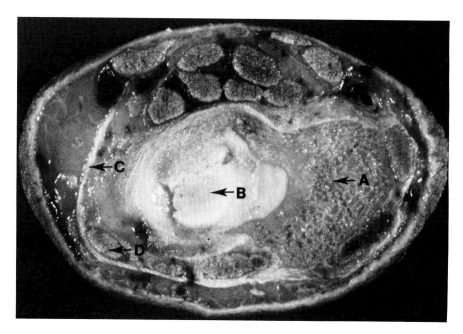

Fig. 2-26. Cross section of the wrist at the level of the distal radioulnar styloid. *C*: Supratendinous retinaculum along ulnar aspect of flexor carpi ulnaris (*D*). (From Taleisnik J, Gelberman RH, Miller BW, Szabo RM: The extensor retinaculum of the wrist. J Hand Surg 9A:495, 1984.)

Fig. 2-27. Central insertion of supratendinous retinaculum (C). *A*: Extensor carpi radialis longus tendon. *B*: Extensor pollicis brevis and abductor pollicis longus tendons.

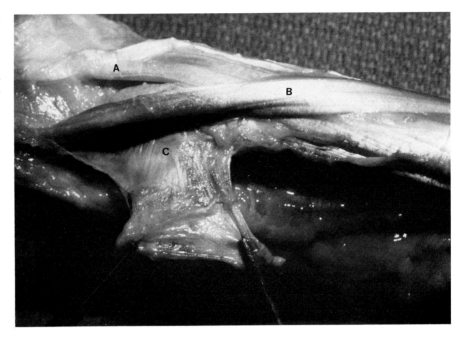

Fig. 2-28. Ulnar insertion of supratendinous retinaculum. P, proximal; C, central; D, distal.

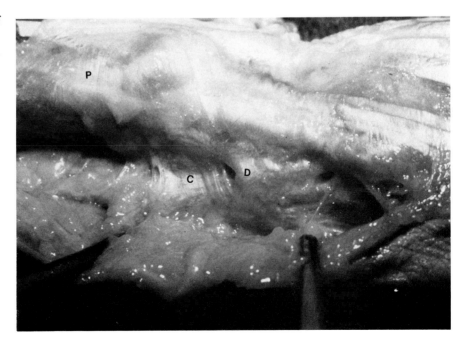

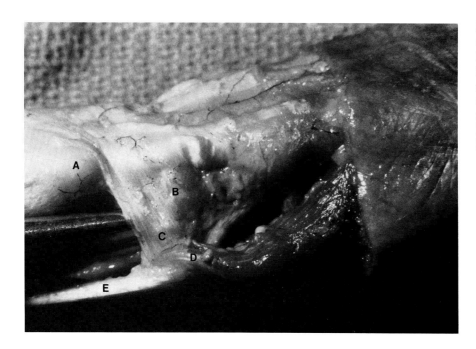

Fig. 2-29. Central insertion of supratendinous retinaculum. *A:* Ulnar head. *B:* Central portion of supratendinous retinaculum attaching on the triquetrum. *C:* Attachment on pisiform. *D:* Origin hypothenar muscles. *E:* Flexor carpi ulnaris tendon.

of 50 specimens. The floor of this tunnel is the periosteum of the distal radius and the insertion of the brachioradialis tendon.

The *second compartment* is occupied by the extensor carpi radialis brevis and longus. The floor is the radius covered by periosteum.

The *third compartment* contains the extensor pollicis longus. It crosses diagonally over the radial wrist extensors, although still contained within its own separate sheath (Fig. 2-32). The floor of this tunnel is a very thin, adherent periosteum, almost impossible to elevate if subperiosteal exposure of

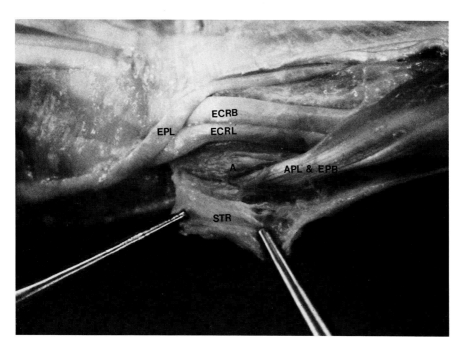

Fig. 2-30. Triangular bone prominence on distal radius (A) for attachment of second retinacular septum. STR, supratendinous retinaculum; EPL, extensor pollicis longus; ECRL and ECRB, extensor carpi radialis longus and brevis; APL, abductor pollicis longus; EPB, extensor pollicis brevis.

Fig. 2-31. Sixth septum is held by forceps (arrow). ECU, extensor carpiulnaris; EDQ, extensor digiti quinti; EDC, extensor digitorum communis.

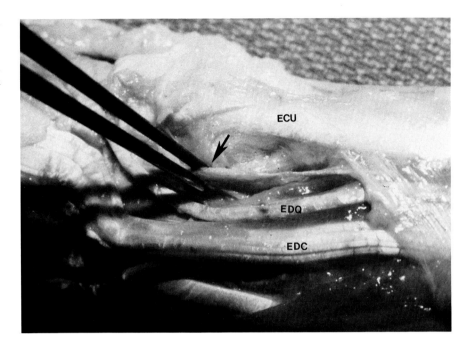

the radius at this level should be needed. A few fibers from the infratendinous retinaculum cross the periosteum transversely.

The *fourth compartment* for the extensor indicis proprius and extensor digitorum communis is a fibrous tunnel: the supratendinous retinaculum is the roof, the fourth and fifth septa the lateral and medial walls, and the infratendinous retinaculum the floor (Fig. 2-32).

The *fifth compartment* is also a fibrous tunnel created by both layers of the dorsal retinaculum, and extending from the distal radius to the midcar-

Fig. 2-32. Cross section of wrist at the level of the proximal carpal row. *A:* Compartment for extensor pollicis longus crossing over second compartment. *B:* Septum in first compartment between abductor pollicis longus and extensor pollicis brevis. *C:* Radial artery. *D:* Extension of supratendinous retinaculum to radial palmar fascia. *E:* Flexor carpi radialis tendon. *F:* Supratendinous retinaculum over *G,* flexor carpi ulnaris. *H:* Infratendinous retinaculum.

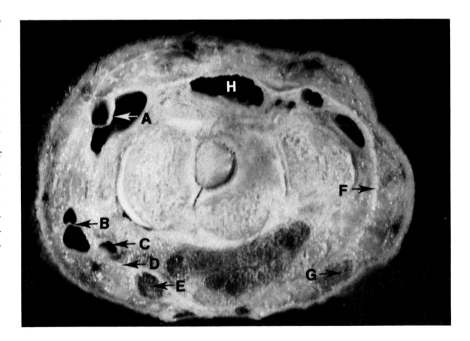

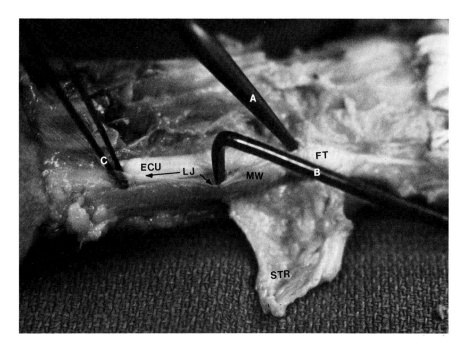

Fig. 2-33. Ulnar aspect of right wrist specimen. Probe A is inserted into fibrous tunnel (FT) for extensor carpi ulnaris tendon (ECU); probes B and C elevate the linea jugata (LJ); STR is supratendinous retinaculum.

pal joint level. It hugs the head of the ulna as it changes direction toward the base of the fourth metacarpal.

The *sixth compartment* contains within the space covered by the supratendinous retinaculum a separate fibrous tunnel for the extensor carpi ulnaris, a dependence of the infratendinous retinaculum (Fig. 2-15).

The two layers of the retinaculum are separated by a thin space filled with a loose areolar tissue. The infratendinous fibrous tunnel adheres to the ulnocarpal complex. This gives support to Kauer[18] and Landsmeer,[24] who believe that the ulnocarpal complex participates in the formation of the extensor carpi ulnaris sheath. Medial to the extensor carpi ulnaris tendon, past its fibrous tunnel, the infratendinous retinaculum and the central fibers of the supratendinous retinaculum merge and both in turn blend with the dorsal capsule to insert into the triquetrum and fifth metacarpal.[26,39] Proximal to its own fibrous tunnel, at a level where the infratendinous retinaculum is not yet defined, the proximal fibers of the supratendinous retinaculum wrap around the medial aspect of the wrist to blend with the anterior forearm fascia. Here, the medial wall of the extensor carpi ulnaris is a discrete band of transverse fibers that attach on the palmar lip of the groove for the extensor carpi ulnaris, along the distal 1 cm of ulna and styloid process. These transverse fibers are reinforced by a set of longitudinal fibers called "linea jugata" (Fig. 2-33),[26] best visualized by inspection of the deep surface of the retinaculum covering the extensor carpi ulnaris (Fig. 2-34). This structure originates from the base of the ulnar styloid distally and spreads in an oblique direction proximally, dorsally, and medially to coalesce with the supratendinous retinaculum and the pars profunda of the antebrachial fascia.

Therefore, *proximal to the base of the ulnar styloid* medial containment for the extensor carpi ulnaris is supplied by the linea jugata, tensing up at the extremes of supination, as a "dynamic block" against the tendency of the tendon to sublux in a medial and palmar direction. At the *level of the ulnar styloid* this containment is provided by the medial wall of transverse fibers, and *distal to the ulnar styloid,* by the fibrous tunnel, a part of the infratendinous retinaculum.[26,39] Thus, the extensor carpi ulnaris is the only dorsal tendon without a fixed fibroosseous tunnel, but rather with a fibrous sheath of its own that attaches distally on the carpus (triquetrum).[39] When the supratendinous retinaculum is removed, the extensor carpi ulnaris is still maintained in its position by this fibrous tunnel,[35]

Fig. 2-34. Linea jugata (LJ) seen during surgical exposure of rheumatoid wrist. U, ulnar head. (From Taleisnik J, Gelberman RH, Miller BW, Szabo RM: The extensor retinaculum of the wrist. J Hand Surg 9A:495, 1984.)

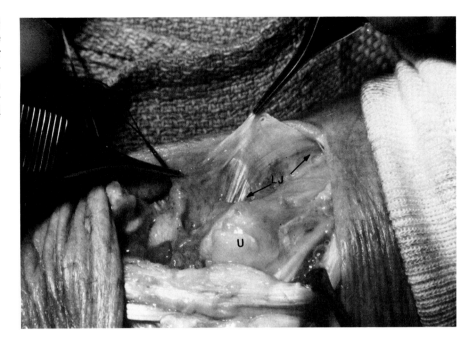

which provides the tendon with a straight approach to the carpus, regardless of the degree of pronation or supination.[39] Obrant[32] noted that in supination, the extensor carpi ulnaris forms an obtuse angle directed medially. The apex of the angle is at the transition between the proximal "dynamic" system (linea jugata) and the distal "fixed" fibrous tunnel. This angle results in an ulnar translation stress during extensor carpi ulnaris muscle contractions,[4] particularly with the forearm in supination and the hand in ulnar deviation (Fig. 2-35). Loss of the medial "dynamic" wall allows pathologic subluxation of the extensor carpi ulnaris to occur.

REFERENCES

1. Anson BJ, Wright R, Ashley F, Dynes Y: The fascia of the dorsum of the hand. Surg Gynecol Obstet 81:327, 1945
2. Berger RA, Blair WF, Crowninshield RD, Flatt AE: The scapholunate ligament. J Hand Surg 7:87, 1982
3. Bryce TH: On certain points in the anatomy and mechanism of the wrist joint reviewed in the light of a series of roentgen ray photographs of the living hand. J Anat 31:59, 1896
4. Burkhart S, Wood M, Linscheid RL: Post-traumatic recurrent subluxation of the extensor carpi ulnaris tendon. J Hand Surg 7:1, 1982

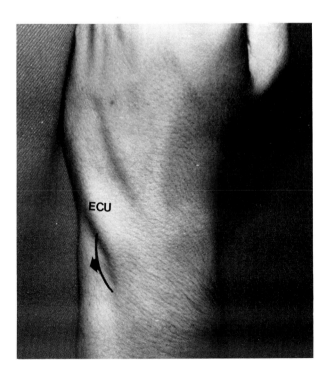

Fig. 2-35. Ulnar translation stress (arrow) on extensor carpi ulnaris (ECU) with the forearm in supination.

5. Dameron TB Jr: Traumatic dislocation of the distal radio-ulnar joint. Clin Orthop 83:55, 1972

6. Destot E: Injuries of the wrist. A radiological study. Ernest Benn, London, 1925

7. Fahrer M: Introduction to the anatomy of the wrist. In Tubiana R (ed): The Hand. Saunders, Philadelphia, 1981

8. Fick R: Handbuch der Anatomie und Mechanik der Gelenke: III. Spezielle Gelenke und Muskelmechanik. G. Fisher, Jena, 1911

9. Fisk GF: Carpal instability and the fractured scaphoid. Ann R Coll Surg Engl 46:63, 1970

10. Ghia C: Contributo allo studio della articolazione della mano. Chir Organi Mov 24:344, 1939

11. Giles K: Anatomical variations affecting the surgery of de Quervain's disease. J Bone Joint Surg [Br] 42:352, 1960

12. Hollinshead WH: Anatomy for surgeons. 2nd Ed. Vol. 3. Hoeber (Harper & Row), New York, 1969

13. Jeanne LA and Mouchet A: Les lésions traumatiques fermeés du poignet. 28th Congrès Français de Chirurgie, 1919

14. Johnston HM: Varying positions of the carpal bones in the different movements at the wrist. Part I. Extension, ulnar and radial flexion. J Anat 41:109, 1907

15. Kaplan EB: Functional and surgical anatomy of the hand. 2nd Ed. Lippincott, Philadelphia, 1965

16. Kauer JMG: The interdependence of carpal articulation chains. Acta Anat 88:481, 1974

17. Kauer JMG: The articular disc of the hand. Acta Anat 93:590, 1975

18. Kauer JMG: The collateral ligament function in the wrist joint. Acta Morphol Neerl Scand 17:252, 1979

19. Kauer JMG: Functional anatomy of the wrist. Clin Orthop 149:9, 1980

20. Kauer JMG, Landsmeer JMF: Functional anatomy of the wrist. In Tubiana R (ed): The Hand. Saunders, Philadelphia, 1981

21. Kaufman L: The dorsal fascia of the hand and the extensor carpi ulnaris tendon. In Tubiana R (ed): The Hand. Saunders, Philadelphia, 1981

22. Kirk JA, Ansell BM, Bywaters EGL: The hypermobility syndrome. Ann Rheum Dis 26:419, 1967

23. Kuhlmann N: Anatomía descriptiva y funcional del carpo en relación con la patologia traumática del mismo. Rev Esp Cir Mano 5:13, 1977

24. Landsmeer JMF: Les coherences spatials et l'equilibre spatial dans le region carpienne. Acta Anat (Basel) [Suppl 54], vol 70, 1968

25. Landsmeer JMF: Atlas of anatomy of the hand. Churchill Livingstone, Edinburgh, 1976

26. Leeuw B de: The stratigraphy of the dorsal wrist region as basis for an investigation of the position of the m. extensor carpi ulnaris in pronation and supination of the forearm. Thesis, Leiden, Luctor et Embergo., 1962

27. Lewis OJ, Hamshere RJ, Bucknill TM: The anatomy of the wrist joint. J Anat 106:539, 1970

28. Lichtman DM, Swafford AR, Mack GR: Ulnar midcarpal instability. Clinical and laboratory analysis. J Hand Surg 6:515, 1981

29. Mayfield JK, Johnson RP, Kilcoyne RF: The ligaments of the human wrist and their functional significance. Anat Rec 186:417, 1976

30. Mayfield JK, Williams WJ, Erdman AC, et al: Biomechanical properties of human carpal ligaments. Orthop Trans 3:143, 1979

31. Navarro A: Anales del Instituto de Clínica Quirúrgica y Cirugía Experimental, Imprenta Artística de Dornaleche, Montevideo, 1935

32. Obrant O: Fall av senluxation i handleden. Nord Med 29:656, 1946

33. Palmer AK, Werner FW: The triangular fibrocartilage complex of the wrist. Anatomy and function. J Hand Surg 6:153, 1981

34. Poirier P, Charpy A: Traité d'anatomie humaine. 3rd Ed. Vol. I. Masson, Paris, 1911

35. Spinner M, Kaplan EB: Extensor carpi ulnaris. Clin Orthop 68:124, 1970

36. Sutro CJ: Hypermobility of bones due to "overlengthened" capsular and ligamentous tissues. Surgery 21:67, 1947

37. Taleisnik J: The ligaments of the wrist. J Hand Surg 1:110, 1976

38. Taleisnik J: Wrist: Anatomy, function and injury. Am Acad Orthop Surgeons Instruct Course Lect 27:61, 1978

39. Taleisnik J, Gelberman RH, Miller BW, Szabo RM: The extensor retinaculum of the wrist. J Hand Surg 9A: 495, 1984

40. Testut L, Latarjet A: Tratado de anatomía humana. Vol. 1, 9th Ed. revised. Salvat Editores, Buenos Aires, 1951

41. Weber ER: Biomechanical implications of scaphoid waist fractures. Clin Orthop 149:83, 1980

42. Wright RD: A detailed study of movement of the wrist joint. J Anat 70:137, 1935

43. Zancolli EA: Structural and dynamic bases of hand surgery. 2nd Ed. Lippincott, Philadelphia, 1979

3 Carpal Kinematics

THE COLUMNAR CARPUS

Michael Lyser was the first to propose names for the carpal bones.[19] He also left detailed instructions on how to articulate carpal bones of skeletal specimens. He recommended that the trapezium, trapezoid, capitate, hamate, triquetrum, and pisiform be joined, in that order, by a single wire drawn through each bone. Only the scaphoid and lunate were left in the proximal row to be strung with a second wire. This division of the carpus into a distal row with six bones, and lunate and scaphoid as only members of the proximal row, was obviously intended for the practical anatomist and is still used today, more than three centuries later, for the preparation of skeletal specimens (Fig. 3-1). In 1929 Von Bonin[38] suggested that for some wrist motions, it was more expedient to think of the carpus as three separate sets of bones: the lunate (the "nearest to the role of the interarticular disc of all wrist bones"), the scaphoid, and "the five distal bones" (triquetrum, hamate, capitate, trapezoid, and trapezium).

Classical textbooks and publications on wrist anatomy, however, have consistently represented the carpus as two horizontal or transverse rows of four bones each[4,9,14,18–20,28,37–39]: scaphoid, lunate, triquetrum, and pisiform in the proximal, or antebrachial, row, and trapezium, trapezoid, capitate, and hamate in the distal, or metacarpal, row. This traditional concept does not conform to the dynamic anatomy of the wrist joint, to its function or to its behavior during and after injury.

In publications spanning the period between 1919 and 1935[26,27,30] Navarro proposed an entirely different concept, that of the vertical or "columnar" carpus. In his opinion, the carpus is not made of transverse condylar articulations, but is made of a central column for flexion and extension and two side columns for rotation. He stressed the fundamental role of the medial column (which he called the triquetropisiform system) in hand rotation, and he agreed with Destot,[9] who had previously pointed out the importance of the scaphoid-trapezium group. Navarro's columnar carpus was comprised of a *central or flexion-extension column,* formed by the lunate, capitate, and hamate, a *lateral* or *mobile column,* comprised of the scaphoid, trapezium, and trapezoid, and a *medial or rotation column,* consisting of the triquetrum and pisiform. Some phylogenetic support for this longitudinal representation of the carpus may be found in the primitive representation of the carpal bones.[19] Earlier anatomists had proposed a scheme of 24 cartilaginous centers, representing the possible number of carpal bones that may develop through independent ossification. The final appearance for different species would depend on the ossification pattern, causing some centers to disappear while others coalesce to form a process or an adjacent carpal bone, or else continue to develop independently as a supernumerary bone.

The ideal primitive carpus is represented as a longitudinal arrangement of bones radiating symmetrically from the axis of the limb toward the different digits. Developmental changes were sec-

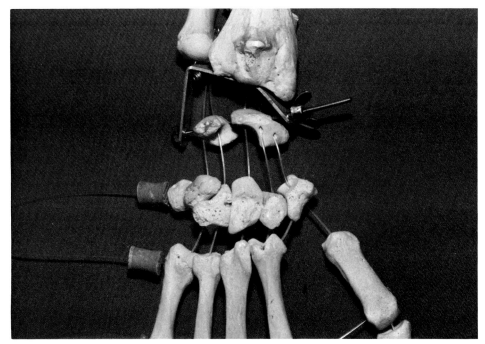

Fig. 3-1. Mounted skeleton. Lunate and scaphoid are only carpal bones in proximal row. All others are part of a single distal row.

ondary to the specialization of the radial digits for grasping and of the ulnar digits for support, stability, and strength. The only part of the primitive carpus disposed transversely was the distal row, called carpalia.[19] The primitive carpalia was composed of five bones, arranged one at the base of each of the five metacarpals. The first modification of this primitive carpus is found in digitate vertebrates, in whom the two ulnar bones are fused into one single carpal, articulating with both the fourth and fifth metacarpals.[3,19] This numerical reduction, represented by the hamate in humans, is consistently seen in mammals and is considered to be another physiologic expression of the need for stability on the ulnar side of manus and pes.[19] This disposition is similar to that in the human carpus, for the trapezium, trapezoid, capitate, and hamate are intimately joined by ligaments and constitute, for all practical purposes, a true transverse functional unit, articulating with all five metacarpals. A modification of Navarro's interpretation[34,35] incorporated this concept, expanding the central column to include the entire distal carpal row along with the lunate. The mobile column was limited to

the scaphoid, and the rotation column to the triquetrum (Fig. 3.2).

In 1202, Leonardo de Pisa, nicknamed Fibonacci, came across a sequence of numbers in connection with the breeding of rabbits.[1] In this sequence, each number is the sum of the previous two (0, 1, 1, 2, 3, 5, 8 ⋯). The Fibonacci pattern is not limited to rabbits. It is also found in the ancestral tree of the male bee and in the world of botany, from the numbers of petals in many flowers, to the scales of fir cones and pineapples. Even electricians cannot escape the obstinate sequence, since certain electrical networks can be analized in Fibonacci's terms. A carpal arrangement of three vertical columns would also fit Fibonacci's concept, for the skeletal sequence for the upper extremity would be one scapula, one humerus, two antebrachial bones, three carpal columns, and five metacarpal-digital units.

Central Flexion Extension Column: The Radiolunocapitate Link

The human wrist may be described as a central flexion-extension, longitudinal link,[13] a double

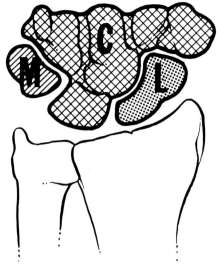

Fig. 3-2. Columnar carpus. L, lateral or mobile column (scaphoid); C, central or flexion-extension column (lunate and distal carpal row); M, medial or rotation column (triquetrum).

trochlea[27] (Fig. 1-9). Such a link mechanism allows greater total motion with flatter joint surfaces for increased stability.[13] Onto this central column attach the two V-shaped ligament structures present between radius, lunate and capitate (Figs. 2-2, 2-19, 2-20). Motions along the radiolunocapitate link are produced by muscles that bypass the carpus on the way from their origin, to their insertion into the bases of the second, third, and fifth metacarpals. Steindler[32] had pointed out that these muscle forces are asymmetrical, and that the resulting plane of dorsiflexion is radialward and that of volarflexion is ulnarward. This plane from dorsal and radial to volar and ulnar is the physiologic axis of wrist activity[3,5] (Fig. 3-3). As early as 1898 Corson[7] had stressed that flexion and adduction (volarflexion and ulnar deviation) and extension and abduction (dorsiflexion and radial deviation) are "supplementary movements." In Jeanne and Mouchet's interpretation it is the volar and ulnar angle of the distal radius that favors volarflexion during ulnar deviation.[15] Within this link system, the distal row of carpal bones, firmly attached to the capitate, moves with the hand, to which it is connected by strong interosseous ligaments. Within this radiolunocapitate system, the position of the lunate, the

potentially unstable intercalated segment, varies in response to the pull of its ligaments, the contact pressures of other carpals, and the shape of the lunate, a wedge with a larger volar pole, favoring dorsiflexion[21] (Fig. 1-8). In this type of link, stabilization is needed in only one direction and is provided by the mobile column, the scaphoid.

Lateral Mobile Column: The Scaphoid

In 1941, MacConaill[25] proposed a subdivision of the carpus that stressed the functional role of the scaphoid, a concept previously suggested by Ghia[12] and by Von Bonin.[38] MacConaill grouped the carpals into the scaphoid, then the lunate and triquetrum, and finally the trapezoid, capitate, and hamate. The trapezium was excluded, possibly because of its independent role in thumb motions. The pisiform was also excluded, because it was considered to be "part of the apparatus by which the wrist is moved," rather than part of the wrist itself. The value of this concept was that it singled out the scaphoid as an intercalated rod between proximal and distal carpals. Without the scaphoid, the central radiolunocapitate link would be very unstable under compression loads: it would tend to crumple.[10,13,23] MacConaill[25] compared the carpal function to a screw-clamp device: as dorsiflexion is completed, the scaphoid becomes one with the distal carpal row, in fact behaving as the fixed jaw of a carpal screw-vice. In further dorsiflexion, opposing the scaphoid, the hamate acts as an actual screw, pushing the triquetrolunate mass against the fixed scaphoid. At the end of dorsiflexion, the carpal bones are closely packed or locked, a position of support, stability, and strength.

The proximal pole of the scaphoid is, in a sagittal cut, wedge-shaped like the lunate,[21] with a tendency to dorsiflex similar to that of the lunate. This tendency is controlled, however, by the influence exerted by the trapezium and trapezoid on the distal pole of the scaphoid (Fig. 1-8).[12,16,17,21] Thus, during wrist volarflexion, the scaphoid is made to volarflex against this dorsiflexing tendency; during wrist dorsiflexion, the scaphoid dorsiflexes in response to its own bias, but only as far as allowed by the position of the trapezium and trapezoid and its ligamentous restraints. More complex intercarpal motions occur in ulnar and radial deviation, when

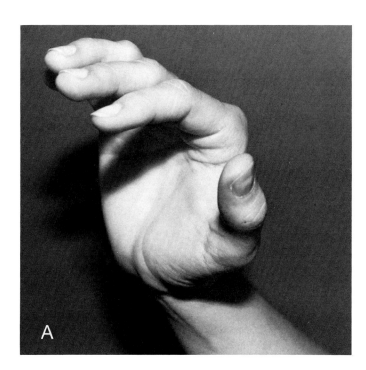

Fig. 3-3. Greatest range of motion of the wrist takes place from radial deviation and dorsiflexion *(A)* to ulnar deviation and palmarflexion *(B)*.

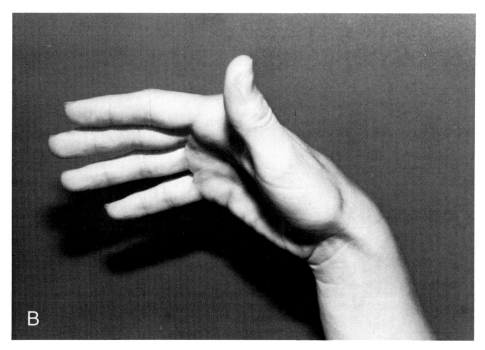

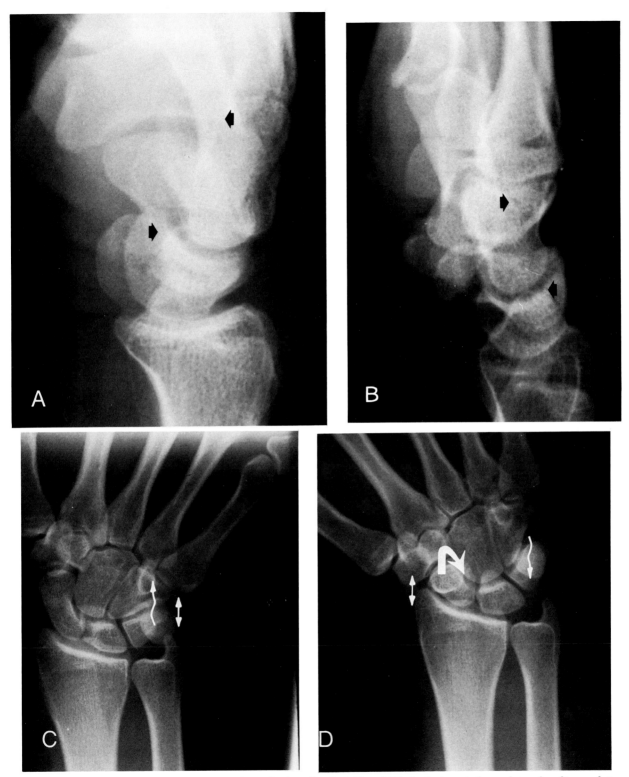

Fig. 3-4. Intercarpal relationships in ulnar (*A* and *C*) and radial (*B* and *D*) deviation. *A* shows lateral radiograph in ulnar deviation. Lunate is dorsiflexed and capitate palmarflexed to restore radiometacarpal alignment. In radial deviation (*B*) the opposite motions take place. Posteroanterior radiograph in ulnar deviation (*C*) shows dorsiflexion of the proximal carpal row: scaphoid is elongated (longitudinal), lunate is trapezoidal and triquetrum distal in relation to the hamate (wavy arrow) to accommodate for shortening of ulnocarpal distance (double arrow). In radial deviation the proximal carpal row is palmarflexed (*D*). The triquetrum is proximal in relation to the hamate (wavy arrow), lunate is triangular in shape, and scaphoid is palmarflexed to accommodate for shortening of radiocarpal distance (double arrow). (See Fig. 1-10.)

equal but opposite rotations of proximal (lunate) and distal (capitate) carpal rows can be observed (Meyer, quoted by Bryce[5]). Lateral roentgenographs of the wrist in ulnar deviation (Fig. 3-4A) show volarflexion of the capitate, and a corresponding dorsiflexion of the lunate. The opposite occurs in radial deviation (Fig. 3-4B). Divergent lunocapitate rotations create a zigzag alignment at the extremes of ulnar and radial deviation, very similar to abnormal patterns found in volar and dorsal carpal collapse deformities.[36] Volarflexion of the lunate during radial deviation is induced by the scaphoid.[12,16,17] In turn, the scaphoid is made to volarflex by the lever action of the trapezium and trapezoid,[16,17] obligated to ride dorsal to the distal pole of the scaphoid, in response to the pull of the extensor carpi radialis longus and brevis on the second and third metacarpals. As the scaphoid volarflexes, its longitudinal axis becomes perpendicular to that of the radius. In anteroposterior roentgenographs (Fig. 3-4D) the perpendicular, volarflexed scaphoid appears foreshortened, its distal pole seen end-on. This allows the radial carpal height to shorten, and the trapezium to translate very close to the tip of the radial styloid. At the same time, the triquetrum is pulled proximally, near the apex of the hamate. The coexistence of a volarflexed perpendicular scaphoid and a triquetrum in a proximal position is therefore normal (Fig. 1-10).

Medial Rotation Column: The Triquetrum

It was Navarro who first stressed the importance of the triquetropisiform system in wrist function.[26] He believed that the influence of the radius on the carpus ended on the scaphoid, "while the disposition of bones and ligaments in the medial column explained the continuation along the medial column of the movements of the forearm." In 1896 Meyer (quoted by Bryce[5]) and later on Capener[6] and Cyriax[8] suggested that there is intrinsic carpal rotation independent from forearm pronation and supination. Clinical observations during wrist dorsiflexion and ulnar deviation demonstrate a tendency of the hand to pronate, a tendency enhanced by the dorsal extension of the fourth and fifth metacarpals. In dorsiflexion and radial deviation, there is supination of the hand (Fig. 3-5). This additional

degree of wrist motion may be a factor in the mechanism of wrist injuries and their treatment.

In 1939, Ghia[12] observed that, because scaphoid displacement in a volardorsal (flexion-extension) direction was greater than that of the lunate, and nonexistent for the triquetrum, the proximal row showed a "rotation movement around a proximal-distal axis which passes through the pyramidal (triquetrum) bone." Two years later MacConaill[25] pointed out that, in the opposite motions of ulnar and radial deviation, it is the triquetrum that moves the most, and the scaphoid the least, the movement of the lunate around the head of the capitate being intermediate in amounts between those of its neighboring bones. In effect, the triquetrum does move, as stated by MacConaill, but strictly along the proximal-distal axis described by Ghia, in a pistonlike manner, up and down the hamate, from a high (proximal) to a low (distal) position (Fig. 3-4C,D).[40] This concept of the triquetrum as a movable, pistonlike pivot point is further reinforced by the disposition of the carpal ligaments in relationship to this bone, and by the shape of the joint surface that the hamate offers to the triquetrum. Volar ligament fascicles inserting on the triquetrum attach in a central area around the base of the pisiform facet (Fig. 2-2). From here they radiate toward the ulnocarpal complex, the lunate and the capitate. In the dorsum the two main ligaments related to the triquetrum approach it at right angles to each other (Fig. 2-18). This radiating ligament distribution adapts well to the proximal-distal and rotary motions of the triquetrum. This pattern of triquetral displacement is further facilitated by the helicoidal shape of the corresponding articular surface of the hamate. Ulnar deviation and the consequent shortening of the ulnar carpus are accompanied by a rotation of the medial column.[27] At the completion of ulnar deviation, when the triquetrum has descended to a distal position on the hamate, its articular surface for the hamate has rotated to face dorsally and radially: the triquetrum is dorsiflexed (Fig. 2-22). Johnston believed that dorsiflexion of the lunate in ulnar deviation was induced by the triquetrum, which was made to dorsiflex in turn by the distal carpal row carrying the triquetrum volarward along the screwlike surface of the hamate.[17] This telescoping of the triquetrum on the hamate allows the ulnar side of the wrist to shorten, as the base of the fifth metacarpal gets

Fig. 3-5. Intrinsic hand rotation during ulnar *(A)* and radial *(B)* deviation.

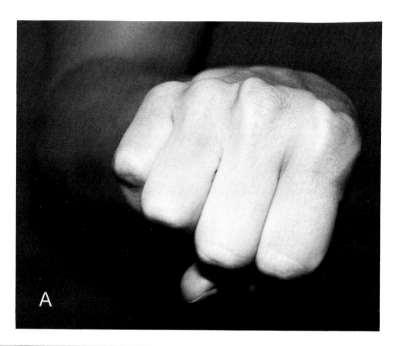

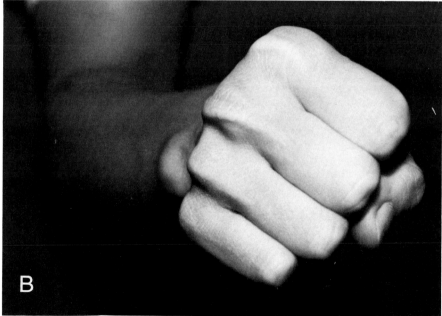

closer to the ulnar head in full ulnar deviation (Fig. 3-4C). At the same time, the scaphoid is pulled along into dorsiflexion, its long axis becoming almost parallel to that of the radius. Therefore, coexistence of a dorsiflexed triquetrum in the low, distal position and a dorsiflexed, longitudinal scaphoid is normal.

Summary

The wrist may be described as a longitudinal central flexion-extension link,[13] composed of the radius, the lunate, and the human carpalia, onto which attach two V-shaped ligament structures. Wrist motions are produced by muscles that attach

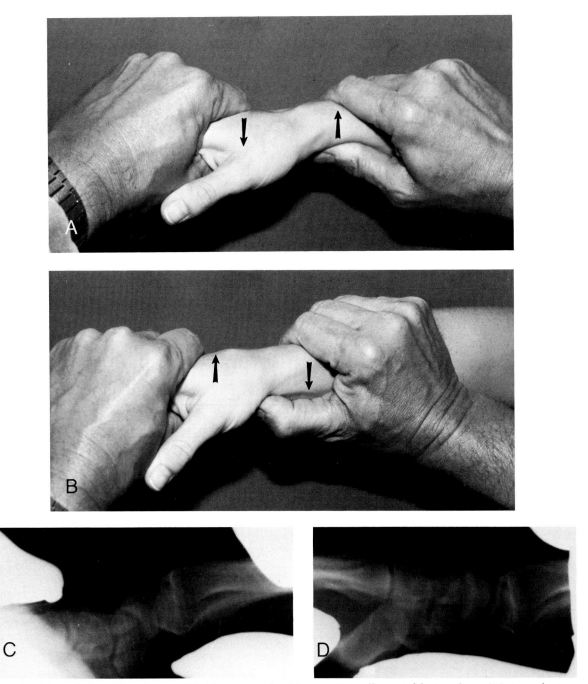

Fig. 3-6. Palmar *(A)* and dorsal stress *(B)*. Most normal wrists are minimally unstable to palmar *(C)* stress, but are stable to dorsal *(D)* stress.

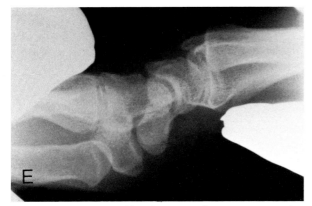 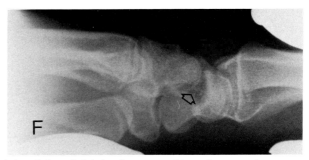

Fig. 3-6 (cont.) Normal but lax wrist shows greater palmar *(E)* and dorsal *(F)* displacement. Note the space between lunate and head of capitate after dorsal stress (arrow). Carpal alignment is similar to a dorsiflexed intercalated segmental instability (DISI).

beyond this column into the metacarpals and occur along a physiologic plane that goes from dorsal and radial to volar and ulnar. The distal carpal row moves with the hand through firm carpometacarpal attachments. These motions influence scaphoid and triquetrum behavior. In ulnar deviation, shortening of the ulnar length of the wrist is allowed by a distal telescoping of the triquetrum on the hamate, during which the triquetrum becomes dorsiflexed. In radial deviation, shortening of the radiocarpal height is made possible by volarflexion of the scaphoid into a perpendicular, foreshortened attitude. Both the radiocarpal and the midcarpal (lunocapitate) joints contribute to the total range of wrist motion, their relative participation dictated partly by the location and orientation of the scaphoid.[35] When the scaphoid is *longitudinal*, in dorsiflexion and in ulnar deviation, midcarpal motion is largely eliminated, the carpus effectively changed into a single functional unit moving on the radius at the radiocarpal joint. When the scaphoid becomes *perpendicular* to the long axis of the radius, in volarflexion and in radial deviation, the midcarpal joint "unlocks," and the distal carpal row is allowed to migrate radially. Volarflexion and radial deviation take place predominantly at the midcarpal joint level. The lunate is the intercalated segment with a morphologic, built-in tendency to dorsiflex, neutralized by the scaphoid and enhanced by the triquetrum.

THE UNSTABLE WRIST

An area of weakness in the volar aspect of the wrist may be found, caused by the absence of a volar lunocapitate ligament (Fig. 2-19). When this fascicle is present, the long intrinsic V ligament is changed into a more continuous radiate or deltoid structure. Conversely, the absence of this capitolunate support may be responsible for some forms of wrist instability. Fisk[10] believed that stability of the carpus depended on the integrity of the volar capsule between capitate and lunate. He stated that the midcarpal joint did not become unstable until this capsule was divided.

Systemic articular hypermobility in otherwise normal individuals may predispose them to joint instability.[22,33] Abnormal joint laxity may explain Nicolo Paganini's devilish virtuosity as a violinist.[31] Traumatic synovitis of the wrist was recently described in a classical guitarist.[2] The hypermobility syndrome may be at the near-normal end of a continuous range of conditions showing progressive joint laxity. This includes the hyperelastic joint disease syndrome[11] and culminates in the clearly pathologic Marfan's and Ehlers-Danlos syndromes. The combination of ligamentous deficiency and systemic joint hypermobility may explain why some normal wrists are somewhat unstable to manipulation.[34] Most normal wrists are minimally unstable when volar stress is applied to the hand (Fig.

3-6A,C), while the distal forearm is supported, but they are stable to dorsal stress (Fig. 3-6B,D). However, other wrists are not only more lax on volar stress but are also unstable on dorsal stress, especially at the midcarpal level where the capitate can almost be displaced dorsally on the lunate (Fig. 3-6E,F).[34,35] Volar stress applied to such a "lax" wrist, which is otherwise normal, reproduces the volar intercalated segment instability (VISI) deformity described by Linscheid and coworkers.[24] In addition, on dorsal stress, a dorsiflexed intercalated segmental instability (DISI) deformity is produced. Therefore pathologic patterns of instability can be reproduced in "lax" but otherwise normal wrists that are subjected to stress. The response of a wrist to injury probably depends upon its intrinsic stability, and this in turn depends not only on the bony elements, but also on the musculotendinous and ligamentous supports and their relative strength or laxity. Excessive dorsal midcarpal laxity is frequently found in the uninjured wrist of patients with carpal subluxations or dislocations and may need to be present for an injury to produce a carpal dislocation or subluxation, rather than a fracture without ligament disruption.

REFERENCES

1. Archibald RC: Golden Section, Am Math Month 25:232, 1918
2. Bird HA, Wright V: Traumatic synovitis in a classical guitarist: A study of joint laxity. Ann Rheum Dis 40:161, 1981
3. Boyes JH: Bunnell's Surgery of the Hand. 5th Ed. Lippincott, Philadelphia, 1970
4. Brash JC, Jamieson EB: Cunningham's Text-Book of Anatomy. 8th Ed. Oxford University Press, New York, 1943
5. Bryce TH: On certain points in the anatomy and mechanism of the wrist joint reviewed in the light of a series of roentgen ray photographs of the living hand. J Anat 31:59, 1896
6. Capener N: The hand in surgery. J Bone Joint Surg [Br] 38:128, 1956
7. Corson ER: An x-ray study of the normal movements of the carpal bones and wrist. Proc Assoc Am Anat 11:17, 1898
8. Cyriax EF: Some new facts in the anatomy of certain movements. J Anat 51:396, 1917
9. Destot E: Injuries of the Wrist. A Radiological Study. Ernest Benn, London, 1925
10. Fisk GF: Carpal instability and the fractured scaphoid. Ann R Coll Surg Engl 46:63, 1970
11. Gardner RC: The hyperelastic joint disease syndrome. JAMA 236:1115, 1976
12. Ghia C: Contributo allo studio della articolazione della mano. Chir Organi Mov 24:344, 1939
13. Gilford WW, Bolton RH, Lambrinudi C: The mechanism of the wrist joint with special reference to fractures of the scaphoid. Guys Hosp Rep 92:52, 1943
14. Hollingshead WH: Anatomy for Surgeons. 2nd Ed. Vol. 3. Harper & Row, New York, 1969
15. Jeanne LA and Mouchet A: Les lésions traumatiques fermées du poignet. 28th Congrès Français de Chirurgie, 1919
16. Johnston HM: Varying positions of the carpal bones in the different movements at the wrist. Part I. Extension, ulnar and radial flexion. J Anat 41:109, 1907
17. Johnston HM: Varying positions of the carpal bones in the different movements at the wrist. Part II, (a) Palmar and dorsal flexion, (b) radial and ulnar flexion combined with palmar and dorsal flexion. J Anat 41:280, 1907
18. Johnston TB, Whillis J: Gray's Anatomy: Descriptive and Applied. 30th Ed. Longmans, Green, New York, 1949
19. Jones FW: The Principles of Anatomy as Seen in the Hand. 2nd Ed. (Reprint). Baillière, Tindall, London, 1949
20. Kaplan EB: Functional and Surgical Anatomy of the Hand. 2nd Ed. Lippincott, Philadelphia, 1965
21. Kauer JMG: Functional anatomy of the wrist. Clin Orthop 149:9, 1980
22. Kirk JA, Ansell BM, Bywaters EGL: The hypermobility syndrome. Ann Rheum Dis 26:419, 1967
23. Landsmeer JMF: Studies in the anatomy of articulation. The equilibrium of the "intercalated" bone. Acta Morphol Neerl Scand 3:287, 1961
24. Linscheid RL, Dobyns JH, Beabout JW, Bryan RS: Traumatic instability of the wrist. J Bone Joint Surg [Am] 54:1612, 1972
25. MacConaill MA: The mechanical anatomy of the carpus and its bearing on some surgical problems. J Anat 75:166, 1941
26. Navarro A: Luxaciones del carpo. An Fac Med (Montevideo) 6:113, 1921
27. Navarro A: Anatomia y fisiologia del carpo. An Inst Clin Quir Cir Exp. Montevideo, 1935
28. Rouviere H: Anatomie Humaine, Descriptive et Topographique. 5th Ed. Vol. 2. Masson, Paris, 1940
29. Sarrafian SK, Melamed JL, Goshgarian GM: Study of

wrist motion in flexion and extension. Clin Orthop 126:153, 1977

30. Scaramuzza RFJ: El movimiento de rotación en el carpo y su relacion con la fisiopatologia de sus lesiones traumaticas. Bol Trabaj Soc Argentina Ortop Traum 34:337, 1969

31. Smith RD, Worthington JW: Paganini, the riddle and connective tissue. JAMA 199:156, 1967

32. Steindler A: Postgraduate Lectures in Orthopedics, Diagnosis and Indications. Charles C Thomas, Springfield, IL, 1950

33. Sutro CJ: Hypermobility of bones due to "over-lengthened" capsular and ligamentous tissues. Surgery 21:67, 1947

34. Taleisnik J: The ligaments of the wrist. J Hand Surg 1:110, 1976

35. Taleisnik J: Wrist: Anatomy, function and injury. Am Acad Orthop Surgeons Instruct Course Lect 27:61, 1978

36. Taleisnik J: Post-Traumatic carpal instability. Clin Orthop 149:73, 1980

37. Testut L, Latarjet A: Tratado de anatomía humana. 9th Ed. Vol. 1, revised. Salvat Editores, Buenos Aires, 1951

38. Von Bonin G: A note on the kinematics of the wrist joint. J Anat 63:259, 1929

39. Von Lanz T, Wachsmuth W: Praktische Anatomie. Springer-Verlag Berlin, 1959

40. Weber ER: Biomechanical implications of scaphoid waist fractures. Clin Orthop 149:83, 1980

4 The Vascular Anatomy of the Wrist

PERICARPAL ARTERIAL NETWORK

THE CLASSIC ANATOMIC NORM

The blood supply to the wrist derives from branches of the radial, ulnar, and interosseous arteries. The following is a schematic representation of the classic descriptions of the extraosseous circulation to the carpus.[15-17,34,35,42] (See Figs. 4-1 and 4-2.)

The Radial Artery

The radial artery is the smaller of the two terminal branches of the brachial artery. Proximal to the radiocarpal joint, this artery rests on the pronator quadratus muscle, on the volar-radial quadrant of the wrist. As it reaches the radial styloid, the artery changes its direction to proceed dorsally and distally, first around and then just beyond the tip of the styloid process of the radius. It continues deep to the abductor pollicis longus and extensor pollicis brevis tendons, across the anatomic snuffbox and under the extensor pollicis longus tendon, to reach the apex of the first dorsal interosseous space. It passes between the two heads of the first dorsal interosseous muscle in a volar direction to reach the palm of the hand, where it joins the deep palmar branch of the ulnar artery to form the deep palmar arch.

The Ulnar Artery

The ulnar artery originates from the brachial artery at a rather sharp angle. Between its inception and the branching out of its interosseous division, the ulnar artery is rather large, and has been called the ulnointerosseous (cubitointerosseous) trunk, a denomination that appears to be embryologically correct.[41] Upon reaching the distal third of the forearm the ulnar artery lies on the pronator quadratus muscle between the flexor carpi ulnaris and the flexor digitorum superficialis tendons. At the level of the wrist, the artery courses on the transverse carpal ligament, deep to the volar carpal ligament. It enters the canal of Guyon, between the pisiform medially and the hook of the hamate on its radial side. It terminates, joining the superficial palmar branch of the radial artery, to form the superficial palmar arch.

The Common Interosseous Artery

The common interosseous artery is short and substantial. It originates in the proximal forearm from the dorsal aspect of the ulnar artery. Upon reaching the proximal border of the interosseous membrane in the proximal forearm, it bifurcates into anterior and posterior interosseous arteries. The anterior interosseous descends on the interosseous membrane, between the flexor pollicis longus radially and the flexor digitorum profundus medially. Upon reaching the pronator quadratus, it gives off two branches: a small *volar* division, which

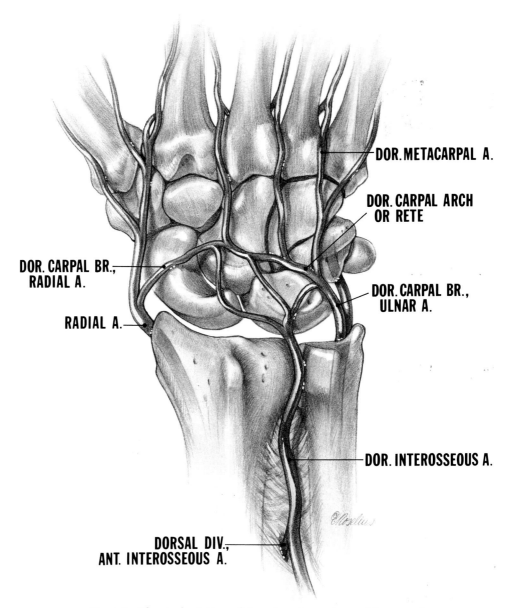

DOR. METACARPAL A.

DOR. CARPAL ARCH
OR RETE

DOR. CARPAL BR.,
RADIAL A.

DOR. CARPAL BR.,
ULNAR A.

RADIAL A.

DOR. INTEROSSEOUS A.

DORSAL DIV.,
ANT. INTEROSSEOUS A.

Fig. 4-1. Classic depiction of dorsal pericarpal arterial network.

passes deep to the pronator quadratus and anastomoses with the volar carpal network, and a larger *dorsal* division,[15] considered by many to be a continuation of the main anterior interosseous trunk. This dorsal division perforates the interosseous membrane to enter the dorsum of the wrist, running alongside the posterior interosseous nerve after that point. It is then joined by the termination of the posterior interosseous artery, which had descended along the interosseous space, in a plane between the superficial and the deep muscle layers of the extensor compartment of the forearm. This terminal common interosseous dorsal vessel bifurcates into lateral and medial branches, which in turn anastomose with ascending rami from the dorsum of the carpus, the lateral division with vessels

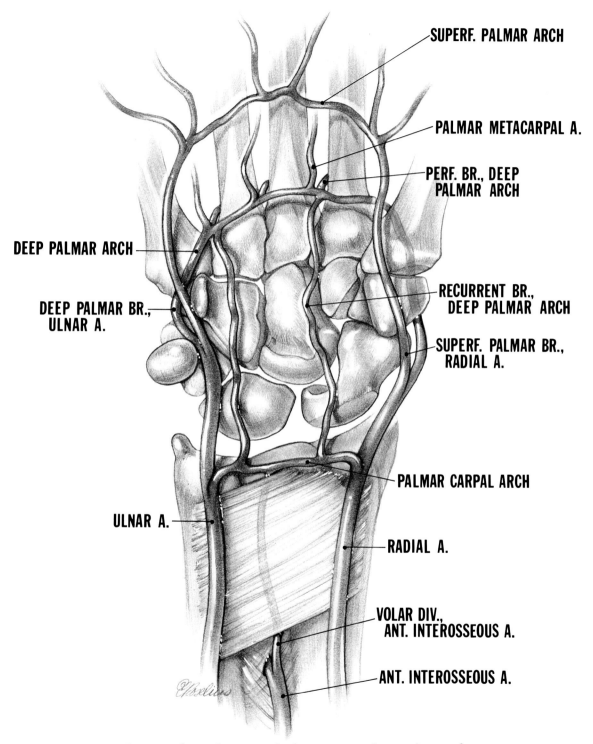

Fig. 4-2. Classic depiction of palmar pericarpal arterial network.

arising from the dorsal carpal branch of the radial artery, and the medial division with vessels from the dorsal carpal branch of the ulnar artery.[42] One additional artery, the *median*, a slender branch of the distal portion of the anterior interosseous vessel, which accompanies the median nerve, ends in the superficial palmar arch, and is occasionally large enough to be a meaningful contributor.[16]

Branches of the Main Arteries

Branches of these main arterial trunks supply the carpus. Just before the radial artery leaves its anterior location to reach the dorsum of the hand, it gives off a palmar carpal branch that anastomoses with the analogus ulnar palmar carpal branch to form a *palmar carpal* or *transverse arch*,[16] running along the distal border of the pronator quadratus. Likewise, a dorsal carpal artery (ramus carpeus dorsalis[26]) originates from the radial artery within the anatomic snuff box, at a point level with the lunocapitate joint. It then courses along the dorsum of the carpus in a medial direction, to join a similar branch from the ulnar artery, both constituting a *dorsal carpal arch*. The two contributing vessels from the ulnar artery, the dorsal and volar carpal branches, originate from the main trunk as it passes along the base of the ulnar styloid. From the convex distal side of the dorsal arch arise small descending (distal) interosseous arteries, which join perforating metacarpal vessels arising from the deep palmar arch. From the concave side of the arch arise several ascending (proximal) rami, which join with the common dorsal termination of the interosseous vessels. This vascular plexus dorsal to the carpus has been called "dorsal carpal rete."

On the palmar aspect, distal to the palmar carpal arch, two additional vascular loops are traditionally described as the superficial and the deep palmar arches. The first, formed by the anastomosis of the superficial palmar branch of the radial artery and the termination of the ulnar artery proper, does not share in the blood supply of the carpus. The second, the deep palmar arch, is an important contributor to the vascularity of the carpal bones. It is formed by the deep palmar branch of the ulnar artery and by the radial artery after it pierces the first dorsal interosseous muscle to enter the palm. The deep palmar arch lies directly on the interosseous plane, deep to the adductor pollicis and to all the flexor tendons. It traverses the hand immediately distal to the metacarpal bases, approximately 1.5 to 2 cm proximal to the superficial palmar arch. Ascending (recurrent or articular) branches arise from the deep palmar arch and traverse on the volar surface of the carpus in a proximal direction to join descending vessels from the volar carpal arch and from the volar division of the anterior interosseous artery. There are four descending (metacarpal or volar interossei) arteries arising from the convexity of the deep palmar arch. The princeps pollicis may be included in this group. From the posterior or deep surface of the deep palmar arch arise three posterior (dorsal or perforating) branches for the second, third, and fourth interosseous spaces. These vessels anastomose with the dorsal metacarpal arteries[6] and are important contributors to the blood supply of the dorsum of the hand. The branch perforating the first interosseous space is, of course, the radial artery itself.

In summary, a classic description of vessels of the wrist shows the ulnar, radial, and interosseous arteries contributing to form four main vascular arches: palmar and dorsal carpal and superficial and deep palmar.

ARTERIAL VARIATIONS

McCormack et al.[24] reported 18.53 percent major variations in the brachial and antebrachial arterial patterns of 750 consecutive upper extremity specimens. Departures from the anatomic norm involved the radial artery in 81.3 percent of all variations encountered. The ulnar artery was anomalous in only 12.22 percent. In most cases, the significant aberration was a high origin for the radial artery.

Closer to the hand, unusual terminal branches of the radial artery were comparatively rare. Six specimens in the series of McCormack and coworkers[24] presented a duplication into a dorsal branch, reaching the first dorsal interosseous space, and a palmar branch terminating within the palm as the radial contributor to the deep palmar arch. Frequently, the ulnar artery was seen to give off two, instead of one, deep palmar branch. Some authors[6,45] have described superior and inferior deep palmar arteries arising from the ulnar. Either of these independently, or both simultaneously, can anastomose with the terminal radial artery to form the deep palmar arch. The superior ramus may be found running alongside the deep branch of the ulnar nerve and contributing to the deep palmar arch in approximately one third of specimens. The inferior deep branch completed the deep palmar arch more frequently, and was seen in 49 percent of cases in Coleman and Anson's[6] series, but in only 34 percent of specimens in a similar study by Weathersby.[44] In Weathersby's opinion, when the ulnar contribution to the deep palmar artery failed to occur, the arch was completed by a perforating branch from a dorsal metacarpal artery.[44] Several studies[6,26,27] describe significant contributions to the carpus from both the dorsal and volar interosseous arteries. Most discrepancies are found in the distribution of the posterior interosseous artery. Some authors[14,22,38] give this artery an active role in the formation of the dorsal carpal arterial plexus. Others[16] show this artery stopping short of the carpus. Travaglini believes that the posterior interosseous artery actually exhausts its supply on the superficial dorsal network of the carpus, mainly on the dorsal retinaculum and adjacent soft tissues.[42] The distribution of the artery beyond this point has traditionally been extremely difficult to follow. In Travaglini's[42] opinion, this artery does not reach the carpus which is, therefore, supplied only by the anterior interosseous with its dorsal and volar branches for both dorsal and volar carpal surfaces. In 1923 Lawrence and Bachuber[18] described an anastomosis between the volar terminal branches of the anterior interosseous artery and recurrent carpal rami from the volar carpal arch. This was again reported by Lawrence in 1937,[19] and by Quiring in 1949.[33] Reports of preservation of hand viability following ligation of both the radial and ulnar arteries, depend to a considerable extent on the completeness of this volar anastomosis.[13] Variations from the classic description of the deep palmar arch and the dorsal carpal arch have also been described. Coleman and Anson[6] classified deep palmar arches into two groups (Fig. 4-3). In group I the arch was complete. Most specimens (97 percent of 200) presented this configuration. In group I, subgroups depended on whether the superior ramus of the ulnar artery, or the inferior ramus, or

both, contributed to the formation of the deep palmar arch. Group II consisted of those specimens with an incomplete arch, without anastomosis between the deep palmar branches of the ulnar and the similar branches from the radial artery. Within these groups, Coleman and Anson[6] described two types, according to anatomic characteristics. In type A the radial artery was the sole contributor to the thumb and the radial side of the index finger, while the ulnar artery ended in an anastomosis with the second perforating vessel. In type B the second perforating stayed with the radial artery, while the ulnar artery ended in an anastomosis with the third perforating artery.

The dorsal blood supply to the carpus has been the subject of some controversy. In 1881 Von Meyer[25] stated that the dorsal carpal rete was of only secondary importance in supplying the dorsum of the hand. Anseroff[2] attempted to compare the volume of dorsal versus palmar supply to the carpus and concluded that the dorsal predominates in some areas, but that there was palmar preponderance for most carpal bones. Logroscino and De Marchi[22] believed that the dorsal carpal supply was functionally more important than the palmar. Some reports have stressed the importance of the dorsal vascularity,[26,42] although in most investigations only a single significant dorsal carpal arch has been described.[6,34,41]

A review of the literature suggests that the palmar blood supply to the carpus is rudimentary. This opinion may be due to the difficulty in exposing the palmar network, while the more accessible dorsal vessels are easier to demonstrate. Coleman and Anson[6] showed that all dorsal blood supply is heavily dependent on the passage of branches from the palmar arteries to the dorsum, the main volar contributors being the anterior interosseous and both ulnar and radial arteries. The classic description of the dorsal carpal arch is actually far from constant.[6,26,27] Coleman and Anson[6] studied the dorsal carpal vessels in 75 specimens. The dorsal carpal branch of the radial artery (ramus carpeus dorsalis[26]) contributed to the dorsal carpal rete in 93.3 percent of their specimens. The participation of the ulnar branch was more rare, seen in only 38.6 percent of these dissections. Frequently (82.7 percent) a common contribution arose from the volar and dorsal interosseous arteries. Six arterial pat-

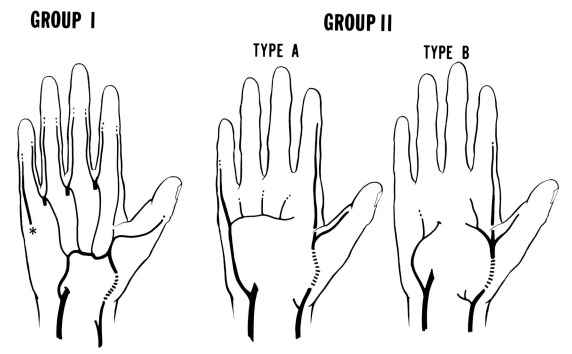

Fig. 4-3. Coleman and Anson's classification of variations of deep palmar arch. Group I: complete. Group II: incomplete. In type A, radial artery is sole contributor to thumb and radial side of index; ulnar artery anastomoses with second perforating vessel. In type B, radial artery anastomoses with second perforating, and ulnar artery with third. (Modified by permission from Surgery, Gynecology & Obstetrics from Coleman SS, Anson LJ: Arterial patterns in the hand, based upon study of 650 specimens. Surg Gynecol Obstet 113:1409, 1961.)

terns were found, all resulting in the formation of a single carpal arch (Fig. 4-4). In type I, the dorsal plexus resulted from anastomosis of radial and interosseous branches. In type II, all three arteries, radial, interosseous, and ulnar, were contributors. This, the classic configuration, was actually second in frequency and present in approximately one third of all specimens. Type III was formed exclusively by the radial branch alone, and type IV by radial and ulnar rami without any participation from the interosseous artery. In type V, only the ulnar and interosseous arteries contributed to form the dorsal carpal rete. In type VI, there was no discernible dorsal plexus. Mestdagh et al.,[26] in a study limited to the dorsal arterial network of the wrist, agreed in general with Coleman and Anson's findings; the dorsal carpal branch of the radial artery was found to be the most important and constant contributor to the dorsal carpal arch, joining a common dorsal interosseous (in 80 percent of their

specimens) or, rarely, a dorsal ulnar carpal branch, frequently minute and of limited reach. Just as in Coleman and Anson's experience, the plexus formed by radial and interosseous branches, (radial-interosseous arch) was the most prevalent, while the more classical radial-interosseous-ulnar system was second in frequency.

RECENT STUDIES[*]

The use of standard dissecting techniques, even with the help of magnification for the study of these small vessels and their anastomoses, is diffi-

* The author wishes to thank R.H. Gelbermian and Drs. W.H. Akeson, T.D. Bauman, M. Baumgaertner, J. Menon, and J.S. Panagis for the material included in this chapter, updating the extra- and intraosseous arterial anatomy of the carpus.

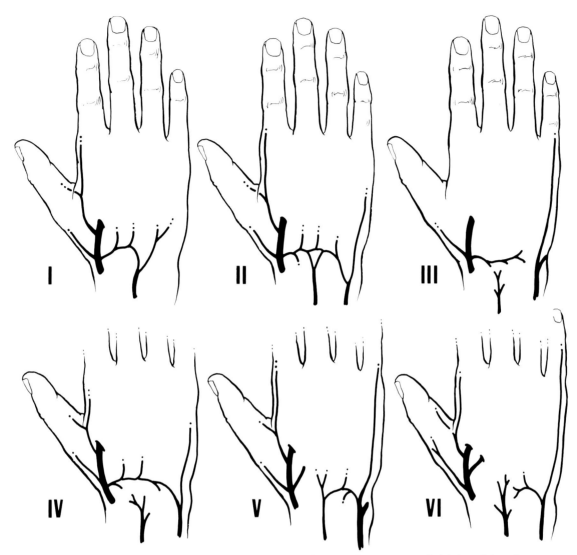

Fig. 4-4. Variations in the formation of the dorsal carpal network. Type I: Radial (R) and dorsal interosseous (DI) arch. Type II: R, DI, and ulnar (U) arch. Type III: R arch. Type IV: R and U arch. Type V: U and DI arch. In type VI there was no discernible dorsal plexus. (Modified by permission from Surgery, Gynecology & Obstetrics from Coleman SS, Anson LJ: Arterial patterns in the hand, based upon a study of 650 specimens. Surg Gynecol Obstet 113:1409, 1961.)

cult[4,6,26,42] and may produce results that are frequently contradictory,[6,26,27,34,40,42] and at times confusing. This is in part due to their small size and to their location, embedded deeply within the joint capsule and ligaments, and in part to the vascular arrangement into a tridimensional lattice around the wrist, extremely difficult to expose intact by dissecting techniques alone. Fracassi[10] reported on

the successful use of corrosion of perivascular tissues to produce striking specimens of vascular trees. Technical improvements involving the use of chemical debridement of perivascular soft tissues, have allowed a more accurate study of fine extraosseous arteries. These techniques make dissection of minute vessels penetrating through capsule and ligamentous structures unnecessary. By debriding the fibrous tissues surrounding the vessels of wrist specimens, their tridimensional orientation can be preserved[11,12,13] and their access to each carpal bone may be more precisely determined. Gelberman et al.[13] and Panagis et al.[29] injected specimens with either diluted Ward's blue latex, or Batson's compound (Polyscience Incorporated, Warrington, PA). Batson's compound sets up as a rigid material which maintains its three-dimensional orientation. Injected specimens are treated in full-strength household bleach (sodium hypochloride). Both latex and Batson's compound resist bleach digestion, allowing the tridimensional vascular pattern to emerge virtually intact. These techniques were particularly useful in studying the ulnar artery's variable and fragile branches to the midcarpus. The pericarpal arterial network was found to be formed by the anastomosis of three dorsal and

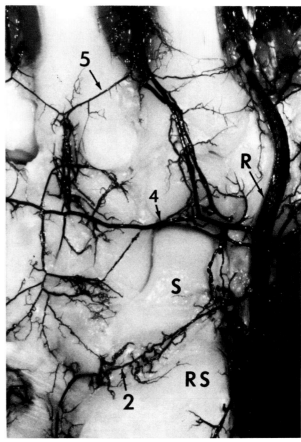

Fig. 4-6. View of the three dorsal transverse arches. RS, Radial styloid; S, scaphoid; R, radial artery; 2, dorsal radiocarpal arch; 4, dorsal intercarpal arch; 5, basal metacarpal arch. (From Gelberman RH, Panagis JS, Taleisnik J, Baumgaertner M: The arterial anatomy of the human carpus. Part I: The extraosseous vascularity. J Hand Surg 8:367, 1983.)

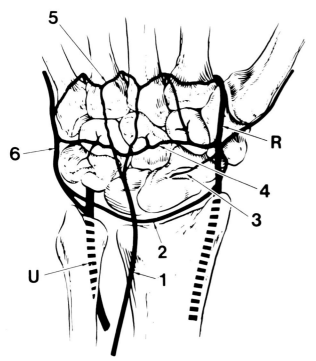

Fig. 4-5. Schematic drawing of the arterial supply of the dorsum of the wrist. R, radial artery; U, ulnar artery; 1, dorsal branch, anterior interosseous artery; 2, dorsal radiocarpal arch; 3, branch to the dorsal ridge of the scaphoid; 4, dorsal intercarpal arch; 5, basal metacarpal arch; 6, medial branch of the ulnar artery. (From Gelberman RH, Panagis JS, Taleisnik J, Baumgaertner M: The arterial anatomy of the human carpus. Part I: The extraosseous vascularity. J Hand Surg 8:367, 1983.)

three volar arches, connected longitudinally along their medial and lateral borders by the ulnar and radial arteries, with additional longitudinal anastomoses provided by the dorsal and volar branches of the anterior interosseous artery. The radial and ulnar arteries at this level are 3 to 4 mm in diameter, the arches are approximately 1 mm, and their branches are less than 1 mm in diameter.

The Dorsal Arches

The three dorsal arches (Figs. 4-5, 4-6) are located at the radiocarpal, intercarpal, and basal metacarpal levels. Of these, the radiocarpal and intercarpal arches are most constant.

The more proximal *radiocarpal arch* courses deep to the extensor tendon layer, at a level even with the radiocarpal joint. It is present in most specimens (80 percent) and usually results from the anastomosis of branches of the radial, ulnar, and interosseous arteries. In less than one third of specimens, only two arteries contributed to the radiocarpal arch, either a radial-ulnar or a radial-interosseous combination. The dorsal interosseous artery itself was not found to contribute significantly.

The *intercarpal arch* was present in all specimens, running transversely across the wrist, at the midcarpal joint level. Unlike previous reports[6,26] the classic configuration with contributions from the radial, ulnar, and interosseous arteries was found most consistently, in 53 percent of specimens. In 20 percent, a radioulnar arch was present, in 20 percent a radial-interosseous arch, and in 7 percent an ulnar-interosseous configuration.

The distal or *basal metacarpal arch* was complete in 27 percent of specimens. It was absent in 27 percent and was partially present (on its radial portion alone) in 46 percent. It was supplied by the second, third, and fourth perforating vessels, arising from the deep palmar arch, and by a small branch from the first perforating (the radial artery) given off as the radial artery pierced the two heads of the first dorsal interosseous muscle. The basal metacarpal arch extended across the bases of the second through fifth metacarpals, just distal to the carpometacarpal joint level. It was the smallest of the three dorsal systems. Longitudinal anastomosis between the arches were provided by the radial and ulnar arteries, and by the dorsal branch of the anterior interosseous artery. The intercarpal arch was generally the largest, corresponding to the single dorsal carpal arch of classic descriptions.

The Volar Arches

The three *volar arches* (Fig. 4-7) are the radiocarpal, the intercarpal, and deep palmar.[29]

The *volar radiocarpal* was present in all specimens, formed by the volar carpal branches of the radial and ulnar arteries, together with the anterior interosseous artery in 87 percent of specimens. In 13 percent, only radial and ulnar arteries contributed to its formation. It traverses the wrist within the volar capsule, 5 to 8 mm proximal to the radio-

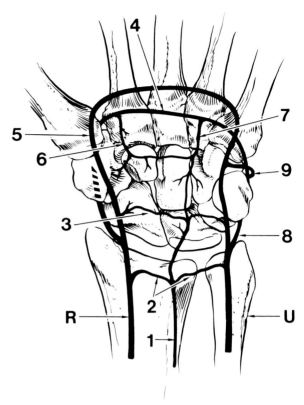

Fig. 4-7. Schematic drawing of the arterial supply of the palmar aspect of the wrist. R, radial artery; U, ulnar artery; 1, palmar branch, anterior interosseous artery; 2, palmar radiocarpal arch; 3, palmar intercarpal arch; 4, deep palmar arch; 5, superficial palmar arch; 6, radial recurrent artery; 7, ulnar recurrent artery; 8, medial branch, ulnar artery; 9, branch off ulnar artery contributing to the dorsal intercarpal arch. (From Gelberman RH, Panagis JS, Taleisnik J, Baumgaertner M: The arterial anatomy of the human carpus. Part I: The extraosseous vascularity. J Hand Surg 8:367, 1983.)

carpal joint. It is the volar carpal arch of the classic anatomist.

The *intercarpal arch* was seen in only 53 percent of specimens, the smallest and most variable of the three. Three fourths of volar intercarpal arches received contributions from the radial, ulnar, and interosseous arteries; the other fourth from the radial and ulnar arteries alone.

The *deep palmer arch* was present in 100 percent of specimens. There are three systems of vessels arising from this arch: proximal, deep, and distal. Of these, the two proximal vessels, called radial and ulnar recurrent arteries, were found to be most important. The three volar arches are connected longitudinally by the radial, ulnar, and interosseous arteries, and by these deep palmar recurrent arteries.

The Radial Artery

The *radial artery* is the most consistent of all major arterial contributors to the carpal arches (Fig. 4-8). Seven branches arise from the radial artery, of which the second, third, and sixth contribute to the formation of the carpal arches. While still coursing on the anterior aspect of the wrist, between the flexor carpi radialis and the brachioradialis, the radial artery gives off a first branch, the superficial palmar artery, which is the radial contribution to the formation of the superficial palmar arch (Fig. 4-9). The second branch is the volar carpal artery, arising 5 mm distal to the first, the tributary to the volar radiocarpal arch. The third branch supplies the dorsal radiocarpal arch and originates as the radial artery changes its course toward the dorsum. The fourth and fifth branches are direct suppliers to the scaphoid and trapezium (Fig.

4-10). The sixth branch is analogous to the dorsal carpal artery classically described, the ramus carpeus dorsalis, a rather large vessel arising directly from the radial artery in most specimens, frequently (56 percent) at the midcarpal level, and rarely (12 percent) as the radial artery enters the first interosseous space. In 22 percent, this branch was seen to originate from a more medial branch of the radial artery, directed toward the second interosseous space. Mestdagh et al.[26] have also described a bifurcation of the radial artery into two branches, one medial and the other lateral, perforating the first two interosseous spaces to reach the palm. In 28.5 percent of their specimens the dorsal carpal branch was seen to arise from the most medial of the two divisions of the radial artery. The last or seventh branch of the radial artery is a direct supplier for the trapezium and for the first metacarpal.

The Ulnar Artery

In general, the contributions from the *ulnar artery* are smaller, more fragile, and less well-de-

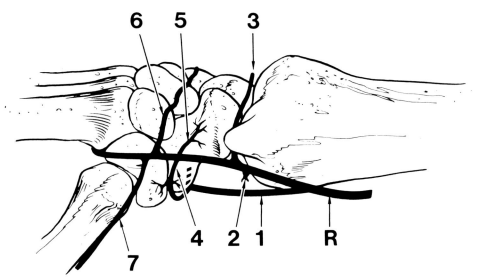

Fig. 4-8. Schematic drawing of the arterial supply of the lateral aspect of the wrist. R, radial artery; 1, superficial palmar artery; 2, palmar radiocarpal arch; 3, dorsal radiocarpal arch; 4, branch to the scaphoid tubercle and trapezium; 5, artery to the dorsal ridge of the scaphoid; 6, dorsal intercarpal arch; 7, branch to the lateral trapezium and thumb metacarpal. (From Gelberman RH, Panagis JS, Taleisnik J, Baumgaertner M: The arterial anatomy of the human carpus. Part I: The extraosseous vascularity. J Hand Surg 8:367, 1983.)

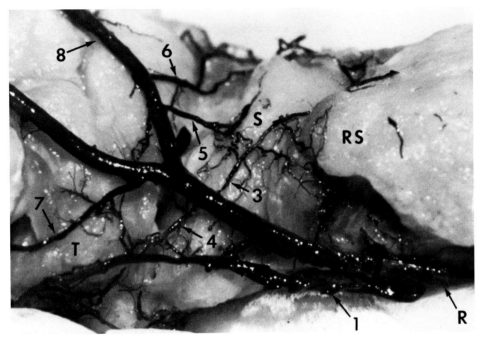

Fig. 4-9. Vascularity to the lateral aspect of the wrist. RS, radial styloid; S, scaphoid; T, trapezium; R, radial artery; 1, superficial palmar branch of radial artery; 3, dorsal radiocarpal arch; 4, branch to the tubercle of the scaphoid and trapezium; 5, artery to dorsal ridge of scaphoid; 6, dorsal intercarpal arch; 7, branch to the lateral trapezium and thumb metacarpal; 8, medial branch of radial artery (seen in 22% of the specimens) penetrating the base of the index-long web space. (Note, in this view, 2, the palmar radiocarpal arch, cannot be seen). (From Gelberman RH, Panagis JS, Taleisnik J, Baumgaertner M: The arterial anatomy of the human carpus. Part I: The extraosseous vascularity. J Hand Surg 8:367, 1983.)

fined. The first level of branches includes those tributaries to the dorsal and the volar radiocarpal arches, arising either independently, or from a common trunk given off proximal to the ulnar styloid (Fig. 4-5). The ulnar contribution to the intercarpal arch arises most frequently (in 60 percent of specimens) as the ulnar artery faces the lateral aspect of the pisiform. Distal to the pisiform several smaller vessels are seen, directly supplying the pisiform and the hamate and contributing in many specimens to the formation of the dorsal intercarpal arch. The most distal branches of the ulnar artery are the contributions to the basal (dorsal) metacarpal arch and the deep palmar artery for the deep palmar arch (Figs. 4-7 and 4-11). In 42 percent of specimens a medial branch of the ulnar artery was seen to arise proximal to the ulnar styloid, as a common trunk for the ulnar tributaries to the

dorsal radiocarpal, dorsal intercarpal, and basal metacarpal arches.

The Anterior Interosseous Artery

The *anterior interosseous artery* (Figs. 4-5, 4-7) is the third major contributor to the blood supply of the carpus. Its volar division continues deep to the pronator quadratus. In most specimens at least one of its terminal branches connected with the volar radiocarpal arch, and terminated joining the recurrent vessels of the deep palmar arch. The dorsal division joined the dorsal radiocarpal arch in 89 percent of specimens, proceeded to bifurcate into two branches for the intercarpal arch (83 percent) and in 69 percent of specimens terminated further distally by anastomosing with recurrent vessels

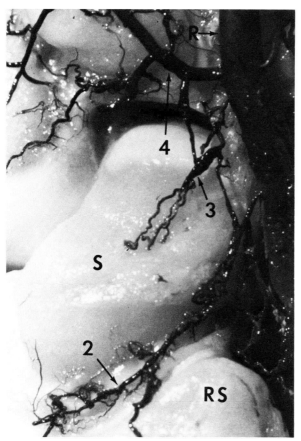

Fig. 4-10. Close-up view of the dorsoradial aspect of the wrist, demonstrating nutrient vessels entering the scaphoid. RS, radial styloid; S, scaphoid; R, radial artery; 2, dorsal radiocarpal arch; 3, branch to the dorsal ridge of the scaphoid; 4, dorsal intercarpal arch. (From Gelberman RH, Panagis JS, Taleisnik J, Baumgaertner M: The arterial anatomy of the human carpus. Part I: The extraosseous vascularity. J Hand Surg 8:367, 1983.)

from the basal metacarpal arch, at the third and fourth interosseous spaces (Fig. 4-12).

The Recurrent Arteries

The *radial* and *ulnar recurrent arteries* from the deep palmer arch are a fourth major source of blood supply to the carpus (Fig. 4-7). These vessels are responsible for the primary volar arterial supply to the distal carpal row. The radial recurrent originates from the deep palmar arch just lateral to the base of the index metacarpal. In 45 percent of specimens the smaller radial recurrent anasto-

mosed with the ulnar recurrent. The latter originates from the deep palmar arch between the bases of the long and ring finger metacarpals. This ulnar recurrent artery courses proximally along the capitohamate articulation. In 75 percent of specimens both recurrent branches anastomosed with the volar intercarpal arch and with the volar radiocarpal arch. In 80 percent these recurrent vessels joined the terminal branches of the volar division of the anterior interosseous artery. In 27 percent of specimens there was an accessory ulnar recurrent, originating from the deep palmar arch 5 to 10 mm medial to the proper ulnar recurrent. Survival of the hand following major arterial injury proximal to the wrist may depend on the efficacy of this volar system of recurrent vessels connecting the deep palmar arch with the more proximal arterial circulation.

A comparison of the size and number of the vessels on the volar and dorsal aspects of the wrist showed a rather balanced distribution, with no significant difference based on gross anatomic observation.

THE EXTRAOSSEOUS ARTERIAL CIRCULATION

From the pericarpal arterial network that surrounds the wrist originate a system of vessels that reach the carpal bones. This extraosseous arterial carpal system has been particularly difficult to demonstrate by mechanical dissection alone. Several studies have been published designed to outline the immediate extraosseous supply and its relationship to the intraosseous circulation, either by injection of vessels and their observation as they enter specimens made translucent, or by injection of radiopaque materials followed by x-ray examination, or by the study of the vascular foramina in dried carpal bone specimens.[2,4,9,14,21–23,26,40,42] It is this portion of the arterial anatomy of the carpus that is particularly suitable to study by techniques involving the treatment of perivascular tissues by chemical means. In most textbooks of anatomy the actual carpal circulation, between the pericarpal vascular plexus and the intraosseous distribution, is summarily referred to as volar or dorsal carpal rete.[16]

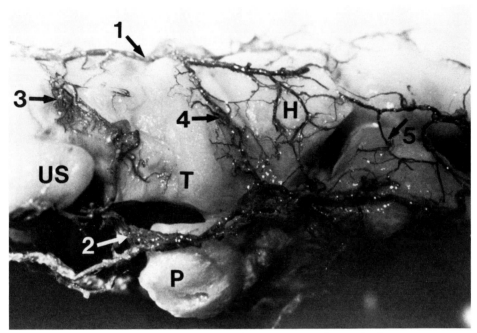

Fig. 4-11. Vascularity of the medial aspect of the wrist. US, ulnar styloid; T, triquetrum; P, pisiform; H, hamate; 1, dorsal branch of anterior interosseous artery; 2, medial branch of ulnar artery; 3, dorsal radiocarpal arch; 4, dorsal intercarpal arch; 5, basal metacarpal arch. (From Gelberman RH, Panagis JS, Taleisnik J, Baumgaertner M: The arterial anatomy of the human carpus. Part I: The extraosseous vascularity. J Hand Surg 8:367, 1983.)

Carpal bones receive their blood supply in areas without cartilaginous cover, nonarticular, where ligaments or capsule attach. In 1937 Anseroff catalogued the vascular foramina of 32 series of carpal bones, and concluded that there is a dorsal preponderance of foramina for the trapezoid and hamate, a lateral preponderance for the triquetrum and pisiform, and a volar preponderance for all other carpal bones.[2] Anseroff believed that vascularization for each carpal bone was proportionate to its functional stresses. In 1959 Travaglini[42] noted that the volar carpal branches of the radial and ulnar arteries, augmented by a contribution of the volar division of the interosseous artery, irrigated the bones of the proximal carpal row, while the more important dorsal carpal branches supplied the distal row (but also contributed to the radial and ulnar aspects of the proximal row). The blood supply to the triangular fibrocartilage derived from the volar division of the anterior interosseous artery.

In summary, in Travaglini's opinion, the *volar carpal arch* supplies the proximal carpal row from the volar aspect, the triangular fibrocartilage, and the distalmost ulna. The *dorsal carpal arch,* more important than the volar, supplies the lower (distalmost) radius, the distal carpal row from the dorsum, and the side aspects of the proximal row.

In 1973 Minne et al.[27] proposed a general plan of distribution of the extraosseous arterial supply to the carpus arising from carpal arches disposed according to the classical description (see p. 51). They observed that certain branches are common to more than one bone: scapholunar, triquetrolunar, scaphostyloid, scaphotrapezium, and pisotriquetral arteries. In these authors' opinion, the thumb-column (lateral) is irrigated by vessels originating from the radial artery or its main branches. The column in relationship to the fifth digit (medial) is vascularized by arteries from the ulnar, or from one of its deep divisions converging into circles formed around the pisiform and hook of the hamate. The intermediate carpal bones receive a mixed supply, as a transition between the lateral and medial patterns: (1) trapezoid, capitate, and

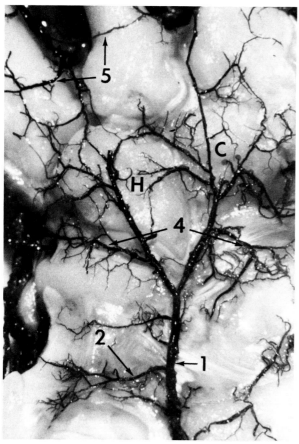

Fig. 4-12. Dorsal view of the wrist, showing contributions of the dorsal branch of the anterior interosseous artery to the three dorsal arches. H, hamate; C, capitate; 1, dorsal branch of the anterior interosseous artery; 2, dorsal radiocarpal arch; 4, dorsal intercarpal arch; 5, basal metacarpal arch. (From Gelberman RH, Panagis JS, Taleisnik J, Baumgaertner M: The arterial anatomy of the human carpus. Part I: The extraosseous vascularity. J Hand Surg 8:367, 1983.)

the lateral portion of the hamate are irrigated by volar branches from the deep palmar arch and dorsal branches from the dorsal carpal arch. These vessels follow the capitohamate and capitotrapezoid interlines as they distribute throughout these bones; and (2) the lunate is linked to both the triquetrum and the scaphoid, with a number of vessels reaching it from the dorsal and volar carpal arches. Minne and coauthors[27] state that, unlike other bones surrounded by a dense vascular network, running within the capsular ligamentous

layer, the lunate is penetrated by a single palmar vessel sometimes surrounded by other very much smaller twigs.[27] Under these conditions, this vessel truly constitutes a pedicle and its foramina is the bone's "hilum." These findings were corroborated in 1977 by Mestdagh and collaborators[26] in a study limited to the dorsal arterial network of the wrist. These investigators found that, while the radial artery itself provided branches to the "outer" carpal bones (scaphoid, lateral lunate, trapezium) and the ulnar artery irrigated triquetrum and hamate, the radial part of the classic dorsal carpal arch and the end branches from the "interosseous arteries" provided twigs to the dorsal scaphoid, the dorsal lunate, and the trapezoid, hamate, and capitate.

In summary, from this review of the literature it is apparent that when considered in a longitudinal (proximal-to-distal) direction, the volar carpal arch is responsible for the proximal carpal row, and the dorsal carpal arch for the distal carpal row, with contributions to the sides of the proximal row as well. In the transverse direction (radial-ulnar), the radial artery, or its direct branches, supplies the thumbside column of the carpus, the ulnar artery, the fifth metacarpal, and the ulnar carpal column, while the intermediate carpals receive blood supply from the connecting dorsal and volar arterial arches. Recent investigations[13] agree that the dorsal intercarpal arch (the dorsal carpal arch of classic descriptions) is the major supplier of the distal carpal row, but also contributes to the lunate and the triquetrum (Fig. 4-13). The more proximal dorsal radiocarpal arch supplies the distal radial metaphysis, the lunate, and the triquetrum. The basal metacarpal arch has, at times, significant branches to the distal carpal row. Of the three volar arches (Fig. 4-14), the main arch, *radiocarpal*, supplies the volar lunate and triquetrum, while the volar intercarpal is not a major contributor to the carpus. In this investigation the radial and ulnar recurrent arteries arising from the deep palmar arch were the main supplier to the distal carpal row. In agreement with Travaglini, the dorsal interosseous artery was not found to directly contribute to the carpal vascularity, but both the volar and dorsal divisions of the anterior interosseous artery did so.

Most carpal bones are exclusively supplied by branches of the transverse arches, rather than by branches of the main arterial trunks. Exceptions are the scaphoid and the pisiform, and to some extent the trapezium, which receive their arterial supply from the radial and ulnar arteries. Vessels to the scaphoid come directly from the radial artery in 70 to 80 percent of specimens or from its superficial palmar and dorsal intercarpal branches in the wrist.[12] When this supply originated from the superficial palmar arch, consistent anastomosis were shown with branches from the volar division of the anterior interosseous artery. Although the ulnar artery did not appear to participate in scaphoid supply, the dorsal and volar divisions of the anterior interosseous artery were significant contributors. Preiser[31] had observed that branches from anastomosis between radial artery and the dorsal division

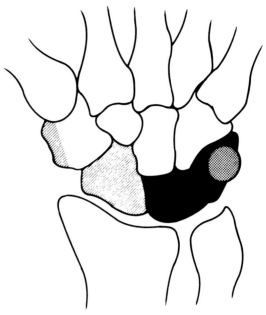

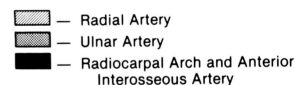

— Radial Artery

— Ulnar Artery

— Radiocarpal Arch and Anterior Interosseous Artery

— Recurrent arteries off Deep Palmar Arch

Fig. 4-14. Schematic drawing of the palmar aspect of the wrist, showing the contributions to carpal bones. (From Gelberman RH, Panagis JS, Taleisnik J, Baumgaertner M: The arterial anatomy of the human carpus. Part I: The extraosseous vascularity. J Hand Surg. 8:367, 1983.)

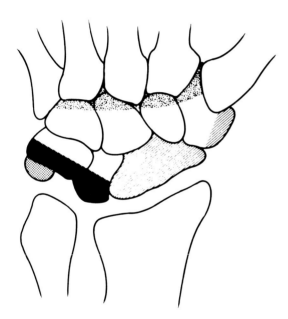

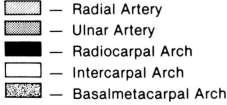

— Radial Artery

— Ulnar Artery

— Radiocarpal Arch

— Intercarpal Arch

— Basalmetacarpal Arch

Fig. 4-13. Schematic drawing of the dorsum of the wrist, showing contributions to the carpal bones. (From Gelberman RH, Panagis JS, Taleisnik J, Baumgaertner M: The arterial anatomy of the human carpus. Part I: The extraosseous vascularity. J Hand Surg 8:367, 1983.)

of the interosseous artery entered the dorsum of the scaphoid. Vessels to the pisiform arise predominantly from the ulnar artery and those to the trapezium partly from the radial artery, and partly from the radial recurrent branch of the deep palmar arch. In general, none of the carpal bones is totally dependent upon a single arch or artery. Extensive anastomoses exist, both volar and dorsal, which would ensure the vascularity of individual carpal bones in case of injury to a major artery. The major collateral circulation about the wrist is provided by an anastomosis between the radial and ulnar recurrent arteries, joining both volar and dorsal divisions of the anterior interosseous artery. This anastomotic pattern was first described by Lawrence and Bachuber[18] in a doctoral thesis published in 1923. It was again mentioned by Lawrence in 1937,[19] and by Quiring in 1949.[33] Preservation of hand viability following major injury to the radial and ulnar arteries in the forearm may relate to the completeness of this volar anastomosis.

THE INTRAOSSEOUS CIRCULATION

In 1904 Lexer, Kuliga, and Turk[21] published a classic study of arteries of bones injected for radiographic visualization. These studies were mostly limited to long tubular bones in different age groups, to "flat" bones (pelvis, ribs, scapula), and to some "short" bones (vertebra, calcaneus, and talus). Prior to 1910 there were no investigations of carpal circulation.[8,21] In 1910 and 1911 Preiser[31,32] reported 24 fractures of the scaphoid and five additional cases of cystic scaphoids, as well as postmortem studies of upper extremity specimens that

he had injected with radiopaque material. He called attention to what has become known as posttraumatic osteitis, posttraumatic cyst, or rarefying osteitis of the scaphoid. Aware of the work of Lexer and colleagues, Preiser asked Lexer to inject and photograph a scaphoid. Drawings based on this specimen have been reproduced repeatedly.[5,30,36,37,43] Following Preiser's contributions, numerous studies of the intraosseous blood supply to individual carpal bones were published. Because of the frequency of scaphoid and lunate involvement in conditions resulting in arterial compromise, the investigation of the circulation of these two bones has received particular emphasis.[3,9,11,12,20,22,23,27,29,40,42]

Scaphoid

The scaphoid receives its supply through ligamentous attachments. The lateral bundle of the intrinsic V ligament originates from the tuberosity. Proximal and lateral to this is the insertion of the radial collateral ligament. The dorsal radiocarpal ligament attaches to the spiral groove, called the waist. Two additional ligaments are only precarious vehicles for vascular access, because their

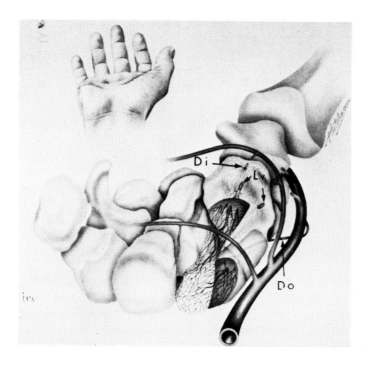

Fig. 4-15. Schematic representation of extraosseous and intraosseous blood supply of the scaphoid, according to Taleisnik and Kelly. Lv, laterovolar vessels; Do, dorsal vessels; and Di, distal vessels. (From Taleisnik J, Kelly PJ: The extraosseous and intraosseous blood supply of the scaphoid bone. J Bone Joint Surg [Am] 48:1125, 1966.)

scaphoid attachments are either tenuous (radio-capitate ligament) or very localized to a small fossa or fovea (deep radioscapholunate ligament). Most studies point out that the distal half of the scaphoid receives a more abundant arterial supply. This coincides with the overall ligamentous arrangement. The proximal half of the scaphoid is essentially an intraarticular pole or head, comparable to the head of the femur, and covered by articular hyaline cartilage. Only one ligament, the deep radioscapholunate, attaches on this proximal pole, in a manner reminiscent of the attachment of the ligamentum teres on the head of the femur (Fig. 2-9). Like the ligamentum teres, it inserts into a very limited, localized fovea of minimal significance for the survival of the proximal pole should this pole become

isolated by a fracture. In 1955 Grettve[14] showed that the main scaphoid supply entered a narrow area curving around the radial border of the carpus divided into three groups: dorsal, proximal, and volar. Taleisnik and Kelly[40] also described three groups of vessels responsible for the supply to the scaphoid (Fig. 4-15). The *laterovolar* vessels approach the scaphoid immediately distal and lateral to the radial articular surface. The *dorsal* group pentrates the dorsum of the scaphoid along the spiral waist, and the *distal* vessels enter it on the volar aspect of the distal pole. The laterovolar and dorsal systems anastomose freely, while the distal group supplies a circumscribed area of the tuberosity only. In these authors' opinion, the laterovolar system is the main contributor to the intraosseous

Fig. 4-16. Microangiogram of the terminal intraosseous vascular pattern. *A* (×5) and *B* (×40) show vascular arcades becoming smaller and smaller as vessels spread out toward the periphery of the bone. (From Taleisnik J, Kelly PJ: The extraosseous and intraosseous blood supply of the scaphoid bone. J Bone Joint Surg [Am] 48:1125, 1966.)

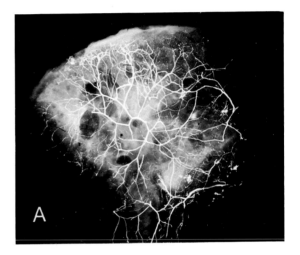

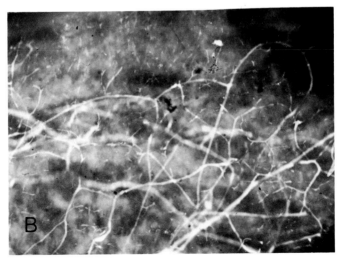

blood supply. After penetration of the bone, these vessels divide into branches which spread proximally and medially toward the articular surfaces of the scaphoid for the radius and capitate. The laterovolar arteries provide most of the blood supply to the proximal two thirds of the scaphoid. There are profuse anastomoses among its branches and with similar branches from the dorsal system, ending in subperiosteal and subchondral vascular arcades, typical of the vascular pattern of cancellous bone (Fig. 4-16). Dorsal vessels were usually of the same size or at times slightly smaller than the laterovolar arteries. The dorsal vessels contribute to the blood supply of the proximal two thirds of the scaphoid, anastomose with similar branches from the laterovolar arteries, and terminate by forming the typical vascular arcades described. The distal arterial group is the smallest of the three, but supplies a much more restricted area limited to the tuberosity, without anastomosing with the rest of the intraosseous arterial system.

Minne and coauthors[27] described a similar pattern of three arterial groups: dorsal, along the dorsal groove or waist, distal, and external or lateral. The dorsal pedicle was distributed throughout the spiral groove of the scaphoid. The distal and lateral vessels were unequally allocated to the lateral and volar aspects, although predominantly within the distal half of this bone. In contrast with these findings, Gelberman and Menon, in a more recent study,[12] describe two vascular systems instead of three: *dorsal*, along the spiral ridge or groove of the scaphoid, and *volar*, limited to the scaphoid tubercle and comparable to the distal group in Taleisnik and Kelly's description.[40] Gelberman and Menon agreed that there are no intraosseous anastomoses between the arteries to the tuberosity and the remainder of the intraosseous vessels. They pointed out that several small vessels, which did not penetrate bone, were seen in the region of the proximal pole, undoubtedly related to the deep radioscapholunate ligament. This observation was also made by Preiser in 1910.[31] A comparison of some of the illustrations in Gelberman and Menon's paper, with those in Taleisnik and Kelly's, shows a striking similarity, suggesting that their dorsal system and the lateral volar group are very likely the same (Fig. 4-17).

In a study of dried specimens, Obletz and Halbstein[28] catalogued 297 scaphoids according to the location of foramina for their blood vessels. In 13 percent there were none proximal to the waist of the bone. The specimens depicted as representative of this group showed two clusters of foramina, one on the tuberosity, and the second just radial to it, corresponding to the point of entry of the laterovolar system in Taleisnik and Kelly's study.[40] This 13 percent figure is almost identical to the 14 percent of specimens in Gelberman and Menon's investigation,[12] which showed the blood supply entering distal to the waist. Therefore, approximately one out of seven specimens in either series would have shown a significant loss of blood supply to the proximal pole following a fracture through the waist. In 20 percent of the scaphoids in Obletz and Halbstein's series there was one arterial foramen proximal to the wrist, while 67 percent showed two or more foramina.

Lunate

Investigations of blood supply to the lunate have yielded conflicting results. Its supply by a predominant volar source was suggested by Cordes.[7] In 1947 Ståhl[39] studied 31 cadaver specimens with stereoscopic roentgenograms, after the injection of a radiopaque contrast material. In only one was there evidence of a dorsal vessel. All other specimens showed an exclusively volar supply. Except for these two investigations, a review of the literature indicates that, in most cases, there are important volar *and* dorsal arterial contributions to the lunate, with abundant intraosseous anastomoses. In 1938 Logroscino and DeMarchi[22] found intraosseous anastomosis of dorsal and volar vessels. Grettve[14] also described a rather symmetrical pattern: a large central and a smaller distal artery, entering both volar and dorsal poles. These vessels anastomosed in the center of the lunate, with branches radiating to cover the entire bone. Unfortunately, Grettve's findings and descriptions may be incomplete, for he injected his specimens distal to the origin of the intraosseous artery. Travaglini[42] found vascular foramina equally distributed on the nonarticular volar and dorsal surfaces of the lunate. On the volar side, the volar carpal branches of the

Fig. 4-17. Comparison of specimens of scaphoid injected to delineate the intraosseous blood supply. (*A* from Taleisnik J, Kelly PJ: The extraosseous and intraosseous blood supply of the scaphoid bone. J Bone Joint Surg 48A: 1125, 1966; *B* from Gelberman RH, Menon J: The vascularity of the scaphoid bone. J. Hand Surg 5:508, 1980.)

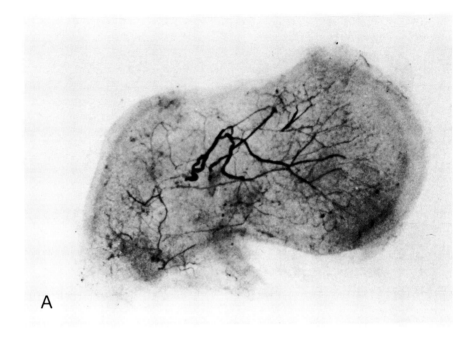

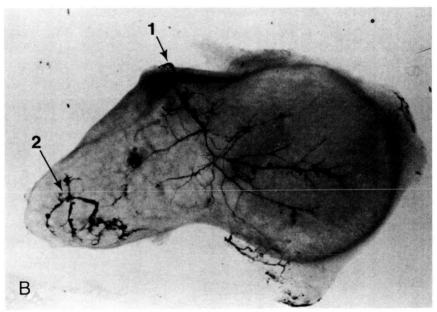

radial artery follow the deep radioscapholunate ligament, while the volar division of the anterior interosseous artery follows the volar radiolunate ligament to reach the lunate. On the dorsum, branches from the radial artery approach the lunate progressing along the dorsal radiocarpal ligament, while branches from the dorsal division of the anterior interosseous artery reach the lunate with the fibers of the radiolunotriquetral ligament. Both networks appeared to be of equal importance.

In 1963 Lee[20] published his now classical study of the intraosseous arterial pattern of the lunate. In

66 percent of 53 normal lunate specimens, volar and dorsal vessels were present, which anastomosed within the bone. In 26 percent there was a single volar or a single dorsal vessel, and 7.5 percent were supplied by volar and dorsal arteries that fail to connect with each other. In a fascinating doctoral thesis on the pathogenesis of lunatomalacia, Antuña Zapico[1] studied in depth the architectural characteristics of the lunate. He observed that the volar aspect, in many lunates, is not grossly rectangular as classically described, but rather trapezoidal in shape. The proximal (radial) and medial (triquetral) surfaces converge to a prominent proximal vertex or apex (Fig. 1-7). Consequently, the two diagonal lines that can be traced bisecting this surface are of unequal length, one longer ("major axis"), the other shorter ("minor axis") (Fig. 4-18). The minor axis divides the volar surface into two triangles. Antuña Zapico pointed out that perforations for blood vessels, when present, were contained within the triangle proximal to the minor axis, which he chose to call "the vascular triangle." In 72 percent of 50 lunates, this triangle contained either a large orifice for a single blood vessel or three or four good-sized foramina, or multiple smaller openings. In 14 percent the blood supply was more abundant, and in 14 percent there was only a minimal supply or actually no evidence at all of vascular penetration. The dorsal pole or aspect could also be subdivided into two triangles, and here again vascular imprints were localized to the proximal triangle, although their disposition and number were not as clear as on the volar side. However, all of the 50 specimens studied showed dorsal foramina. Antuña Zapico[1] found a compensatory relationship between the size and quantity of the volar and dorsal arteries: Scarce volar vascularity coincided with a more abundant dorsal supply, and vice versa. In his experience, all volar vessels to the lunate originated from the radial and interosseous arteries, or their anastomoses (volar radiocarpal arch?); dorsal vessels were frequently recurrent branches from a vascular arch akin to the dorsal intercarpal arch. Similar findings were published by Minne and collaborators: volar vessels arising from the volar (radiocarpal) arch were larger, while dorsal vessels were smaller but twice as numerous.[27] In many instances, these were common arteries to contiguous bones, that is, scapholunate or lunotriquetral branches both volar and dorsal.

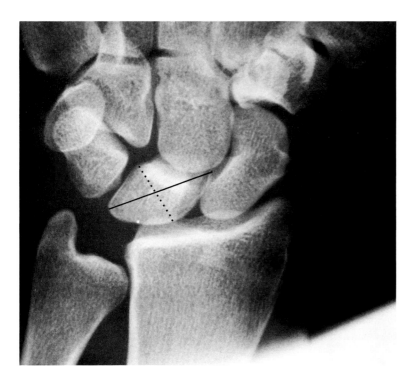

Fig. 4-18. Major (full line) and minor (dotted line) axes of lunate. Area proximal to minor axis is called "vascular triangle" by Antuña Zapico.[1]

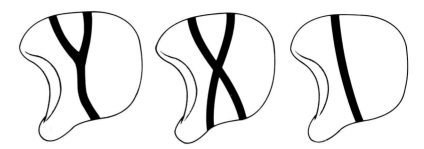

Fig. 4-19. Patterns of intraosseous blood supply to the lunate. (From Gelberman RH, Bauman TD, Menon J, Akeson WH: The vascularity of the lunate bone and Kienböck's disease. J Hand Surg 5:272, 1980.)

A recent investigation[11] showed that the major contributions to the dorsal supply of the lunate arose from the intercarpal branch of the radial artery. A second, less frequent, contributor was a radiocarpal branch traversing from the radial artery across the carpus to the lunate. Anastomoses between these branches created a dorsal lunate plexus, also supplied by the dorsal divisions of the anterior interosseous artery. From this plexus originated one or two vessels that entered the dorsal surface of the lunate. A similar volar rete was formed by radiocarpal branches of the radial and ulnar arteries, and contributions from the anterior interosseous and a recurrent branch of the deep palmar arch. From this arose one or two nutrient vessels that penetrated the lunate through foramina on its volar surface. The volar arteries were slightly larger, and anastomosed with the dorsal just distal to the midportion of the lunate. Three major intraosseous vascular patterns were described, and identified on account of their configuration as Y, X, or I (Fig. 4-19). The Y pattern was the most common, found in 59 percent of specimens. The stem of the Y was either volar or dorsal in roughly equal numbers. The I pattern was seen in 31 percent of lunates, a singe dorsal system in a straight line across the bone. The X pattern was noted in 10 percent of specimens, and consisted of two dorsal and two volar vessels joined at the center of the lunate. Branches from these central intraosseous systems reached subchondral areas; the proximal region adjacent to the radial articular surface was found to be the least vascular zone, an interesting observation in view of Antuña Zapico's findings of preponderance of vascular foramina in the superior "vascular" triangle. The correlation of extraosseous and intraosseous vascularity in the study of Gelberman and coauthors substantiates

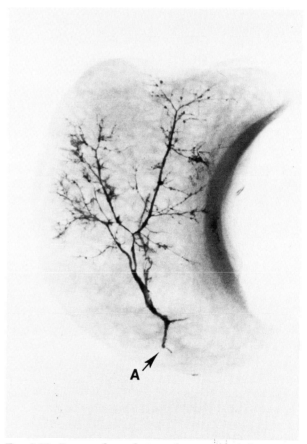

Fig. 4-20. Lunate: lateral view, showing single large vessel entering palmar surface and branching within the bone to provide the sole blood supply. This pattern was seen in 20% of the specimens. (From Panagis JS, Gelberman RH, Taleisnik J, Baumgaertner M: The arterial anatomy of the human carpus. Part II. The intraosseous vascularity. J Hand Surg 8:375, 1983.)

the findings of simultaneous, consistent dorsal and volar nutrient vessels.[11] In a more recent study from the same laboratory 20 percent of lunates showed only volar vessels spreading to supply the entire lunate (Fig. 4-20).[29]

Triquetrum

The triquetrum is pyramidal in shape, its long axis oblique from proximal to distal and ulnar. The base is occupied by a facet for the articulation with the lunate. The distal and proximal surfaces are articular (for the hamate and triangular fibrocartilage, respectively). It has two mostly nonarticular surfaces through which it receives its blood supply: volar (contains the small facet for the pisiform) and dorsal. According to Travaglini,[42] most of the triquetral circulation is related to that of the lunate, through common volar and dorsal branches of the anterior interosseous artery that follow ligaments to reach both bones, and through recurrent vessels from the dorsal carpal (intercarpal) arch. There is no mention of a contribution from the ulnar artery. Minne et al.[27] described three groups of vessels: superior, palmar, and dorsal, the first two fed by tributaries from the ulnar artery, the third by branches of the dorsal carpal (intercarpal) arch. Our investigations have shown that on the dorsum both dorsal intercarpal and radiocarpal arches supply the triquetrum.[29] The dorsal surface is traversed from medial to lateral by a ridge.[41] Two to four vessels entered the triquetrum through this ridge in most specimens (Fig. 4-21). The dorsal supply produced 60 percent of the intraosseous circulation. On the volar aspect, the triquetrum received branches from the ulnar artery, and from the volar radiocarpal arch reinforced, at this level, by communications from the volar branch of the anterior interosseous artery.[13] One to two small or medium-sized vessels enter the anterior aspect of the bone, proximal to the articular facet for the pisiform. These vessels supply the volar 40 percent of the bone. In 86 percent of specimens there are significant anastomoses between both systems (Fig. 4-22). In 60 percent the dorsal supply is predominant, in 20 percent the volar supply is greater, and in the remaining 20 percent both systems contributions are essentially equal.

Pisiform

The pisiform receives one to three small vessels directly from the ulnar artery entering the bone at the proximal and distal poles.[13,29] Vessels running parallel and just beneath the articular surface of the pisiform anastomose with each other, assuming a vascular ring pattern that is consistently seen in all specimens (Fig. 4-23). Other branches reach the areas under the volar cortex. Extensive anastomosis occur, with approximately equal participation of the proximal and distal vascular pedicles in supplying this bone.

Trapezium

The trapezium articulates with the scaphoid proximally, the trapezoid medially and the first metacarpal distally. Three other surfaces and nonarticular: dorsal and lateral, for ligament attachments, and volar, for the thenar musculature and the groove for the tendon of the flexor carpi ra-

(Text continues on page 76)

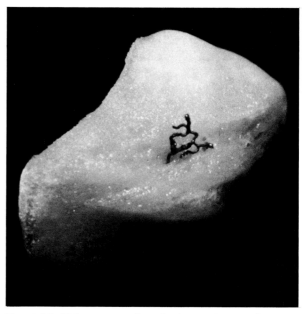

Fig. 4-21. Triquetrum: dorsal view prior to clearance with Spalteholz technique, showing a branching nutrient vessel entering the center of the obliquely running dorsal ridge. (From Panagis JS, Gelberman RH, Taleisnik J, Baumgaertner M: The arterial anatomy of the human carpus. Part II. The intraosseous vascularity. J Hand Surg 8:375, 1983.)

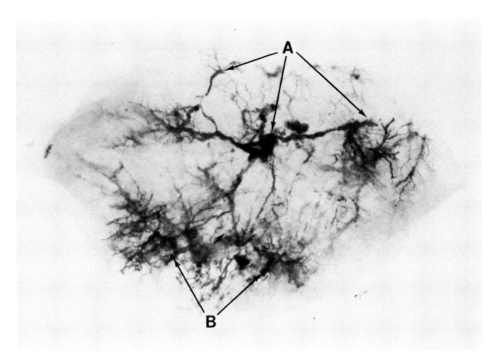

Fig. 4-22. Triquetrum: lateral view, showing three dorsal *(A)* and two palmar *(B)* nutrient vessels with intraosseous anastomoses in the middle one third of the bone. This pattern was seen in 80% of the specimens. (From Panagis JS, Gelberman RH, Taleisnik J, Baumgaertner M: The arterial anatomy of the human carpus. Part II: The intraosseous vascularity. J Hand Surg 8:375, 1983.)

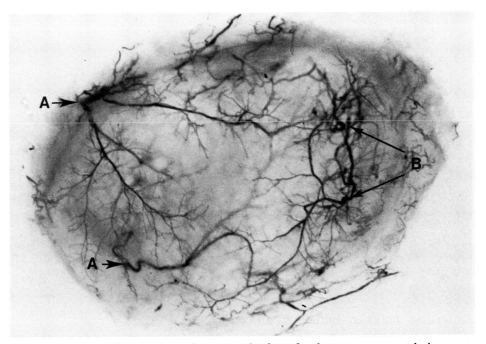

Fig. 4-23. Pisiform: dorsal view looking onto the facet for the triquetrum, with the proximal superior *(A)* and distal superior *(B)* vessels forming an arterial ring beneath the facet. The ring was seen in all specimens. (From Panagis JS, Gelberman RH, Taleisnik J, Baumgaertner M: The arterial anatomy of the human carpus. Part II: The intraosseous vascularity. J Hand Surg 8:375, 1983.)

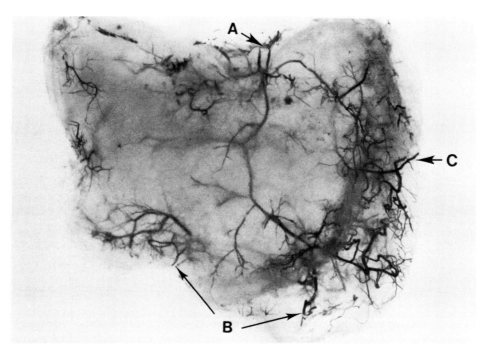

Fig. 4-24. Trapezium: distal view from articular surface at thumb trapeziometacarpal joint, showing dorsal *(A)*, palmar *(B)*, and lateral *(C)*, nutrient vessels, with anastomosis of the three. (From Panagis JS, Gelberman RH, Taleisnik J, Baumgaertner M: The arterial anatomy of the human carpus. Part II: The intraosseous vascularity. J Hand Surg 8:375, 1983.)

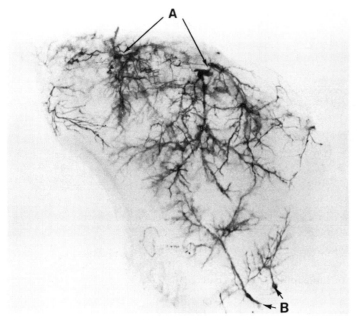

Fig. 4-25. Trapezoid: lateral view, showing dorsal nutrient vessels *(A)*, supplying dorsal 70% of the bone, and palmar vessels *(B)*, supplying palmar 30%. There were no intraosseous anastomoses. (From Panagis JS, Gelberman RH, Taleisnik J, Baumgaertner M: The arterial anatomy of the human carpus. Part II: The intraosseous vascularity. J Hand Surg 8:375, 1983.)

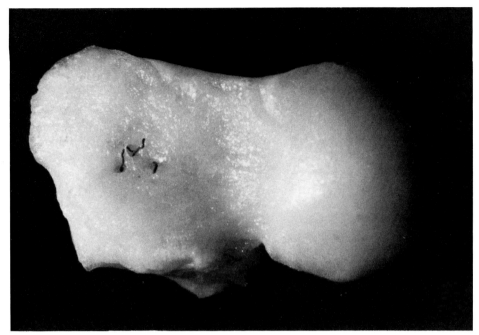

Fig. 4-26. Capitate: dorsal view prior to clearance with the Spalteholz technique, showing three arteries entering nutrient foramina in the distal one third of the bone *(A)*. (From Panagis JS, Gelberman RH, Taleisnik J, Baumgaertner M: The arterial anatomy of the human carpus. Part II: The intraosseous vascularity. J Hand Surg 8:375, 1983.)

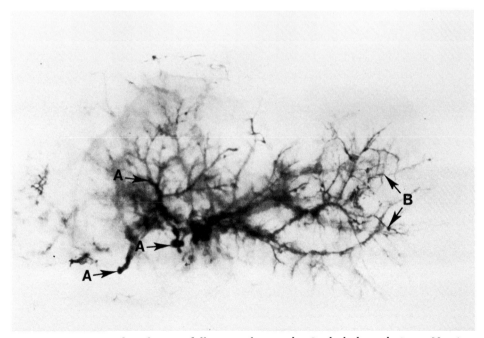

Fig. 4-27. Capitate: dorsal view, following clearing by Spalteholz technique. Nutrient vessels enter distal third *(A)*, with retrograde course toward the proximal articular surface. *B;* terminal vessels in the head of the capitate. (From Panagis JS, Gelberman RH, Taleisnik J, Baumgaertner M: The arterial anatomy of the human carpus. Part II: The intraosseous vascularity. J Hand Surg 8:375, 1983.)

dialis. The trapezium receives vessels directly from the radial artery on its dorsal and lateral surfaces.[13,27] There is some controversy as to the origin of the branches that approach the bone on its volar aspect. Travaglini had stated that the trapezium is the only carpal bone not supplied by recurrent volar branches from the deep palmar arch. Our investigation[13] showed, however, that the volar aspect is supplied by the radial recurrent artery from the deep palmar arch and by direct vessels from the radial artery. There are one to three dorsal and one to three volar vessels entering the trapezium, joined by three to six very fine branches from the lateral surface (Fig. 4-24). All three systems anastomose freely in at least 35 percent of specimens, although in all cases the dorsal vascular supply predominate.

Trapezoid

All blood vessels reach the trapezoid through its two very small nonarticular facets: volar and dorsal.

The volar supply originates from the deep palmar arch via its radial recurrent artery. The dorsum is supplied by branches from the dorsal intercarpal arch.[29] The dorsal 70 percent of the intraosseous circulation originated from three to four small vessels entering the center of the dorsal nonarticular surface (Fig. 4-25).[29] The remaining volar 30 percent was supplied by one to two smaller volar vessels that did not anastomose with the dorsal circulation.

Capitate

The nonarticular areas for vascular access to the capitate are limited to the volar and dorsal facets. Although volar arteries may be larger in size,[14] dorsal vessels are more numerous and predominate in supplying the capitate.[29] Most arteries enter the capitate distally, and follow a retrograde, proximal course to supply the rest of the bone. Travaglini described an additional system of smaller vessels entering the neck of the capitate and distributing in

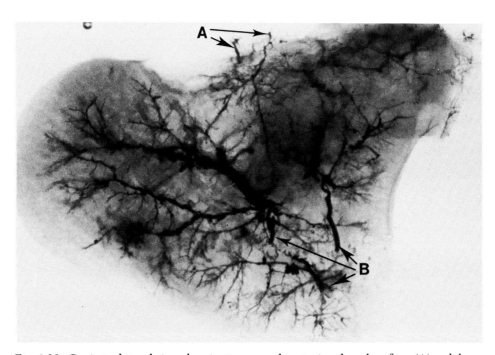

Fig. 4-28. Capitate: lateral view showing two vessels entering dorsal surface *(A)* and three entering palmar surface *(B)*, with intraosseous anastomosis of the two supplies. This specimen also shows blood vessels to the head of the capitate originating from the palmar surface, seen in 33% of the specimens. (From Panagis JS, Gelberman RH, Taleisnik J, Baumgaertner M: The arterial anatomy of the human carpus. Part II: The intraosseous vascularity. J Hand Surg 8:375, 1983.)

a distal direction.[42] Dorsally, two to four medium-sized branches of the dorsal intercarpal arch enter the distal two thirds of the capitate (Fig. 4-26), course in a volar, proximal, and slightly ulnar direction (Fig. 4-27) to supply the body and head of the capitate in 67 percent of specimens in the series of Panagis and coauthors.[29] On the volar aspect, one to three medium-sized vessels enter the distal half of the capitate, arising from the ulnar and radial recurrent branches of the deep palmar arch.[27,29,42] In 33 percent of specimens[29] the blood distribution to the head of the capitate originates entirely from this volar supply (Fig. 4-28). Volar-dorsal anastomoses were significant in 30 percent of specimens. In the remainder there were no intraosseous anastomosis seen.

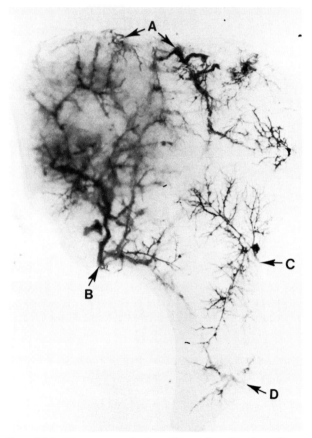

Fig. 4-29. Hamate: end view from the distal surface, demonstrating dorsal *(A)* and palmar *(B)* supplies. Vessels to the hook enter at the medial base *(C)* and the tip of the hook *(D)*. (From Panagis JS, Gelberman RH, Taleisnik J, Baumgaertner M: The arterial anatomy of the human carpus. Part II: The intraosseous vascularity. J Hand Surg 8:375, 1983.)

Hamate

Most of the volar supply to the hamate originates from the ulnar recurrent branch of the deep palmar arch, which courses in a retrograde direction as a common capitohamate trunk, along the volar capitohamate interspace. Direct branches from the ulnar artery supply the most medial portion of the volar aspect and the medial aspect of the hook of the hamate.[27,29] In some 27 percent of specimens in Panagis' series, circulation to the medial hamate was provided instead by an independent accessory ulnar recurrent branch of the deep palmar arch.[29] The dorsal circulation is entirely provided by three to five vessels from the dorsal intercarpal arch. These branched in all directions (Fig. 4-29) after entering the bone, and supplied 30 to 40 percent of the hamate. Rarely, a significant contribution was found arising from the dorsal basal arch to the distalmost portion of all four bones of the distal carpal row. Of the volar vessels, one large artery predominated,[14,29] entering the hamate through the radial base of the hook. It branched intraosseously and anastomosed with the dorsal vessels in 50 percent of specimens. The vascularity of the hook was found to be largely independent from that of the body by most authors.[24,42]

REFERENCES

1. Antuña Zapico: Malacia del semilunar. Tesis Doctoral. Universidad de Valladolid. Industrias y editorial Sever-Cuesta. Valladolid, 1966
2. Anseroff NJ: Die Arterien der Skelets der Hand und der Fusses des Menschen. Z Anat Entwicklungsgesch 106:193, 1937
3. Barber H: The intraosseous arterial anatomy of the adult human carpus. Orthopaedics 5:1, 1972
4. Belou P: Revision anatomicá del sistema arterial. Libreria Editoria El Ateneo, Buenos Aires, 1934
5. Böhler L: The Treatment of Fractures. 4th Ed. William Wood, Baltimore, 1935
6. Coleman SS, Anson LJ: Arterial patterns in the hand, based upon a study of 650 specimens. Surg Gynecol Obstet 113:1409, 1961
7. Cordes E: Über die Entstehung der subchondralen Osteonekrosen A.: Die Lunatum Nekrosen. Beitr Klin Chir 149:28, 1930
8. Delskamp G: Das Verhalten der Knochenarterien bei Knochenerkrankungen und Frakturen. Fortschr Geb Röntgenstr Nuklearmed 10:219, 1906–1907

9. Fajardo JC: Irrigación del hueso escafoides de la mano. Rev Med Rosario 51:3, 1962

10. Fracassi H: Arterias interóseas de la mano. Prensa Med Argent 32:27, 1945

11. Gelberman RH, Bauman TD, Menon J, Akeson WH: The vascularity of the lunate bone and Kienböck's disease. J Hand Surg 5:272, 1980

12. Gelberman RH, Menon J: The vascularity of the scaphoid bone. J Hand Surg 5:508, 1980

13. Gelberman RH, Panagis JS, Taleisnik J, Baumgaertner M: The arterial anatomy of the human carpus. Part I: The extraosseous vascularity. J Hand Surg 8:367, 1983

14. Grettve S: Arterial anatomy of the carpal bones. Acta Anat 25:331, 1955

15. Hollinshead WH: Anatomy for Surgeons: The Back and Limbs. 2nd Ed. Vol. 3. Harper & Row, New York, 1969

16. Kaplan EB: Functional and Surgical Anatomy of the Hand. 2nd Ed. Lippincott, Philadelphia, 1965

17. Lanz Titus von, Wachsmuth W: Praktische Anatomie: Ein Lehr- und Hilfsbuch der anatomischen. Grundlagen artzlichen Handelns. 2nd Ed. p. 232. Springer-Verlag, Berlin, 1959

18. Lawrence HW, Bachuber AE: The collateral circulation after ligature of both radial and ulnar arteries at the wrist. Thesis. University of Wisconsin, 1923

19. Lawrence HW: The collateral circulation in the hand. Indust Med 6:410, 1937

20. Lee MLH: The intraosseous arterial pattern of the carpal lunate bone and its relation to avascular necrosis. Acta Orthop Scand 33:43, 1963

21. Lexer E, Kuliga Turk W: Untersuchungen über Knochenarterien mittelst Röntgenaufnahmen injizierter Knochen und ihre Bedeutung für einzelne pathologische Vorgänge am Knochen System. August Hirschwald, Berlin, 1904

22. Logroscino D, DeMarchi E: Vascolarizzazione e trofopatie delle ossa del carpo. Chir Organi Mov 23:499, 1938

23. Lützeler H: Die Entstehungsursache der Pseudoarthrose nach Bruch des Kahnbeins der Hand. Dtsch Z Chir 235:450, 1932

24. McCormack LJ, Cauldwell EW, Anson BJ: Brachial and antebrachial arterial patterns. A study of 750 extremities. Surg Gynecol Obstet 96:43, 1953

25. Meyer, H. von.: Der Grundtypus des Rete Dorsale der Handwurzel und der Fusswurzel. Arch Anat Physiol 5:378, 1881

26. Mestdagh H, Bailleul JP, Chambon JP, Laraki A: The dorsal arterial network of the wrist with reference to the blood supply of the carpal bones. Acta Morphol Neerl Scand 17:73, 1979

27. Minne J, Depreux R, Mestdagh H, Lecluse P: Les pédicules artériels du massif carpien. Lille Med 18:1174, 1973

28. Obletz BE, Halbstein BM: Non-union of fractures of the carpal navicular. J Bone Joint Surg 20:424, 1938

29. Panagis JS, Gelberman RH, Taleisnik J, Baumgaertner M: The arterial anatomy of the human carpus. Part II: The intraosseous vascularity. J Hand Surg 8:375, 1983

30. Pfab B, Zöllner F: Zur Pathologie der Handgelenkverletzungen: Naviculare-Frakturen, bzw. Pseudarthrosen mit Cystenbildung Lunatum Lunationen. Lunatum Malacien. Dtsch Z Chir 233:355, 1931

31. Preiser G: Eine typische Posttraumatische und zur spontannfraktur führende Ostitis des Naviculare Carpi. Fortschr Geb Röntgenstr Nuklearmed 15:189, 1910

32. Preiser G: Zur Frage der typischen traumatischen Ernährungsstörungen der kurzen Hand und Fusswurzelknochen. Fortschr Geb Röntgenstr Nuklearmed 17:360, 1911

33. Quiring AP: Collateral Circulation. Lea & Febiger, Philadelphia, 1949

34. Robinson A (ed): Cunningham's Manual of Practical Anatomy. 8th Ed. Vol. 1. Oxford University Press, New York, 1933

35. Rouvière H: Anatomie Humaine: Descriptive et Topographique. 5th Ed. Vol. 2: Membres, Système Nerveux Central. Masson, Paris, 1940

36. Schneck F: Zur Entstehung, Behandlung und Verhütung der sogenannten posttraumatischen Navicularezyste. Fortschr Geb Röntgenstr Nuklearmed 39:1016, 1929

37. Schneck F: Die Verletzungen der Handwurzel. Ergeb Chir Orthop 23:1, 1930

38. Scholder P: Vascularisation osseuse et pseudokystes du poignet. Rev Chir Orthop 39(Suppl 1):1, 1953

39. Ståhl F: On lunatomalacia (Kienböck's disease). Acta Chir Scand 45(Suppl 126):3, 1947

40. Taleisnik J, Kelly PJ: The extraosseous and intraosseous blood supply of the scaphoid bone. J Bone Joint Surg 48A:1125, 1966

41. Testut L: Traité d'anatomie Humaine, Anatomie Descriptive, Histologie, Développement. Vol. 8. Octave Dion, Paris, 1889–1894

42. Travaglini F: Arterial circulation of the carpal bones. Bull Hosp Joint Dis (NY) 20:19, 1959

43. Watson-Jones R: Fractures and Joint Injuries. 4th Ed. Vol. 2. Williams and Wilkins, Baltimore, 1955

44. Weathersby NT: The volar arterial arches. Anat Rec 118:365, 1954 (Abstract)

45. Zuckerkandl E: Ueber die tiefen hohlhandaste der arteria ulnaris. Anat Hefte 6:533, 1896

5 Radiographic Examination of the Wrist

In 1895 Wilhelm Conrad Röntgen, a professor of physics at the University of Würzburg, Germany, discovered radiations which he called x-rays because of their uncertain nature. Few events in history have had so powerful an impact in the progress of science. Within a year after he first obtained an x-ray, that of his wife's hand, at least 49 books and pamphlets and more than 1,000 original articles were published on the subject. By February 1896, Destot was "equipped with all the necessary apparatus," and had begun the extensive study of the normal wrist, of experimental carpal injuries, and of the abnormal wrist, which culminated in the publication of his monumental work *Traumatismes du Poignet et Rayons X* in 1923.[13] Less than one year after Röntgen's discovery, Bryce, a lecturer on anatomy at Queen Margaret's College at the University of Glasgow, presented a report to the Anatomical Society of London on the use of the "new photography" in a study of the wrist.[10] He realized that the normal wrist showed "a degree of incongruity" of the carpal articulations that had not been represented in textbooks of that time. Bryce's paper showed anteroposterior radiographs of his own hand in pronation, and in supination, and in ulnar and radial deviation. He accurately pointed out that the ulnar styloid is closer to the center of the wrist in supination and closer to the margin of the head of the ulna in pronation. He also described the foreshortening or perpendicularization of the scaphoid in radial deviation and the extension (dorsiflexion) of lunate and triquetrum in ulnar deviation. In 1898 the first detailed radiographic study

of the wrist "in profile" was presented by Eugene R. Corson of Savannah, Georgia.[12] The exposure time for these x-rays was eight minutes. Corson was aware of the difficulty in reading "the composite shadows obtained from the profile view," and solved this problem by tracing bony outlines on negatives placed on a white surface at an angle of 45 degrees before a shaded Welsbach lamp, the first published account of a workable x-ray viewer!

Until Röntgen's discovery, the diagnosis of wrist injuries depended on the very detailed study of surface landmarks. X-rays introduced a new era. Today, roentgenography continues to be the most frequently used diagnostic tool for the study of skeletal injuries and disease.

ROUTINE PROJECTIONS

For many years, only the classic "frontal" and lateral projections were used in radiographic examinations of the wrist.[20] Three views, posteroanterior, lateral, and oblique, are now routinely advised (Fig. 5-1). The hand should be in neutral alignment in both the posterior anterior and lateral projections, the longitudinal axis of the third metacarpal parallel to that of the radius. Minor deviations from neutral can produce changes of alignment that may be erroneously interpreted as abnormal. A careful clinical evaluation should precede the request for roentgenograms. Extra ossicles, congenital variations, and different types of carpal coalitions should be kept in mind and corre-

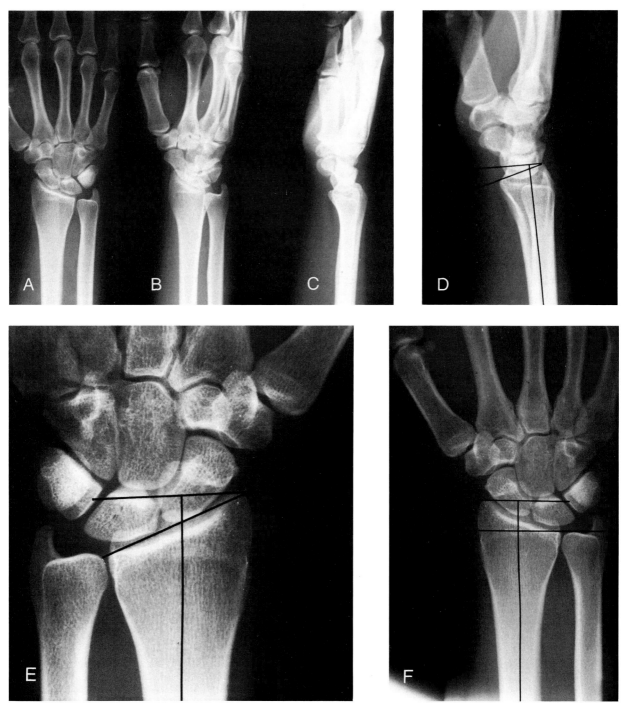

Fig. 5-1. Routine radiographic study of the wrist. *A:* Posteroanterior view. *B:* Oblique. *C:* Lateral. *D:* Palmar tilt of distal articular surface of radius. *E:* Radial inclination or angulation. *F:* Radial length.

lated with clinical findings.[5,15,19,24,28,31,40,46,54] The routine posteroanterior projection is obtained with the hand and forearm in pronation on the x-ray plate. In the routine lateral and posteroanterior views, three radiographic measurements are significant: palmar tilt, radial inclination or angulation, and radial length.

Palmar tilt (Fig. 5-1D) is determined by the angle between the plane of the distal articular surface of the radius as seen on lateral radiographs and a perpendicular to the long axis of the shaft of the radius. When this angle is 90 degrees, the tilt is zero degrees. Palmar tilt is identified with a plus (+) sign and dorsal tilt with a minus (−) sign. Normally, the palmar tilt averages +11 degrees.

Radial inclination or *angulation* (Fig. 5-1E) is represented by the angle between a line tangential to the distal articular surface of the radius as seen in posteroanterior roentgenograph, and a perpendicular to the shaft of the radius. It averages 22 degrees.

Radial length (Fig. 5-1F) is expressed by the distance in millimeters between two parallel lines that are perpendicular to the central axis of the radius, the first traced at the tip of the radial styloid, and the second tangential to the head (not the styloid process) of the distal ulna as seen in posteroanterior radiographs: it averages 9 mm. Gilula[17] proposed a systematic approach to analyze posteroanterior radiographs based on three major radiographic features to be surveyed sequentially. First, the three normal carpal arcs, drawn to define normal carpal relationships (Fig. 5-2): Arc I is traced along the smooth proximal convex outline of scaphoid, lunate, and triquetrum. Arc II outlines the distal concave curvatures of these bones. Arc III is drawn on the convex condylar surface created by capitate and hamate. A broken arc usually indicates disruption of joint integrity at that site. Second, the width and symmetry of joint spaces, and third, the correct shape of individual carpal bones, particularly the scaphoid and the lunate. In the posteroanterior view (Fig. 5-1) the scaphoid is seen in a slightly volarflexed attitude. The triquetrum is aligned with the ulnar facet of the hamate, without excessive overlap across the triquetrohamate space. The lunate has a trapezoidal shape, (a four-sided geometrical figure with two parallel sides).[17] The lunate becomes triangular with extremes of volarflexion or dorsiflexion. In the normal posteroanterior projection in neutral, the lunate strad-

Fig. 5-2. Normal carpal arcs, according to Gilula. (See Ref. 18.)

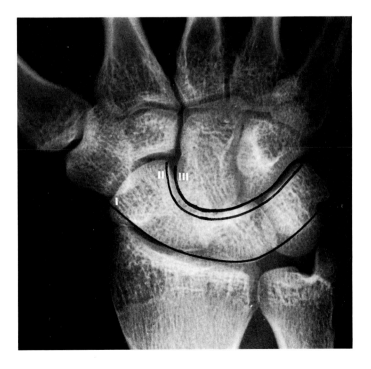

dles the radioulnar joint[10] (Fig. 5-1). This was first reported in the medical literature in 1890 by Shepherd, five years before Röntgen discovered x-rays.[50] Shepherd noted that in the primitive carpus the "intermedium" articulates with radius and ulna, the "radiale" with the radius and the "ulnare" with the ulna. In the human carpus the scaphoid (radiale) articulates with the radius, the triquetrum (ulnare) with the ulna and the lunate (intermedium) with the radius and the cartilaginous complex that separates it from the ulna. This was a departure from classical descriptions where both scaphoid and lunate were shown articulating with only the radius. Shepherd had also noticed that in those specimens showing a perforation of the triangular fibrocartilage a kissing lesion was found on the lunate and not on the triquetrum (Fig. 5-3).

Recent kinematic studies[34,56] of the wrist provide us with a reproducible method for measuring carpal height, and for the determination of radiocarpal alignment in the posteroanterior projection, both in the normal and under pathologic conditons. Youm, McMurtry and collaborators[57] defined car-

pal height as the distance from the base of the third metacarpal to the distal articular surface of the radius, measured along the proximally projected axis of the third metacarpal in posteroanterior views (Fig. 5-4). This distance was found to remain constant throughout radial and ulnar deviation of the normal wrist, executed in a fixed plane. The ratio of this height to the length of the third metacarpal is 0.54 ± 0.03. Carpal-ulnar distance is also measured in posteroanterior roentgenograms and is defined as the perpendicular distance between the distally projected longitudinal axis of the ulna, and the axis of rotation of the wrist (located within the head of the capitate) during radial and ulnar deviation (Fig. 5-5). This distance is also constant in the normal wrist in all positions of radial and ulnar deviation in a fixed plane. The ratio of the carpal-ulnar distance to the length of the third metacarpal is normally 0.30 ± 0.03. These measurements aid in the diagnosis of the pathologic loss of carpal alignment that may be seen after injury or disease (Kienböck's disease, rheumatoid arthritis).[34]

An *anteroposterior* projection obtained with the hand and forearm in full supination is helpful in the

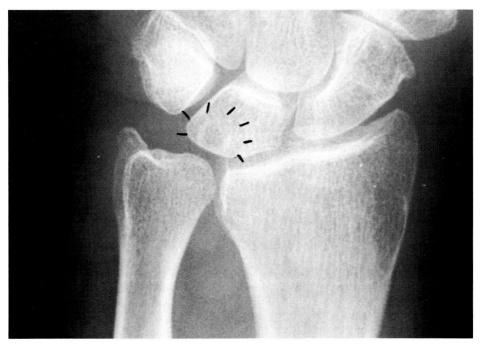

Fig. 5-3. Lunate lesion opposite ulnar head, in patient with arthrographic perforation of triangular fibrocartilage and ulnocarpal impingement.

radius.[25] In patients with an unstable scaphoid, forearm supination exerts a volarflexing action on the dissociated scaphoid through the radioscapho-capitate ligament,[16] accentuating the abnormal foreshortened appearance of the subluxed scaphoid, and causing a widening of the scapholunate gap. The routine posteroanterior projection, however, should be preferred when a fracture of the scaphoid is suspected. Additional views may be required as well.

Lateral views are extremely important for the evaluation of radiolunocapitate alignment, and for the assessment of radioscaphoid, lunoscaphoid,

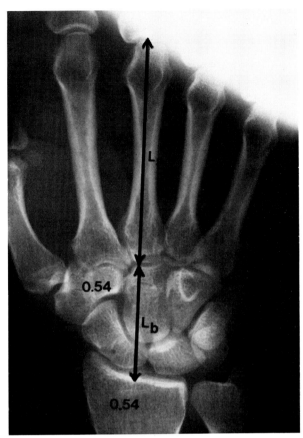

Fig. 5-4. Carpal height ratio calculated as L_b/L_a. L_a is the length of the third metacarpal and L_b is the carpal height (normal 0.54 ± 0.03). (Data from Youm Y, McMurtry RY, Flatt AE, Gillespie TE: Kinematics of the wrist. I. An experimental study of the radial-ulnar deviation and flexion-extension. J Bone Surg [Am] 60:423, 1978.)

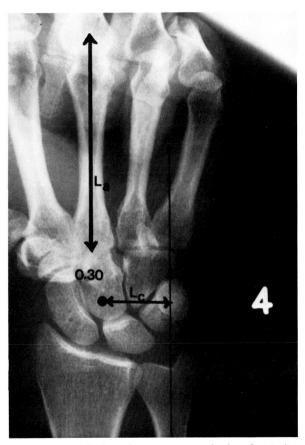

Fig. 5-5. Carpal-ulnar distance ratio calculated as L_c/L_a. L_c is the carpal-ulnar distance and L_a the length of the third metacarpal (normal 0.3 ± 0.03). (Data from Youm Y, McMurtry RY, Flatt AE, Gillespie TE: Kinematics of the wrist. I. An experimental study of the radial-ulnar deviation and flexion-extension. J Bone Joint Surg 60-A:423, 1978.)

diagnosis of rotatory subluxation of the scaphoid[2,11] and has been proposed to replace the routine posteroanterior projection.[52] The anteroposterior view in supination is very similar to that obtained in pronation. As routinely obtained, it can be recognized by the central position of the ulnar styloid on the head of the ulna, as compared to the medial position of the styloid[10] in line with the pisiform[25] in the posteroanterior views (Fig. 5-6). The capitohamate articulation can be visualized better because the overlap between capitate and hamate is no longer present.[20] In some cases the lunate shifts radialward and articulates completely with the

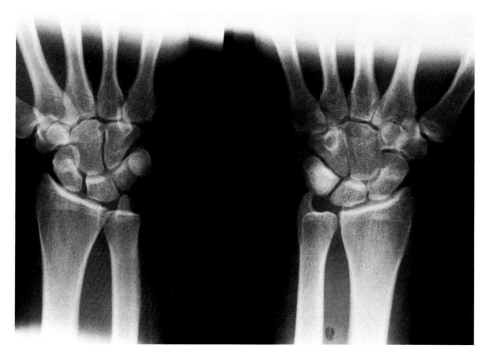

Fig. 5-6. Anteroposterior (left) and posteroanterior (right) projections of the same wrist.

and capitoscaphoid relationships (Fig. 5-7). The head of the capitate should fit concentrically within the distal concavity of the lunate, and the lunate into the slight concavity of the distal radius. In a radiologic study of wrist motion in flexion and extension, Sarrafian et al.[47] observed that with the wrist in neutral position, a lateral roentgenograph shows that the lunate is more frequently volarflexed (71 percent of the subjects in their study). In only 11 percent was the radiolunate alignment coaxial. The average volarflexion was only 11.9 degrees, but could be as much as 31 degrees. This may be an important predisposing factor for the development of some forms of wrist instability (see Chapter 12). Conversely, in most cases (73 percent), the capitate was found to be dorsiflexed. However, in only 11 percent did the capitate angle neutralize that of the lunate. Most lateral roentgenograms (51 percent) showed a slight flexion of the radiocapitate axis, averaging 11 degrees. The longitudinal axis of the scaphoid was found to average 58 degrees of volarflexion in relationship to the longitudinal axis of the radius (Fig. 5-7A). Linscheid et al.[32] stressed the value of the determination of the angle between the longitudinal axis of lunate and scaphoid (Fig. 5-8A). The lunate axis connects the midpoint of the proximal and distal articular surfaces; according to Gilula and Weeks,[18] the lunate axis is best determined by finding the perpendicular to a line joining the palmar and dorsal poles of the lunate. When the lunate is symmetric, this method is very accurate. However, the lunate is frequently asymmetric because the palmar pole is larger than the dorsal.[26] Therefore, an axis line perpendicular to a line tangential to the poles of the lunate may not coincide with the central axis of the lunate.[18] In spite of this objection, this method of drawing the lunate axis is very advantageous because of its reproducibility.[18] The scaphoid axis is traced tangential to the palmar outlines of the proximal and distal poles. This line is parallel to the true central axis of the scaphoid, or it may be off just a few degrees, not enough to invalidate the method (Figs. 5-7A, 5-8B). The lunate axis is normally colinear with the long axes of radius and third metacarpal in true lateral views. Normally, the scapholunate angle averages 47 degrees, and ranges from 30 to 60 degrees in normal wrists (Fig.

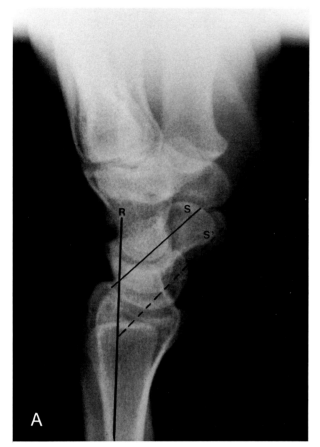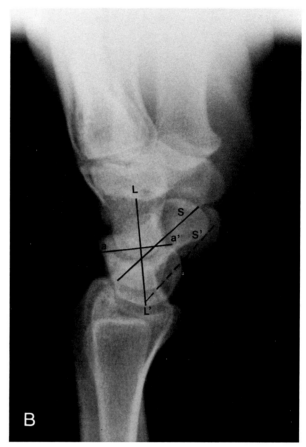

Fig. 5-7. Normal radioscaphoid and scapholunate angles. *A:* Radioscaphoid angle. R, longitudinal axis of radius; S, true central axis of scaphoid: S′, traced tangential to palmar outlines of proximal and distal poles. *B:* scapholunate angle. S, true central axis of scaphoid; S′, palmar tangential axis of scaphoid. Lunate axis LL′ traced perpendicular to line aa′ traced touching dorsal and palmar poles of lunate.

5-7B).[32] An angle greater than 70 degrees indicates carpal instability with scapholunate dissociation, the lunate being dorsiflexed and the scaphoid volarflexed (Fig. 5-8). Identical lateral views of the uninjured side may assist to evaluate the alignment of the injured wrist properly. A capitolunate angle of greater than 20 degrees is also strongly suggestive of carpal instability. A rapid evaluation of a lateral view of the wrist can be made by locating the longitudinal axis of the scaphoid and its volar concave outline.[52] Normally the longitudinal axis of the scaphoid and a line tangential to the volar flare of the distal radius are nearly parallel. In the normal wrist the volar outline of the scaphoid and that of the radial styloid make up a C or a bracket shape

(Fig. 5-9A). In rotatory sublaxation of the scaphoid, the volarflexed scaphoid can be quickly detected in lateral views, because its longitudinal axis and the tangent to the volar radial flare intersect at an acute angle, and the volar scaphoid-to-styloid outline has collapsed into a V (Fig. 5-9B). Lateral roentgenographs are obtained placing the ulnar border of the hand on the film. It has been suggested that for injuries of the radial carpus, particularly the scaphoid, a magnified distortion is thus produced. Instead, a lateral projection can be obtained placing the radial border of the pronated hand against a vertically held film with the rays directed from the ulnar side.[51]

The routine *oblique* view is obtained with the

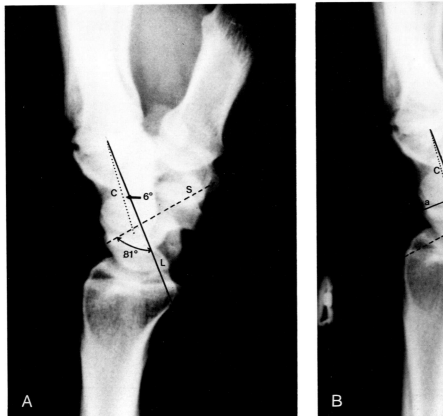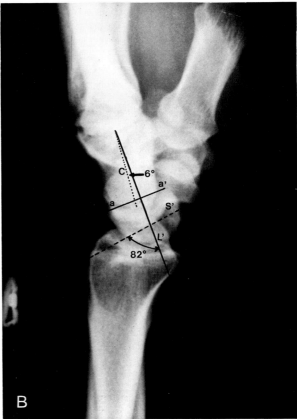

Fig. 5-8. Scapholunate angle in wrist with scapholunate dissociation. *A:* Determined using true central axes, S (scaphoid) and L (lunate). Lunocapitate angle (LC) is also shown. *B:* Determined using tangential axes S′ (scaphoid) and L′ (lunate) (see Fig. 5-7B). Lunocapitate angle (L′C) is also shown; aa′ is line traced touching dorsal and palmar poles of lunate.

ulnar border of the hand resting on the film and the forearm and hand pronated 45 degrees. This gives the examiner a different profile of structures on the volar-radial and on the dorsal-ulnar quadrants of the wrist (Fig. 5-10A). For the evaluation of the areas diagonally opposed the reverse, "ball-catcher" or semisupination oblique view is helpful[8,18,55] (Fig. 5-10B). This was one of 16 projections described by Graziani[20] for the radiologic evaluation of the wrist, and had been proposed by Nørgaard[39] for the study of early roentgenographic changes in inflammatory polyarthritis. The ulnar border of the hand rests on the film but hand and forearm are *supinated* 45 degrees from neutral (Fig. 5-10C). This allows injuries and anomalies on the volar-ulna and on the dorsal-radial quadrants to stand out. This view may be modified by adding some dorsiflexion or volarflexion for enhanced viewing of the hook of the hamate, the pisiform or the dorsum of the carpus and carpometacarpal areas, respectively. A variation of this reverse oblique view, obtained with the forearm and hand hyperpronated 30 degrees from the routine posteroanterior (pronated) position, was proposed by Bora and Didizian[6] for the visualization of fractures of the carpometacarpal joint of the little finger.

SPECIAL PROJECTIONS

SCAPHOID VIEWS

Although the diagnosis of fracture of the scaphoid may be suspected clinically, it can only be con-

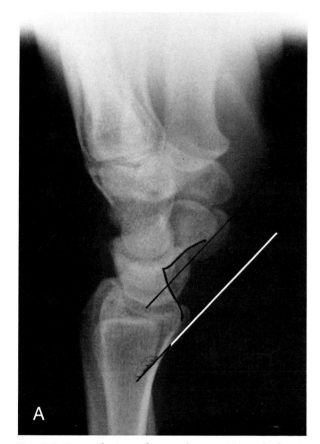 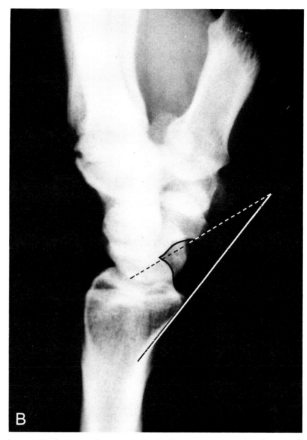

Fig. 5-9. Lateral view of normal wrist *(A)* and of wrist with scapholunate dissociation *(B)*. *A:* Longitudinal axis of scaphoid and line drawn tangential to palmar flare of distal radius are nearly parallel. Palmar outlines of scaphoid and radial styloid make up a C or bracket. *B:* Axis of scaphoid and line along flare of distal radius intersect at an acute angle. Palmar scaphoid-radial styloid outline is collapsed into a V.

firmed by radiographic examination. Special views have been proposed, designed to align the beam with the plane of the fracture line. Because these fractures are predominantly transverse, and occur across the waist of the normally volar flexed scaphoid, the beam-to-fracture alignment could be obtained by either angling the x-ray tube or dorsiflexing the scaphoid. Stecher[51] recommended that the hand be placed prone, with the fist clenched (Fig. 5-11A). He further suggested that this maneuver may "tend to widen a fracture line" for easier detection. The addition of ulnar deviation may further improve visualization of the scaphoid fracture[20] although Russe[45] cautioned against this, lest it should produce unwanted distraction of the fracture fragments. In 1949, Bridgman[9] proposed that

the hand in ulnar deviation be placed on a 17-degree (or 23-degree) angle board, with the wrist in neutral flexion. Conversely, the hand may remain flat, but the beam could be angled 17 to 23 degrees (Fig. 5-11B). Ulnar deviation could be omitted if too painful.

Carpal Tunnel View

The carpal tunnel view (Fig. 5-12) is most useful for the detection of fractures of the hook of the hamate. The carpal tunnel profile view was described by Hart and Gaynor;[22] it provides an end-on, axial view of the carpal canal. The anterior aspect of the forearm and wrist are on the film, a

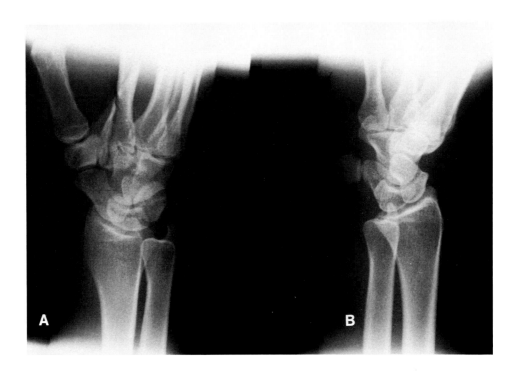

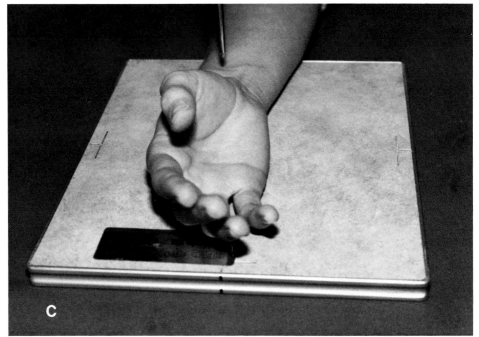

Fig. 5-10. Routine *(A)* and reversed or supinated *(B* and *C)* oblique projections.

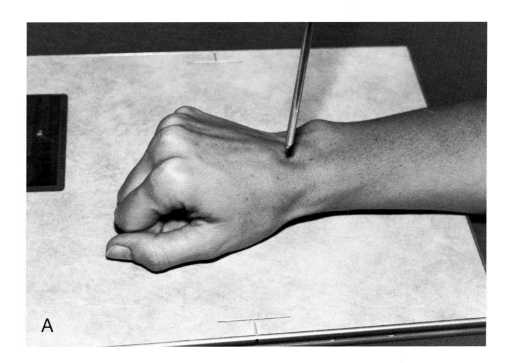

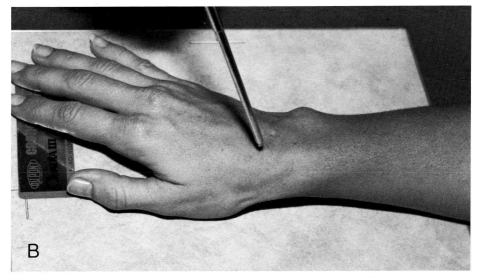

Fig. 5-11. Stecher's *(A)* and Bridgman's *(B)* projections of the wrist for improved visualization of the scaphoid. (See Refs. 51 and 9.)

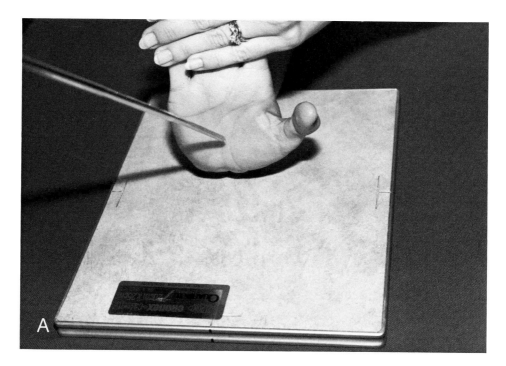

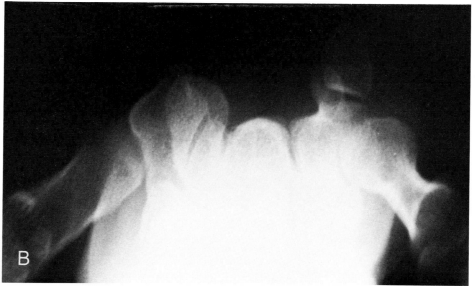

Fig. 5-12. Carpal tunnel projection *(A)* and radiographic appearance *(B)*.

small sponge may be placed under the wrist; the wrist, hand, and fingers are hyperextended by the patient's other hand. The beam is directed 1 inch distal to the base of the fourth metacarpal, at 25 to 30 degrees to the long axis of the hand.[35]

DYNAMIC VIEWS

Dynamic views are routine anteroposterior, posteroanterior, or lateral projections with the wrist in volar- and dorsiflexion, or in ulnar and radial deviation. These views are helpful for the diagnosis of dynamic forms of carpal instability (see Chapters 10, 11, 12, 13) to accentuate carpal dissociation patterns, such as scapholunate gap in rotatory subluxation of the scaphoid, or to bring into view fractures of the scaphoid. The examiner should be aware of the normal changes that may be seen in the carpus in radial and ulnar deviation (Fig. 5-13). In radial deviation the scaphoid is foreshortened, volarflexed, its long axis perpendicular to the long axis of the radius. The lunate appears to be triangular in shape, and the triquetrum comes to rest at the top of the hamate in a "high" or proximal alignment (see Chapter 3). In ulnar deviation the scaphoid appears elongated; it is in a longitudinal position; the triquetrum is now in a "low," distal alignment; there is total triquetrohamate contact and triquetral dorsiflexion. The lunate shape is trapezoidal.

Lateral views obtained with the forearm pronated, the radiographic beam approaching the wrist from the side, and the wrist in ulnar (or radial) deviation against the x-ray plate placed vertically are helpful for the diagnosis of dynamic midcarpal instability (Fig. 5-14). Normally, in ulnar deviation, the lunate dorsiflexes and dips in a palmar direction to allow the capitate to remain colinear with the radius. The loss of this compensatory mechanism allows the capitate to displace dorsal to the radius, (see Chapters 12 and 13). The opposite takes place during radial deviation.

TANGENTIAL POSTEROANTERIOR RADIOGRAPH

The tangential posteroanterior radiograph (Fig. 5-15) allows direct viewing of the scapholunate space and is helpful in the diagnosis of scapholunate dissociation.[37] In routine posteroanterior radiographs, scaphoid and lunate overlap. When the ulnar border of the hand is elevated 20 degrees off the table, the beam then is aligned with the scapholunate articulation. Normally, the width of this space should not exceed 2 mm or be greater than any other intercarpal space.

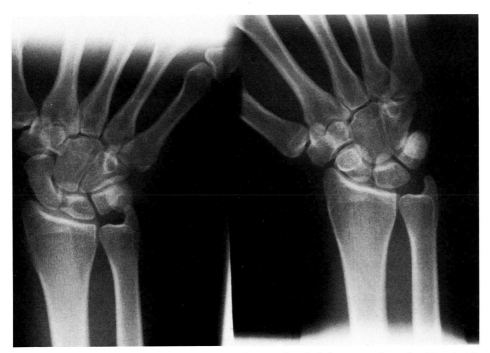

Fig. 5-13. Posteroanterior radiographs in ulnar and radial deviation (see also Fig. 3-4C, D).

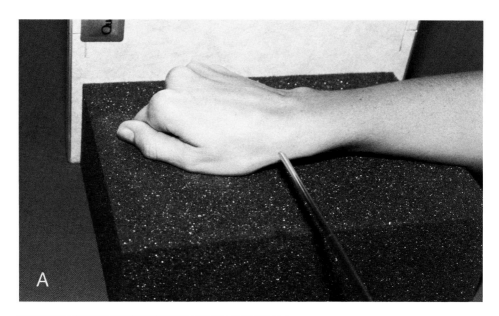

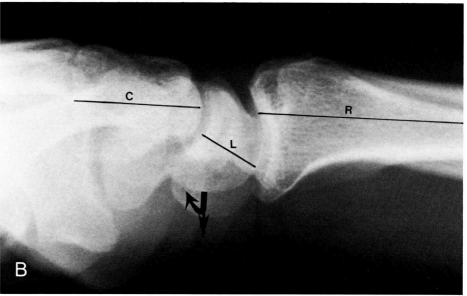

Fig. 5-14. Lateral view of wrist in ulnar deviation. *A:* Position of the hand in relation to x-ray beam and plate. *B:* Lunate (L) dorsiflexes and translates palmarward; longitudinal axes of radius (R) and capitate (C) remain colinear.

CARPAL BRIDGE VIEW[29]

This view was designed to study the dorsum of the wrist. The name "carpal bridge view" was chosen to indicate that this view is precisely opposite to the carpal tunnel view. It is obtained with the patient sitting, the arm abducted at a right angle to the body and the elbow flexed 90 degrees to allow the forearm to approach the table in a perpendicular direction. The wrist is fully volarflexed, allowing the dorsum of the hand to be placed on the x-ray cassette. The central beam approaches the hand at a 45-degree angle, directed to an area 2 inches proximal to the plane of the plate. This view was

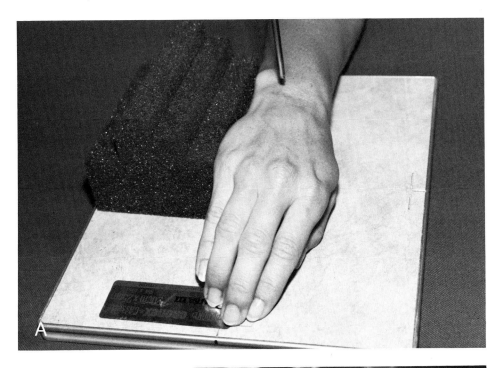

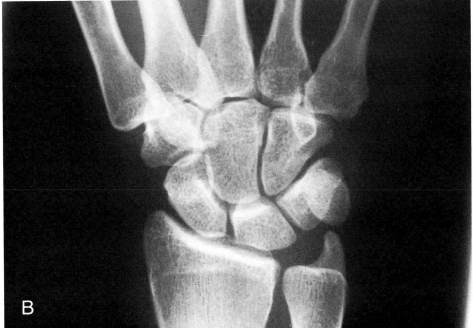

Fig. 5-15. A and B: Tangential posteroanterior radiograph (See Ref. 37.)

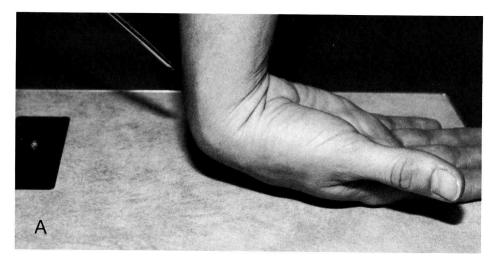

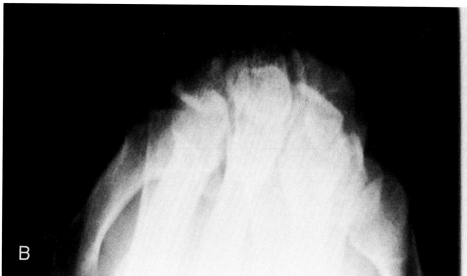

Fig. 5-16. A and *B:* Carpal bridge view.

proposed for the diagnosis of some lunate dislocations, fractures of the scaphoid, and foreign bodies
or calcifications of the dorsum of the wrist. It may
be helpful to further detect small chip fractures of
the dorsum of the carpus, and in some cases of
scapholunate dissociation when the scapholunate
gap may be wider than normal, or else the proximal
pole of the scaphoid displaced dorsally, breaking
the smooth outline of the dorsal "carpal bridge"
(Fig. 5-16).

CLENCHED-FIST RADIOGRAPH

Dobyns and coworkers[14] proposed that a longitudinal compression load applied to the wrist by
the patient making a fist may enhance detection of
scapholunate dissociations that would otherwise be
missed. The head of the capitate would be driven in
a proximal direction, prying apart the scaphoid
from the lunate, when a ligamentous injury is
present.

TRAPEZIUM VIEW

The routine radiographic examination of the trapezium does not show its entire outline or its relationship to the scaphoid and trapezoid. A better view may be obtained by placing the hand palm-down on a radiolucent support, at a 35-degree angle to the film. The wrist is held in ulnar deviation, the forearm supported on a bolster, and the thumb abducted and extended.[7]

For the past three years, we have used a slight modification of this technique (Bett view*). The entire outline of the trapezium is projected without overlap from the surrounding bones. The wrist is placed in the lateral position, with the elbow raised from the cassette. The thumb is extended and abducted and the hand slightly pronated. The center beam is directed to the scaphotrapezium-trapezoid joint. (See Fig. 5-17).

SPECIAL PROCEDURES

TOMOGRAPHY

Tomography may be of help in the detection of small, occult, or very early fractures, mostly those involving the scaphoid, and the hook of the hamate (Fig. 5-18A). It is also helpful to determine the degree of healing in cases of troublesome carpal fractures, particularly of the scaphoid.

CINERADIOGRAPHY

Cineradiography has been valuable in understanding the dynamics of carpal function in normal and abnormal wrists.[1] It is particularly useful in those patients with a normal wrist alignment, who can voluntarily assume a position of carpal collapse, at which point cinegradiography may detect a sudden abnormal carpal shift, accompanied by a

painful, loud "snap." These are dynamic forms of voluntarily recurrent carpal instability[53] (see Chapters 10, 11, 12, and 13).

ARTHROGRAPHY

Arthrography (Fig. 5-19) has been of help in the evalution of the painful wrist with negative roentgenographs[27] and may assist in finding areas of cartilaginous or ligament tear not otherwise apparent.[42] It has also been proposed for the preoperative evaluation of ligament disruptions in the more severe complex carpal injuries.[38] In the early involvement of the wrist by rheumatoid disease[41] abnormal infolding of synovium or corrugated appearance of the synovial cavity may assist to establish a diagnosis. The technique of arthrography can be modified to allow a more precise study of the multiple carpal joints. It is important that the flow of opaque material be followed in an image intensifier to find leaks and abnormal communications.[48] Recently, digital fluorography has been used advantageouly for the same purpose. This technique allows continuous digital recording following injection; successive frames show the progress of the opaque material. The use of subtraction techniques enhances the visualization of subtle amounts of contrast material. This information can be stored and retrieved for repeated evaluation and study (Fig. 5-20). Multiple arthrograms may also be helpful, if different wrist compartments (i.e., radioulnar, radiocarpal, midcarpal) are injected on different occasions (Fig. 5-19). Arthrotomography may assist to pinpoint a ligamentous or bone defect that may otherwise be lost in the single radiographic projection of the entire wrist. Communications between the different compartments of the wrist are not necessarily the result of trauma or disease. Most frequently the radiologic material may leak from the radiocarpal into the distal radioulnar joint. Kessler and Silberman noted this in 7 percent of radiocarpal arthograms.[27] Lewis et al.[30] demonstrated abnormal communications between the radiocarpal and distal radioulnar joints, between radiocarpal and midcarpal joints, and between radiocarpal and pisotriquetral joints in at least one third of cadaver dissections. The inci-

---

* Woodard, Bette J, R.T., Hartford Orthopaedic and Hand Surgeons, Inc., Hartford, Connecticut. March 1, 1981.

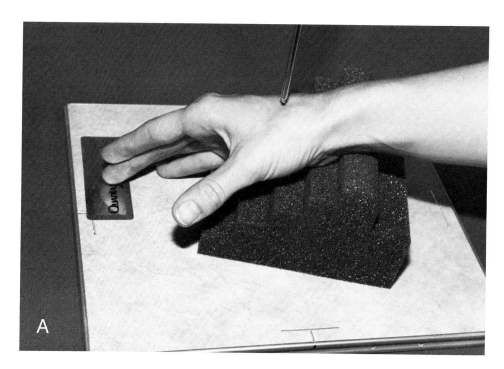

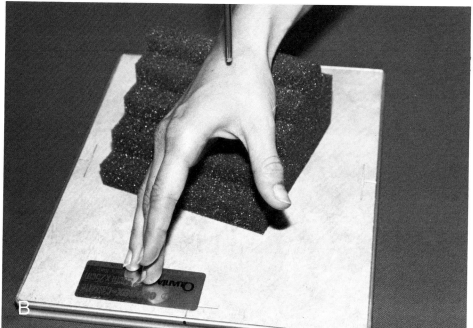

Fig. 5-17. Trapezium views (see text). *A* and *B:* Position of the hand and wrist (Bett's view).

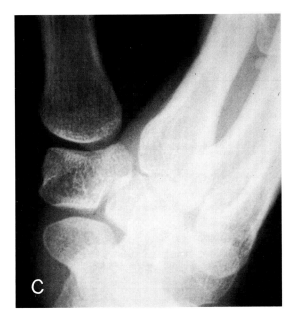

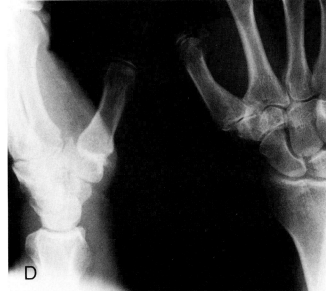

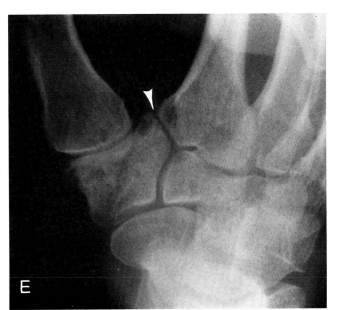

Fig. 5-17 (cont.) C: Normal appearance. *D:* Routine posteroanterior and lateral projections of trapezio-metacarpal joint. *E:* Bett's view shows impingement between trapezium and base of second metacarpal (arrow).

dence of degenerative changes allowing these abnormal communications increases with age.[43]

COMPUTED TOMOGRAPHY

Computed tomography may prove to be a most useful diagnostic tool for wrist problems. The wrist is particularly suitable for this type of investigation, especially for those problems for which conventional radiologic modalities offer only limited help, such as in the evaluation of the ulnar half of the carpus (because of bony overlap), and for the detection of subtle alterations of distal radioulnar joint alignment[36,49] (Fig. 5-21). It has also been proposed as a diagnostic aid for problems involving the carpal tunnel.[58]

(Text continues on page 102.)

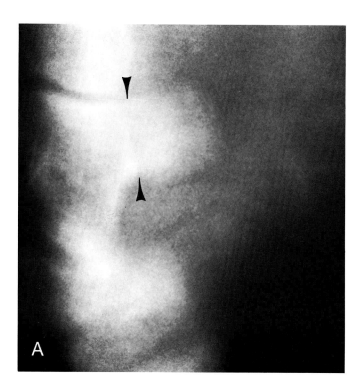

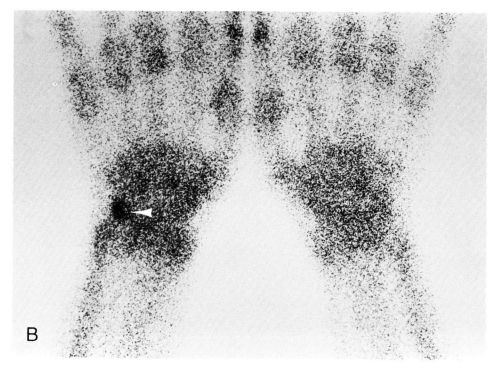

Fig. 5-18. Tomography *(A)* and bone scan *(B)* of wrist with fracture of hook of hamate (arrow).

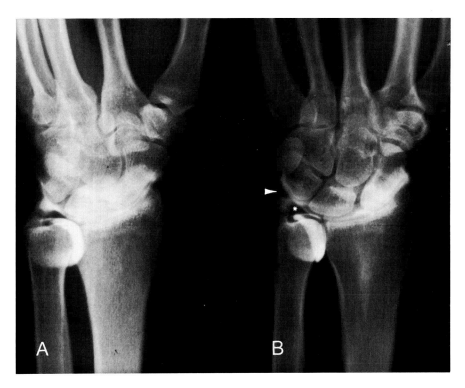

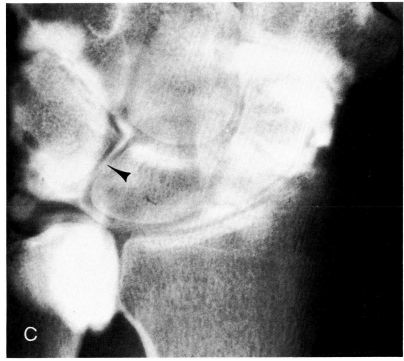

Fig. 5-19. Arthrography of wrist following injection of opaque material into radioulnar and radiocarpal spaces. *A* and *B:* Normal initial appearance. Arrow points to outline of ulnocarpal meniscus homologue. Asterisk is placed on triangular fibrocartilage. *C:* Later flow of opaque material into midcarpal space due to abnormal tear of lunotriquetral ligaments (arrow).

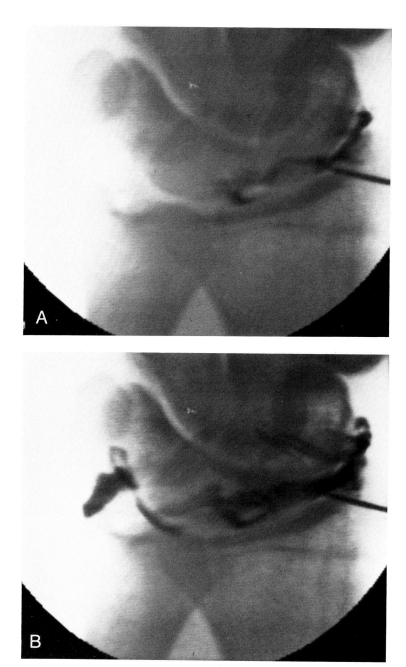

Fig. 5-20. Digital fluorography.

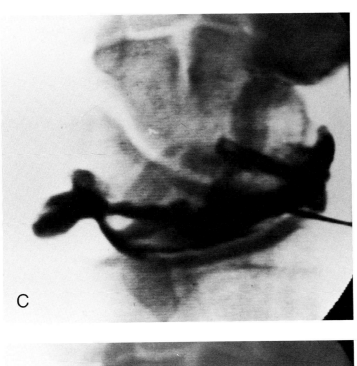

C

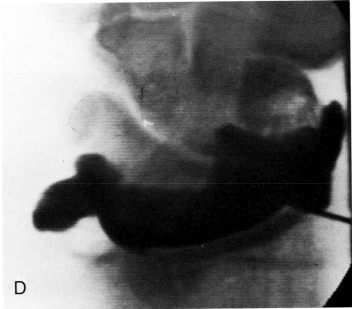

D

Fig. 5-20 *(cont.)*

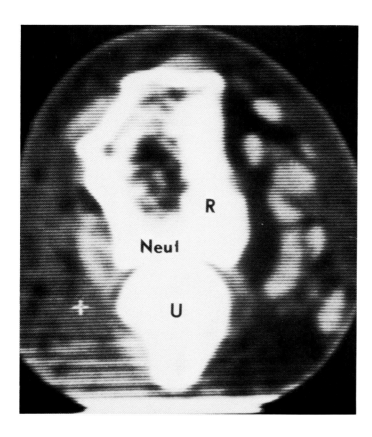

Fig. 5-21. Computed tomography of normal radioulnar joint in neutral rotation of the forearm.

Bone Scintigraphy

Increased accumulation of radioactive tracers may be associated with a neoplasm, infection, arthritis, and occasionally blunt trauma.[4] Technetium-99m pyrophosphate bone scans have been useful in the early diagnosis of occult fractures[3] (Fig. 5-18B). Fractures may be detected by bone scan as early as 6 to 7 hours following injury.[33] A negative bone scan 3 to 5 days later is a strong indication that a fracture has not occurred.[44] Because skeletal scans lack specificity, they should not be used as isolated diagnostic techniques, but rather be adjuncts to information obtained by classic clinical and radiographic means.

Other radioactive isotopes may prove more accurate for the diagnosis of inflammation or infection. Gallium scans will usually be positive in septic arthritides at a time when the bone scan is still negative.[21] Early uptake of gallium also occurs in the initial stages of osteomyelitis, when bone scans may still be negative.[23]

REFERENCES

1. Arkless R: Cineradiography in normal and abnormal wrists. Am J Roentgenol Radium Ther Nucl Med 96:837, 1966
2. Armstrong GWD: Rotational subluxation of the scaphoid. Can J Surg 11:306,1968
3. Bastillas J, Vasilas A, Pizzi WF, Gokcebay, T: Bone scanning in the detection of occult fractures. J Trauma 21:564, 1981
4. Belsole RJ, Eikman EA, Muroff LA: Bone scintigraphy in trauma of the hand and wrist. J Trauma 21:163, 1981
5. Bogart FB: Variations of the bones of the wrist. Am J Roentgenol Radium Ther Nucl Med 28:638, 1932
6. Bora FW, Didizian NH: The treatment of injuries to the carpometacarpal joint of the little finger. J Bone Joint Surg [Am] 56:1459, 1974
7. Boyes JH: More accurate diagnosis of hand and wrist injuries. Consultant 13:144, 1973
8. Brewerton DA: The rheumatoid hand. Proc R Soc Med. 59:225, 1966
9. Bridgman CF: Radiography of the carpal navicular bone. Med Radiogr Photogr 25:104, 1949

10. Bryce TH: On certain points in the anatomy and mechanism of the wrist joint reviewed in the light of a series of rontgen ray photographs of the living hand. J Anat 31:59, 1896

11. Campbell RO Jr, Thompson TC, Lance EM, Adler JB: Indications for open reduction of lunate and perilunate dislocations of the carpal bones. J Bone Joint Surg (Am) 47:915, 1965

12. Corson ER: An x-ray study of the normal movements of the carpal bones and wrist. Proc Assoc Am Anat 11:67, 1898

13. Destot E: Traumatismes du Poignet et Rayons X. Masson, Paris, 1923

14. Dobyns JH, Linscheid RL, Chao EYS, et al: Traumatic instability of the wrist. Am Acad Orthop Surgeons Instruct Course Lect 24:182, 1975

15. Faulkner DM: Bipartite carpal scaphoid. J Bone Joint Surg 10:284, 1928

16. Ghigi C: Contributo allo studio della articolazione della mano. Chir degli organi mov. 24:344, 1939

17. Gilula LA: Carpal injuries: Analytic approach and case exercises. Am J Roentgenol 133:503, 1979

18. Gilula LA, Weeks PM: Posttraumatic ligamentous instability of the wrist. Radiology 129:641, 1978

19. Graham CE: Bilateral congenital carpal fusion in a champion golfer. Clin Orthop 83:70, 1972

20. Graziani A: L'esame radiologica del carpo. Radiol Med 27:382, 1940

21. Handmaker H, Giammona ST: "Hot Joint": Increased diagnostic accuracy using combine 99m-Tc phosphate and 67-gallium citrate imaging in pediatrics. (Abstract). J Nucl Med 17:554, 1976

22. Hart VL, Gaynor V: Roentgenographic study of the carpal canal. J Bone Joint Surg 23:382, 1941

23. Hoffer PB: The use of gallium in diagnosing inflammatory disease. p 39. In Hoffer PB, Bekerman C, Kenkin RE: Gallium-67 Imaging. Wiley, Wiley, New York, 1978

24. Jerre T: Bipartite carpal scaphoid bone. Acta Orthop Scand 17:70, 1947

25. Johnson MK, Cohen MJ: The Hand Atlas. Charles C Thomas, Springfield, IL, 1975

26. Kauer JMG: Functional anatomy of the wrist. Clin Orthop 149:73, 1980

27. Kessler I, Silberman Z: An experimental study of the radiocarpal joint by arthrography. Surg Gynecol Obstet 112:33, 1961

28. Koostra G, Huffstadt AJC, Kauer JMG: The styloid bone. A clinical and embrylogical study. Hand 6:185, 1974

29. Lentino, W, Lubetsky HW, Jacobson HG, Poppel MH: The carpal-bridge view. A position for the roentgenographic diagnosis of abnormalities in the dorsum of the wrist. J Bone Joint Surgery [Am]39:88, 1957

30. Lewis OJ, Hamshere RJ, Bucknill TM: The anatomy of the wrist joint. J Anat 106:539, 1970

31. Lindgren E: On os naviculare bipartitum. Acta Radiol 22:511, 1941

32. Linscheid RL, Dobyns JH, Beabout JW, Bryan RS: Traumatic instability of the wrist. Diagnosis, classification and pathomechanics. J Bone Joint Surg [Am] 54:1612, 1972

33. Matin P: The appearance of bone scans following fractures, including immediate and long-term studies. J Nucl Med 20:1227, 1979

34. McMurtry RY, Youm Y, Flatt AE, Gillespie TE: Kinematics of the wrist. II. Clinical applications. J Bone Joint Surg [Am] 60:955, 1978

35. Merrill V: Atlas of Roentgenography Positions and Standard Roentgenographic Positions. 4th Ed. Vol. 1. CV Mosby, St. Louis, 1975

36. Mino DE, Palmer AK, Levinsohn EM: The role of radiography and computerized tomography in the diagnosis of subluxation and dislocation of the distal radioulnar joint. J Hand Surg 8:23, 1983

37. Moneim MS: The tangential posteroanterior radiograph to demonstrate scapholunate dissociation. J Bone Joint Surg [Am] 63:1324, 1981

38. Moneim MS, Omer GE, White RE: Wrist arthrography in complex carpal injuries. Presented at the 35th Annual Meeting of the American Society for Surgery of the Hand, Atlanta, Georgia, Feb. 6, 1980

39. Nørgaard F: Earliest reontgenological changes in polyarthritis of the rheumatoid type: Rheumatoid arthritis. Radiology 85:325, 1965

40. O'Rahilly R: A survey of carpal and tarsal anomalies. J Bone Joint Surg [Am] 35:626, 1953

41. Ranawat CS, Frieberger RH, Jordan LR, Straub, LR: Arthrography in the rheumatoid wrist joint (a preliminary report). J Bone Joint Surg [Am] 51:1269, 1969

42. Ranawat CS, Harrison MO Jordan LR: Arthrography of the wrist joint. Clin Orthop 83:6, 1972

43. Resnick D: Rheumatoid Arthritis of the wrist. The Compartmental Approach-Medical radiography and Photography 52:50, 1976

44. Rosenthal L, Hill RO, Chuang S: Observation on the use of 99mTc-phosphate imaging in peripheral bone trauma. Radiology 119:137, 1976

45. Russe O: Fracture of the carpal navicular. Diagnosis non-operative treatment, and operative treatment. J Bone Joint Surg [Am] 42:759, 1960

46. Sandzen SC Jr: Atlas of Wrist and Hand Fractures. PSG Publishing, Littleton, MA, 1979

47. Sarrafian SK, Melamed JL, Goshgarian GM: Study of

wrist motion in flexion and extension. Clin Orthop 126:153, 1977

48. Schwartz AM, Ruby LK: Wrist arthrography revisited Orthopedics 5:883, 1982

49. Sclafani SJA: Dislocation of the distal radioulnar joint. J Comput Assist Tomogr 5:450, 1981

50. Shepherd FJ: A note on the radiocarpal articulation. J Anat 25:349, 1890

51. Stecher WR: Roentgenography of the carpal navicular bone. Am J Roentgenol 37:704, 1937

52. Taleisnik J: Wrist: Anatomy, function, and injury. Am Acad Orthop Surgeons Instruct Course Lect 27:61, 1978

53. Taleisnik J: Post-traumatic carpal instability. Clin Orthop 419:73, 1980

54. Waugh RL, Sullivan RF: Anomalies of the carpus, with particular reference to the bipartite scaphoid (navicular). J Bone Joint Surg [Am] 32:682, 1950

55. Weston WJ: Functional anatomy of the pisi-cuneiform joint. Br J Radiol 46:692, 1973

56. Youm Y, Flatt AE: Kinematics of the wrist. Clin Orthop 149:21, 1980

57. Youm Y, McMurtry RY, Flatt AE, Gillespie TE: Kinematics of the wrist. I. An experimental study of radial-ulnar deviation and flexion-extension. J Bone Joint Surg [Am] 60:423, 1978

58. Zucker-Pinchoff B, Hermann G, Srinivasan R: Computed tomography of the carpal tunnel: A radioanatomical study. J Comput Assist Tomogr 5:525, 1981

6 Fractures of the Scaphoid

Until Röntgen's discovery of x-rays, injuries to the scaphoid were part of a large, nondescript group of "wrist sprains." Prior to 1895 several isolated cases of fractures of the scaphoid were reported during autopsy examinations.[27,93] Today, among all wrist injuries, the incidence of these fractures is second only to fractures of the distal radius.[12-14,16,17,20,37,38,166,168] Despite a voluminous literature on the subject, the treatment of the fractured scaphoid is still controversial, both for the acute as well as for the old injury.

DIAGNOSIS

This fracture is most frequent in the young adult male and usually involes the waist of the scaphoid. Because of this age preference, the incidence of scaphoid fractures is greater than that of fractures of the distal radius among military personnel[9,20,32,49,80,110,124,156,171] and athletes ("fracture du gymnaste"[89,179]). It is a rare injury in children in whom the most common variety is the fracture of the distal third.[56,109,185] Eddeland et al.[56] reviewed 196 fractures of the scaphoid and found only 13 in children 12 to 15 years of age. In the Vahvanen and Westerlund series[185] most patients were 10 years of age or older. They stressed that, although rare and usually without complications, scaphoid fractures in children should be kept in mind for they may progress to nonunion if neglected. Recently, a rare case of osteochondritis dissecans of the scaphoid was reported[3] involving the proximal pole, in a 19-year-old patient whose original injury was sustained at age 13. There is frequently a history of a fall, usually against the palm of the hand in dorsiflexion. This may seem an insignificant injury, one easily dismissed as "just a sprain," except for the persistence of symptoms, pain and swelling. Initially there is surprisingly little limitation of motion[91,140] and minimal loss of grip strength. This explains the frequent delay in seeking medical attention. On examination, the most consistent finding is tenderness in the anatomic snuffbox area. Pain in this location can be aggravated by axial compression along the index and long fingers, the Vaughan's test (quoted by Cole[36]), by percussion on the tip of the abducted[164] or extended[72,73] thumb, by forced dorsiflexion[89,184] or by active pronation of the hand against manual resistance.[186,187] All these maneuvers are of doubtful clinical value, since only a thorough radiographic examination can confirm the diagnosis. Conversely, in the presence of tenderness over the anatomic snuffbox, without deformity, a fracture of the scaphoid should always be presumed until radiographic examination proves negative beyond doubt.[64,194] After Röntgen's discovery and for more than 20 years thereafter, only posteroanterior and lateral x-rays were routinely used. There were some exceptions. In 1905 Codman and Chase[34] recommended to radiograph both wrists in the same plate, in pronation and in supination and in ulnar deviation, for this "extends the scaphoid bone, that is, it lifts the distal end so that it comes nearer the plane of the proximal end." In 1921 Todd[180] proposed that the wrist be examined radiographically "anteroposteriorly and laterally, and sometimes obliquely as well," and mentioned "Codman and Chase's" view. Toward 1930 it became obvious that posteroanterior and lateral views alone were not sufficient, and that many fractures of the scaphoid could be missed shortly after injury, only to be diagnosed too late, when pseudoarthrosis had developed (Fig. 6-1). Additional views were emphasized, both to better visualize the scaphoid and to better detect its most common fracture, transversely across the waist (Fig. 5-11). Ulnar deviation[153] and some dorsiflexion of the wrist designed to bring the normally volarflexed scaphoid to a

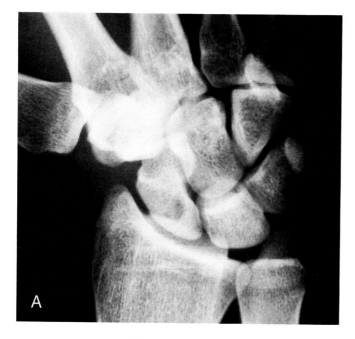

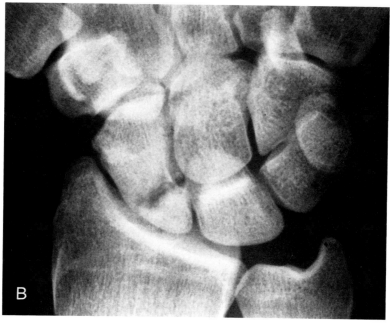

Fig. 6-1. Initial radiograph of wrist after injury fails to show a fracture *(A)*. Because of persistent pain, a second radiograph six months later shows a fracture with resorption and early cystic changes *(B)*.

plane parallel to the x-ray plate[129,142,170] were found to be useful. This culminated in a paper by Graziani[77] who in 1940 proposed 16 views for an exhaustive study of wrist injuries. Actually, only four routine views are recommended: posteroanterior, lateral, and two obliques (see Chapter 5). Of these, the posteroanterior and routine oblique (semipronated) views are most reliable for visualization of the fracture.[102] In only 2.6 percent of all cases in Leslie and Dickson's[102] series was the fracture visible in only the lateral view, the reverse oblique view or both. When a scaphoid fracture is strongly suspected on clinical grounds, and routine projections fail to show it, additional views are justified, designed to align the plane of the fracture with the central rays (Fig. 6-2). Ulnar deviation alone may be all that is required,[80,120,159,168] although Russe[155] cautioned that ulnar deviation may cause distraction of the fracture fragments.

A consistent and accurate radiographic recording of the scaphoid may be obtained using Bridgman's[21] guidelines: the hand in ulnar deviation

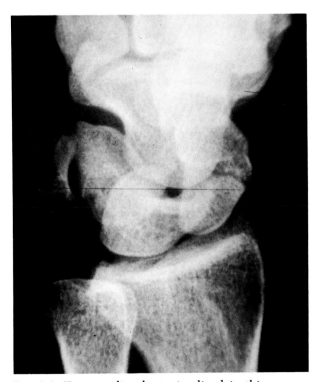

Fig. 6-2. Fracture line best visualized in this reverse oblique view.

rests on a 17-degree angle board, the central ray projected perpendicularly through the scaphoid. A similar appearance results if the hand is left horizontal, but the central ray is projected 17 degrees cephalad. This angle of approach may be changed to 20 or even 30 degrees, when a fracture is strongly suspected and still not visualized. Scaphoid fractures are not usually visible in the lateral projection. This, however, is a most important view, for it allows the examiner to evaluate carpal alignment, and to detect the presence of a possible carpal instability pattern (Fig. 6-3). Because the usual lateral roentgenograms are obtained with the ulnar border of the hand resting on the film, a magnified distortion of the scaphoid may be produced. This can be corrected when indicated by placing the radial aspect of the pronated hand against a vertical x-ray plate, and projecting the beam from the ulnar side.[170] If initial studies are negative, it is prudent to immobilize the wrist in a splint and repeat radiographs in two to three weeks.[6,20,25,26,32,85,92,120,127,155,164,167,168,179,194] Resorption between the fracture fragments may produce enough widening of the fracture line to allow its detection at that time. This widening of the fracture line, clearly demonstrating fractures not visible on initial films, had led to the erroneous belief that "spontaneous" fractures of the scaphoid can occur several weeks or even months after an injury to the wrist with "negative" initial radiographs.[129] In a recent review of 222 consecutive fresh scaphoid injuries, Leslie and Dickson[102] pointed out that two percent of fractures that became radiographically visible after treatment had begun were incomplete, across the compression (concave) side of the scaphoid, and were better visualized on routine oblique radiographs with the hand semipronated 45 degrees. If symptoms persist, this radiographic study may be repeated once more. Dickson[49] stressed that the diagnosis of sprain of the wrist should be made with the greatest of caution, and only after an injury to the scaphoid has been positively excluded. Terry and Ramin[178] have called attention to a small radiolucent area normally present next to the scaphoid in the frontal projection, (also visible in the oblique view), which they named *navicular fat stripe* (Fig. 6-4). A fracture on the radial side of the wrist (radial styloid, scaphoid, base of first metacarpal) can either dis-

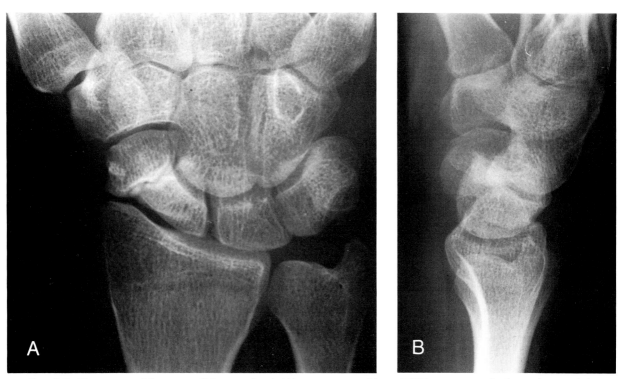

Fig. 6-3. Nonunion of fracture of the scaphoid *(A)* accompanied by a DISI pattern in the lateral view *(B)*.

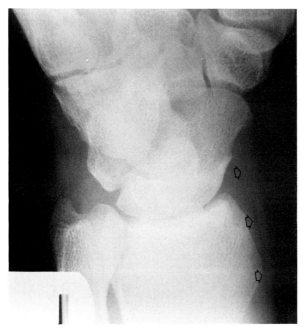

Fig. 6-4. Scaphoid ("navicular") fat stripe (arrows), seen in oblique projection. (See Ref. 178.)

place or obliterate this space. Conversely, a preserved fat stripe is a strong indication that a fracture has not occurred. Cetti and Christensen[30] found an abnormal fat stripe in 73 of 78 fractures of the scaphoid reviewed retrospectively. Because the scaphoid fat stripe may reappear as early as five days following a fracture, this sign is valuable only in fresh injuries. In difficult cases, laminographs, trispiral tomography,[39] and isotope scanning may be used (Fig. 6-5). A normal scan excludes the fracture. Increased focal activity suggests that injury to the scaphoid has occurred, even if the fracture is not visible in roentgenographs at that time.[67,97] Bone scans may also provide information on the vascularity of the fracture fragments.[103]

Although bipartition of the scaphoid is now considered to be a rare entity,[127,151] it is mentioned in the differential diagnosis of the injured scaphoid. Many authors consider bipartition the most frequent malformation in the carpus.[40,88] Actually, this is a rare condition that becomes meaningful only because of its similarity with old ununited

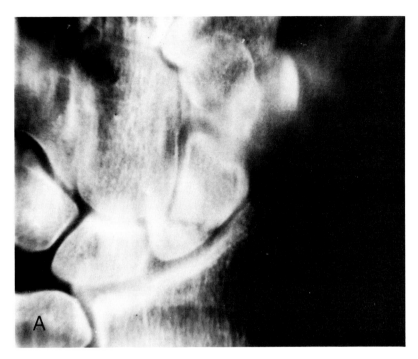

Fig. 6-5. Laminogram *(A)* and isotope scanning *(B)* are useful to demonstrate a persistent nonunion of a fracture of the scaphoid.

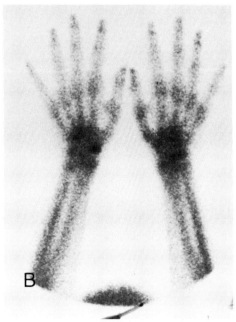

fractures of the scaphoid (Fig. 6-6). It is thought that bipartition may develop consequent to a persistent but separate os centrale[194] (an unlikely theory) or as a result of ossification from two independent cartilaginous anlages[145,146] or two ossification centers that fail to fuse within the same pri-

mordial cartilage,[60,94,180] although Troll (quoted by Blencke[15]) never encountered a bipartition of the scaphoid in an examination of hundreds of serial sections of the wrists of human embryos of various ages. In 1905 Codman and Chase[34] flatly denied the existence of scaphoid bipartition having failed

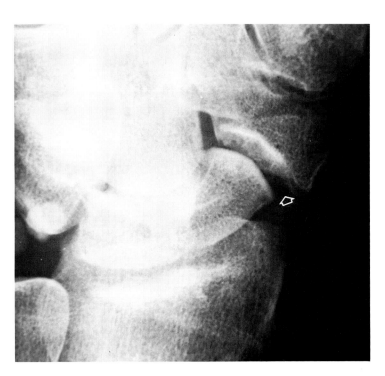

Fig. 6-6. Nonunion presenting as a bipartite scaphoid (arrow).

to show a single "divided scaphoid" without a clear-cut history of an injury, in a review of 1040 radiographs of the wrist. Scaphoid development from more than one center has been reported in diseases involving abnormal ossification.[84,104,138] The differential diagnosis can be extremely difficult, particularly because true nonunions of the scaphoid may develop following trivial injuries, with very minimal and transient disability long forgotten by the patient. Gollasch's[74] report of bipartite scaphoids in several members of a family must be accepted as a true instance of this unusual condition. Other reports[19,31,60,94,104,161] show radiographic changes very reminiscent of nonunions rather than congenital abnormal partitions, in spite of negative histories for previous injury. A diagnosis of bipartite scaphoid must be based on a foolproof negative history, on radiographs showing two fragments of near normal density, although not necessarily of equal size,[40] with clear-cut edges, separated by a smooth jointlike space, with rounded corners.[20,138] Bilaterality is supportive of the diagnosis but does not exclude fracture.[50] There should not be periscaphoid degenerative

changes, and the patient must either be asymptomatic, or return to an asymptomatic state after a short period of splinting. This last condition may, however, be found in asymptomatic nonunions. If the wrist is surgically explored, the interface between the bone fragments should be covered by hyaline articular cartilage, rather than by the dense sclerotic bone found in nonunions.[15] Under these strict guidelines, bipartition of the scaphoid becomes an extremely rare possibility indeed. Fractures with nonunion should always be considered as the likely diagnosis. An old fracture or nonunion may show a space between fragments similar to a normal carpal space. There is sclerosis of the bony outline at the fracture line, surrounding degenerative and cystic changes and variations in the width of the interfragmentary gap during motions.[50] The cystic appearance, however, may be misleading because it can be simulated at times by x-ray projections[104] as was shown experimentally in freshly induced scaphoid osteotomies.[72] The need to establish an accurate diagnosis, however, may be of academic interest only, for if the condition is symptom-free, no treatment is required, but should it be symptomatic and disabling, whether a nonunion or bipartite scaphoid, the treatment indicated will be identical.

MECHANISM OF INJURY

Fractures of the scaphoid have been interpreted as bone failures caused by compressive or tension loads.[160] Destot[48] attributed this injury to "the shape and function of the bone." He was the first to propose that the scaphoid breaks by bending or compression. He theorized that during a fall on the hand in dorsiflexion, the scaphoid becomes wedged "between the radius and the ground"; fractures occur "by exaggeration of its curve." He was able to reproduce scaphoid fractures by placing the hand in radial deviation and directing the force of injury to the thenar eminence. In 1918 Jeanne and Mouchet[93] suggested that the scaphoid may also fail by "opening of the angle" (that is, under tension loads), and could reproduce fractures experimentally by hyperpronation of the hand. Two years later, Todd[180] called this injury a "snapped waist" fracture, similar to the response of a sugar lump subjected to a tension load. Dickinson and Shannon[49] suggested that in falls on the hand in dorsiflexion the proximal scaphoid is fixed against the radius, and that all further stress takes place at the midcarpal level, causing the scaphoid to "snap." The location of the fracture within the scaphoid may vary according to the radial or ulnar deviation of the wrist at the time of injury, for in full radial deviation only the distal one third of the scaphoid is exposed, while in progressive ulnar deviation increasing portions of this bone become destabilized. In 1933 Hopkins[89] suggested that scaphoid fractures are produced by a mechanism similar to that found in Colles fractures: a fall on the dorsiflexed hand, usually in radial deviation, the loads being transmitted through the third metacarpal to the capitate, which causes an impingement of the narrow portion of the scaphoid against the radius. Frykman[65] subjected cadaver wrists to static loading and observed that the greater the dorsiflexion of the wrist, the larger the force required to produce a fracture, and the more distal the location of the injury. Thus, with the wrist dor-

siflexed 35 degrees of less, fractures of the forearm could be produced with loads lower than those required to produce a fracture of the distal radius, with dorsiflexion of 90 degrees or more, injury occurred to the carpal bones, and consistently to the scaphoid when radial deviation was added. Loads were greater than for fractures of the distal radius. Static intermediate loading with the wrist in 40 to 90 degrees dorsiflexion resulted in fractures of the distal radius. Coby and White[33] agreed that the scaphoid breaks because of compression rather than tension loads, and that compression is exerted against the concave surface of the scaphoid by the head of the capitate. Torsion or rotation have also been considered important,[61,72,93,158] both pronation and supination. An additional factor is the point of application of the floor reaction force at the time of impact.[48,176] This was confirmed experimentally by Weber and Chao[195] in fresh cadaver specimens. They demonstrated that for a fracture of the scaphoid to be consistently reproduced under experimental conditions, the load applied to the hand had to be concentrated on the radial half of the palm, with the wrist in 95 to 100 degrees of dorsiflexion. While the proximal half of the scaphoid is stabilized between radius, capitate, and volar capsular ligaments, bending loads are applied to the distal half, causing the fracture to occur between the supported and unsupported zones (Fig. 6-7).

TREATMENT

There is a considerable difference of opinion regarding treatment of the fractured scaphoid, from the length and position of immobilization, to the indications for surgery in the recent and old injuries, and the need for bone grafts and internal fixation. If any agreement is found in a review of the extensive literature on the subject, is that most fresh fractures of the scaphoid will heal if properly immobilized for a long enough period. This is in contrast to early opinions[48] that considered osseous consolidation exceptional, and pseudoarthrosis between fragments the rule, and advised against rigid immobilization.[114] For those fractures with "little displacement of the fragments" expectant treat-

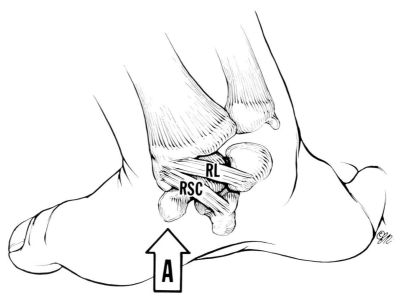

Fig. 6-7. Mechanism of fracture of the scaphoid according to Weber and Chao. Force applied to the radial half of the palm (arrow **A**) with the wrist in 95 to 100 degrees of dorsiflexion, produces bending loads to the unprotected distal half of the scaphoid. The proximal half is protected between the radius and the palmar radiocarpal ligaments (RL, radiolunate; RSC, radioscaphocapitate). (See Ref. 195.)

ment, consisting of massage, and "the limitation of active movements, but not passive" was advised.[114]

FRACTURES OF THE MIDDLE THIRD

This is the most common fracture of the scaphoid, comprising 62.7 to 87 percent of all scaphoid fractures.[37,49,56,140,155] Like most intraarticular injuries, it is notorious for a high percentage of slow or delayed unions or nonunions. This has been attributed to the action of synovial fluid[28,61,132,157] to the pattern of blood supply to the scaphoid[137,155,159,188] and the absence of periosteal healing.[42,95] There is, however, enough blood supply and endosteal callus to achieve union in 95 to 100 percent of fresh fractures, if properly treated.[16,54,56,103,108,111,134,153,159,160,164,171] Lützeler[111] demonstrated that smooth transverse fracture lines through the middle third of the scaphoid are subjected to mechanical "traction of the tight joint capsules and ligaments, even when the wrist joint is in the resting state, but even more so with movements." He agreed with previous reports stressing the value of complete immobilization in the treatment of this injury. A valid reason for the development of delayed or nonunion may be the lack of recognition of asssociated carpal instability once the obvious fracture is diagnosed.[62] In these cases the wrist is managed for the isolated scaphoid fracture, rather than for the most extensive carpal involvement. Loss of scaphoid support renders the carpus unstable.[62,72,100] The lunate assumes a dorsiflexed position, and the colinear radiolunocapitate alignment is lost. The resultant collapse deformity has been called "crumpling"[72] "concertina,"[62] or DISI (dorsal intercalated segment instability (Fig. 6-3)).[105] Less frequently a **VISI** (volar intercalated segment instability), pattern accompanies the fracture (Fig. 6-8).[105] This type of instability should be carefully evaluated, for it may actually represent a reduced transscaphoid perilunate fracture dislocation. The most consistent cause of nonunion, how-

Fig. 6-8. Displaced fracture of scaphoid accompanied by volar carpal instability (VISI). *A*: Original radiographs. (From Taleisnik J: Fractures of carpal bones. In Green DP (ed): Operative Hand Surgery. Vol. 1. Churchill Livingstone, New York, 1982.) *B*: Persistent VISI after the fracture healed.

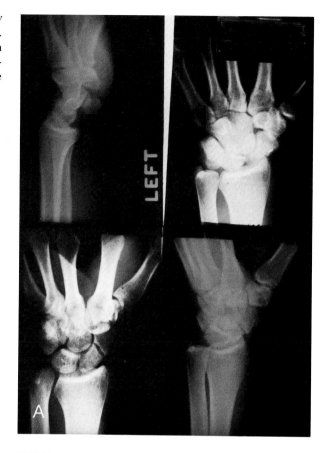

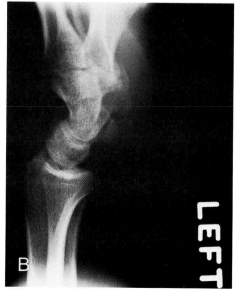

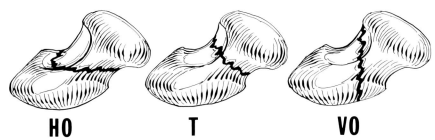

HO   **T**   **VO**

Fig. 6-9. Classification of fractures of the scaphoid (Russe). HO, horizontal oblique; T, transverse; VO, vertical oblique.

ever, continues to be the lack of recognition of the severity of the injury and, consequently, the delay in initiating proper treatment.

NONOPERATIVE TREATMENT

Scaphoid fractures may be classified into three types according to the relationship of the fracture line to the long axis of the scaphoid (Fig. 6-9).[17,155] The most frequent, *horizontal oblique* fractures, are oblique to the long axis of the scaphoid, but occur along a plane that is perpendicular to the longitudinal compressive forces acting across the wrist (Fig. 6-10A). These are the most stable, offer the best prognosis and are expected to heal in six to eight weeks. Next in frequency, the *transverse fractures*, are perpendicular to the long axis of the scaphoid, but slightly oblique in relationship to the longitudinal axis of the radiocapitate link (Fig. 6-10B). These fractures are subject to some shear, and should heal in six to twelve weeks, if properly immobilized. The rare *vertical oblique fractures* run almost parallel to the long axis of the forearm, have a high longitudinal shear component, are relatively unstable, and require longer immobilization (Fig. 6-10C).

Undisplaced fractures are stable, and, for the most part, free of problem. When the fracture is angulated, regardless of the direction of the fracture line, some degree of carpal instability should be suspected.[196] McLaughlin and Parkes[123] grouped scaphoid fractures into *Class A*, incomplete fractures that could be treated by splinting for just a few weeks, *Class B*, complete but stable fractures treatable in plaster casts for longer periods, and *Class C*, displaced or unstable fractures

requiring internal fixation. Cooney et al[38] further refined this treatment concept and suggested a management program similar to that proposed by Herbert[81] in 1974, based on a clinical assessment of fracture stability. Stable fractures are undisplaced. Unstable fractures showed an offset greater that 1 mm between the fragments or a lunocapitate angle greater than 15 degrees or a scapholunate angle greater than 45 degrees. According to these authors, acute stable fractures do well treated in short arm thumb spica casts with the wrist held in radial deviation and slight volarflexion. Unstable fractures are best treated in a long arm cast or by open reduction and internal fixation, if closed casting fails to provide a satisfactory reduction. Old stable nonunions may be treated by bone grafting. If unstable, internal fixation should be added to the bone graft.

There is now universal agreement that the vast majority of these fresh or acute fractures will heal if immobilized properly and for long enough, even in the presence of avascular changes.[16,54,56,108,133,134,151,152,159,163,164,171] The type and duration of immobilization are controversial. There is disagreement as to the position of the wrist in plaster, the need to immobilize joints other than the wrist in the casts, and the duration of immobilization. On a review of the literature regarding the position of immobilization, there is enough lack of uniformity to suggest that immobilization itself is important, rather than the position in which the limb is placed.[20] Accurate, prolonged immobilization should be attained, either by skin-tight plaster casts that are changed repeatedly or by the use of the newer, resined fiberglass material.[6] The need for rigid immobilization was stressed by Farquharson[59] who proposed a special metal palmar splint attached to an above-the-wrist forearm cast for the treatment of this injury. It is important to allow the hand to function, for this seems to enhance the healing potential and reduce the degree of atrophy. In my opinion, the best position of the wrist is that which allows anatomic coaptation in radiographs taken after the plaster is applied. This position usually includes some radial deviation, either neutralflexion or slight volarflexion and pronation. When a DISI pattern is present, correction of the lunate dorsiflexion should be attempted by full radial deviation of the wrist.[196]

Regarding immobilization of joints other than the wrist, and in spite of reports to the contrary,[92] I believe that there is nothing to be lost, and much to be gained by inclusion of the proximal joint of the thumb in the cast. The distal joint is left free and within range of the fingers to allow for prehension. The scaphoid is functionally related to the thumb; its immobilization effectively eliminates any potential disruptive action particularly from the abductor pollicis longus[171] and brevis.[163,164] The inclusion of the elbow in the scaphoid has also been suggested. Verdan[186] placed great emphasis on eliminating the action of the volar radiocarpal ligament on the scaphoid during pronation and supination,[188] despite Stewart's report[171] (also in 1954) of 436 fractures treated in the U.S. Army Medical Corps in a short arm thumb spica cast with a union rate approaching 95 percent. The benefit from immobilization in a long arm cast was further suggested by an independent study from Borås, Sweden. The results of treatment with short and long arm casts in comparable series of scaphoid fractures were evaluated, showing a statistically significant reduction in the time needed for fracture healing when immobilization included the elbow.[22] I believe that elbow immobilization is important and that a long arm thumb spica circular plaster dressing is ideal for the initial six weeks of treatment, followed by the application of a short-arm, thumb-spica circular plaster dressing. Recovery of motion in all uninvolved joints is very prompt following removal of the cast, and even wrist motion can return to near normal in one to five weeks.[16,56,171] If there is a strenuous objection from the patient, or a contraindication to elbow immobilization for this prolonged period, an epicondylar bearing cast may be fashioned to restrict pronation and supination, while allowing some degree of elbow flexion and extension.[125]

Immobilization of the fingers was first proposed by Bürkle-de-la-Camp (cited by Rehbein[149,150]), who used a short arm cast including the proximal joints of the index and long fingers. Nitsche, also quoted by Rehbein, immobilized the thumb in addition to the index and long fingers. Rehbein himself first suggested that the thumb and all fingers be included, from elbow to fingertips. Nenninger[136] and Düben and Gelbke[53] reported excellent results using Rehbein's "fist cast." I have had limited experience with this type of immobilization, and abandoned it altogether because of patient dissatisfaction, mostly secondary to poor hygiene. In my opinion, the three-digit cast[47] is less objectionable. It should be reserved for the potentially unstable scaphoid fractures in good alignment and for the postoperative care of the unstable nonunion during the initial or vascular period of fracture healing (Fig. 6-11).

The duration of immobilization was rather brief in early reports on the treatment of fractures of the scaphoid.[48,111] As experience accumulated, it became clear that longer periods of immobilization for fresh fractures produced higher percentages of union. Plaster immobilization may also be used for the treatment of previously untreated or poorly managed ununited fractures in the absence of carpal collapse or fracture displacement. In 1938 Moore[128] reported a three-year-old untreated, ununited fracture of the scaphoid, in a heavy laborer, which went on to heal after six months immobilization in a molded leather-covered aluminum volar splint. He emphasized the importance of hand use during immobilization. Luxardo[112] reported a 15 month old nonunion which healed after 210 days in a cast. Speed[165] concluded that some ancient fractures may indeed yield to prolonged immobilization, as shown by Rehbein and Düben, who report healing of ununited fractures as old as five years using ther fist cast. The immobilization time is frequently longer than for fresh fractures[103] and may be shortened by the application of pulsing electromagnetic field treatment (Fig. 6-12).[66] In 1960, however, Russe[155] stated that "since the period of immobilization may, in some cases, require many months, operative treatment by an experienced surgeon may be considered preferable."

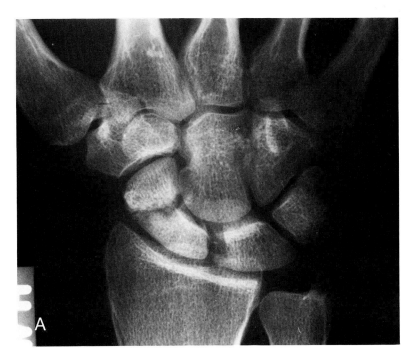

Fig. 6-10. Fractures of the scaphoid. *A:* Horizontal oblique. *B:* Transverse.

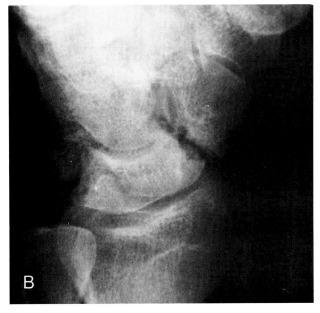

OPERATIVE TREATMENT

Fresh displaced fractures imply a more severe ligamentous damage.[196] With few exceptions[190] there is agreement that these displaced fractures are best treated by open reduction and internal fixation with Kirschner wires or screws (Fig. 6-13).[61,63,81,82,105,118,123,182,188] Most surgical procedures, however, have been devised for ununited fractures. Frustration with the management of this problem injury produced some unusual forms of treatment. For instance, injection into the fracture

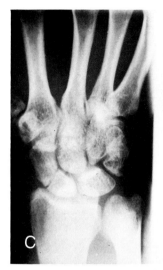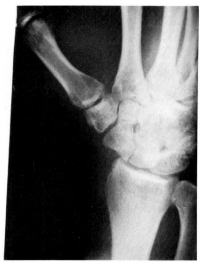

Fig. 6-10 (cont.)   C: Vertical oblique.

of "germinal tissue" from extracts of bone was suggested in 1937 in order to stimulate new bone formation.[87] For many years surgical ablation of the scaphoid was the only procedure recommended for nonunions.

Many patients with ununited scaphoids may not require any treatment, for they can remain essentially symptom-free.[20,49,98,107,120,121,156] This is the case with stable fractures, when there is no associated carpal collapse (Fig. 6-14). Not infrequently, these injuries are surprising findings following minor trauma and respond well to a brief period of splinting, returning to their previous, nondisabling state. Furthermore, there is no clear-cut evidence to suggest that the incidence of post-traumatic arthrosis is increased in these patients. Prolonged immobilization has been shown to produce a reversal of the nonunion process in a high percentage of patients.[112,150,171] However, this would currently seem to be a rather radical approach. Therefore, the potential for economic hardship caused to young adults by prolonged immobilization and the availability of more reliably successful surgical techniques have been justification for many authors to also recommend surgery for older, ununited fractures as well as more recent fractures that remain symptomatic and fail to unite after three to four months of adequate nonsurgical treatment.[20,25,33,37,45,51,57,85,123,182,184] Surgery is a reasonable alternative and a rather conservative

approach to the management of this injury under those circumstances. There is little justification for immobilization to continue beyond three to four months in the presence of a symptomatic scaphoid fracture that has not been treated previously. When nonunion is accompanied by periscaphoid degenerative changes, replacement of the scaphoid with silicone implants, partial and total wrist fusions or proximal row carpectomies may be indicated.

In summary, surgical treatment is indicated for all painful delayed unions and nonunions that have failed to heal or become symptom free after a reasonable trial of adequate immobilization, regardless of the presence of degenerative, avascular, or cystic changes. In their evaluation of treatment of nonunions of the scaphoid, the Pennsylvania Orthopaedic Society[140] concluded that "no one method of treatment can be used for types of disability caused by an ununited fracture of the carpal navicular." It was further stated that "a well stocked surgical armamentarium ready for any contingency does exist." The choice of procedure will vary with the surgeon's preference and experience, the type of fracture, the patient's age, the presence of carpal instability or avascular changes of the scaphoid, and the degree and location of periscaphoid arthrosis. Following is a discussion of frequently used surgical techniques for the treatment of nonunions of the middle third of the scaph-

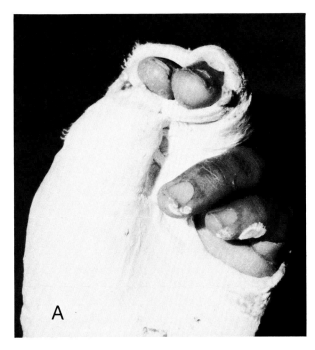

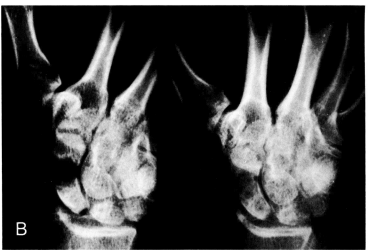

Fig. 6-11. A: For very unstable fractures and after re-operations, a three-digit cast is preferred for the initial postoperative immobilization. *B*: Preoperative (left) and postoperative radiographs (right). (*B* from Taleisnik J: Fractures of the carpal bones. In Green DP (ed): Operative Hand Surgery. Vol. 1. Churchill Livingstone, New York, 1982.)

oid. Procedures no longer in use[10] will not be discussed.

Bone Graft

Bone grafts for the scaphoid were first advocated by Adams[1] in 1928. He used an autogenous graft carefully slotted across the fracture. In 1934 Murray[133] presented his initial satisfactory results with tibial bone pegs inserted into holes drilled across the fracture. Burnett's[25,26] experience was similar. In 1946 Murray[134] reviewed 100 operations using his technique and reported a union rate of 96 percent. A simple, mostly cortical, graft was preferred because it combined the advantages of drilling,[10] with the osteogenic properties of the graft and the internal fixation effect of the bone pegs. Similar satisfactory results were published by others.[139,181] Cobey[33] reported on the use of a triple-peg bone graft obtained from the radius, rather than the tibia.

In 1929 Matti[116] first published his experience with "autoplastically transplanted spongy tissue as 'bone mortar' for the filling up of bone defects of any kind." In 1937 Matti[117] reported on the use of spongiosa (cancellous) bone grafts obtained from the greater trochanter for the treatment of nonunions of the scaphoid and patella. He showed that healing can be achieved by cancellous bone chips packed into the excavated scaphoid fracture site through a dorsal approach. In spite of Cole and Williamson's[34] admonition that bone grafting "will never be a successful method of choice for routine procedure and is mainly a surgical stunt," Matti's technique proved quite successful. It was later modified by Russe,[154] who proposed a volar approach to fill an egg-shaped cavity created within the scaphoid and across the fracture site with a cancellous bone plug and additional cancellous bone chips. Most recent publications favor Russe's anterior approach,[43,51,54,56,62,84,123,130,182,184,188] although the shape of the graft, its donor site, and the bone grafting technique itself have not been consistent among different authors. Russe's original procedure is effective even in those ununited scaphoids with volar angulation. Fisk[62] observed that in these cases, a wedge-shaped defect is present anteriorly, which responds well to an anterior or volar bone graft. This technique is indicated for all symptomatic established nonunions, symptomatic delayed unions after unsuccessful casting, and fresh fractures that require immobilization beyond three to four months. Cystic and avascular changes are not contraindications.[130] The avascular appearance of the proximal fragment actually recedes after union occurs.[38] Periscaphoid arthrosis[49] is a contraindication to the use of this technique.

Bone Graft Technique (Russe) (Fig. 6-15).[155] A 4- to 5-cm longitudinal incision is made along the radial border of the flexor carpi radialis tendon, centered at a level even with the tip of the radial styloid, which usually corresponds to the level of the fracture itself. The capsule is divided longitudinally, and the underlying deep volar radiocarpal ligaments are either divided partially and retracted or completely severed and tagged for later suture. An egg-shaped cavity is created well into both fracture fragments without using power tools. Care is taken to hinge this cavity on the dorsal cortex, which is visualized through the defect and carefully coapted before insertion of the bone graft. A strictly cancellous bone graft is then obtained from the ipsilateral iliac crest and fashioned into an ovoid plug large enough to fit snugly into the scaphoid cavity. The graft is actually jammed into both fragments, as these are forcibly distracted by traction and angulation of the fragments. Coaptation of the dorsal surfaces can still be checked on both sides of the inserted graft. The gaps surrounding the cancellous plug are then filled with cancellous bone chips. Once the cavity is full, both fragments and the graft itself are further impacted manually to produce a satisfactory degree of stability. Stability is checked and the wrist is taken through a full range of motion. If the scaphoid's mechanical behavior as a unit has been restored, no further fixation is utilized. Internal fixation is reserved for only those cases when instability persists after the bone graft is in place (Fig. 6-16). A pair of Kirschner wires are preferred for this purpose, carefully inserted parallel to each other and to the longitudinal axis of the scaphoid. For those fractures with severe resorption of the palmar-scaphoid, palmarflexion of the distal fragment and evidence of dorsal carpal instability in lateral radiographs, realignment of the fracture fragments produces a large palmar defect. For these patients, a wedge-shape corticocancellous bone graft is preferred, accompanied by internal fixation (Figs. 6-17, 6-18). The volar radiocarpal ligaments are repaired, and the hand and wrist are immobilized in a compression-type dressing incorporated into a long arm circular plaster cast. This cast is changed to a long arm thumb spica cast at six weeks postoperatively. In those cases when the fracture is very unstable, or after reoperation, I prefer to use a three-digit cast with the thumb in opposition and the index and long fingers in an intrinsic-plus position (Fig. 6-11). After three postoperative weeks, a long arm thumb spica cast is applied, followed by a short arm thumb spica cast at six weeks. The total immobilization time for this procedure has averaged 12 to 14 weeks in my experience. Union in ≥90 percent of patients can be expected.

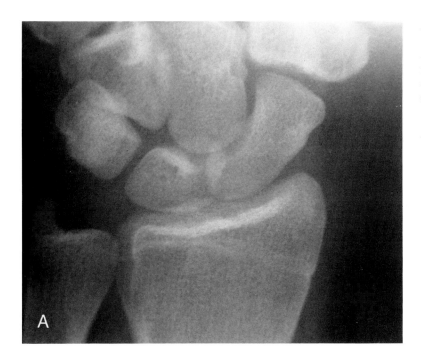

Fig. 6-12. Nonunion of fracture of the scaphoid treated with immobilization and the application of pulsing electromagnetic field treatment. *A*: Initial radiograph. *B* and *C*: After six months immobilization.

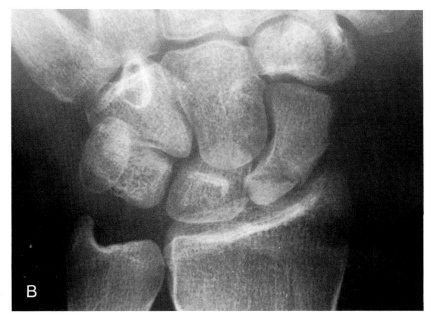

Osteosynthesis

Internal fixation of scaphoid fractures with screws, Kirschner wires or staples[191] is indicated following the treatment of transscaphoid perilunate fracture-dislocations, and for those fractures accompanied by more subtle forms of carpal insta-

bility.[62,68,118] Screw fixation was proposed by Maatz[113] in 1943, Buhlmann[24] in 1948, and McLaughlin[122] in 1954, and again more recently by several other authors.[62,78,81,82,118,144] The technique of screw osteosynthesis should be precise and meticulous to avoid unwanted complications,

Fig. 6-12 (cont.) D: Localizer radiograph for the application of pulsing electromagnetic field treatment.

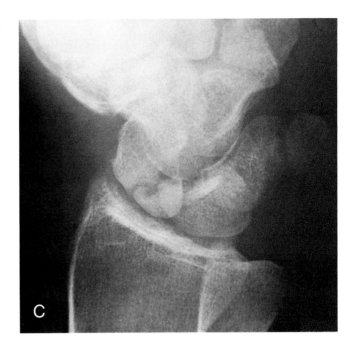

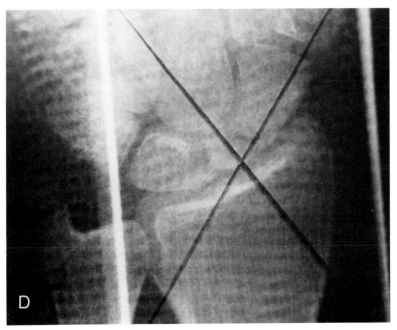

such as delayed union or nonunion perpetrated by poor screw insertion. Such fixation frequently requires a radial styloidectomy to facilitate exposure and may need special instrumentation. With the exception of the Herbert screw,[82] a second operative procedure is required for the removal of the screw (Fig. 6-19). Screw fixation is usually reserved for those scaphoids with fractures through the middle third, without comminution, and provided the proximal fragment does not show evidence of avascular changes.[24,68] Results may not be consistently reliable, if one is to judge by the ASIF

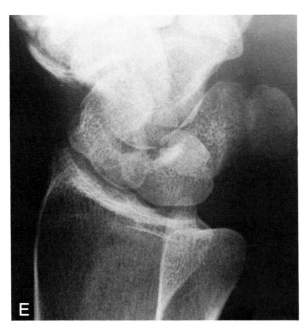

Fig. 6-12 (cont.) E: Four months later, the fracture is healed.

experience[78]: three of four screw fixations for delayed unions, and 3 of 22 used for primary osteosynthesis required a subsequent bone graft to achieve union. A similar discouraging experience was published by Koob et al.[99] At times, a satisfactory result may be seen with screw fixation even if nonunion persists, probably because of the increased stability produced by the insertion of the screw (Fig. 6-20).[118]

The use of Kirschner nails to immobilize fractures of the scaphoid was first proposed by Geissendörfer.[69,70] Prior to this, "wiring" of scaphoid fragments was thought to be highly impractical.[114] Kirschner wires, in my opinion, are easier to insert and remove, do not require a radial styloidectomy to facilitate exposure, and provide satisfactory stability. They can be used in the presence of avascular changes of the proximal fragment, when screws are formally contraindicated, and may actually be the only form of fixation possible in those comminuted fractures most in need of internal support. For the open reduction and internal fixation of the complex transscaphoid perilunate fracture dislocation, a longitudinal dorsal approach to the wrist is preferred. Displaced recent fractures of the scaph-

oid can be satisfactorily exposed using a lazy-S incision along the long axis of the anatomic snuffbox. The serrated edges of the fracture can be carefully coapted, and at least two Kirschner wires are introduced from distal to proximal across the fracture plane, and along the longitudinal axis of the scaphoid. The Kirschner wires should not cross the radiocarpal joint, if at all possible. This would provide a safety valve for the dissipation of stress exerted against those other joints that are rigidly fixed. Bone grafts may be used in conjunction with any type of internal fixation.

Scaphoid Arthroplasties

All reports of fractures of the scaphoid published shortly after the turn of this century and into the 1930s, stress that the prognosis for this injury was very poor. For this reason, excision of the scaphoid was recommended. Kaufman was the first to remove the entire scaphoid, a procedure reported in 1902 (quoted by Codman and Chase).[35] Codman and Chase[35] in 1905 and MacLennan[114] in 1911 recommended excision of one or preferably both fragments of the scaphoid as the treatment of choice. Codman and Chase reserved excision for the nonunited fractures but were among the first to realize that in acute injury it is possible to obtain union by immobilization.[34,35] They stressed, however, that when treatment is delayed as little as three weeks, the fracture would tend to go into nonunion. A few decades later Böhler[16] demonstrated conclusively that fractures of the scaphoid do unite, with excellent functional results, provided the fracture fragments are reduced and held in a plaster cast until healed. In addition, Böhler condemned excision of the scaphoid as an "absurd operation," leading to deformity and weakness. In 1935 Hirsch[86] attributed Böhler's poor results to errors in technique rather than to the procedure itself, and continued to favor complete excision because this allowed patients to return to work sooner. The earlier the surgery the better the results, prompting Hirsch to recommend that the procedure be done "preferably initially" following injury, rather than for nonunions alone. Periscaphoid arthritis was considered a contraindication. In spite of Hirsch's opinion, excision of the scaphoid

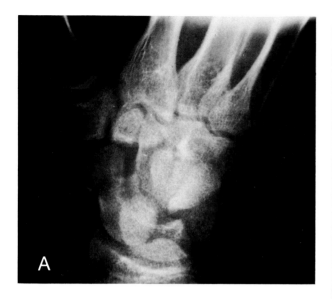

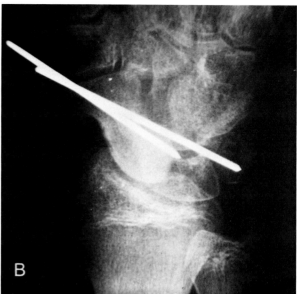

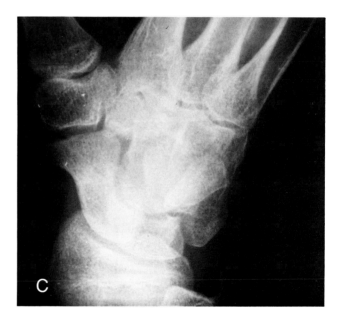

Fig. 6-13. *A*: Displaced horizontal oblique fracture of the scaphoid. *B*: The same fracture 6 weeks following open reduction and internal fixation with Kirschner wires. *C*: Follow-up radiograph at three months. The fracture is healed. (From Taleisnik J: Fractures of the carpal bones. In Green DP (ed): Operative Hand Surgery. Vol. 1. Churchill Livingstone, New York, 1982.)

for the treatment of fresh fractures was largely abandoned after Böhler's publications. It continued to be the surgical treatment of choice, however, for nonunions or old fractures with "malacia of the scaphoid.[129] After bone grafting procedures became popular and proved successful, excision of the scaphoid fragments rapidly lost popularity,[16,17,139,153,164,169,172,179,183,189] although it was still proposed as a viable surgical alternative as re-

cently as 1949,[55] particularly for comminuted fractures,[29,44,156] and after complete dislocation of the scaphoid.[80] Although excision of the entire distal fragment alone has been reported,[52] most advocates of this technique have emphasized complete and early removal of all scaphoid fragments without damaging surrounding bony articular surfaces. The main criticism of this procedure was the disruption it could create in the function of the rest

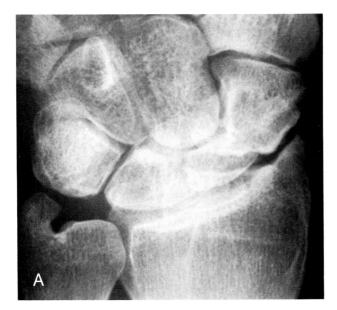

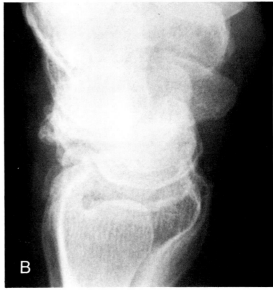

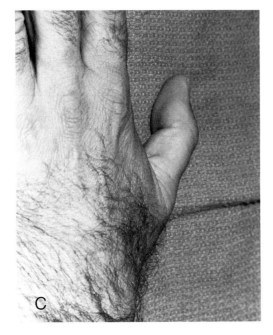

Fig. 6-14. Asymptomatic nonunion of a fracture of the scaphoid (*A* and *B*). The patient was examined and his wrist radiographed after the sudden loss of extension to his thumb *(C)*.

of the carpus. In an attempt to preserve wrist architecture, prosthetic replacements were proposed, made with vitallium,[101,126] acrylic,[2,4,147] or Teflon.[135] In 1974 Barber[7] published a follow-up on the use of acrylic replacements, and noted that in spite of acceptable clinical results, scaphoid replacement alone had not, for the most part, been effective in preserving the normal anatomy of the remaining carpus.

In 1970 Swanson[173] presented his initial experience using a silicone rubber implant, anatomically shaped and sized to specifications based on the morphologic study of numerous cadaver specimens, and on roentgenographic evaluations of mul-

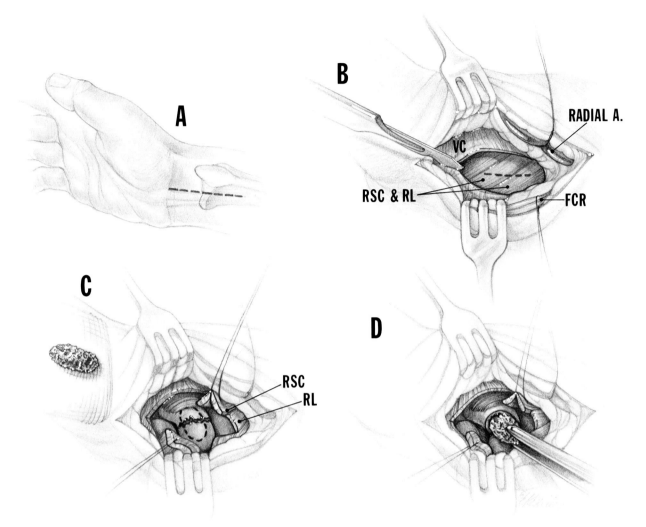

Fig. 6-15. Bone graft technique (Russe). *A*: Incision. *B*: Exposure. *C*: Division of radioscaphocapitate (RSC) and radiolunate (RL) ligaments. *D*: A cancellous bone graft is used to fill a cavity carved within the scaphoid.

tiple wrists.[173,174] For initial stabilization, the implant was designed with a stem arising from the distal pole, for insertion into the trapezium. Long term support relies on implant encapsulation. Further initial fixation by sutures or Kirschner wires, without fragmentation of the implant, became possible after High Performance Silicone Elastomer° was developed,[175] thus reducing the potential for reactive particulate synovitis. Scaphoid replacement arthroplasties are indicated for those patients

with or without nonunion, but with extensive arthrosis strictly limited to the periscaphoid joints, provided carpal alignment is satisfactory (Fig. 6-21). Herndon and collaborators[83] reported a long-term evaluation of 607 cases of lunate and scaphoid arthroplasties. The main complication was related to subluxation of the implant. These authors stressed the importance of good carpal stability in achieving a satisfactory, long-lasting result. Therefore, when carpal collapse is present, provisions should be made during surgery for a load-bearing column to transmit forces across the wrist directly to the radius, bypassing the implant.

(Text continues on page 130.)

°Dow Corning, Midland, Michigan.

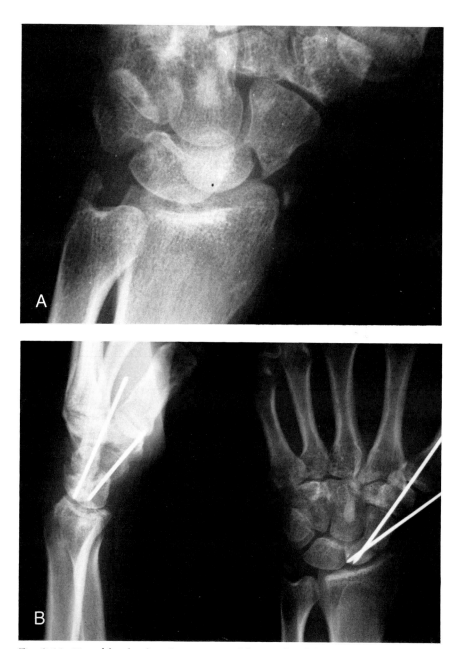

Fig. 6-16. Unstable, displaced nonunion of the scaphoid *(A)* required bone grafting and internal fixation for stabilization *(B)*.

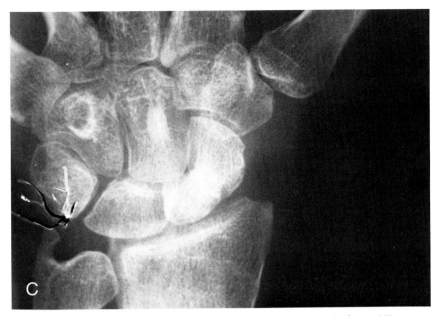

Fig. 6-16 (cont.) Appearance of fracture four months later *(C)*.

Fig. 6-17. A: Schematic representation of normal alignment between scaphoid (S) lunate (L) and capitate (C). *B:* Nonunion of a fracture of the scaphoid with palmar flexion of the distal fragment, and a dorsal intercalated carpal instability (DISI) pattern. *C:* The scaphoid alignment is corrected. *D:* It is maintained by the insertion of a palmar wedge-shaped bone graft.

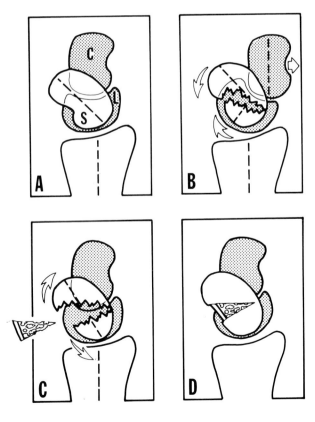

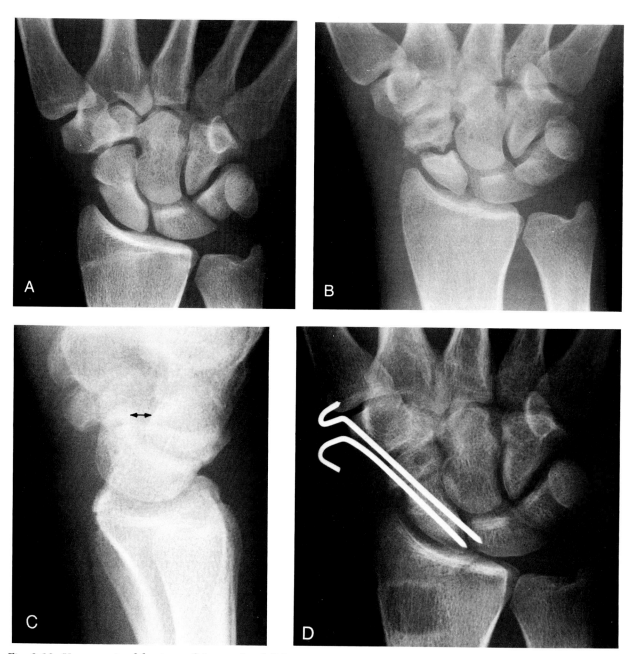

Fig. 6-18. Unrecognized fracture of the scaphoid *(A)* progressing to nonunion *(B)* with DISI *(C:* arrow). Immediate postoperative radiograph shows wedge-shaped bone graft and internal fixation with Kirschner wires *(D).*

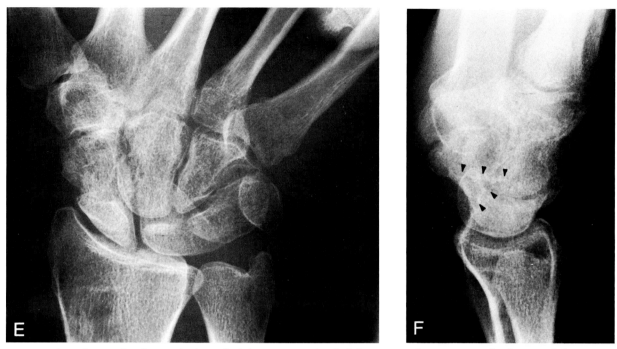

Fig. 6-18 (cont.)   Final radiographs (*E* and *F*) demonstrate healed fracture and restoration of radiocarpal alignment. Outline of bone graft is highlighted in *F*.

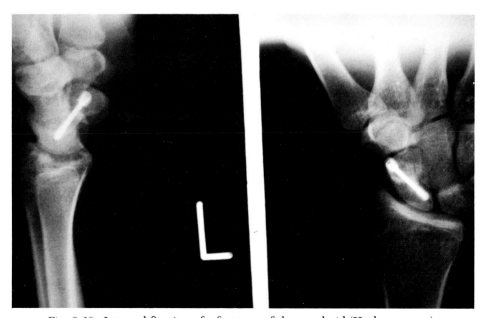

Fig. 6-19. Internal fixation of a fracture of the scaphoid (Herbert screw).

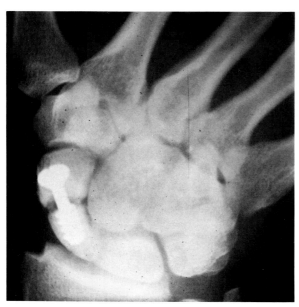

Fig. 6-20. Persistent but asymptomatic nonunion of a fracture of the scaphoid, following internal fixation with a screw.

This can be accomplished by supplementing scaphoid excision and its replacement with a limited arthrodesis performed across the midcarpal joint (Fig. 6-22).[193]

Scaphoid Implant Technique (Swanson) (Fig. 6-23). An oblique incision on the dorsoradial aspect of the wrist is preferred. It is traced immediately ulnar to Lister's tubercle, and is directed proximally and medially. Its distal end may be prolonged transversely and radially for better exposure of the scaphotrapezium-trapezoid joint. Cutaneous branches from the radial nerve should be isolated and protected. The radial artery may have to be mobilized to allow full access to the distal scaphoid and the scaphotrapezial joint. The extensor pollicis longus tendon, which crosses the area diagonally, is unroofed and retracted radialward. At this point, one may follow one of two approaches. The extensor carpi radialis longus and brevis tendons may be mobilized and retracted radialward and the capsule may be detached from the dorsal rim of the radius, dissected distally and carefully preserved. My preference, however, is to incise the floor of the extensor pollicis longus tendon tunnel longitudinally, and elevate both capsular flaps from the underlying carpus, and subperiosteally from the radius, without disturbing the extensor tendon compartments. The scaphoid is removed. A thin wafer of distal pole may be preserved to provide a buttress for the implant against the palmar capsule (Figs. 6-21, 6-22, 6-23, 6-24). Different implant sizes and designs are available for preliminary fitting. If a midcarpal fusion is required, it is completed at this point, prior to the insertion of the implant. A hole is then drilled into the scaphoid surface of the trapezium along the direction of the stem in the implant. A smaller trial size may be used to accurately place the drill-hole on the surface of the trapezium. The implant itself must be thoroughly washed prior to insertion, and should be handled with instruments, rather than with gloved fingers. Further fixation may be obtained by tying the proximal pole to the lunate by means of a synthetic absorbable suture, passed through a small drill-hole in the lunate, and through the proximal pole of the implant itself. A fine Kirschner wire may be used instead. The dorsal capsule, whether divided transversely or longitudinally, must be carefully repaired and reattached to the dorsal rim of the radius, using nonabsorbable sutures passed through drill-holes in the radius if necessary. The extensor pollicis longus tendon may be left outside its tunnel and the extensor retinaculum repaired deep to the tendon. Initial postoperative immobilization is provided in a voluminous compression dressing reinforced with plaster splints. This is usually removed at four to six days postoperatively, at which time roentgenograms may be obtained. A short arm thumb spica is then applied and worn for a total postoperative immobilization period of five to six weeks. Gradual motion is then allowed. Protection with a removable splint may be continued intermittently for an additional two- to three-week period, or until satisfactory function is regained. All splinting is usually discontinued after nine weeks. When a simultaneous midcarpal fusion was performed, postoperative immobilization in a long arm plaster circular cast is required for at least four weeks followed by a short arm thumb spica for an additional four-week period.

Proximal Row Carpectomy. Proximal row carpectomy has not been a popular procedure, in spite of favorable reports.[90] There is uncertainty as to

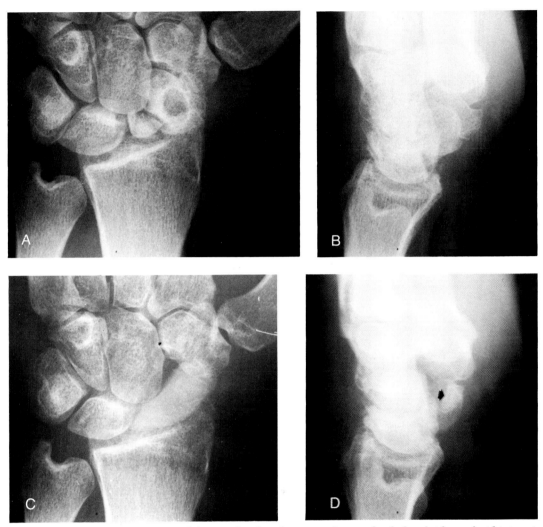

Fig. 6-21. Nonunion of fracture of the scaphoid with osteoarthritis of radial styloid-scaphoid joint. *A:* Posteroanterior view. *B:* Lateral view shows satisfactory radiocarpal alignment. *C:* Posteroanterior view after excision of scaphoid and insertion of implant. *D:* Postoperative view. Radiocarpal alignment is satisfactory. Arrow points to thin wafer of distal pole of scaphoid left in situ as a buttress for the implant.

the long-term result. The postoperative recovery until a stable condition is reached is rather prolonged and the residual weakness of grip may be of concern. This procedure may be used for the treatment of the ununited fracture of the scaphoid. Although Hill[85] finds it indicated in older patients with a symptomatic nonunion who do not wish to accept a long period of immobilization, others[41,90,96] have used this treatment with very good functional and clinical results, even in younger, active, heavy workers. Proximal row carpectomies may be preferable to fusions in some cases when motion is required or desired by the patient, even at the expense of grip strength. It is contra-indicated in the presence of radiocarpal arthrosis.

Technique of Proximal Row Carpectomy. For proximal carpectomies done in traumatic cases, a transverse dorsal skin incision is preferred along the radiocarpal joint projected immediately distal

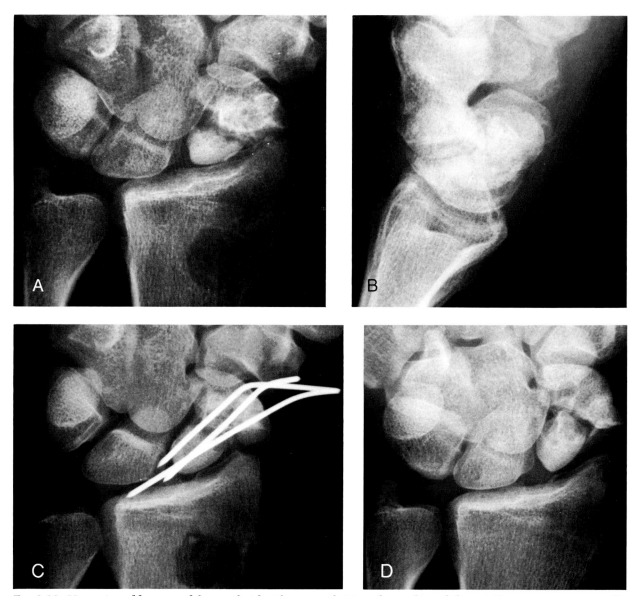

Fig. 6-22. Nonunion of fracture of the scaphoid with osteoarthritis and carpal instability. *A*: Posteroanterior view. *B*: Lateral view shows a dorsal carpal instability patter (DISI). *C*: Immediate postoperative appearance following insertion of a palmar wedge-graft and internal fixation. *D* and *E*: persistent nonunion.

to Lister's tubercle (Fig. 6-25). A longitudinal incision, however, can be used when additional procedures are planned, for example, tendon transfers and synovectomy in the rheumatoid patient. The dorsal retinacular ligament is exposed, and the cutaneous branches of the radial and ulnar nerves are identified and retracted. The dorsal retinaculum is incised over the extensor pollicis longus tunnel. This tendon is unroofed, lifted, and retracted. The retinacular system separating this third dorsal wrist compartment from the extensor indicis proprius and the extensor digitorum communis tendons is incised, and the entire dorsal retinaculum is reflected ulnarward together with the contents of the

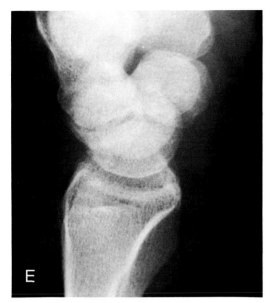
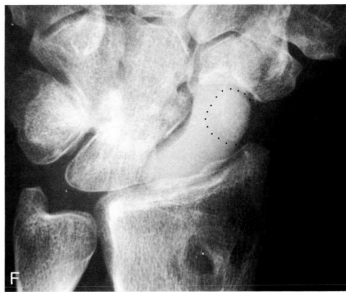

Fig. 6-22 (cont.)　*F*: Final appearance following excision of scaphoid, insertion of implant and midcarpal fusion. Dots delineate wafer of distal pole of scaphoid left behind to support the implant.

fourth dorsal extensor compartment. The entire lunate and triquetrum are removed, usually in this order. The scaphoid can be excised in its entirety, although the distal one third may be left attached to the trapezium and the trapezoid for additional support to the thumb ray, particularly in the wrist with rheumatoid arthritis. The proximal pole of the capitate is seated into the lunate concavity of the radius (Fig. 6-26); if stability is questionable a temporary Kirschner wire is used for three to four weeks to maintain this position. I routinely divide the posterior interosseous nerve since this has been implicated as a possible cause of postoperative pain. The nerve can be found lying beneath the deep fascial layer, on the interosseous membrane along the ulnar border of the radius. It is divided at least 1 inch proximal to the articular surface of the radius. The pisiform is not excised. Closure is performed in layers. Postoperatively, immediate immobilization is provided in a bulky compression dressing enclosed in plaster. At four to six days postoperatively this is replaced by a short arm circular plaster cast that is worn for a total postoperative immobilization of four to six weeks. Full strong flexion and extension of all fingers and thumb are encouraged while in plaster. At the end of this pe-

riod, gradual motion is allowed, while intermittent protection is provided by a removable splint, worn for two to four weeks, or until the patient is capable of free use of his wrist.

Partial Arthrodesis

In 1946 Sutro[172] proposed to treat nonunions of the scaphoid by arthrodesing both fragments to the capitate. He recommended the procedure for those cases with extensive resorption or sclerosis of one or both fragments, or in the presence of degenerative changes between scaphoid and capitate. Helfet[79] resurrected Sutro's procedure in 1952. He emphasized that this operation was indicated for scaphoid nonunions before the development of radiocarpal arthrosis. In 1961 Gordon and King[75] reported seven patients treated by partial wrist arthrodesis. In four of these, radioscapholunate fusions were performed for nonunions of the scaphoid with satisfactory results: relief of pain, restoration of strength and stability, and an average range of flexion-extension of 42 degrees, and of radial-ulnar deviation of 30 degrees. The fourth edition of Watson-Jones' treatise *Fractures and Joint Injuries*,[194] contains a similar example of radioscapho-

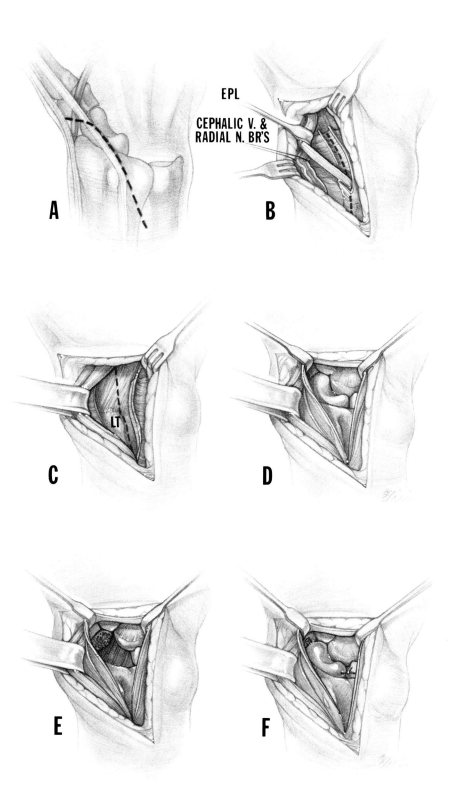

Fig. 6-23. Scaphoid implant technique. *A:* Incision. *B:* The extensor pollicis longus tendon (EPL) is lifted from its tunnel and is retracted radially. Interrupted line shows incision along the floor of the EPL tendon tunnel. *C:* Distal radius and dorsal capsule exposed. LT, Lister's tubercle. *D:* Scaphoid exposed. Carpal bones surrounding the scaphoid should be visualized. *E:* Appearance after excision of the scaphoid. A thin wafer of distal pole is left behind to maintain the integrity of the palmar capsule and support the implant. *F:* Implant inserted.

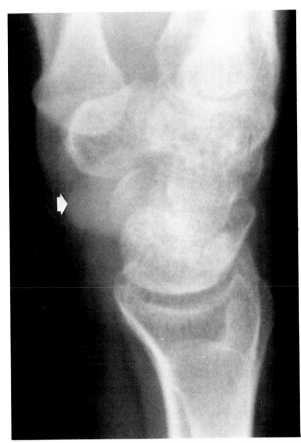

Fig. 6-24. Lateral radiograph after scaphoid silastic implant arthoplasty (arrow: distal pole of scaphoid).

lunate fusion (omitted from the fifth edition published in 1976[197]). Peterson and Lipscomb[143] utilized yet another type of limited arthrodesis for nonunions of the scaphoid, fusing the scaphoid to the lunate, across the proximal, avascular scaphoid fragment, in the belief that blood supply could then reach the smaller proximal fragment from two sources. In 1966 Graner and coauthors[76] published a series of partial fusions used for the treatment of a variety of wrist conditions. Six of their patients were treated for nonunion of the scaphoid by arthrodesis across the midcarpal joint, usually to include at least the scaphoid, lunate, capitate, and hamate, leaving the radiocarpal joint undisturbed. In these six patients, postoperative volarflexion range averaged 25 degrees, and dorsiflexion 31 degrees.

Watson[192] pointed out that patterns of motion in the normal wrist no longer apply to wrists following limited arthrodesis. New patterns are created, and for several months following surgery, adaptation through use maximizes the function of the residual joints, to eventually achieve greater motion. The optimal example may be found in congenital fusions, which are asymptomatic, cause minimal limitation of motion, and frequently are incidental findings in roentgenographs taken following injuries or for comparison purposes.

In my opinion, most nonunions of the scaphoid are amenable to satisfactory treatment using techniques other than limited arthrodesis. These procedures are indicated, however, in some circumstances. They are useful for the exceptional long-standing nonunions, particularly after a failed bone graft procedure, in a heavy laborer, or for the young and active. A partial arthrodesis may offer relief of pain and restoration of stability, with preservation of some useful wrist motion. In these patients there is usually collapse of the scaphoid or resorption of the fracture fragments, and arthrosis involving a variable extension of the scaphocapitate joint. A scaphocapitate fusion, as advocated by Sutro,[172] will be helpful. A second indication for limited arthrodesis for nonunion presents when a scaphoid implant is inserted in a wrist with a collapse deformity (Fig. 6-22). Together with the insertion of the implant, alignment should be restored and maintained by a fusion across the midcarpal joint. This provides a load-bearing column for the transmission of forces from the hand to the radius. A third indication for limited arthrodesis is found after the nonunion has healed, when late degenerative changes produce disabling pain. Here again, a very careful evaluation of actual joint involvement should be made preoperatively to include in the fusion mass only those joints with actual or potential arthrosis.

Technique of Limited Arthrodesis (Watson). A transverse skin incision is usually used. This is placed over the projection of the joint to be fused. Superficial nerves are protected. The extensor retinaculum is exposed and divided longitudinally and the underlying tendons are retracted to either side to expose the capsule overlying the degenerative joint. Once the capsule is divided the joint is exposed and the surfaces to be fused are individual-

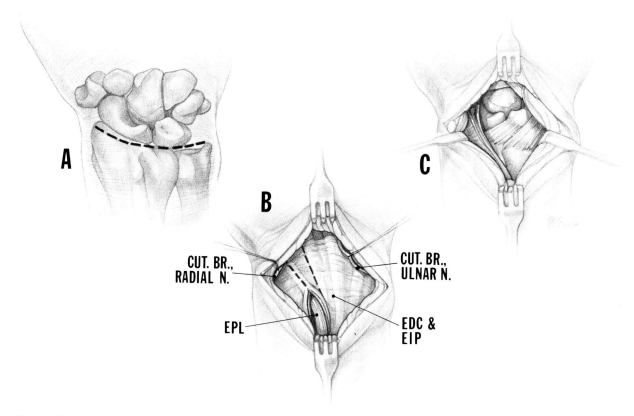

Fig. 6-25. Dorsal approach to the wrist using a transverse incision. *A:* Incision. *B:* The extensor pollicis longus tendon is exposed (**EPL**); **EDC**, extensor digitorum communis; **EIP**, extensor indicis proprius, *C:* Subcapsular and subperiosteal exposure of the joint through longitudinal retinacular and capsular incision between third and fourth dorsal extensor compartments.

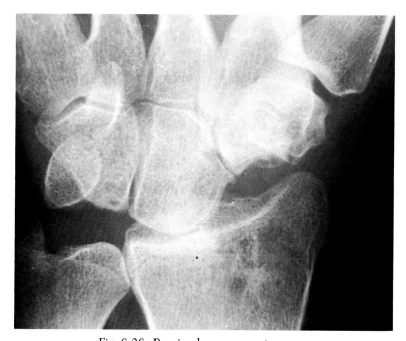

Fig. 6-26. Proximal row carpectomy.

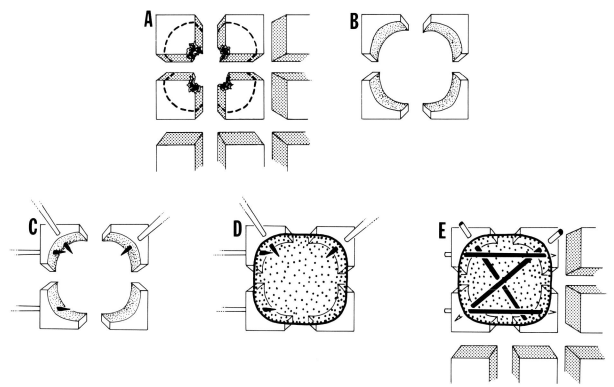

Fig. 6-27. Diagrammatic representation of principles and technique of limited intercarpal arthrodesis. *A*: Articular surfaces are excised down to healthy cancellous bone. *B*: Carpal segments to be fused are not compressed, in order to preserve overall dimension and outer shape of fused unit. *C*: Kirschner wires are introduced until their tips are just visible at the fusion site. *D*: The space to be arthrodesed is packed with cancellous bone chips. *E*: The Kirschner wires are driven across the fused segments; joints not fused are not traversed by the wires if possible; outer dimension, shape, and relationship of arthrodesed unit with neighboring carpal bones and/or radius should remain unchanged.

ized and excised to underlying healthy appearing cancellous bone. A bone graft is now obtained from the distal radius. A second transverse incision may be required for this purpose. The radius is exposed subperiosteally between the tendons of the first and second dorsal wrist compartments (extensor pollicis brevis and extensor carpi radialis longus) or between the extensor carpi radialis longus and brevis within the second compartment. In either location, the radius is flat and can be used as a donor site for both, cortical and cancellous grafts. Kirschner wires, 0.045 inches in diameter, are inserted in a retrograde fashion until their tips are precisely at the fusion surface. The bones to be fused are held in their normal relationship: compression is not applied. This avoids distortions in those carpal joints which are not to be arthrodesed.

The outside shape and dimensions of the fused unit should remain identical to the shape and dimensions of the comparable unit in the normal wrist (Fig. 6-27). Cancellous bone is packed tightly into the fusion space. A cortical graft may be fitted across the fusion site. The wounds are closed in layers. A well-padded compression dressing, reinforced with a long arm plaster splint, is applied. At one week postoperatively, these dressings are removed and replaced by a long arm cast. The thumb may or may not need to be immobilized, depending on the site of fusion. If immobilization of the distal carpal row is required (i.e., for luno- or scaphocapitate fusions) it is advisable to use a three-digit type of immobilization during these initial four weeks. At this point, the elbow is left free to move. At the end of eight weeks immobilization is discon-

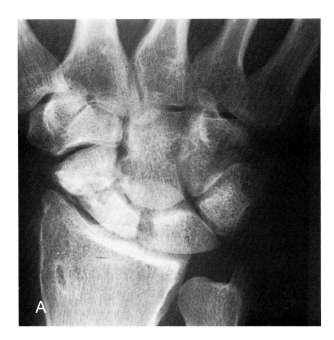

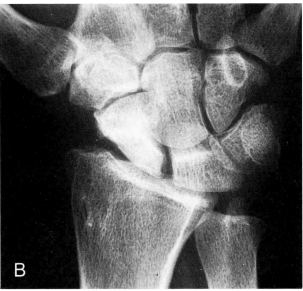

Fig. 6-28. Radial styloidectomy and bone graft for nonunion of fracture of the scaphoid with localized styloid-scaphoid osteoarthritis. *A*: Preoperative radiograph. *B*: Final appearance.

tinued if roentgenographic evidence of healing exists. A splint may be worn for the transition period until satisfactory wrist motion is regained.

Radial Styloidectomy

Radial styloidectomy is performed subperiosteally through the anatomic snuff box. With few exceptions[162] radial styloidectomies performed alone, as isolated procedures, have been unsuccessful.[126] In Mazet and Hohl's series[120] only two single styloidectomies were satisfactory out of a total of eleven. The reason for a successful styloidectomy may reside on the elimination of degenerative styloid-scaphoid contact areas[182] or, according to Verdan, on the release of the origin of the radio-

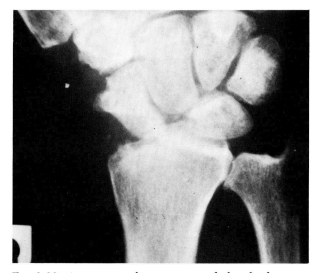

Fig. 6-29. An excessively generous radial styloidectomy may result in carpal instability. (From Taleisnik J: Fractures of the carpal bones. In Green DP (ed): Operative Hand Surgery. Vol. 1. Churchill Livingstone, New York, 1982.)

capitate ligament, thus reducing shear-stress on the scaphoid, during pronation and supination.[186]

Styloidectomies have enjoyed more success when combined with bone grafts with or without internal fixation.[8,37,38,46,119,120,140] Although some authors consider styloidectomy an essential part of the treatment of nonunions,[168] the procedure does not seem to improve on the results of bone grafting alone, except in cases with localized scaphostyloid arthrosis (Fig. 6-28). It may also be a factor of instability if performed carelessly, and may preclude the subsequent use of a scaphoid implant (Fig. 6-29).

Bentzon's Procedure

This operation was initially used by Bentzon[11] in 1939 and was first reported in 1941. In 1944 Bentzon and Madsen[12] reviewed their experience and found the procedure uniformly successful. Its indications are limited to those nonunions of the scaphoid with two equal size fragments and without degenerative changes of the periscaphoid joints. Painful nonunions are converted to pain-free pseudoarthrosis by the introduction between the frac-

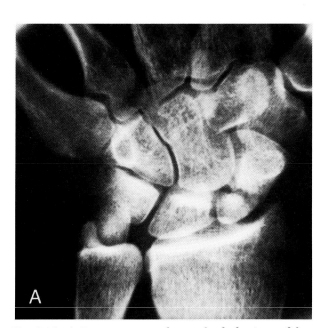
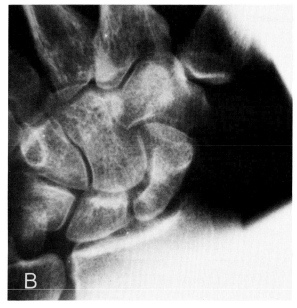

Fig. 6-30. A: Preoperative radiograph of a fracture of the proximal third of the scaphoid. B: Postoperative appearance five months following a palmar bone graft procedure (Russe). (From Taleisnik J: Fractures of the carpal bones. In Green DP (ed): Operative Hand Surgery. Vol. 1. Churchill Livingstone, New York, 1982.)

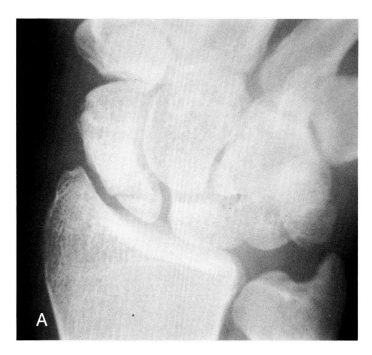

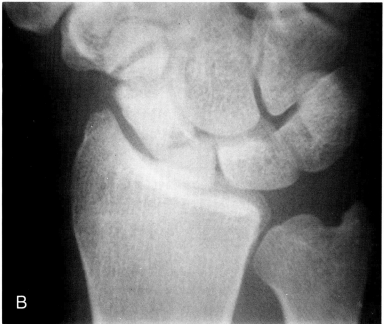

Fig. 6-31. Ununited fracture of proximal pole of scaphoid treated by excision of fracture fragment and insertion of silicone spacer. *A*: Preoperative radiograph. *B*: Postoperative appearance.

ture fragments of a soft tissue flap based on the dorsoradial aspect of the wrist. A similar method had apparently been proposed in 1914 by Gaza (quoted by Scaglietti and Perazzini[157]). In spite of its attractive simplicity, with very few excep-

tions[23,43] Bentzon's procedure has failed to become popular outside Scandinavian countries[5,141,148] and is no longer utilized for fractures of the scaphoid at the Orthopaedic Hospital in Aarhus, Denmark, where it was first used.[131]

FRACTURES OF THE PROXIMAL THIRD

Fractures of the proximal third of the scaphoid show a very high incidence of nonunion and of avascular necrosis of the proximal fragment.[120,121,171] In their study of the vascular foramina in dried scaphoids, Obletz and Halbstein[137] found 13 percent of specimens without vascular perforations and 20 percent with only a single small foramen proximal to the waist. Therefore, in their opinion, 30 percent of middle third fractures could be expected to interfere with the blood supply to the proximal fragment and lead to avascular necrosis or nonunion. This potential is higher the more proximal the fracture. The diagnosis of avascular necrosis is strictly roentgenographic and should be made with caution. It is subjective to a considerable degree.[62] The increased density of the proximal fragment may be more apparent than real, produced by rotation to a position of greater thickness.[72] For a valid diagnosis of avascular necrosis, this should be visualized in all projections. Studies of intraosseous blood supply to the scaphoid[58,71,177] have supplied sufficient experimental

data to explain the high incidence of nonunions and avascular necrosis of the proximal fragment among fractures of the proximal third of the scaphoid (see Chapter 4). These fractures comprise 11 to 34.8 percent of the total number of scaphoid fractures in different series.[37,56,62,140,155] Fractures in this location take an average of 6 to 11 weeks longer to heal than those in the middle third[124,154,171] and have demonstrated an incidence of avascular necrosis of 14 to 39 percent.[37,38,140,171] Although avascular necrosis may delay union in fresh fractures, it is not necessarily a sign of impending nonunion.

Fresh injuries are treated by prolonged long arm cast immobilization. Rehbein and Düben[150] report proximal third fractures healing with the use of their fist-cast. For those that fail to unite after six months, particularly for the fragments that are smaller than 30 percent of the scaphoid, pulsing electromagnetic field stimulation (PEMF) has added a viable alternative to surgical treatment (Fig. 6-12). In a recent report[66] 67 percent of established nonunions of the proximal third went on to heal in an average of 4.3 months, after starting electrical stimulation. PEMF is a pain-free method, that requires a very strict compliance from the pa-

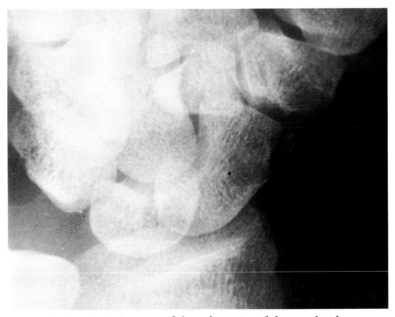

Fig. 6-32. Fracture of the tuberosity of the scaphoid.

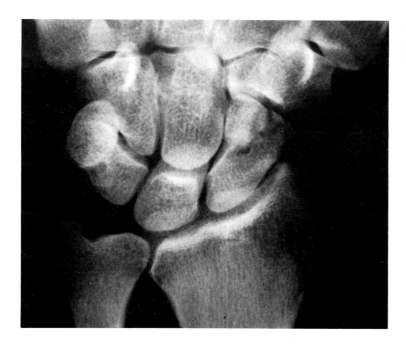

Fig. 6-33. Vertical fracture of distal pole of scaphoid, intraarticular into scaphotrapezium joint.

tient for its success. It is not invasive, and may be used in the presence of infection. In my opinion, this noninvasive technique is preferable to other forms of electrical treatment that require the transcutaneous insertion of electrodes in the fracture site under radiographic control.[18]

The surgical method to be used in the treatment of proximal third fractures is chosen according to the size of the fragment. When this fragment is a full one third of the scaphoid, a bone graft using Russe's or Matti's technique may be successful (Fig. 6-30). For smaller fragments, Matti's original technique[117] may be preferable. For this type of fracture, fixation from the lunate to the distal scaphoid with a staple or Kirschner wires inserted across the proximal fragment may be of considerable help to enhance the chances of healing and increase stability for the fracture fragment. In either case, if union fails to occur, or if the fragment is too small for any conceivable reconstruction, and in the absence of carpal instability, it may be excised.[8,12,13,20,85,112,115,128,164,171,189] I prefer to insert a silastic spacer in place of the excised fragment (Fig. 6-31). This may be carved from a silastic block, or cut out of a silastic scaphoid implant, attempting to reproduce the size and shape of the excised fragment. When there is carpal instability accompanying a proximal third fracture, nothing short of a partial fusion will succeed.[76]

FRACTURES OF THE DISTAL THIRD

Fractures in this location occur infrequently.[49,85,112,140] Fractures of the tuberosity are extraarticular and usually stable and have a generous blood supply (Fig. 6-32).[71,106,137,177] They tend to heal promptly and are best treated in a short arm thumb spica cast worn for three to six weeks. In Russe's classification[155] fractures of the distal third are commonly of the transverse stable type and tend to unite rapidly, usually after four to eight weeks in a short arm thumb spica cast. Vertical fractures into the scaphotrapezium joint have been described (Fig. 6-33).[39] They may be difficult to detect, requiring special views and special techniques (trispiral tomography). Plaster immobilization is usually successful. Here, as in other locations, displacement should not be accepted and if alignment is not anatomic, open reduction and internal fixation with Kirschner wires should be considered.

REFERENCES

1. Adams JD: Fracture of the carpal scaphoid. A new method of treatment with a report of one case. N Engl J Med 198:401, 1928

2. Agerholm JC, Lee MLH: The acrylic scaphoid prosthesis in the treatment of the ununited carpal scaphoid fracture. Acta Orthop Scand 37:67, 1966

3. Aghasi M, Rzetelni V, Axer A: Osteochondritis dissecans of the carpal scaphoid. J Hand Surg 6:351, 1981

4. Agner O: Treatment of ununited navicular fractures by total excision of the bone and the insertion of acrylic prostheses. Acta Orthop Scand 33:235, 1963

5. Agner O, Rasmussen KB: Treatment of ununited fractures of the carpal scaphoid by Bentzon's operation. p. 131. In Stack HG, Bolton H (eds): Proceedings of the Second Hand Club, 1956–67. British Soc For Surg of the Hand, London, 1975

6. Archambault JL: Resined fiberglass cast for carpal navicular fractures. Physician Sports Med 8(1):83, 1980

7. Barber HM: Acrylic scaphoid prostheses: A long-term follow up. Proc R Soc Med 67:1075, 1974

8. Barnard L, Stubbins SG: Styloidectomy of the radius in the surgical treatment of nonunion of the carpal navicular. J Bone Joint Surg 30A:98, 1948

9. Barr JS, Ellison WA, Musnick H, et al: Fracture of the carpal navicular (scaphoid) bone. An end-result study in military personnel. J Bone Joint Surg 35A:609, 1953

10. Beck A: Zur Behandlung der Verzogerten Konsolidation bei Unterschenkelbruchen. Ibl. Chir 56:2690, 1929

11. Bentzon PGK: Redergørelse for virksomheden paa samfundet og hjemmet for vanføres orthopaediske hospital i Aarhus i 4-aarsperioden September 1936-September 1940. Nord Med 11:2366, 1941

12. Bentzon PGK, Madsen AR: Surgical therapy of pseudarthrosis following fractures of carpal scaphoid bone. Nord Med 21:524, 1944

13. Bentzon PGK, Madsen AR: On fracture of the carpal scaphoid: Method of operative treatment of inveterate fractures. Acta Orthop Scand 16:30, 1945

14. Bizarro AH: Traumatology of the carpus. Surg Gynecol Obstet 34:574, 1922

15. Blencke H: Ein Fall von Naviculare Carpi Bipartum. Monatschr Unfallheilk Leipzig 33:75, 1926

16. Böhler L: Técnica del tratamiento de las fracturas, 3rd ed., translated from the German. 7th ed., by Schneider G, and Jimeno Vidal F, vol. 1: Editorial Labor S.A. Barcelona, 1954

17. Böhler L, Trojan E, and Jahna H: Behandlungsergebnisse von 734 Frischen Einfachen Brüchen des Kahnbeinkörpers der hand. Wiederherchir, Traum, 2:86, S Karger, Basel-New York.

18. Bora FW, Osterman AL, Brighton CT: The electrical treatment of scaphoid nonunion. Clin Orthop 161:33, 1981

19. Boyd GI: Bipartite carpal navicular bone. Br J Surg 20:455, 1933

20. Boyes JH: Bunnell's Surgery of the Hand. 5th Ed. Lippincott, Philadelphia, 1970

21. Bridgman CF: Radiography of the carpal navicular bone. Med Radiogr Photogr 25:104, 1949

22. Broomé A, Cedell CA, Colléen S: High plaster immobilization for fracture of the carpal scaphoid bone. Acta Chir Scand 128:42, 1964

23. Brueckman FR: The Bentzon procedure for nonunion of the carpal navicular. Presented at the 1st meeting, Surg-Hands, Indianapolis, Indiana, 1975

24. Buhlmann E von: Über die Behandlung der Navikularepseudarthrose mit Verschraubung. Z Unfallmed Berufskr 41:253, 1948

25. Burnett JH: Fracture of the (navicular) carpal scaphoid. N Engl J Med 211:56, 1934

26. Burnett JH: Further observations on treatment of fracture of the carpal scaphoid (navicular). J Bone Joint Surg 19:1099, 1937

27. Callender M: Fracture of the carpal end of the radius, and of the scaphoid bone. Trans Pathol Soc London 17:21, 1866

28. Callow FH McC: Nonunion of the carpal navicular bone. Med J Aust 1:391, 1939

29. Cave EF: The carpus, with references to the fractured navicular bone. Arch Surg 40:54, 1940

30. Cetti R, Christensen S-E: The diagnostic value of displacement of the fat stripe in fracture of the scaphoid bone. Hand 4:75, 1982

31. Childress HM: Fracture of a bipartite carpal navicular. Report of a case. J Bone Joint Surg 25:446, 1943

32. Cleveland M: Fracture of the carpal scaphoid. Surg Gynecol Obstet 84:769, 1947

33. Cobey MC, White RK: An operation for non-union of fractures of the carpal navicular. J Bone Joint Surg 28:757, 1946

34. Codman EA, Chase HM: The diagnosis and treatment of fracture of the carpal scaphoid and dislocation of the semilunar bone. Ann Surg 41:321, 1905

35. Codman EA, Chase HM: The diagnosis and treatment of fracture of the carpal scaphoid and dislocation of the semilunar bone. Part II. Ann Surg 41:563, 1905

36. Cole WH, Williamson GA: Fractures of the carpal navicular bone. Minn Med 18:81, 1935
37. Cooney WP, Dobyns JH, Linscheid RL: Non-union of the scaphoid. Analysis of the results from bone grafting. Orthop Transl 4:18, 1980
38. Cooney WP, Dobyns JH, Linscheid RL: Fractures of the scaphoid: a rational approach to management. Clin Orthop 149:90, 1980
39. Cooney WP, Ripperger RR, Linscheid RL: Distal pole scaphoid fractures. Orthop Trans 4:18, 1980
40. Cotta J: Ein Beitrag zur Differentialdiagnose Navicularpseudoarthrose — Os Naviculare Bipartitum Carpi. Arch Orthop Unfall Chir 52:581, 1961
41. Crabbe WA: Excision of the proximal row of the carpus. J Bone Joint Surg 46B:708, 1964
42. Cravener EK: Fractures of the carpal (navicular) scaphoid. Am J Surg 44:100, 1939
43. Danyo JJ: Open navicular bone grafting and styloidectomy. Orthop Rev 1:21, 1975
44. Davidson AJ, Horowitz MT: An evaluation of excision in the treatment of ununited fractures of the carpal scaphoid bone. Ann Surg 108:291, 1938
45. Dawkins AL: The fractured scaphoid: A modern view. Med J Aust 1:332, 1967
46. Decoulx P, Razemon J.-P, Lemerle P: Les fractures et pseudathroses du scaphoïde carpien. A propos de 56 cas. Lille-Chir 13:113, 1959
47. Dehne E, Deffer PA, Feighney RE: Pathomechanics of the fracture of the carpal navicular. J Trauma 4:96, 1964
48. Destot E: Injuries of the wrist. A radiological study. Translated by Atkinson FRB, Ernest Benn, London, 1925
49. Dickinson JC, Shannon JG: Fractures of the carpal scaphoid in the Canadian Army. Surg Gynecol Obstet 79:225, 1944
50. Dobyns JH, Linscheid RL: Fractures and dislocations of the wrist. p. 345. In Rockwood CA Jr, Green DP (eds): Fractures. Lippincott, Philadelphia, 1975
51. Dooley BJ: Inlay bone grafting for non-union of the scaphoid bone by the anterior approach. J Bone Joint Surg [Br] 50:102, 1968
52. Downing FH: Excision of the distal fragment of the scaphoid and styloid process of the radius for non-union of the carpal scaphoid. West J Surg Obstet Gynecol 59:127, 1951
53. Düben W, Gelbke H: The conservative treatment of the pseudarthrosis of the os naviculare of the hand. Acta Orthop Scand 26:25, 1956
54. Dunn AW: Fractures and dislocations of the carpus. Surg Clin North Am 52:1513, 1972
55. Dwyer FC: Excision of the carpal scaphoid for ununited fracture. J Bone Joint Surg [Br] 31:572, 1949
56. Eddeland A, Eiken O, Hellgreen E, Ohlsson NM: Fractures of the scaphoid. Scand J Plast Reconstr Surg 9:234, 1975
57. Edelstein JM: Treatment of ununited fractures of the carpal navicular. J Bone Joint Surg 21:902, 1939
58. Fajardo JC: Irrigación del hueso escafoides de la mano. Rev Med Rosario 51:3, 1961
59. Farquharson EL: A splint for fracture of the carpal navicular. J Bone Joint Surg 24:922, 1942
60. Faulkner DM: Bipartite carpal scaphoid. J Bone Joint Surg 10:284, 1928
61. Fisk G: Carpal injuries. p. 101. In Pulvertaft RG (ed): Clinical Surgery: The Hand. Butterworths, Washington, 1966
62. Fisk G: Carpal instability and the fractured scaphoid. Ann R Coll Surg Engl 46:63, 1970
63. Fisk G: Unusual fractures of the carpal scaphoid, p. 129. In Stack HG, Bolton H (eds): Proceedings of the Second Hand Club, 1956–67. British Society for Surgery of the Hand, London, 1975
64. Fisk G: Treatment of fractures and joint injuries of the hand, p. 274. In Stack HG, Bolton H (eds): Proceedings of the Second Hand Club, 1956–67. British Society for Surgery of the Hand, London, 1975
65. Frykman G: Fractures of the distal radius including sequelae—shoulder-hand-finger syndrome, disturbances in the distal radio-ulnar joint and impairment of nerve function. A clinical and experimental study. Acta Orthop Scand Suppl 108, 1967
66. Frykman GK, Helal B, Kaufman R, et al: Pulsing electromagnetic field treatment of nonunions of the scaphoid. A preliminary report. Presented at the 37th Annual Meeting of the American Society for Surgery of the Hand, New Orleans, LA, January, 1982
67. Ganel A, Engel J, Oster Z, Farine I: Bone scanning in the assessment of fractures of the scaphoid. J Hand Surg 4:541, 1979
68. Gasser H: Delayed union and pseudoarthrosis of the carpal navicular: Treatment by compression-screw osteosynthesis. A preliminary report on 20 fractures. J Bone Joint Surg [Am]:249, 1965
69. Geissendörfer H: Welche Veralteten Kahnbeinbrüche der Hand Eignen sich zur Nagelung? Zentralbl Chir 69:421, 1942
70. Geissendörfer J: Erfahrungen und Ergebnisse mit der Nagelung bei 21 Veralteten Kahnbeinbrüchen der Hand. Zentralbl Chir 75:906, 1950

71. Gelberman RH, Menon J: The vascularity of the scaphoid bone. J Hand Surg 5:508, 1980

72. Gilford WW, Bolton RH, Lambrinudi C: The mechanism of the wrist joint, with special reference to fractures of the scaphoid. Guy's Hospital Rep. 92:52, 1943

73. Goeringer CF: Follow-up results of surgical treatment for nonunion of the carpal scaphoid bone. Report of nineteen cases. Arch Surg 58:291, 1949

74. Gollasch W: Congenital bipartite carpal scaphoid bones. Arch Orthop Unfallchir 40:269, 1939

75. Gordon LH, King D: Partial wrist arthrodesis for old ununited fractures of the carpal navicular. Am J Surg 102:460, 1961

76. Graner O, Lopes EI, Costa Carvalho B, Atlas S: Arthrodesis of the carpal bones in the treatment of Kienböck's disease, painful ununited fractures of the navicular and lunate bones with avascular necrosis, and old fracture-dislocations of carpal bones. J Bone Joint Surg 48A:767, 1966

77. Graziani A: L'esame radiologico del carpo. Radiol Med 27:382, 1940

78. Heim U, Pfeiffer KM: Small fragment set manual. p. 87. Technique recommended by the ASIF Group. Springer Verlag, New York, 1974

79. Helfet AJ: A new operation for ununited fracture of the scaphoid. J Bone Joint Surg [Br] 34:329, 1952

80. Henry MG: Fractures of the carpal scaphoid bone in industry and in the military service. Arch Surg 48:278, 1944

81. Herbert TJ: Scaphoid fractures and carpal instability. Proc R Soc Med 67:1080, 1974

82. Herbert TJ, Fisher WE: Management of the fractured scaphoid using a new bone screw. J Bone Joint Surg [Br] 66:114, 1984

83. Herndonk JH, Acevedo M, Hecht O, et al: A long term evaluation of 607 cases of lunate and scaphoid arthroplasty. Presented at the 32nd Annual Meeting. Amer Soc for Surg of the Hand, Las Vegas, NV, February, 1977

84. Herness D, Posner MA: Some aspects of bone grafting for nonunion of the carpal navicular. Analysis of 41 cases. Acta Orthop Scand 48:373, 1977

85. Hill NA: Fractures and dislocations of the carpus. Orthop Clin North Am 1:275, 1970

86. Hirsch M: Konservative oder Operative Therapie der Fraktur des Os Naviculare Carpi? Wien Med Wochenschr 29/30:803, 1935

87. Hoffmeister W: Behandlung von Kahnbeinbrüchen und Pseudarthrosen. Zentralbl Chir 51:2960, 1934

88. Hopf A: 4-Das Naviculare Bipartitum. p. 477. In Hohmann G, Hackenbroch M, Lindeman K (eds): Handbuch der Orthopedie. Vol. 3. Georg Thieme, Stuttgart, 1959

89. Hopkins FS: Fractures of the scaphoid in athletes. N Engl J Med 209:687, 1933

90. Inglis AE, Jones EC: Proximal-row carpectomy for diseases of the proximal row. J Bone Joint Surg 59A:460, 1977

91. Jaekle RF, Clark AG: Acute fractures of the Carpal scaphoid. Surg Gynecol Obstet 68:820, 1939

92. Jahna H: Behandlung und Behandlungsergebnisse von 734 Frischen Einfachen Brüchen des Kahnbeinkörpers der Hand. Wien Med Wochenschr 51/52:1023, 1954

93. Jeanne LA, Mouchet A: Les lésions traumatique fermées du poignet. 28th Congrés Français de Chirurgie, 1919

94. Jerre T: Bipartite carpal scaphoid bone. Acta Orthop Scand 17:70, 1947

95. Johnson RW Jr: A study of the healing processes in injuries to the carpal scaphoid. J Bone Joint Surg 9:482, 1927

96. Jorgensen EC: Proximal-row carpectomy: An end result study of 22 cases. J Bone Joint Surg 51A:1104, 1969

97. Jørgensen TM, Andresen J-H, Thommesen P, Hansen HH: Scanning and radiology of the carpal scaphoid bone. Acta Orthop Scand 50:663, 1979

98. Kessler I, Heller J, Silberman Z, Pupko L: Some aspects in nonunion of fractures of the carpal scaphoid. J Trauma 3:442, 1963

99. Koob E, Goymann V, Hass HG: Ergebnisse nach Verschraubungen der Kahnbeinpseudarthrose an der Hand. Handchirurgie 2:205, 1970

100. Landsmeer JM: Studies in the anatomy of articulation. I. The equilibrium of the "intercalated" bone. Acta Morphol Neerl Scand 3:287, 1961

101. Legge RF: Vitallium prosthesis in the treatment of fracture of the carpal navicular. West J Surg 59:468, 1951

102. Leslie IJ, Dickson RA: The fractured carpal scaphoid. Natural history and factors influencing outcome. J Bone Joint Surg [Br] 63:225, 1981

103. Lichtman DM, Alexander CE: Decision making in scaphoid nonunion. Orthop Rev 11:55, 1982

104. Lindgren E: On os naviculare bipartitum. Acta Radiol 22:511, 1941

105. Linscheid RL, Dobyns JH, Beabout JW, Bryan RS: Traumatic instability of the wrist: Diagnosis, classification, and pathomechanics. J Bone Joint Surg 54A:1612, 1972

106. Logroscino D, DeMarchi E: Vascolarizzazione e

trofo-patie delle ossa del carpo. Chir Organi Mov 23:499, 1938

107. London PS: The broken scaphoid bone. The case against pessimism. J Bone Joint Surg 43B:237, 1961

108. London PS: Ununited fracture of the scaphoid bone, p. 131. In Stack HG, Bolton N (eds): Proceedings of the Second Hand Club, 1956–67. British Society for Surgery of the Hand, London, 1975

109. Lucero B: Fractura del carpo en un niño. Bol Trab Soc Arg Cirujanos 10:260, 1943

110. Luck JV, Smith HMA, Lacey HB, Shands AR: Orthopedic Surgery in the Army Air Forces during World War II. Recurrent dislocation of the shoulder and ununited fractures of the carpal scaphoid. Arch Surg 57:801, 1948

111. Lützeler H: Die Enstehungsursache der Pseudarthrose nach Bruch des Kahnbeins der Hand. Dtsch Z Chir 235:450, 1932

112. Luxardo JC: Consideraciones sobre ciento noventa fracturas de escafoides carpiano. Rev Sanid Mil Argentina 55:420, 1956

113. Maatz R: Schrabung der Kahnbeinpseudarthrose. Zentralbl Chir 48:1720, 1943

114. MacLennan A: The treatment of fracture of the carpal scaphoid and the indications for operation. Br Med J 2:1089, 1911

115. Margo MK, Seely JA: A statistical review of 100 cases of fracture of the carpal navicular bone. Clin Orthop 31:102, 1963

116. Matti H: Über modellierende Osteotomie und Spongiosa Transplantation. Schweiz Med Wochenschr 49:1254, 1929

117. Matti H: Über die Behandlung der Navicularefraktur und der Refractura Patellae durch Plombierung mit Spongiosa. Zentralbl Chir 64:2353, 1937

118. Maudsley RH, Chen SC: Screw fixation in the management of the fractured carpal scaphoid. J Bone Joint Surg 54B:432, 1972

119. Mazet R Jr, Hohl M: Radial styloidectomy and styloidectomy plus bone graft in the treatment of old ununited carpal scaphoid fractures. Ann Surg 152:296, 1960

120. Mazet R Jr, Hohl M: Conservative treatment of old fractures of the carpal scaphoid. J Trauma 1:115, 1961

121. Mazet R Jr, Hohl M: Fractures of the carpal navicular. Analysis of 91 cases and review of the literature. J Bone Joint Surg 45A:82, 1963

122. McLaughlin HL: Fracture of the carpal navicular (scaphoid) bone: Some observations based in treatment by open reduction and internal fixation. J Bone Joint Surg 36A:765, 1954

123. McLaughlin HL, Parkes JC: Fracture of the carpal navicular (scaphoid) bone: Gradations in therapy based upon pathology. J Trauma 9:311, 1969

124. Meekison DM: Some remarks on three common fractures: 1. Fractures of the carpal scaphoid; 2. Fractures of the head of the radius; 3. Fractures of the medial malleolus. J Bone Joint Surg 27:80, 1945

125. Melone CP Jr: Scaphoid fractures: Concepts of management. Clin Plast Surg 8:83, 1981

126. Metcalfe JW: The vitallium sphere prosthesis for non-union of the navicular bone. J Int Coll Surg, 22:459, 1954

127. Milford L: The Hand. Ch. 3, p. 110. In Edmonson AS, Crenshaw AH (eds): Campbell's Operative Orthopaedics. Vol. 1. Mosby, St. Louis MO, 1980

128. Moore AE: Treatment of delayed union of the carpal scaphoid. Br Med J 2:990, 1938

129. Mouchet A: Fractures isolées du scaphoïde carpien. La Presse Med 6:122, 1934

130. Mulder JE: Pseudoarthrosis of the scaphoid bone (Abstract). J Bone Joint Surg 45B:621, 1963

131. Munck J: Personal communication. 1980

132. Murray CR: Delayed and non-union in fractures in adult. Ann Surg 93:961, 1931

133. Murray G: Bone graft for non-union of the carpal scaphoid. Br J Surg 22:63, 1934

134. Murray G: End results of bone grafting for non-union of the carpal navicular. J Bone Joint Surg 28:749, 1946

135. Myrin SO: Fractures of the scaphoid. p. 133. In Stack HG, Bolton H (eds): Proc. of the Second Hand Club. 1956–67, Brit. Soc. for Surg. of the Hand, London. 1975

136. Nenninger W: Über die Behandlung vo Khanbeinfrakturen der Hand. Dsch Med 6:224, 1955

137. Obletz BE, Halbstein BM: Non-union of fractures of the carpal navicular. J Bone Joint Surg 20:424, 1938

138. O'Rahilly R: A survey of carpal and tarsal anomalies J Bone Joint Surg 35A:626, 1953

139. Palmer I, Widen A: Treatment of fractures and pseudarthrosis of the scaphoid with central grafting (autogenous bone-peg). Acta Chir Scand 110:206, 1955

140. Pennsylvania Orthopedic Society, Scientific Research Committee: Evaluation of treatment for non-union of the carpal navicular. J Bone Joint Surg 44A:169, 1962

141. Perey O: A re-examination of cases of pseudarthrosis of the navicular bone operated on according to Bentzon's technique. Acta Orthop 23:26, 1954

142. Perschl L: Zur röntgenologischen Diagnostik der frischen Kahnbeinbrüche der Hand. Röntgenpraxis 10:11, 1938

143. Peterson HA, Lipscomb PR: Intercarpal arthrodesis. Arch Surg 95:127, 1967

144. Pfeiffer KM: Zur Frage der primären Schraubenosteosynthese von Navikularefrakturen. Helv Chir Acta 39:471, 1972

145. Pfitzner W: Variations in the structure of the bones of the hand. Morphol Arb 4:349, 1895

146. Pfitzner W: Die morphologischen elemente des menschlichen handskelets. Z Morphol Anthropol 2:77, 365, 1900

147. Picaud A: Traitement d'une pseudarthrose ancienne du scaphoïde carpien par prosthèse acrylique. Mem Acad Chir 79:200, 1953

148. Rasmussen KB: Bentzon's operation for pseudarthrosis of the scaphoid bone (Abstract). J Bone Joint Surg 45B:621, 1963

149. Rehbein F: Zur konservativen Behandlung der veralteten Kahnbeinbrüches und der Kahnbeinpseudarthrose der Hand. Arch Klin Chir 260:356, 1948

150. Rehbein F, Düben W: Zur Konservativen Behandlung des Veralteten Kahnbeinbrüches und der Kahnbeinpseudarthrose. Arch Orthop Unfall Chir 45:67, 1952

151. Ritter U: Anzeige, erfolgsaussichten und miberfolge bei der Behandlung Veralteter Kahnbeinbrüche und Kahnbeinpseudarthrosen. Der Chirurg, 24:212, 1953

152. Robertson JM, Wilkins RD: Fracture of the carpal scaphoid. Br Med J 1:685, 1944

153. Rothberg AS: Fractures of the carpal navicular. Importance of special roentgenography. J Bone Joint Surg 21:1020, 1939

154. Russe O: Behandlungsergebnisse der Spongiosaauffüllung bei Kahnbeinpseudarthrosen. Z Orthop 81:466, 1951

155. Russe O: Fracture of the carpal navicular. Diagnosis, non-operative treatment and operative treatment. J Bone Joint Surg 42A:759, 1960

156. Sashin D: Treatment of fractures of the carpal scaphoid. A report of sixty-four cases. Arch Surg 52:445, 1946

157. Scaglietti O, Perazzini F: Die Kahnbeinpseudarthrosen. Wiederherchir Traum 2:112, 1954

158. Scaramuzza RFJ: El movimiento de rotacion en el carpo y su relacion con la fisopatologia de sus lesiones traumaticas. Bol Trabajos Soc Argent Ortop Traumatologia 34:337, 1969

159. Sgrosso JA: Traumatismos del carpo: Tratamiento. p. 1–140. Decimosexto Congreso Argentino de Cirugia, Buenos Aires, 1944

160. Sgrosso JA, Añaños V: Sobre el mecanismo de las fracturas del escafoide carpiano. Rev Ortop traumatol 18:183, 1948

161. Shively RA, Sundaram M, Riaz MA: Bilateral bipartite carpal navicular. Contemp Orthop 1:49, 1979

162. Smith L, Friedman B: Treatment of ununited fracture of the carpal navicular by styloidectomy of the radius. J Bone Joint Surg. 38A:368, 1956

163. Soto-Hall R, Haldeman KO: Treatment of fractures of the carpal scaphoid. J Bone Joint Surg 16:822, 1934

164. Soto-Hall R, Haldeman KO: The conservative and operative treatment of fractures of the carpal scaphoid (navicular). J Bone Joint Surg 23:841, 1941

165. Speed K: Fractures of the carpal navicular bone J Bone Joint Surg 7:682, 1925

166. Speed K: Injuries of the carpal bones. Surg Clin North Am 25:1, 1945

167. Speed K: Fractures and dislocations of the carpus. Calif Med 72:93, 1950

168. Sprague B, Justis EJ: Nonunion of the carpal navicular. Modes of treatment. Arch Surg 108:692, 1974

169. Stack JK: End results of excision of the carpal bones. Arch Surg 57:245, 1948

170. Stecher WR: Roentgenography of the carpal navicular bone. Am J Roentgenol 37:704, 1937

171. Stewart MJ: Fractures of the carpal navicular (scaphoid). A report of 436 cases. J Bone Joint Surg 36A:998, 1954

172. Sutro CJ: Treatment of nonunion of the carpal navicular bone. Surgery 20:536, 1946

173. Swanson AB: Silicone rubber implants for the replacement of the carpal scaphoid and lunate bones. Orthop Clin North Am 1:299, 1970

174. Swanson AB: Flexible implant resection arthroplasty in the hand and extremities. Mosby, St. Louis, MO, 1973

175. Swanson AB: Implant arthroplasty in the hand and upper extremity and its future. Surg Clin North Am 61:369, 1981

176. Taleisnik J: Wrist, anatomy, function and injury. Am Acad Orthop Surgeons Instruct Course Lect 27:61, 1978

177. Taleisnik J, Kelly PJ: The extraosseous and intraosseous blood supply of the scaphoid bone. J Bone Joint Surg 48A:1125, 1966

178. Terry DW, Ramin JE: The navicular fat strip. A useful roentgen feature for evaluating wrist trauma. Am J Roentgenol 124:25, 1975

179. Thorndike A Jr, Garrey WE: Fractures of the carpal scaphoid. N Engl J Med 222:827, 1940

180. Todd AH: Fractures of the carpal scaphoid. Br J Surg 9:7, 1921

181. Törngren S, Sandqvist S: Pseudarthrosis in the scaphoid bone treated by grafting with autogenous bone peg: A follow up study. Acta Orthop Scand 45:82, 1974

182. Trojan E: Grafting of ununited fractures of the scaphoid. Proc R Soc Med 67:1078, 1974

183. Trojan E, de Mourgues G: Fractures et pseudarthroses du scaphoïde carpien. Conclusions du Deuxième Rapport. Société Française d'orthopédie et de Traumatologie. Rev Chir Orthop 45:926, 1959

184. Unger HS, Stryker WC: Nonunion of the carpal navicular. Analysis of 42 cases treated by the Russe procedure. South Med J 62:620, 1969

185. Vahvanen V, Westerlund M: Fracture of the carpal scaphoid in childern. A clinical and roentgenological study of 108 cases. Acta Orthop Scand 51:909, 1980

186. Verdan C: Le rôle du ligament anterieur radio-carpien dans les fractures du scaphoïde: Deductions thérapeutiques. Z Unfallmed Berufskr 54:299, 1954

187. Verdan C: Fractures of the scaphoid. Surg Clin North Am 40:461, 1960

188. Verdan C, Narakas A: Fractures and pseud-arthrosis of the scaphoid. Surg Clin North Am 48:1083, 1968

189. Wagner CJ: Fractures of the carpal navicular. J Bone Joint Surg 34A: 774, 1952

190. Wagner CJ: Fracture-dislocations of the wrist: Clin Orthop 15:181, 1959

191. Warner WC, Freeland AE, McAndrew JC: The scaphoid staple for stabilization of selected fractures and nonunions. Presented at the 35th annual meeting, American Society for Surgery of the Hand, Atlanta, 1980

192. Watson HK: Limited wrist arthrodesis. Clin Orthop 149:126, 1980

193. Watson HK: Goodman ML, Johnson TR: Limited arthrodesis. Part II: Intercarpal and radiocarpal considerations. J Hand Surg 6:223, 1981

194. Watson-Jones R: Fractures and joint injuries. 4th Ed. Vol. 2. Williams and Wilkins, Baltimore, 1960

195. Weber ER, Chao EY: An experimental approach to the mechanism of scaphoid wrist fractures. J Hand Surg 5:320, 1980

196. Weber ER: Biomechanical implications of scaphoid waist fractures. Clin Orthop 149:83, 1980

197. Wilson JN: Watson-Jones fractures and joint injuries. 5th Ed. Vol. 2. Churchill Livingstone, New York, 1976

7 Isolated Injuries to Carpal Bones Other Than Scaphoid and Lunate

In 1890, in his *Traité de Chirurgie*, Ricard stated that "clinically one might say, simple fractures of the carpus do not exist. The only sign that has any value whatever and permits affirmation of fractures is crepitus." Pain, limitation of motion and tenderness, although frequently localized to the carpus, were not enough. "Tumor," that is, a palpable abnormal bony mass, was also important in clinical diagnosis although it was rarely interpreted correctly before roentgenography became available.[16] Codman and Chase flatly state that "in the absence of crepitus and tumor, we believe, in no recorded case previous to the use of x-rays has a correct diagnosis been made of a simple fracture of a carpal bone."[16] Only after roentgenography demonstrated the relative frequency of these injuries were additional clinical signs described, particularly changes in comparison measurements between bony landmarks in the injured and uninjured wrists. In 1901 Hofliger (quoted by Codman and Chase[16]) proposed that shortening of the distance between the tip of the radial styloid and the end of the second metacarpal, amounting to 0.5 to 1.5 cm, was suggestive of fracture of the scaphoid. It was, of course, the advent of roentgenography that allowed practitioners to diagnose carpal injuries. Many types of fractures, dislocations, subluxations and fracture-dislocations, and instability patterns of the carpus have since been described, including the isolated injuries to individual carpal bones, a potential cause of significant disability. Most of these are confined to a "vulnera-ble zone,"[39] an area contained between two paths of common carpal injury, a proximal "lesser arc" around the lunate (perilunate dislocations and dislocations of the lunate), and a "greater arc." Many of the major fracture–dislocations of the carpus occur between these arcs (Fig. 7-1). In addition the vulnerable zone also includes the entirety of the radial carpals: the distal scaphoid and the trapezium.

TRIQUETRUM

Fractures of the triquetrum are more commonly associated with other carpal injuries.[21,36] Isolated fractures are much less frequent, although they are reported to represent the second[6,9,23,33,58] or third[13,71] most common group of carpal bone fractures. Dislocations are extremely rare. In most instances, the triquetrum dislocates volarward.[27,58,61] Fractures of the triquetrum have been reported to be anywhere from 1 to 18 percent of carpal lesions in different series.[55]

MECHANISM OF INJURY

Triquetrum fractures may occur by compression or impingement, or may be secondary to traction or avulsion.[10,55] Fractures through the body of the triquetrum, either transverse (Fig. 7-2) or involving the lunate aspect (Fig. 7-3), should be carefully

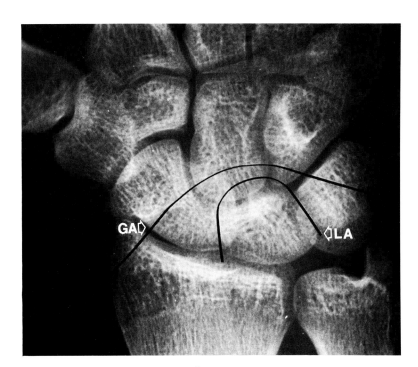

Fig. 7-1. Vulnerable zone of carpus contained between greater (GA) and lesser arcs (LA). (See Ref. 39.)

evaluated, for they may be part of a more complex fracture-dislocation of the carpus, not infrequently the residual of a transscaphoid, transtriquetral perilunate fracture-dislocation that was reduced prior to initial roentgenograms. The mechanism of injury may be a rotation or twisting motion, particularly if resisted, such as when lifting heavy weights,[6] or a shear force applied by impingement of the hamate on the posteroradial projection of the triquetrum, during falls with the wrist in dorsiflexion and ulnar deviation[10,13,20,21,58] or a direct blow to the dorsum of the carpus.[6,36] Avulsion fractures at the site of triquetral attachment of radiotriquetral ligaments (Fig. 7-4) may also occur through an entirely different mechanism of injury, should the hand be forced into volarflexion and radial deviation[21] during a fall. Some degree of carpal supination may also need to be present.[36]

Diagnosis

There are two main types of triquetral fractures. The dorsal cortical fractures (Fig. 7-5) are produced by either avulsion,[6,58] or shear forces.[13] The second type of fracture involves the main body of

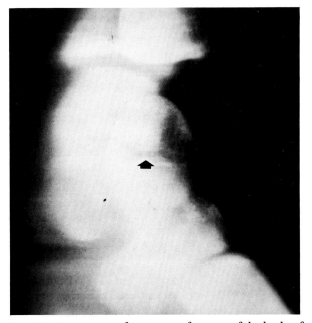

Fig. 7-2. Tomogram of transverse fracture of the body of the triquetrum.

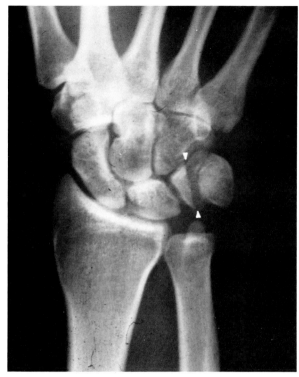

Fig. 7-3. Fracture of the body of the triquetrum involving lunate aspect. (From Taleisnik J: Fractures of the carpal bones. In Green, DP (ed): Operative Hand Surgery. Vol. 1. Churchill Livingstone, New York, 1982.)

the triquetrum (Figs. 7-2, 7-3)[6] and may be linear or comminuted. This type occurs less frequently than the dorsal cortical fracture and is usually undisplaced. On clinical examination the usual findings of tenderness and swelling are localized to the ulnar side of the dorsum of the carpus. Range of motion is decreased, particularly when tension or traction is applied to the triquetrum, such as in radial deviation and volarflexion. The diagnosis is established, however, by thorough radiographic studies. Multiple views in different projections and also planograms may be required before a diagnosis is made. Dorsal cortical fractures are better visualized in oblique and lateral radiographs (Figs. 7-5, 7-6). If the routine views fail to demonstrate the injury, it may be helpful to rotate the wrist to place the area of maximum tenderness tangential to the direction of the beam. Bonnin and Greening[10] point out that dorsal cortical fractures of the triquetrum may frequently be misdiagnosed as fractures of the dorsal pole of the lunate, and that radiographs in different degrees of obliquity assist in localizing the lesion. Fractures of the body of the triquetrum may be difficult to visualize. It is for these that additional radiographic studies such as planograms are helpful (Fig. 7-2).

Fig. 7-4. Avulsion fracture of the triquetrum.

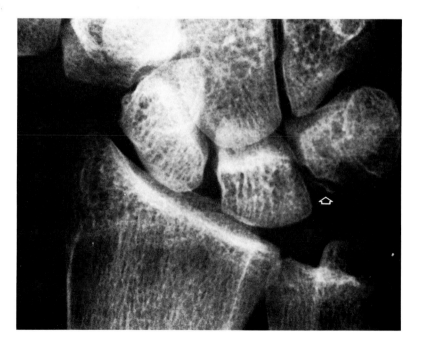

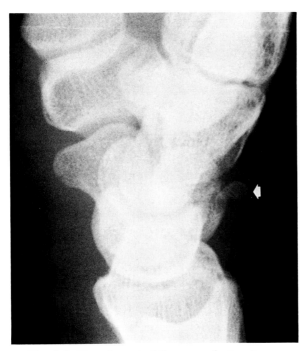

Fig. 7-5. Dorsal cortical fracture of triquetrum.

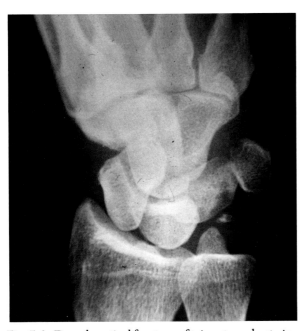

Fig. 7-6. Dorsal cortical fracture of triquetrum best visualized in reverse-oblique projection. (From Taleisnik J: Fractures of the carpal bones. In Green DP (ed): Operative Hand Surgery Vol. 1. Churchill Livingstone, New York, 1982.)

TREATMENT

In my experience, cortical fractures become asymptomatic even in those cases with dorsal cortical fragments that remain ununited. A period of two to four weeks of protective splinting is all that is required in most cases. It is extremely rare to find a cortical fracture with symptoms that are severe enough to require excision of the avulsed fragment and reattachment of ligaments into the bony defect. Fractures of the body can be treated successfully by cast immobilization for four to six weeks. Nonunion may occur,[24] but is exceedingly rare. Avascular necrosis has not been reported. For the very rare dislocation of the triquetrum, excision has been the recommended treatment[27,61] although my personal preference would be to attempt reduction, open if necessary, followed by internal fixation if required and plaster immobilization (Fig. 7-7).

PISIFORM

Jeanne and Mouchet credit Guibout with the first description of a fracture of the pisiform.[36] This was not an isolated injury, but was associated with simultaneous fractures of the scaphoid, triquetrum, and capitate. The first known report of an isolated fracture of the pisiform was published by Alsberg[2] in 1908. The earliest report in the English literature was that of Deane[19] in 1911.

MECHANISM OF INJURY

The pisiform is generally injured during a fall on the dorsiflexed, outstretched hand.[68] The most frequent mechanism of injury seems to be direct trauma on the pisiform, firmly held against the triquetrum by the tension of the flexor carpi ulnaris during a fall. Avulsion injuries may occur by the muscle pull of the flexor carpi ulnaris exerted against a sudden hyperextension motion of the wrist. The distal portion of the pisiform may fracture off, or a vertical fracture or osteochondral fracture of the articular surface may occur.[21] Subluxations or dislocations have been described, and are produced by either a direct blow or by severe muscular violence.[35] Subluxation at the pisotriquetral joint may accompany displaced fractures of the distal radius[68] and should be kept in mind when reading roentgenograms for what would otherwise appear to be an isolated fracture of the distal radius. Posttraumatic degenerative changes in the pisotriquetral joint following intraarticular fractures of the pisiform have been reported.[37,43]

DIAGNOSIS

Injury to the pisiform is suspected because of the mechanism of injury and the localization of tenderness to the base of the hypothenar eminence. In fresh injuries there may be abrasions or discoloration overlying this area. Relaxation of the flexor carpi ulnaris by passive volarflexion of the wrist allows the examiner to "rock" the pisiform on the underlying hamate, at which time crepitation may be felt and heard accompanied by exacerbation of pain (Fig. 7-8). The diagnosis of subluxation or dislocation of the pisiform may be easier to make on clinical grounds, through palpation, than on a radiologic basis, because in some positions of the wrist, the normal pisiform may appear subluxated (Fig. 1-13). Comparison views with the opposite uninjured side, obtained in exactly the same position, must be available before a diagnosis of subluxation or dislocation is made.[68,69] Occasionally, there may be symptoms suggestive of irritation of the ulnar nerve or artery,[34] either secondary to fractures or dislocations of the pisiform.

Roentgenographic examination for a suspected injury to the pisiform should include the routine projections obtained in accurate neutral position, to avoid fictitious changes of alignment and parallelism between the articular surfaces of triquetrum and pisiform or artificial variations in the width of the articular space between the two bones.[68] In addition, a lateral radiograph is helpful when obtained with the hand resting on its ulnar border and with enough added supination to place the outline of the pisiform in the path of the x-ray beam without obstruction or superimposition. The carpal tunnel projection should also be obtained when this injury is suspected. Vasilas[68] studied the radiographic characteristics of the pisotriquetral joint. In the vast majority of normal wrists, the pisiform

and triquetral articular surfaces should be parallel, or deviate from parallelism 15 degrees or less. If radiographs are obtained with the wrist in some flexion or extension, the parallelism may be lost, although 30 to 60 percent of joints actually remain grossly parallel even in dorsiflexion or volar flexion. The width of the normal pisotriquetral joint space was reported by these authors to be 2 mm or less in 85 percent of their cases, but it could be as wide as 4 mm in some normal instances. The space is wider in volar flexion and narrower in dorsiflexion. Both joint surfaces were found to align symmetrically with no pisotriquetral override in 90 to 95 percent of cases. Slight asymmetry was not believed to be an indication of subluxation. Overriding was normally seen with the wrist in volar flexion or dorsiflexion. Vasilas and coauthors established the following criteria for the roentgenographic diagnosis of subluxation of the pisotriquetral joint in radiographs obtained with the wrist in neutral position: (1) the joint space should be 4 mm wide or more; (2) there must be loss of parallelism of the pisotriquetrum joint surfaces greater than 20 degrees; and (3) proximal or distal overriding of the pisiform on the triquetrum, amounting to more than 15 percent of the extent of the joint surface, must exist.

TREATMENT

Fresh fractures of the pisiform are treated by protective splinting. The vast majority of these injuries become asymptomatic. Some may go on to develop persistent pain and localized tenderness, particularly during tight gripping or grasping. For these patients, excision of the pisiform, is a gratifying procedure.[54] The pisiform is best approached by a longitudinal incision overlying its radial border. The incision is slightly curved, the concavity facing medially (Fig. 7-9). It is best to gain immediate control of the ulnar neurovascular bundle prior to proceeding with the actual surgical exposure. The pisiform is exposed by longitudinally spreading all the overlying fibers of the flexor carpi ulnaris tendon and the origin of the abductor digiti minimi muscle. The excision is performed subperiosteally,[32,54] although this may be somewhat tedious and difficult at times. Once the pisiform has

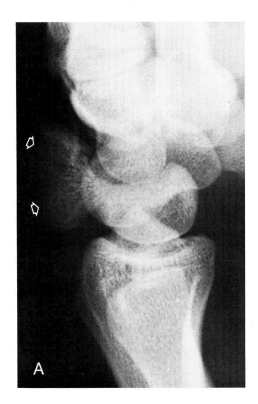

Fig. 7-7. Dislocation of the triquetrum. *A*: Lateral radiograph. *B*: Posteroanterior radiograph.

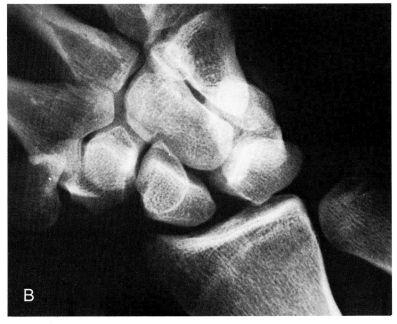

Fig. 7-7(cont.) C: Appearance after successful closed reduction. (Courtesy of Dr. Bertram Goldberg, Englewood, Co.)

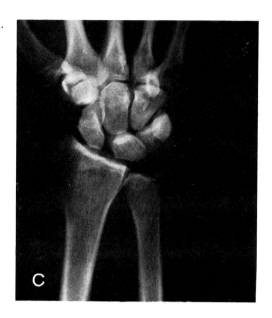

been excised, the soft tissue defect is carefully repaired. Postoperatively, the wrist is splinted in slight volarflexion. Gradual protected range of motion is allowed within the first postoperative week, and increased as permitted by the level of discomfort. Usually, all splinting may be discontinued at three to four weeks following operation.

TRAPEZIUM

Fractures of the trapezium comprise approximately 5 percent of all carpal fractures.[17] Isolated fractures are exceedingly rare (Fig. 7-10). Simultaneous fracture of the first metacarpal is the most frequently associated bony injury and fractures of

Fig. 7-8. Examination of piso-triquetral joint.

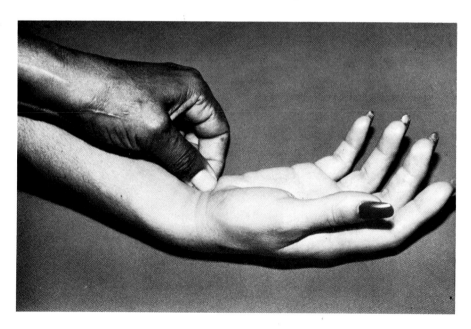

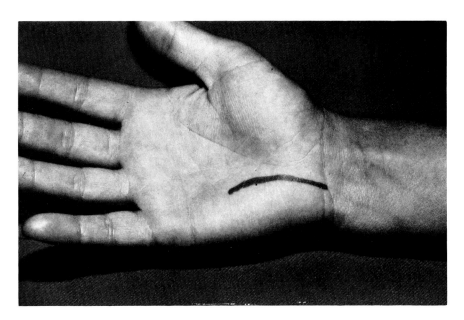

Fig. 7-9. Surgical incision for excision of pisiform.

the distal radius are next most common. Dislocations of the trapezium, usually carrying the first metacarpal, are extremely rare (Fig. 7-11).[57]

MECHANISM OF INJURY

Jeanne and Mouchet[36] showed that the trapezium fractured when subjected to strong compression by the radial styloid and by the base of the first metacarpal with the wrist in full radial deviation. Frequently, these injuries are produced by direct injury. It is conceivable that as part of this mechanism the first metacarpal may be driven into the articular surface of the trapezium causing it to split into radial and ulnar fragments. Avulsion fractures caused by capsular ligaments during forceful deviation of the thumb rarely occur.[21] Direct injury to the heel of the hand during falls or by severe loading of the palm under extremely heavy weight may also result in fractures of the ridge of the trapezium, probably representing partial avulsions of the attachment of the transverse carpal ligament.[47]

DIAGNOSIS

As in all carpal fractures, some measure of localization can be obtained by the presence of tenderness and swelling overlying the projection of the

involved bone. The range of motion of the thumb is relatively unrestricted, although passive attempts to bring the thumb to full adduction or abduction are painful and resisted by the patient. There is weakness of pinch. Occasionally symptoms suggestive of compression of the median nerve may be

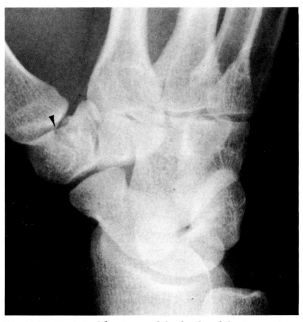

Fig. 7-10. Isolated fracture of the body of the trapezium. (Courtesy Dr. William D. Dixon, Orange, CA.)

Fig. 7-11. Dislocations of the trapezium are rare, and usually carry the first metacarpal.

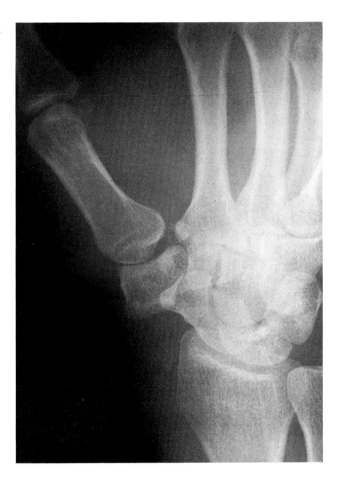

present[47] in those cases of fractures of the volar ridge of the trapezium. These patients also show tenderness to direct pressure on the volar tubercle of the trapezium, palpable very close and immediately distal to the distal tuberosity of the scaphoid. As in other carpal injuries, the diagnosis may be suspected clinically, but it is proven only by radiographic examination. It is important to separate the shadow of the trapezium from the overlying profiles of the trapezoid and the first and second metacarpals. The trapezium view is particularly helpful[12] (see Chapter 5). Fractures of the ridge of the trapezium can only be seen in the carpal tunnel projection.[31,47,70]

TREATMENT

Undisplaced fractures need only be treated in a thumb-spica cast for a period of four to six weeks.

Displaced fractures, particularly vertical intra-articular injuries entering the carpometacarpal joint, are best managed by open reduction and internal fixation. The procedure may be done through a volar hockey stick or longitudinal incision similar to that used for the exposure of the first carpometacarpal joint. Care should be taken to gain control of the radial artery, which crosses the proximal portion of the operative field (Fig. 2-21A), and of the cutaneous branches of the ulnar nerve. Visualization of the fracture requires that traction be applied to the thumb. The radial fragment may be difficult to control. It is best to drive a small Kirschner wire through it, to be used as a handle to manipulate the fragment into reduction.[17] While this position is held by an assistant, a couple of additional Kirschner wires are driven across from radial to ulnar. Postoperatively, the hand is placed in a short arm thumb-spica with the thumb in some abduction. Continuous immobilization need only last for three weeks, and is replaced by intermittent splinting for an additional two to three weeks. The Kirschner wires may be removed sequentially, beginning at three weeks. Fractures of the ridge of the trapezium that continue to be symptomatic after a period of splinting may be excised using a volar, carpal tunnel type of approach.[47]

TRAPEZOID

Fractures of the trapezoid are rare because of its well-protected position, unless the fracture occurs as part of a more complex injury.

MECHANISM OF INJURY

The trapezoid is usually injured as a result of forces applied through the second metacarpal.[21]

Dislocations may occur. Dorsal dislocations are more frequent, although volar dislocations have also been reported (Fig. 7-12).[21,44,57,63] The preponderance of dorsal dislocations is explained by the wedge shape of the trapezoid. Its dorsal surface is larger than the volar and, in spite of strong volar ligaments, this asymmetry favors extrusion dorsally.[63]

DIAGNOSIS

The roentgenographic diagnosis of a dislocation of the trapezoid requires a considerable degree of clinical suspicion and a careful evaluation of the trapezoid relationship in the routine posterior anterior projections. Additional views as well as planograms may be required before a definitive diagnosis is made.

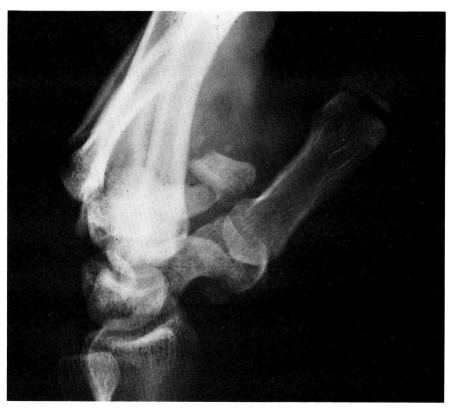

Fig. 7-12. Rare palmar dislocation of the trapezoid.

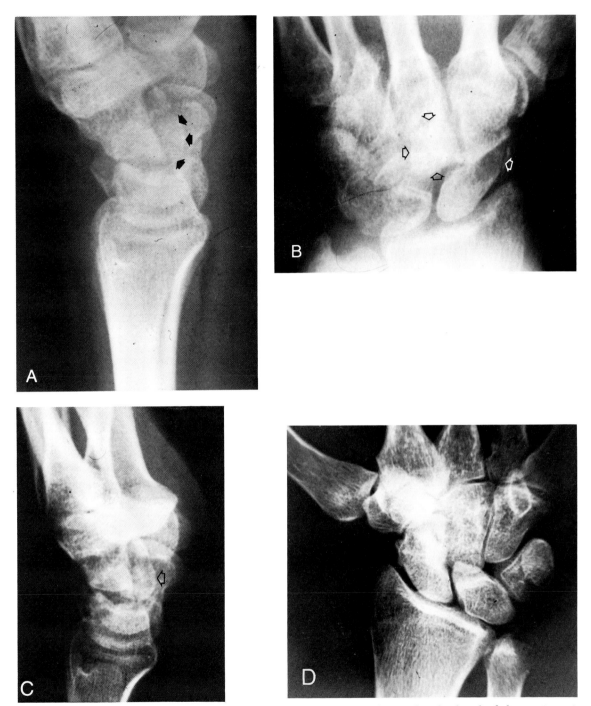

Fig. 7-13. Scaphocapitate fracture syndrome. *A*: Initial lateral radiograph. The head of the capitate is rotated 90 degrees and lies palmar to the body (arrows). *B*: Initial posteroanterior radiograph. Arrows point to the head of the capitate and the scaphoid fracture. *C and D*: Two-year follow-up. The scaphoid fracture is healed. The head of the capitate remains displaced (arrow). The patient is free of symptoms. Wrist motion and grip strength are almost normal. (From Taleisnik J: Fractures of the carpal bones. In Green DP (ed): Operative Hand Surgery. Vol. 1. Churchill Livingstone, New York, 1982.)

The very rare isolated fractures of the trapezoid may be managed by immobilization in plaster for a period of three to four weeks followed by a period of splinting until pain-free function is restored. If proximal migration of the second metacarpal occurs this may have to be corrected by surgical means including the use of a bone graft or even a partial fusion if the carpometacarpal joint is severely involved. When accompanied by other fractures or fracture-dislocations of the carpus the treatment of the trapezoid is only a part of the overall management of the entire carpal injury. In case of isolated dislocations, if the injury is seen fresh and the trapezoid is easily palpable dorsally, a closed manipulation may be attempted. It is unlikely, however, that a stable reduction could be obtained, in which case either an open or a blind pinning through the trapezoid into the surrounding bones (second metacarpal, capitate, trapezium) should be attempted. If a reduction is unsuccessful or when the patient is seen several days or weeks after the injury occurred, an open reduction should be attempted followed by internal fixation and plaster immobilization for a period of four weeks. In most instances, a dorsal surgical approach, centered at the level of the trapezoid is preferred. A volar approach, either alone or with a dorsal incision, is reserved for the more complex injury or for the volar dislocations. Although excision of the trapezoid has been reported, this may lead to a loss of carpal alignment, significant enough to be symptomatic. Therefore, even in the more difficult volar dislocations of the trapezoid, an attempt should be made to replace the bone in its original position.

CAPITATE

Fractures of the capitate may be found in combination with other major carpal fractures or as isolated injuries. Before the advent of roentgenography the diagnosis of fracture of the capitate was extremely rare. Robert in 1845 and Guibout in 1847 are credited with the earliest descriptions.[36] A longitudinal fracture of the body was described by Guermonprez (quoted by Destot).[20] Bizarro[7] included six "incomplete" fractures of the os mag-

num in his series of carpal injuries, of which at least five were located within the body of the bone. In Böhler's review of 826 carpal injuries from 1926 to 1936,[9] only seven fractures of the capitate were found, a frequency of 0.8 percent. This incidence is somewhat lower than that reported by Snodgrass[60] (1.2 percent of 170 carpal fractures) or that found by Rand and coauthors[56] in a review of 978 patients treated for carpal fractures at the Mayo Clinic. During a 13-year period, these authors encountered two ununited and 11 acute fractures of the capitate for an overall incidence of 1.3 percent. In 1962 Adler and Shaftan[1] reviewed 79 cases found in the literature and added 12 of their own. Forty-eight of these cases were isolated body fractures, 11 the so-called scaphocapitate syndrome, and 32 accompanying other carpal injuries. In general, strictly isolated capitate fractures are less frequent than those found in combination with other carpal injuries, for instance, the scaphocapitate syndrome (Fig. 7-13), or with multiple carpal fractures and dislocations (Fig. 7-14).

MECHANISM OF INJURY

In 1898 Auvray[4] published the result of an experimental study of wrist injuries. He reported that falls against the palm of the hand produced fractures of the scaphoid, while falls against the dorsum resulted in fractures of the capitate. Most capitate fractures occur, however, after falls on the outstretched hand with the wrist in dorsiflexion. The magnitude of the injury force applied to the wrist is frequently substantial.[33,56] Rarely are these fractures caused by direct blows. In Adler and Shaftan's review of 79 cases, 44 were due to falls.[1] Of these, 29 occurred on the palm of the hand, 9 on the dorsum, and 6 against the heads of the second and third metacarpals. The capitate is more susceptible to fractures through the neck, frequently found in association with fracture-dislocations of the carpus.[21] Rand and coauthors[56] point out that, during radial deviation and ulnar deviation, maximum tensile stresses are found at the level of the neck of the capitate. Jeanne and Mouchet[36] could consistently reproduce fractures of the capitate in cadavers always occurring at the level of the neck, attributed by them to be opposite actions of the

Fig. 7-14. This fracture of the head of the capitate (arrows), was part of a complex carpal and carpometacarpal injury. (Courtesy of Dr. A. Carlier, Liege, Belgium.)

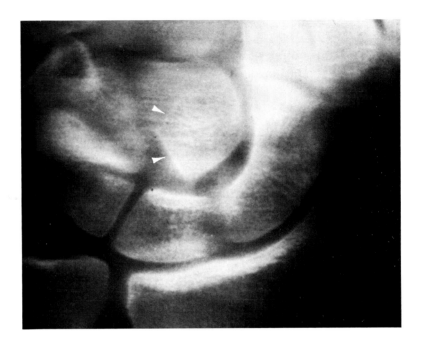

volar capsule, under tension, and the dorsal pole of the lunate acting "on the nape of the capitate." This fracture was consistently transverse in anteroposterior radiographs, but oblique from dorsal and proximal to volar and distal when viewed from the side. Jeanne and Mouchet could also produce a fracture of the capitate by applying impact loads to the dorsum of the hand with the wrist held in full volarflexion. The resulting fracture plane was perfectly transverse "in every direction . . . as if a knife had decapitated the head with a single perpendicular blow." They attributed this injury to the volar pole of the lunate striking the neck of the capitate.

The scapho capitate syndrome consists of a fracture of the neck of the capitate with rotation of the proximal fragment, associated with a fracture of the waist of the scaphoid (naviculo-capitate fracture syndrome (Fig. 7-13)).[1,25,26,40,48,50,64,66,67] The mechanism of this injury may involve a direct blow to the dorsum of the wrist in volar flexion[13,26,67] or, more frequently, a fall on the outstretched hand with the wrist in dorsiflexion.[64] Jeanne and Mouchet[36] produced experimental simultaneous fractures of the neck of the capitate and of the scaphoid, in specimens held in maximum dorsiflexion, "at or nearly at a right angle; in medium ulnar incli-

nation, or better still, combined with a certain degree of pronation." The impact loading was directed to the head of the metacarpals. Most frequently, dorsal perilunate dislocations were produced. In some cases, however, a scapho-capitate type syndrome was produced, a combination which Jeanne and Mouchet believed was clinically "not rare." When the fracture of the capitate occurred at the level of the neck, it was produced, in their opinion, by the abutment of the dorsal pole of the lunate. If the fracture was more distal, then it was preceded by a volar displacement of the lunate, allowing the body of the capitate and the dorsal rim of the radius to come in contact. These authors also produced a fracture through the waist of the scaphoid and through the neck of the capitate in wrist specimens held in dorsiflexion at right angles, and radial deviation. In these cases, a vertical intraarticular fracture of the distal radius frequently coexisted. Fenton postulated that dorsiflexion was accompanied by radial deviation, causing the waist of the scaphoid to be struck by the radial styloid. According to Fenton,[25] the scaphoid fracture occurs first; when the injury force is not fully dissipated on the scaphoid, fracture of the neck of the capitate takes place; the malrotation of the proximal fragment was thought to take place consequent to a continuation of the initial thrust. Stein and Siegel[64] demonstrated in cadaver specimens that the fracture of the capitate could be produced in forced dorsiflexion by the dorsal lip of the radius striking the capitate, while the scaphoid fractured due to the tension created at the midcarpal joint level by the forced dorsiflexion. This mechanism of capitate fracture had already been suggested by Destot.[20] With the loss of stability across the midcarpus secondary to this double fracture, an abnormal range of angulation and dorsiflexion becomes possible. The head of the capitate rotates together with the proximal fragment of the scaphoid. A volarflexion mechanism has also been suggested for some of these injuries.[67] Upon cessation of injury, several radiographic patterns may be found,[67] most commonly a scaphoid-capitate fracture syndrome without dislocation, or less frequently, accompanying a dorsal perilunate dislocation.

Avascular necrosis following fractures of the capitate not associated with a scaphoid-capitate fracture syndrome is extremely unusual.[41,42,45,52] Nonunions may occur, particularly in those cases with severe multiple carpal fractures and dislocations.

DIAGNOSIS

Most capitate fractures produce pain, swelling, and limitation of motion without clear localization of the injury to the capitate. The diagnosis is entirely based on careful radiographic evaluation and may easily be missed. Cave (quoted by Adler[1]) could demonstrate the fracture only by radiographs obtained with the wrist in traction. Laminograms and isotope scanning may be helpful (Fig. 7-14). Just as in the case of the fractures of the scaphoid, a negative scan excludes fracture, but increased local activity may assist to localize the traumatic lesion to the capitate. The scapho-capitate fracture syndrome may erroneously be labeled an isolated fracture of the scaphoid, or a typical transscaphoid perilunate fracture dislocation, while the lesion to the capitate is overlooked. In these cases, although carpal alignment may be restored promptly, either spontaneously or by manipulation, there remains persistent displacement

of the head of the capitate. Despite this, the fracture of the scaphoid can progress to union, and the patient may regain a pain-free wrist with minimal loss of function.[1]

TREATMENT

Undisplaced, isolated fractures should be immobilized in plaster. Four to six weeks are sufficient for healing. A period of protective splinting may be helpful as function of the wrist is restored following immobilization. For the scapho-capitate fracture syndrome, excision of the head fragment has been advised as the treatment of choice.[25,26,46] Other authors,[67] favor an anatomic surgical reduction of the head of the capitate, an opinion with which I concur. For this procedure, a routine dorsal surgical approach is used. The fracture itself may not be well visualized until distraction is applied to the hand and the wrist. The head fragment, frequently devoid of all soft tissue attachments, can be replaced in anatomic alignment. This may require that an assistant apply manual traction to the hand.

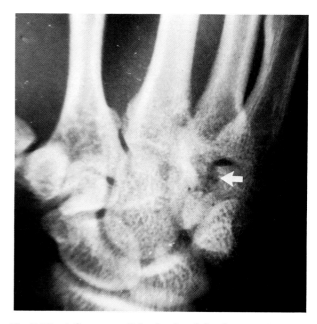

Fig. 7-15. A fracture of the body of the hamate (arrow). (From Taleisnik J: Fractures of the carpal bones. In Green DP (ed): Operative Hand Surgery. Vol. 1. Churchill Livingstone, New York, 1982.)

This allows the fragment to be seated on the neck of the capitate. Upon releasing traction, the stability of the reduction may be tested by taking the wrist through motions. If there is any hint of instability, internal fixation with a couple of fine Kirschner wires should be used. It is easier to insert the wires first distally through the fracture surface of the neck of the capitate, then reduce the head and drill the wires back in a retrograde fashion into the head. It is usually unnecessary to cross the articular surface of the capitate through the lunocapitate joint or into the lunate. At the same time, internal fixation for the fracture of the scaphoid should be performed (see Chapter 6). If this injury is treated within the first three weeks, bone grafting of either scaphoid or capitate is not required. I believe that between three and six weeks following injury, an attempt should still be made to restore anatomic alignment to the capitate, followed by internal fixation and bone grafting. The bone graft may be obtained from the distal radius. The handling of the scaphoid-capitate fracture syndrome that has remained untreated for longer than six weeks is dictated by the patient's condition. In these cases, the main problem is the fracture of the scaphoid rather than the injury to the capitate. If the fracture of the scaphoid is well aligned, and appears to be healing, immediate operative intervention is certainly not needed (Fig. 7-13). If, however, the patient is symptomatic, even with a healed fracture of the scaphoid, surgery becomes indicated. The management of this problem may have to be decided at the time of the operative procedure, and is determined by the condition of the head of the capitate as well as by the appearance and integrity of the articular surfaces of the surrounding carpal bones. If the head can be replaced and appears to be viable, this could be done. Reduction is stabilized by internal fixation with Kirschner wires and a bone graft is used. If the head is obviously avascular, or there are pericapitate degenerative changes, the head may best be excised and a partial fusion across the capitatescapholunate space performed preserving the overall dimensions of the carpus. Kimmel and O'Brien[42] reported treating avascular necrosis of the head of the capitate by excision of the involved area, and its replacement with an anchovy-type soft tissue graft. For those patients whose condition has progressed after several years to painful degenerative arthrosis, midcarpal fusions are indicated.

HAMATE

Isolated fractures of the hamate are rare. In Bizarro's[7] study of 175 cases, only eight involved the hamate. Böhler[9] found 18 among 826 carpal fractures that he reviewed. Hamate injuries are frequent in males in the second and third decades of life.[11] There are two main varieties of hamate frac-

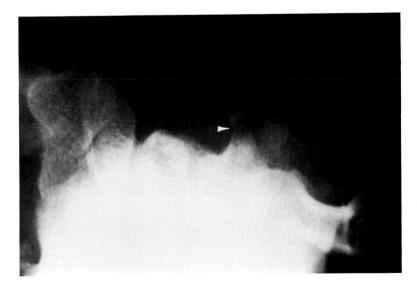

Fig. 7-16. Fracture of the hook of the hamate.

tures: those involving the body (Fig. 7-15) and those localized to the hamular process (Figs. 7-16, 7-17).[49] Fractures of the body also include those entering the distal articular surface and those localized to the proximal pole.[21] From the clinical standpoint, these fractures may be remarkably similar. There is pain on the ulnar half of the wrist, localized swelling and tenderness, usually over the dorsal ulnar projection of the body of the hamate, even for those fractures of the hamulus that do not include the body itself.[15,62] Although involvement of the ulnar nerve is more likely in fractures at the base of the hamulus, ulnar neuropathies have been described following fractures of the body of the

hamate as well, sometimes appearing as tardy forms, and believed to be secondary to perineurofibrosis.[15] Dislocations are rare, but have been reported[22,28,38] as early as 1901 by Oberst and by Eigenbrodt (quoted by Johansson[38]).

MECHANISM OF INJURY

Fractures of the body of the hamate are frequently osteochondral injuries from impaction of the hamate against the lunate during forced dorsiflexion and ulnar deviation. Sheering injuries involving a sudden, violent torque applied to the

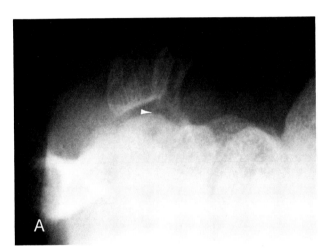

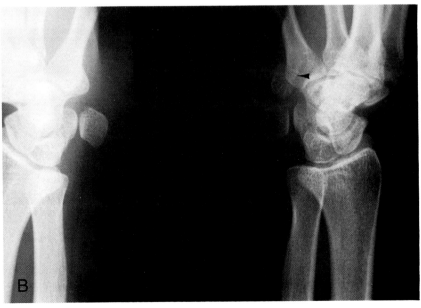

Fig. 7-17. A: Fracture of the hook of the hamate, suspected in a carpal tunnel radiographic projection, is better visualized in a reverse-oblique view. *B:* Left radiograph is of the normal wrist; in the right radiograph the fracture of the hook of the hamate is shown by the arrow.

hand have been described.[21] The fracture may also occur through direct injury or as a result of a force driven along the shaft of the fifth metacarpal as from a fall or a blow on the fist with the wrist in ulnar deviation.[21] The fracture of the hook of the hamate is most likely secondary to a direct blow produced by the butt end of a golf club, baseball bat, or tennis racquet, or following a fall striking the base of the hypothenar area.[14,15,53,62,65]

DIAGNOSIS AND TREATMENT

Fractures of the Body of the Hamate

These fractures are diagnosed by careful radiographic examination, including several oblique projections until the fracture can be clearly visualized (Fig. 7-15). At times, tomography may be helpful. Not infrequently, this type of fracture is accompanied by fractures of the base of the ulnar metacarpals. The fracture line is usually oblique, either ulnar, or, more frequently, radial to the radiographic projection of the hook.[49] Jeanne and Mouchet[36] presented six cases in 1919, of which four had an oblique fracture separating a proximal and lateral third from the rest of the body of the hamate. A fracture in the coronal plane, not diagnosed until surgical exploration, was described by Bowen.[11] Generally, these are stable injuries and become asymptomatic after a period of immobilization of four to six weeks, even if fibrous union is present. This may be because the fracture line remains entirely extraarticular, or if it enters the carpometacarpal joint, it does so between the facets for the articulation of the fourth and fifth metacarpals. Articular fractures with significant displacement may require an open reduction and internal fixation. Painful pseudoarthrosis have not been reported in the modern literature: only Vulpius (quoted by Johansson[38]) reported a case of a painful pseudoarthrosis.

Fractures of the Hamular Process

In 1906 a fracture of the hook of the hamate was reported by Chevrier (quoted by Jeanne and Mouchet[36]). This is the first recorded instance of such an injury in the post-Röntgen era. Fractures of the hook of the hamate may be easily missed. This in-

jury should be strongly suspected, however, when a deep, ill-defined pain is referred to the ulnar half of the wrist, particularly in golfers,[15,53,62,65] but also in tennis, baseball, and squash players.[15,62] Symptoms are aggravated when attempting to swing a golf club, tennis racquet, or baseball bat. Tenderness may be elicited by deep palpation over the tip of the hook of the hamate in the palm and by pressure on the dorsal ulnar aspect of this bone.[15,62] The hook of the hamate is consistently found distal and radial to the pisiform, along a line traced from the pisiform to the head of the third metacarpal.[29] Lateral movements of the little finger against resistance increase the discomfort. Ulnar nerve involvement has been reported[3,34,59] and has been attributed to hemorrhage, edema and intra- or extraneurofibrosis of the nerve within the "loge de Guyon."[34,53,59] Guyon's canal is closely related to the hamulus, which constitutes its lateral and distal wall;[30] the medial and more proximal boundary is the pisiform. The floor of the canal is covered by the deep reflection of the transverse carpal ligament and the pisohamate ligament. The canal is covered by the volar carpal ligament anteriorly. Not only can the ulnar nerve be involved in fractures of the hamulus, but also ruptures by attrition of flexor profundus tendons may occur against the rough irregularity of the fracture site.[18] The diagnosis is confirmed by radiographic demonstration of the fracture. The carpal tunnel profile view described by Hart and Gaynor[31] is particularly helpful (Fig. 7-16). An oblique projection obtained with the hand in 45 degree of supination and the wrist in radial deviation[3] and dorsiflexion is also useful (Fig. 7-17). In both these projections, demonstration of the hamulus may require several radiographs in slightly different degrees of rotation, until a satisfactory profile of the hook is obtained. Although rare, bipartition of the hamulus has been mentioned in the differential diagnosis[29] and carpal tunnel views of the uninjured hand have been recommended to assist in establishing this diagnosis, for bipartition may be suspected if bilateral and without a clear-cut history of injury. Tomograms are helpful when all other views fail to demonstrate the fracture and the diagnosis is still strongly suggested on the basis of the history, the patient's symptoms, and the clinical findings.[8,51]

With few exceptions the recommended treatment has been excision of the ununited hamular fragment, even in fractures through the very base of the hamulus.[8,14,15,23,49,53,62,65,72] The indications for excision are usually pain and symptoms suggestive of ulnar neuropathy. Very rarely the indication for surgical treatment arises from involvement of the flexor tendons either by tenosynovitis or rupture. Excision is carried out through a short palmar incision overlying the projection of the hook. Care should be taken to preserve the integrity of the motor branch of the ulnar nerve, which is in close proximity to the hamular process. In some patients there may be some difficulty localizing the fracture site, but superiosteal dissection and gentle manipulation of the tip of the hamulus should lead to the site of nonunion. The fracture fragment is excised, smoothness to the base of the hook of the hamate is restored, and this is covered by careful repair of the overlying periosteal layer. Postoperative casting immobilization is required only until acute tenderness subsides after which a gradual return to full activities is allowed.

REFERENCES

1. Adler JB, Shaftan GW: Fractures of the capitate. J Bone Joint Surg [Am] 44:1537, 1962
2. Alsberg A: Isolierte Fraktur des Erbsenbeins. Z Orthop Chir 20:299, 1908
3. Andress MR, Peckar VG: Fracture of the hook of the hamate. Br J Radiol 43:141, 1970
4. Auvray M: Fracture de scaphoide de la main avec luxation d'un des fragments sur la face dorsale. Gaz Hop (Paris) 71:377, 1898
5. Baird DB, Freidenberg ZB: Delayed ulnar-nerve palsy following a fracture of the hamate. J Bone Joint Surg [Am] 50:570, 1968
6. Bartone NF, Grieco V: Fractures of the triquetrum. J Bone Joint Surg [Am] 38:353, 1956
7. Bizarro AH: Traumatology of the carpus. Surg Gynecol Obstet 34:574, 1922
8. Blair WF, Kilpatrick WC, Omer GE: Open fracture of the hook of the hamate. A case report. Clin Orthop 163:1801, 1982
9. Böhler L: Tecnica del tratamiento de las fracturas. 3rd Ed. translated from the German. 7th Ed. Schneider G, Jimeno Vidal F (eds). Vol. 1. Editorial Labor S.A. Barcelona, 1954
10. Bonnin JG, Greening SW: Fractures of the triquetrum. Br J Surg 31:278, 1944
11. Bowen TI: Injuries of the hamate bone. Hand 5:235, 1973
12. Boyes JH: More accurate diagnosis of hand and wrist injuries. Consultant 144, 1973
13. Bryan RS, Dobyns JH: Fractures of the carpal bones other than lunate and navicular. Clin Orthop 149:107, 1980
14. Cameron HU, Hastings DE, Fournasier VL: Fractures of the hook of the hamate: a case report. J Bone Joint Surg [Am] 57:276, 1975
15. Carter PR, Eaton PH, Littler JW: Ununited fracture of the hook of the hamate. J Bone Joint Surg [Am] 59:583, 1977
16. Codman EA, Chase HM: The diagnosis and treatment of fracture of the carpal scaphoid and dislocation of the semilunar bone, with a report of thirty cases. Ann Surg 41:863, 1905
17. Cordrey LJ, Ferrer-Torells M: Management of fractures of the greater multangular. Report of five cases. J Bone Joint Surg [Am] 42:1111, 1960
18. Crosby EB, Linscheid RL: Rupture of the flexor profundus tendon of the ring finger secondary to ancient fracture of the hook of the hamate. J Bone Joint Surg [Am] 56:1076, 1974
19. Deane RB: Single fracture of the pisiform bone. Ann Surg 54:229, 1911
20. Destot E: Injuries of the wrist: A radiological study. Translated by Atkinson FRB. Ernest Benn, London, 1925
21. Dobyns JH, Linscheid RL: Fractures and dislocations of the wrist. p.345. In Rockwood CA Jr, Green DP, (eds): Fractures, Lippincott, Philadelphia, 1975
22. Duke R: Dislocation of the hamate bone: Report of a case. J Bone Joint Surg 45B:744, 1963
23. Dunn AW: Fractures and dislocations of the carpus. Surg Clin North Am 52:1513, 1972
24. Durbin FC: Nonunion of the triquetrum. J Bone Joint Surg [Br] 32:388. 1950
25. Fenton RL: The naviculo-capitate fracture syndrome. J Bone Joint Surg [Am] 38:681, 1956
26. Fenton RL, Rosen H: Fracture of the capitate bone: Report of two cases. Bull Hosp Joint Dis 11:134, 1950
27. Frykman E: Dislocation of the triquetrum: Case report. Scand J Plast Reconstr Surg 14:205,1980
28. Geist DC: Dislocation of the hamate bone. J Bone Joint Surg 21:215, 1939
29. Greene MH, Handied AM: Bipartite hamulus with ulnar tunnel syndrome — Case report and literature review. J Hand Surg 6:605, 1981
30. Guyon F: Note sur une disposition anatomique propre a la face anterieure de la region du poignet et nonencore decrite. Bull Soc Anat Paris 6:184, 1861
31. Hart VL, Gaynor V: Roentgenographic study of the carpal canal. J Bone Joint Surg 23:382, 1941

32. Helal B: Racquet player's pisiform. Hand 10:87, 1978
33. Hook FR: Fractures of the carpus. US Naval Med Bull 37:553, 1939
34. Howard FM: Ulnar nerve palsy in wrist fractures. J Bone Joint Surg 43:1197, 1961
35. Immermann EW: Dislocation of the pisiform. J Bone Joint Surg [Am] 30:489, 1948
36. Jeanne LA and Mouchet A: Les lesions traumatiques fermeés du poignet. 28th Congrès Français de Chirurgie, 1919
37. Jenkins SA: Osteoarthritis of the pisiform-triquetral joint. Report of three cases. J Bone Joint Surg [Br] 33:532, 1951
38. Johansson S: Ein Fall von Luxation des Os Hamatum. Acta Radiol 7:9, 1926
39. Johnson RP: The acutely injured wrist and its residuals. Clin Orthop 149:33, 1980
40. Jones GB: An unusual fracture-dislocation of the carpus. J Bone Joint Surg [Br] 37:146, 1955
41. Jonsson G: Aseptic bone necrosis of the os capitatum. Acta Radiol 23:562, 1942
42. Kimmel RB, O'Brien ET: Surgical treatment of avascular necrosis of the proximal pole of the capitate. Case report. J Hand Surg 7:284, 1982
43. LeCocq EA: Traumatic arthritis of the pisiform-triangular joint. Case report. West J Surg 59:357, 1951
44. Lewis HH: Dislocation of the lesser multangular. J Bone Joint Surg [Am] 44:1412, 1962
45. Lowry WE, Cord SA: Traumatic avascular necrosis of the capitate bone. Case report. J Hand Surg 6:245, 1981
46. Lucero B: Fractura del carpo en un niño. Bol Trab Soc Argent Cirujanos 10:260, 1943
47. McClain EJ, Boyes JH: Missed fractures of the greater multangular. J Bone Joint Surg [Am] 48:1525, 1966
48. Meyers MH, Wells R, Harvey JP: Naviculo-capitate fracture syndrome. Review of the literature and a case report. J Bone Joint Surg [Am] 53:1383, 1971
49. Milch H: Fracture of the hamate bone. J Bone Joint Surg 16:459, 1934
50. Monahan PRW, Galasko CSB: The scapho-capitate fracture syndrome. A mechanism of injury. J Bone Joint Surg [Br] 54:122, 1972
51. Murray WT, Meuller PR, Rosenthal DI, Javerner RR: Fracture of the hook of the hamate. Am J Roentgenol 133:899, 1979
52. Newman JH, Watt I: Avascular necrosis of the capitate and dorsal dorsi-flexion instability. Hand 12:176, 1980
53. Nisenfield FG, Neviaser RJ: Fracture of the hook of the hamate: A diagnosis easily missed. J Trauma 14:612, 1974
54. Palmieri TJ: The excision of painful pisiform bone fractures. Orthop Rev 11:99, 1982
55. Pineyro MR, Adaminas AE: Fracturas del Piramidal. pp. 55–65. Primera Sesion Ordinaria, Sociedad Argentina de Ortopedia y Traumatologia, Buenos Aires. April 26, 1966
56. Rand JA, Linscheid RL, Dobyns JH: Capitate fractures: A long-term follow-up. Clin Orthop 165:209, 1982
57. Russell TB: Inter-carpal dislocations and fracture-dislocations: A review of fifty-nine cases. J Bone Joint Surg [Br] 31:524, 1949
58. Sgrosso JA: Traumatismos del carpo: Tratamiento. pp. 1–140. Decimosexto Congreso Argentin de Cirugia, Buenos Aires, 1944
59. Shea JD, McClain EJ: Ulnar nerve compression syndromes at and below the wrist. J Bone Joint Surg [Am] 51:1095, 1969
60. Snodgrass LE: Fractures of the carpal bones. Am J Surg 38:539, 1937
61. Soucacos PN, Hartofilakidis-Garofalidis GC: Dislocation of the triangular bone: Report of a case. J Bone Joint Surg [Am] 63:1012, 1981
62. Stark HH, Jobe FW, Boyes JH, Ashworth CR: Fracture of the hook of the hamate in athletes. J Bone Joint Surg [Am] 59:575, 1977
63. Stein AH: Dorsal dislocation of the lesser multangular bone. J Bone Joint Surg [Am] 53:377, 1971
64. Stein F, Siegel MW: Naviculocapitate fracture syndrome: A case report. J Bone Joint Surg [Am] 51:391, 1969
65. Torisu T: Fracture of the hook of the hamate by a golf swing. Clin Orthop 83:91, 1972
66. Van Cauwenberghe R: Un cas rare de fracture-luxation du carpe. Acta Orthop Belg 23:79, 1957
67. Vance RM, Gelberman RH, Evans EF: Scaphocapitate fractures: Patterns of dislocation, mechanisms of injury, and preliminary results of treatment. J Bone Joint Surg [Am] 62:271, 1980
68. Vasilas A, Grieco V, Bartone NF: Roentgen aspects of injuries to the pisiform bone and pistotriquetral joint. J Bone Joint Surg [Am] 42:1317, 1960
69. Weston WJ, Kelsey CK: Functional anatomy of the pisi-cuneiform joints. Br J Radiol 46:692, 1973
70. Wilson JN: Profiles of the carpal canal. J Bone Joint Surg [Am] 36:127, 1954
71. Wiot JF, Dorst JP: Less common fractures and dislocations of the wrist. Radiol Clin North Am 4:261, 1966
72. Wissin HA: Resection of the hook of the hamate. Plast Reconstr Surg 56:501, 1975

8 Kienböck's Disease

Before the discovery of x-rays by Röntgen, the occurrence of fractures and other traumatic anomalies of isolated carpal bones was believed to be nearly impossible. Abnormal lunate specimens found in anatomic dissections were thought to represent skeletal variations rather than posttraumatic conditions. Thus avulsion or "chip" fractures were diagnosed as supernumerary bones, and were called "epilunatum" when located along the dorsal lunate and "hypolunatum" when on the palmar aspect. Lunates found split into two main, larger pieces, of roughly equal size, were called "bipartitum." More frequently, the proximal dome of the lunate was comminuted with abnormal changes of the overlying cartilaginous articular cover. This was the "lunatum partitum."[56] Fractures of the lunate were recognized as such in exceptional cases, and only when associated with other injuries.[81] Kienböck[56] reviewed these anatomic descriptions, as well as radiographs published between 1895 and 1910, including those of his own patients, and concluded that in most cases there was a "regular localization of the more severe changes in the proximal part" of the lunate. These changes involved both "the shape and the structure" of the lunate. In 1910 he published his study *Traumatic Malacia of the Semilunar Bone.* Kienböck postulated that traumatic lesions of the lunate were not as rare as was suggested by the medical literature of the time. Since this classic description, however, neither the cause nor a reliable treatment for lunatomalacia have been established with certainty.

ETIOLOGY

The cause of lunatomalacia has remained elusive. Many theories have attempted to explain the structural changes that allow lunate collapse, but none has been clearly proven. Kienböck[56] noted that the investigator's background had a lot to do with his interpretation of the problem. Thus the anatomist did not recognize lunatomalacia as a disease and attributed lunate changes to *congenital or developmental disorders*, while surgeons, such as R. Wolff, considered lunatomalacia to be primarily a *traumatic* occurrence. Wolff (quoted by Kienböck[56]) had mentioned that in all probability lunate changes were the result of compression fractures occurring by crushing of the bone between capitate and radius. Radiologists, on the other hand, such as Kienböck himself (and Preisser in the case of the scaphoid) believed that fractures were secondary, occurring within bone made already soft, porous, or sclerotic by the *"primary rupture of the ligaments and blood vessels."* Kienböck postulated that at the moment of injury there is a transient perilunar luxation of the hand, causing perilunar ligamentous tears which "obviously deprive the semilunar bone of important arteries." This concept of traumatic interference with the circulation or ligament injury with subsequent degeneration and collapse has been shared by others,[29,66] in spite of the lack of objective evidence of ligament tears[22,36] and the absence, for the most part, of avascularity following actual dislocation of the lunate.[30,50] Lesire and Allieu[61] point out that lunate subluxation and dislocation with retention of the palmar radiolunate ligament lead to avascular changes in 17 percent of cases. This figure increases to 50 percent in those patients with complete dislocation and displacement of the lunate and tear of all ligamentous attachments. The evolution of this avascular necrosis is, however, different than that found in Kienböck's disease: although there is increased bony density, architectural changes, collapse and fragmentation of the lunate may not occur if prolonged immobilization is continued.

Lunatomalacia has also been attributed to *hematogenous infections,*[46] *primary circulatory deficiency,*[7,60,76] and *median neuropathy*[21] within the carpal tunnel. More frequently, Kienböck's disease is believed to represent the sequela of *single or multiple fractures,* resulting in secondary vascular impairment.   [10,12,13,18,22,27,32,43,45,55,71,79,80,105,111,-112,115] Mueller[72] recognized three types of injury: *anatomical,* produced by an abnormal loading allowed by anatomical anomalies; *occupational,* due to repeated minimal trauma; and *traumatic,* caused by a single acute episode resulting in a fracture of the lunate. He also observed in two of his patients that the ulna was shorter than the radius, an anatomical variation later found by Hultén[50] to be more frequent than normal in patients with Kienböck's disease. Cordes[22] found fissures largely parallel to the proximal articular surface of the lunate in microscopic examinations of relatively fresh cases of lunatomalacia. In a review of 158 radiographs showing lunate abnormalities, Brolin[16] subjected 90 to tomographic examinations and found 27 fractures dividing the lunate into major palmar and dorsal fragments, and only 10 where the fracture plane was parallel to the proximal articular surface. Fractures in the series of Armistead and coauthors[5] were predominantly oriented in the frontal plane. The question of whether lunate fractures or fissures are primary and precede the avascular changes, or occur secondarily in a porotic weakened bone, remains, however, largely unanswered. There is some evidence to suggest that there are actual primary simple major fractures of the lunate, which may or may not lead to avascular changes in one or both of the fracture fragments. These fractures frequently occur on a frontal plane,

producing two major lunate pieces, one volar and one dorsal. They follow clear-cut traumatic episodes, and don't necessarily lead to the collapse seen in the typical lunatomalacia (Fig. 8-1). Conversely, in Kienböck's disease, there may or may not be a definitive traumatic episode preceding the onset of symptoms, and the radiologic features are different than those of a simple fracture. These two types of changes justify the differentiation between the bipartite lunates and the "lunate partitum." Kienböck had described both types, and observed that "it cannot be imagined that a healthy semilunar bone could be flattened by the effects of a force . . . without accompanying injuries to the adjacent bones."[56]

In 1928 Hultén published a comparative study of distal radioulnar relationships in radiographs of normal wrists and in patients with Kienböck's disease.[50] In 51 percent of the normal individuals, the distal articular surfaces of radius and ulna were found to be at the same level; this was referred to as the *zero variant.* The ulna was proximal to the radius, the *ulna-minus variant,* in only 23 percent of 400 normal wrists. In contrast to this normal proportion, the majority of patients wth Kienböck's disease (18 out of 23) showed an ulna-minus stance. Only five cases showed a zero variant. The ulna-plus relationship was not present in this group of patients. Although no simple causative factor could be verified for this disease in Axelsson's extensive review, enough objective data was found to support Hultén's *minus variant theory*[6] Gelberman and coauthors[40] also found a statistically significant association between negative ulnar variants and Kienböck's disease in a comparison study of roentgenograms of normal and affected wrists in randomly selected white and black patients. They were careful to point out, however, that the significant association found between negative ulnar variants and the presence of Kienböck's disease should not be considered a *primary* etiologic association, and that negative ulnar variants must at best be only predisposing factors. Only Köstler[58] disagreed with the importance of a minus variant configuration in the production of Kienböck's disease. In the minus variant wrist the ulnar half of the lunate lacks its normal protective support from the ulna. Because of uneven resistance between the articular surface of the radius and the cartilaginous ulnocar-

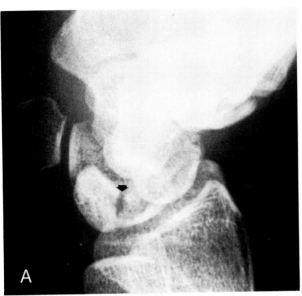
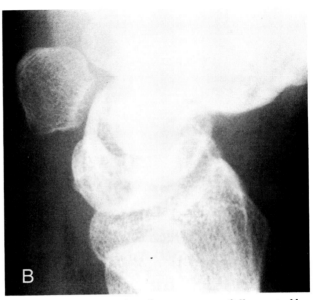

Fig. 8-1. *A*: Lunate fracture (arrow) following a fall on the hand with the wrist in dorsiflexion, successfully treated by immobilization and the application of pulsing electromagnetic field treatment. *B*: Appearance after five months of treatment.

pal complex, loads on the radial half of the lunate are comparatively greater.[16] The lunate is subjected to a "nutcracker" effect between the ulnar border of the radius and the head of the capitate, a mechanism already suggested at the turn of this century by Pfitzner.[82,83] R. Wolff, Wittek, and Ebermayer (quoted by Kienböck[56]) also attributed malacia changes to compression of the lunate "like a nut" between capitate and radius. The increased incidence of Kienböck's disease in adult patients with cerebral palsy, although attributed to disturbances in blood supply, may well be secondary to a chronic nutcracker effect on the lunate, rendered more vulnerable in cerebral palsy patients by their forced habitual volarflexed attitude. In 1966 Antuña Zapico[4] observed a relationship between the shape of the lunate and the length of the ulna. In ulnar-minus wrists the proximal and medial aspects of the lunate, as seen in posteroanterior radiographs, converge into a prominent proximal apex or crest; this is a type I lunate (Fig. 8-2A). Zero and ulnar-plus variants coexist with more square or rectangular lunates, the types II and III (Fig. 8-2B,C). In 1936, Franck[39] established that the trabeculae within the lunate are perpendicular to the articular surfaces and, therefore, related to the ability of the

bone to receive and transmit loads. Antuña Zapico incorporated Franck's concept into his three types of lunates and suggested that the trabecular pattern in type I is the weakest (Fig. 8-2D); compression loads would result in increased intertrabecular angulation and a greater potential for bone fatigue and stress fractures. If a fracture is already present, this trabecular arrangement would interfere with attempts at healing, particularly in the presence of an increased "nutcracker" effect. Lunate fragmentation is more frequent in ulna-minus variants with type I lunates. Razemon[86] directed attention to yet another anatomical peculiarity of the lunate in patients with Kienböck's disease. While in most normal wrists, posteroanterior radiographs in neutral position show the lunate mostly under the radius, in patients with Kienböck's disease the overlap of the lunate with the ulnocarpal complex is significant (Fig. 8-3). In the first case, stresses may be uniformly dissipated throughout the lunate, while in the second, there is an uneven compression, with the radial half of the lunate receiving most of the stress during loading.

In 1967 Rossack[93] also stressed the importance of the ulna minus variant in the pathogenesis of Kienböck's disease. He postulated that the lunate is

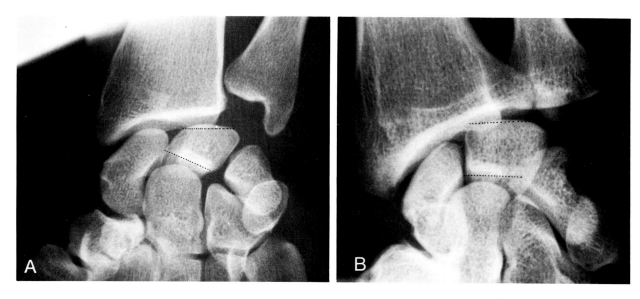

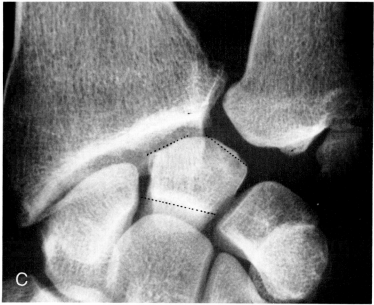

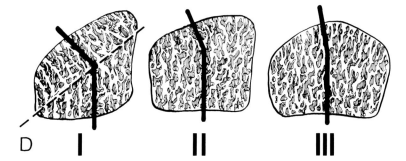

Fig. 8-2. Types of lunate and relationship with ulnar variance according to Antuña Zapico. *A:* Type I lunate coexists with ulna minus variant. *B* and *C:* Types II and III lunates coexist with zero and ulna plus variants. *D:* Trabecular patterns for types I, II and III lunates. (See Ref. 4.)

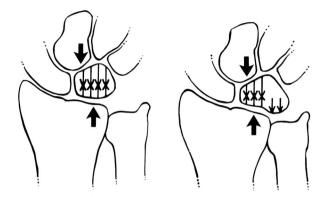

Fig. 8-3. In most normal wrists, lunate is mostly under the radius (left); in patients with Kienböck's disease, lunate is subject to uneven compression between radius and ulnocarpal complex (right). (See Ref. 86.)

subject to greater shear stresses in forced ulnar deviation. In ulna-minus wrists, shear and compression loads on the lunate are greater during ulnar deviation, favoring compression fractures and vascular changes. Study of load stresses on the lunate[55] tend to support Hultén's theory demonstrating concentration of forces on the lunate in dorsiflexion and ulnar deviation,[55] and tensile forces on the distal surface of the lunate that predispose it to fracture.[5,55] Armistead and coauthors[5] suggest that in extreme dorsiflexion, radiolunate and lunotriquetral ligaments become tense. The triquetrum is more likely to shift dorsally and proximally on the lunate because it is supported solely by the softer ulnocarpal cartilaginous complex. Tension through the triquetrolunate ligament is transmitted to the palmar pole of the lunate. This, added to compression between capitate and radius, results in failure, most frequently at the junction of the anterior and middle thirds of the lunate (Fig. 8-4). There are other, more nebulous, factors that must also be implicated in the pathogenesis of Kienböck's disease. For instance, the absolute rarity of Kienböck's disease in the Chinese is difficult to explain, as is the infrequent appearance of other "osteochondritis," such as Legg-Perthe's disease of the hip, Köhler's disease of the tarsal navicular, and Sever's disease of the os calcis. Chan and Huang[19] reported a study of 400 random roentgenograms of the wrist in Chinese patients who were

seen in consultation for other conditions. The study was patterned after that of Hultén's. Contrary to Hultén's findings, there was a majority of plus variant wrists amongst Chinese patients. However, the ulna minus group, although smaller, showed a distribution of radioulnar discrepancies similar to that in Hultén's study. Chan and Huang concluded that the rarity of Kienböck's disease in the Chinese cannot be explained solely on the basis of a radioulnar anatomic variation. Racial and constitutional factors were thought to be more important. A particular hormonal and metabolic makeup that allows local mechanical factors, that is increased intraarticular pressures, to interfere with bone response at the cellular and capillary level, has also been postulated.[4]

From this review of the literature it is apparent that no single cause can be blamed for the production of Kienböck's disease, but that instead, an insidious combination of factors must be required for lunatomalacia to occur. In all likelihood, Kienböck's disease results from repeated compression stresses or, more rarely, from a single severe com-

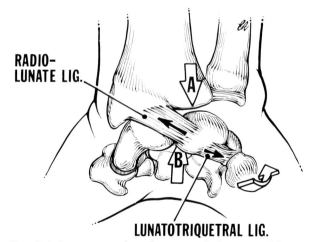

Fig. 8-4. In extreme dorsiflexion, radiolunate and lunotriquetral ligaments become tense producing equal forces of opposite directions acting on the lunate (black arrows). The triquetrum is more likely to shift dorsally and proximally on the more compliant ulnocarpal cartilaginous complex (right arrow). Added compression from radius *(A)* and capitate *(B)* result in lunate failure. (See Ref. 5.)

pression load, possibly associated with tensile forces on the concave distal surface of the lunate, producing a disruption of the intraosseous trabecular pattern in morphologically vulnerable lunates. Disruption of blood supply,[41,59] secondary synovitis, intraarticular effusions,[73] and the unavoidable continuous stress of normal function on this "carpal keystone"[56,65] interfere with attempts at healing. The lunate is rendered susceptible to the "nutcracker" effect between radius and capitate, particularly in those patients exhibiting the ulna-minus variant of radioulnar relationship. A self-perpetuating mechanism is thus set in motion, leading to progressive lunate collapse and fragmentation, and eventual loss of carpal height.

DIAGNOSIS

Although lunatomalacia may be suspected on clinical grounds alone, the actual diagnosis is strictly based on radiographic studies. There may not be a strict correlation between the patient's disability and the severity of the roentgenographic changes; severely disabled patients with minor lunate abnormalities as well as patients with chronic disease and severe fragmentation of the lunate but with only a relatively minimal disability, are not infrequent (Fig. 8-5). The pain may be deceptively mild even initially. This can explain the poor recollection that many patients have for what may have been the precipitating injury. The lack of severe pain may be due to the anatomical characteristics of the lunate, an actual cartilaginous shell devoid of nerve endings with very small areas covered with periosteum.[16,66] The degree of pain may actually be directly proportional to the severity of the reactive mechanical synovitis, rather than to the actual appearance of the lunate in radiographs. This is a disease of the young adult male whose occupation is frequently physically demanding, involving the major dominant wrist in the majority of cases. These patients have limitation of motion of the wrist, and some swelling and tenderness that is localized to the area of the lunate. A specific severe traumatic event predating the onset of symptoms may be absent or forgotten, although some form of injury is described by a significant number of patients. Dorsiflexion is particularly limited,[10] and

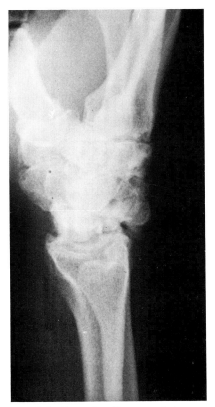

Fig. 8-5. Carpal collapse and degenerative changes 29 years following onset of Kienböck's disease.

there is a striking weakness of grip for the relative paucity of clinical findings. The average grip strength in different series varies between 47 percent[10] and 53 percent[5] of the normal uninvolved hand. Symptoms suggestive of involvement of the median nerve within the carpal tunnel have been reported,[10,21] underlying the importance of radiographic examination of patients with apparent typical carpal tunnel syndromes without complaints specifically referred to the lunate area. Release of the carpal tunnel has been shown effective in relieving symptoms in these patients[10,52] and has been advocated as a treatment of choice for Kienböck's disease by some authors.[21]

Radiographs may show no abnormalities initially except for the presence of the ulna-minus variant and a type I lunate (Fig. 8-6A). Trispiral tomography may be of help in this very early situation. Bone scintigraphy may show an abnormal lunate up-

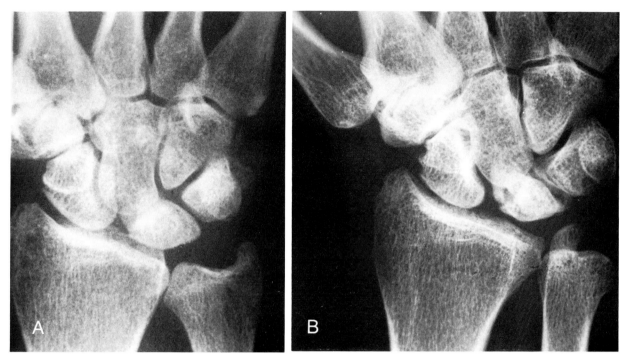

Fig. 8-6. A: Initial radiograph of patient with painful wrist. There is a type I lunate and minimal ulna minus variant. *B*: At three months. There is sclerosis and early fragmentation of the lunate.

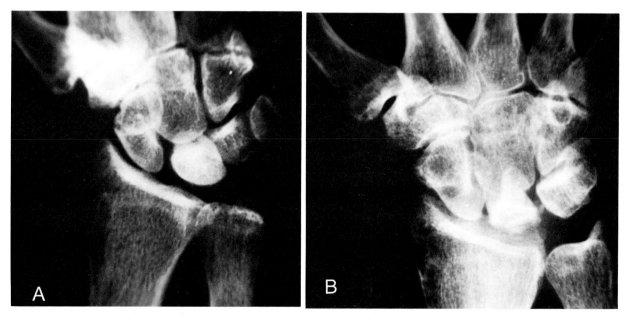

Fig. 8-7. A: Increased density of the lunate. There is no collapse or fragmentation. *B*: Increased sclerosis, collapse, and deformity of the lunate at four months.

take.[11] During the ensuing weeks, more typical radiographic findings such as sclerosis, flattening, eventually fragmentation, and collapse become apparent (Figs. 8-6B, 8-7). Decoulx and coauthors[25] proposed a radiographic classification into four stages: In stage I there is increasing density with preservation of the form of the lunate. Excessive radiodensity of the lunate may be more striking because of decreased radiodensity of the surrounding carpal bones due to disuse and immobilization.[11] Stage II occurs when cystic changes become apparent. In stage III there is collapse and fragmentation, and in stage IV perilunate osteoarthritis is present.[8] Loss of lunate height does not translate into a corresponding loss of carpal height until fragmentation allows the scaphoid to volarflex to a foreshortened perpendicular alignment, with simultaneous dorsiflexion of the triquetrum as it descends to a "low" or distal position on the hamate (see Chapter 3). The simultaneous but opposite rotation of scaphoid and triquetrum within the proximal carpal row is indicative of car-

pal dissociation, except that in Kienböck's disease the dissociation does not take place at a joint interface, but occurs within the substance of the lunate and is allowed by its fragmentation (Fig. 8-8). Armistead et al.[5] studied the degree of carpal collapse by the method proposed by Youm and collaborators[120] (see Chapter 5) and found initial proximal migration of the carpus in 11 of 20 patients. In early cases, a fracture may be seen, most frequently of the anterior pole of the lunate along a frontal plane (Fig. 8-9).

TREATMENT

There are many forms of treatment proposed for Kienböck's disease, designed either to correct one or more of the factors that may cause lunate collapse, or to treat the collapsed lunate itself.[20,23,29,31,47,50,60,64,73,76,79,80,107,108] In his landmark study Kienböck stated that the initial stages of the disease may be managed ". . . according to the usual general principles of massage, of hot

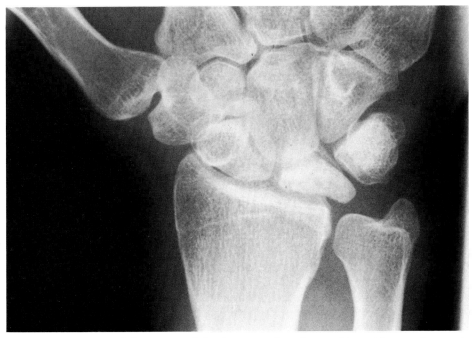

Fig. 8-8. Collapse and flattening of the lunate with radiographic evidence of opposite rotations of scaphoid (foreshortened = palmarflexed) and triquetrum (distal = dorsiflexed).

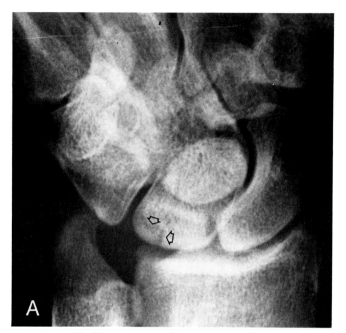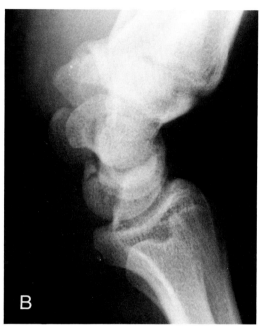

Fig. 8-9. Early fractures may be seen most frequently on the palmar pole of the lunate along a frontal plane. *A:* Posteroanterior radiograph. There is an ulna minus variant. Arrows point to lesion within the lunate. *B:* Lateral view.

compresses, hot air treatments, etcetera."[56] He added that "in the cases with severe disturbances, intense pain and incapacity for work, the semilunar bone is removed." Since then several authors have reported good results following simple excision of the lunate,[18,29,35,44,66,71,95,109] while others have called this procedure, now largely abandoned, "crippling" or "mutilating."[105] MacConaill stressed the importance of side-to-side intercarpal pressures for the normal function of the wrist, particularly between scaphoid and lunate, and triquetrum and lunate.[65] He described the carpus as a screw-vise or clamp; in palmarflexion, scaphoid and lunate tend to separate, while in dorsiflexion, scaphoid lunate and triquetrum are "screwed together." During initial dorsiflexion, as the scaphoid becomes longitudinal, it effectively joins the distal carpal row and continues to move with it. It becomes the fixed jaw of a vise. During the second stage of dorsiflexion, the triquetrum "is screwed toward the navicular, pushing the lunate with it. The resemblance of the whole mechanism to that of a screw-vise or screw-clamp is made more obvious." In MacConaill's opinion, the substitution of fibrous tissue for the lunate after excision destroys the effect of the lateral pressures that are produced by this carpal clamp resulting in progressive carpal disorganization. After lunate excision became obsolete because of its biomechanical drawbacks, other procedures were suggested that attempted to preserve carpal architecture. Konjetzny[57] proposed to remove the dorsal cortex expecting that this would open the core of the lunate to vascular invasion from the surrounding tissues and to eventual replacement with living bone. Müeller,[72] Remijnse,[90] and others[105] showed that enucleation of necrotic bone in early cases with preservation of the lunate shell could lead to satisfactory results. The filling of the collapsing lunate with material that could eventually be replaced by bone (i.e., plaster of paris) was attempted as a substitute for lunate excision.[76] More recently, Tajima has proposed an operation involving a palmar exposure of the lunate, curettage of the necrotic area, and packing of the cavity with autogenous cancellous bone chips.[110] His results, however, have not been published. Replacement of the excised lunates with a lunate filler was the logical next step. This was attempted using soft tissues,[89,113] bone,[47] or else replacement arthroplasties made of Vitallium,[64] acrylic,[1,9] or medical grade silicone rubber.[106,107,108]

Ståhl[105] and others suggested that prolonged immobilization alone may be the treatment of choice for these patients, particularly in the initial stages of the disease.[76,87,99] This concept never gained widespread acceptance.[62] However, recent reports indicate that nonsurgical treatment, although accompanied by pain with use and progressive radiologic osteoarthritis, is rarely accompanied by a change of these patients' occupations, while surgical techniques of different types are actually followed by inability to return to previous occupations in close to one half of cases.[98] In Tajima's own survey of 80 wrists with Kienböck's disease seen during a 42-year period, there was no appreciable difference in the end results of nonoperative versus surgical treatment.[110] Nevertheless, there are continuous attempts at finding a consistently reliable surgical technique for these patients. Revascularization of the necrotic lunate by the direct insertion of a vascular pedicle has been reported. Experimental studies for revascularization of necrotic femoral heads in dogs[49] and necrotic humeral heads in rats[3] have shown active vascular proliferation and attempts at substitution of necrotic bone by new bone. The application of this concept to the lunate is still highly experimental and has shown conflicting results.[38,49] The replacement of the lunate by viable bone grafts has also been suggested, either by the pisiform still attached to its vascular supply and to the flexor carpi ulnaris tendon[28,97,118] or by a bone graft obtained from the radius and left attached to a pronator quadratus pedicle.[15] The results for these procedures are still inconclusive, and do not seem to offer any advantages over other, more accepted techniques. Also proposed for the treatment of Kienböck's disease have been denervation of the wrist joint,[17,42,94,119] decompression of the median nerve,[21,52] proximal row carpectomy,[23,51,53] joint leveling operations, either through ulnar lengthening,[5,26,35,79,80,84,104,112,114] or radial shortening,[2,6,35,50,54,69,70,74,77,88,92,100–102,116] partial and total arthrodeses,[20,31,37,47,75,117] and the already mentioned excision of the lunate followed by the insertion of a lunate implant.[1,10,24,48,62–64,67,68,85,106–108]

Excision of the Lunate and Prosthetic Replacement

In an effort to prevent the shift of the remaining carpal bones after excision of the lunate, the use of a Vitallium implant was proposed in 1949.[64] Two years later, Danis[24] presented a case of Kienböck's disease treated by excision of the lunate and its replacement with an acrylic prosthesis. Agerholm and Goodfellow[1] reported that 12 of 15 patients similarly treated were relieved of their preoperative pain and were able to return to heavy manual labor. They stated that the lunate is particularly suitable for prosthetic replacement, that a well-fitting prosthesis is remarkably stable, "even with the posterior capsule open" and that this procedure minimizes the distortion of the carpus commonly found after excision alone. Vitallium and acrylic prostheses have had only limited clinical trials, and have been superseded by the use of silicone implants. Swanson's design has been extensively used; this is probably the most commonly performed operation for Kienböck's disease in this country. Earlier problems with fitting and easy subluxation or dislocation of the implant (Fig. 8-10) have been corrected to a considerable degree by a change in design to a deep-cup shape,[10,63] by careful reconstruction of the palmar capsule, or preservation of the volar cortex of the lunate,[10,62,107] and by the addition to the insertion of the implant of a limited arthrodesis when carpal instability and collapse are present. Lichtman[62] correlated his results of silicone replacement arthroplasty with four clinical and radiographic stages of the disease that are somewhat different to those proposed by Decoulx.[25] In Lichtman's classification, stage I lunates may show a linear or compression fracture but present otherwise normal architecture and density. In his published series, no patient in this group has received a silicone replacement arthroplasty. In stage II, lunate density is abnormal. There is no lunate or intercarpal collapse. Silicone replacement was uniformly successful in these patients, although other types of treatment, particularly joint leveling procedures could be attempted at this point. Lunate collapse indicated the onset of stage III, and was accompanied by proximal migration of the capitate, distal displacement of the triquetrum on the hamate, and

Fig. 8-10. Subluxation of lunate implant. *A:* Radiographic appearance. Arrow in lateral view points to subluxed lunate implant. *B:* Surgical approach through the carpal tunnel shows lunate implant behind a thin membrane. *C:* Implant exposed. (From Taleisnik J: Fractures of the carpal bones. In Green DP: Operative Hand Surgery. Vol. 1. Churchill Livingstone, New York, 1982.)

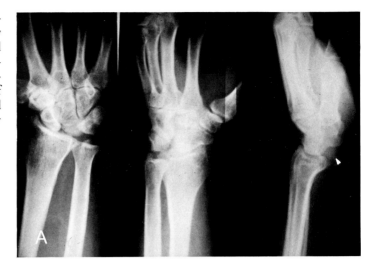

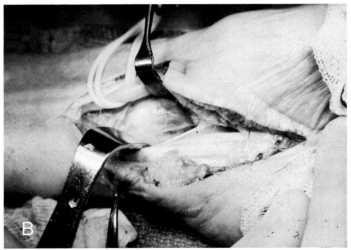

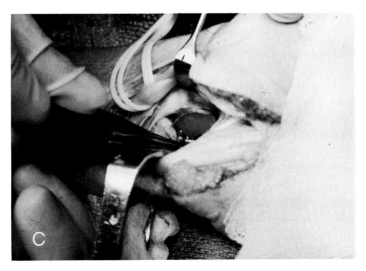

palmarflexion and foreshortening of the scaphoid. In lateral radiographs, the lunate is elongated. In an earlier study Lichtman and coworkers[62] reported a 40 percent failure rate in this group and advised against the use of an implant when carpal collapse and fragmentation of the lunate had occurred. More recently, however, these authors report markedly improved results using the newer, deep-cup, high performance silastic elastomer lunates in stage III.[63] This agrees with Stark and coauthors'[106] satisfactory experience with the use of a hand-carved silicone-rubber spacer for patients with lunate fragmentation and collapse. As a matter of fact, Stark and coauthors' indication for excision of the lunate and its replacement with their hand-carved implant was limited to stage III lunates. They reported that this type of spacer was "reasonably effective in relieving symptoms in 36 patients with advanced Kienböck's disease." Beckenbaugh et al.[10] reviewed the Mayo Clinic experience from 1960 through 1975; 22 patients had had silastic arthroplasties in conjunction with lunate excision; six early cases received lunate implants that were hand-carved from medical grade silicone rubber, but this procedure was later on abandoned in favor a premolded, Swanson-type implant. In stage IV there are generalized osteoarthritic changes of the carpus. Arthrodesis is proposed as a better procedure for this stage.[62]

Silicone replacement arthroplasties are uniformly successful in relieving pain.[10,48,62,63,67,68,85,106–108] Grip strength and range of motion improve when compared to preoperative values,[63,106] but do not reach normal in most patients. Unfortunately, the goal proposed by Lippman[64] in 1949, to prevent carpal shift, is only partially accomplished. In Stark and coauthors'[106] study, carpal collapse beyond that present preoperatively was seen to take place in the majority of their patients after insertion of a hand-carved spacer. A simultaneous intracarpal arthrodesis[20,117] has been proposed as a mechanism to avoid carpal collapse when used in conjunction with the insertion of a lunate implant.

Technique of Lunate Implant with Resection Arthroplasty (Swanson)

The wrist is approached through a longitudinal dorsal incision in line with the axis of the third metacarpal and centered at Lister's tubercle. A transverse skin incision may also be used. A carpal tunnel, palmar approach has been recommended,[68,91] for this would allow reconstruction of the palmar capsule, and at the same time exploration and decompression of the median nerve, a possble source of disabling symptoms in these patients.[21] Published data using this palmar approach shows, however, that the potential for palmar dislocation of the implant persists and, at times, there are postoperative median paresthesias which may have been caused by the exposure and retraction of the median nerve throughout surgery.[91] A dorsal approach is, I believe, preferable. A carpal tunnel decompression may still be done at a later or earlier time, should clear-cut symptoms of involvement of the median nerve arise. Once the dorsal skin flaps have been developed, dorsal sensory nerves are identified and preserved. The dorsal retinaculum is exposed and divided along the roof of the tunnel for the extensor pollicis longus (see Figs. 6-23 and 6-25). This tendon is retracted radially. The fourth dorsal compartment is elevated by sharp dissection between the floor of the tunnel and the underlying joint capsule. This is somewhat of an artificial plane, and care should be taken to preserve a strong, thick capsule. The extensor digitorum communis and extensor indicis proprius tendons are left undisturbed if at all possible, still contained within their retinacular-synovial envelope. The radiocarpal capsule is incised transversely a few millimeters distal to the rim of the radius, leaving, if possible, a short capsular apron for later repair. A vertical capsular incision maybe added if needed. The lunate is exposed. Its ligamentous attachments to the surrounding carpals are divided. The lunate is excised piecemeal if necessary, leaving a thin cortical palmar wafer of bone still attached to the palmar capsule. Rents in this part of the capsule must be avoided, and repaired when created. An attempt should be made to close with nonabsorbable sutures, those naturally occurring "holes" that may present between palmar ligaments. Leaving behind a thin bony layer of palmar lunate, however, obviates these problems. Traction and compression across the wrist at this time will demonstrate potential carpal instability. If this is present a scaphotrapeziotrapezoid fusion should be considered. A proper-sized implant is selected, large enough to fit snugly and be stable, although usually smaller than the space left by removal of the lunate. The implant has a stem designed to enter a hole drilled into the triquetrum. The use of a high performance silicone elastomer allows excision of the stem and suturing of the implant to both the triquetrum and the scaphoid with absorbable sutures, through small (<1 mm) drill holes (Fig. 8-11). A fine Kirschner wire may be used if additional fixation is necessary. The high performance elastomer is four times less apt to tear allowing temporary fixation with Kirschner wires or absorbable sutures.[63] The capsule is repaired with nonabsorbable sutures, to bone if necessary. A firm repair must be secured. If the capsule is not sufficiently strong, it may be reinforced with a strip of extensor carpi radialis brevis tendon or with a portion of the extensor retinaculum that is replaced deep to the extensor tendons directly on the dorsal capsule.

Failure to provide this support may result in implant subluxation and carpal instability (Fig. 8-12). Immediate postoperative immobilization in a compression-type dressing is changed at five to seven days to a short arm plaster cast, which is worn for a total postoperative immobilization of six weeks. The Kirschner wires are removed at 4 to 6 weeks.

Joint Leveling Operations

Joint leveling operations[6] are designed to neutralize the ulna-minus variant seen frequently in these patients, by either ulnar lengthening[5,26,35,79,80,84,104,112,114] or radial shortening.[2,6,33,50,54,69,70,74,77,88,92,100–102,116] Persson[79,80] had suggested that stress fractures of the lunate are more likely to occur in wrists with an ulna-minus relationship because the lunate abuts against surfaces of different hardness: the bony radius laterally and the soft ul-

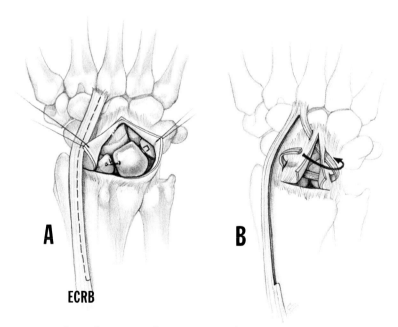

A

ECRB

B

Fig. 8-11. Silastic lunate implant. *A:* Stem of implant is in the triquetrum; further fixation secured by suture of implant to scaphoid with 2-0 nylon suture on an FS needle. *B:* Ulnar third of extensor carpi radialis brevis tendon is used to reinforce the dorsal capsular repair. Avoid tenodesing the tendon slip to the radius to prevent loss of wrist flexion. (Redrawn from Swanson AB: Stabilization Techniques for Carpal Bone Implants (Scaphoid, Lunate, Trapezium). Orthopaedic and Reconstructive Surgeons of Grand Rapids, Grand Rapids, Michigan, 1979.)

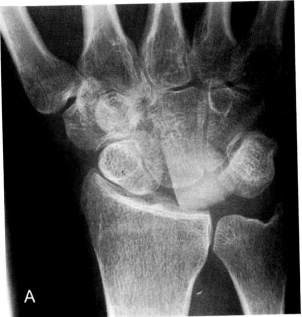 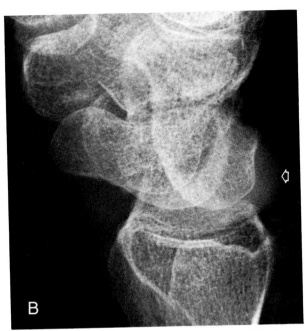

Fig. 8-12. A and B: Lunate implant subluxation (arrow) and carpal instability. Scaphoid is foreshortened (palmar-flexed). Triquetrum is distal (dorsiflexed).

nocarpal complex medially. This produces a stress concentration on the lunate that favors stress or compression fractures (Fig. 8-3). Persson proposed to lengthen the ulna to correct this discrepancy.

Only recently have joint leveling procedures become popular in this country.[2,5,100–102] Their success is explained on the basis of postoperative changes in radiolunate relationship. Although in theory both types of joint leveling operations should produce the same mechanical effect,[5] proponents of radial shortening believe that radial osteotomies heal more readily than ulnar osteotomies, which have a greater percentage of pseudoarthrosis, and that radial shortening reduces compression loads across the wrist by reducing the distance spanned by the muscles crossing this joint. Supporters of ulnar lengthening point out the ease of dissection leading to the ulna, the direct effect on the carpus through the "cushion" provided by the ulnocarpal complex through advancement of the ulnar head, and the greater potential for loss of pronation and supination in patients after radial shortening. It is apparent, however, that either procedure is acceptable and that the final choice depends more on the surgeon's

experience than on the relative merits of each technique. Armistead and collaborators[5] have shown an increased radiolunate joint space in intraoperative arthrograms obtained before and after ulnar lengthening. Partial joint denervation,[33] and circulatory changes together with the benefit of prolonged postoperative immobilization, may also help to explain the success of these procedures. Pain is consistently relieved, although often not completely; many patients continue to complain of some degree of residual discomfort, particularly during strenuous activities. In most cases, there is some improvement of the range of motion, except for ulnar deviation. Concern with disruption of the distal radioulnar relationship has prompted a modification of the ulnar lengthening technique, whereby only the most medial portion of the ulna is lengthened,[103] leaving the radioulnar space undisturbed. However, a review of all reported cases shows that pronation and supination remain full in the vast majority of patients in spite of the change in the radioulnar alignment. The radiologic appearance of the lunate may improve with time, although it does not return to normal[2] (Fig. 8-13). It may remain unchanged.[96] Lunate fragmentation and

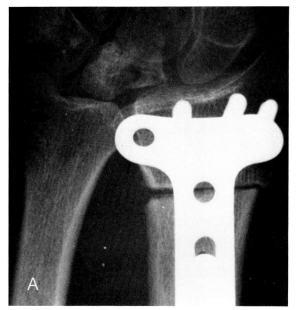
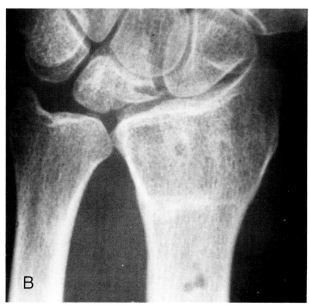

Fig. 8-13. Radial shortening for the treatment of Kienböck's disease. *A:* Initial postoperative radiograph. *B:* Late (two-year) postoperative radiograph. The patient is free of symptoms. The appearance of the lunate is improved. (Courtesy of Dr. J. R. Doyle, Honolulu, Hawaii.)

collapse no longer progress. These procedures are indicated in patients with an ulna-minus variant, with lunate architecture fairly well maintained,[96] a preserved lunocapitate joint,[5] minimal fragmentation and collapse, and absense of degenerative changes. Since the radioulnar relationship is "normalized" by either the shortening of the radius or the lengthening of the ulna, without actual surgical exposure of the carpus, carpal fusions or arthroplasties remain available should the joint levelling procedure fail.

The radiographic determination of the actual ulnar variance requires standardized techniques to be used in different patients for comparison purposes, and on the same patient to determine the exact amount of "leveling" that is indicated.[14,34,78] Epner and coauthors[34] have shown that the radiologic degree of ulnar variance is changed by the position of the wrist when the radiograph is obtained, by whether the forearm is in pronation or in supination at the time, and by the direction of the x-ray beam. These authors proposed a standardized technique for posteroanterior and lateral views obtained in what they called "zero rotation." The recommended posteroanterior view is ob-

tained with the patient's shoulder abducted 90 degrees, the elbow flexed 90 degrees, the forearm in zero rotation, and the wrist in ulnar deviation. For the lateral view, the arm is brought to the patient's side (zero should abduction), the forearm is kept at zero degrees rotation, and the wrist is in normal deviation.

Technique of Ulnar Lengthening (Armistead, Linscheid, Dobyns, Beckenbaugh) (Fig. 8-14)

A longitudinal incision overlying the palpable distal one third of the ulna is recommended. Dissection proceeds along the space between the extensor carpi ulnaris dorsally and the flexor carpi ulnaris. The ulna is exposed subperiosteally. A partial osteotomy is performed through the medial three fourths of the ulna. A plate with four or more slotted holes is placed over the ulna and centered at the level of the osteotomy. All screws are loosely inserted in the position within each slot that is closest to the osteotomy side. The osteotomy is then completed. A laminar spreader is used to distract the fragments to a width 1 to 2 mm greater than the ulnar variant. This technique allows lengthening

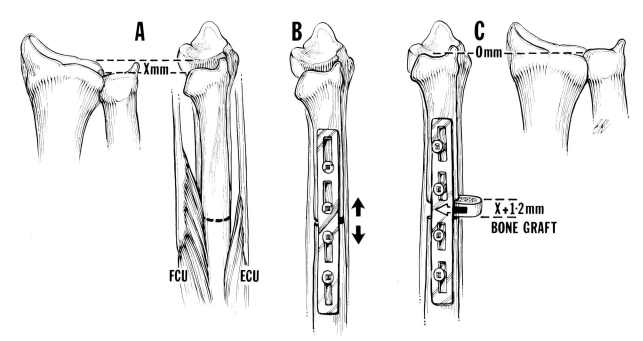

Fig. 8-14. Technique for lengthening the ulna. *A:* Initial ulna-minus variant. *B:* Ulnar osteotomy and stabilization with a slotted plate. Distraction is applied (arrows). *C:* A bone graft is inserted, 1 to 2 mm wider than the ulnar variance. (Redrawn from Armistead RB, Linscheid RL, Dobyns JH, Beckenbaugh RD: Ulnar lengthening in the treatment of Kienböck's disease. J Bone Joint Surgery [Am] 64:170, 1982.)

without loss of rotatory alignment. A bicortical graft of this same width is obtained from the iliac crest and is then wedged in the osteotomy gap. The two screws in the proximal fragment are further loosened to allow tissue elasticity to provide compression across the graft. All screws are then tightened. The graft is trimmed if needed. It is useful to obtain roentgenograms in the operating room. Postoperatively the arm is immobilized in a long arm circular plaster dressing for two weeks, and in a palm-to-elbow circular plaster dressing for an additional four to six weeks. If union is not solid, continuous immobilization is required, often in an orthoplast splint. For delayed unions, the use of pulsing electromagnetic force stimulation may be helpful.

Technique of Radial Shortening

Almquist and Burns[2] recommend a radial-palmar approach to the distal radius. The incision is placed along the distal radius starting distally at the base of the radial styloid and following the projection of

the brachioradialis. The incision is deepened medial to the radial artery. The broad insertions of the pronator quadratus distally and the flexor pollicis longus proximally are exposed. The periosteum is incised along this insertion and the palmar aspect of the radius exposed. This same skin incision could be used to expose the dorsum of the radius by pronating the forearm and incising the periosteum dorsal to the brachioradialis. Care should be taken throughout to preserve the sensory branch of the radial nerve which can be identified along the deep surface of the brachioradialis. A direct dorsal approach may be easier to perform. The incision is longitudinal and in line with the projection of Lister's tubercle. Once the deep forearm fascia is incised the abductor pollicis longus and extensor pollicis brevis are exposed as they cross the field obliquely distally and radially. These muscles are elevated in a distal and medial direction exposing the underlying extensor carpi radialis longus and brevis. The distal shaft of the radius can be felt immediately deep to the wrist movers. It is exposed subperiosteally. With the radius exposed a section is excised of a thickness consistent with the radioulnar length discrepancy. No matter what the approach, care should exercised not to change the actual alignment of the radius following the osteotomy.

Internal fixation is performed with a four- to six-hole compression plate. Bone grafting is usually not necessary (Fig. 8-13). Kapandji proposes an oblique osteotomy of the radius that is performed with the aid of an accurate template and fixation with a sliding compression plate. Closure is performed in the usual manner and immediate postoperative immobilization is provided in a compression-type dressing incorporated into a long arm circular plaster dressing. This is changed at five to seven days into a long arm cast, which is worn until approximately four weeks postoperatively, at which time it is replaced with a short arm circular plaster dressing. The total postoperative plaster immobilization varies from eight to twelve weeks.

Technique of Subperiosteal Wedge Resection of the Distal Radius (Simmons)

A dorsal approach is used to expose the distal radius. After a subperiosteal dissection of the area proximal to the radioulnar joint is completed, a wedge of bone based on the medial cortex of the radius is excised of sufficient width to offset the distal radioulnar length discrepancy. The osteotomy is closed, and fixed with a single compression screw introduced obliquely across, from dorsally and distally, from the radial wall of Lister's tubercle, to engage the opposite cortex (Fig. 8-15). Additional fixation with a Kirschner wire may be required. Postoperative immobilization is provided in a long-arm circular plaster splint.

Intercarpal Arthrodesis

Partial carpal fusions have also been proposed for the treatment of this disease. Chuinard and Zeman[20] suggested that the capitate be fused to the hamate to prevent the proximal migration of the capitate-third metacarpal axis into the defect created by the gradual collapse of the lunate. This should, according to the authors, remove the "nutcracker" effect of the capitate on the lunate. They recommend that the carpal height be measured preoperatively, between the articular surface of the radius and the top of the head of the capitate. When compared to the carpal height in the uninvolved side, if the difference is 2 mm or less, only the capitate-hamate fusion is performed. (Figs. 8-16A,B; 8-17). When the difference is greater than 2 mm, the lunate may be excised. A silicone implant may or may not be inserted (Figs. 8-16C, 8-17, 8-18). In my experience, a fusion across the capitate-hamate joint has not resulted in maintenance of carpal height (Fig. 8-17). In the normal

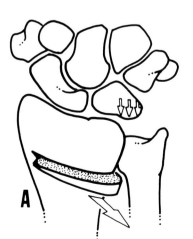 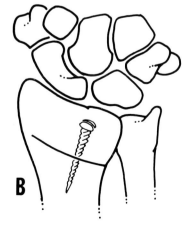

Fig. 8-15. A: Subperiosteal wedge resection of the distal radius. *B*: The osteotomy space is closed with a lag screw. (Redrawn from Simmons EH, Fu F: Kienböck's disease. Orthop Consult 2(11):1, 1981.)

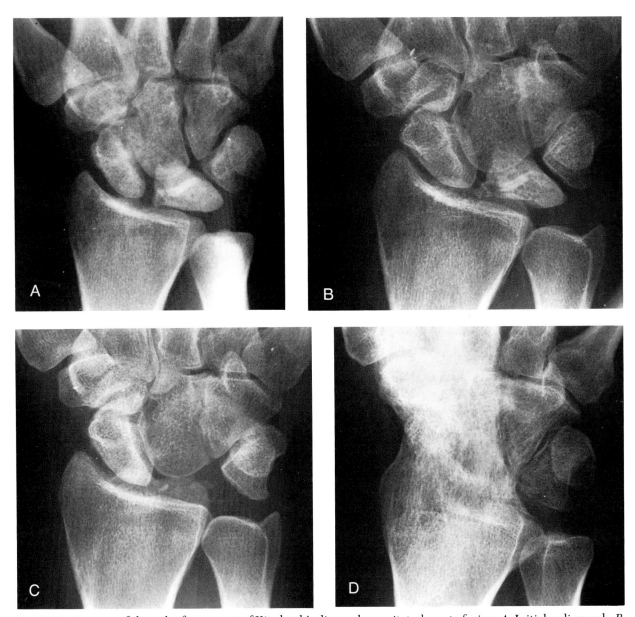

Fig. 8-16. Unsuccessful result of treatment of Kienböck's disease by capitate-hamate fusion. *A:* Initial radiograph. *B:* Progressive lunate collapse following capitate-hamate fusion. *C:* After the lunate is excised, there is further carpal collapse and disabling pain. *D:* Final appearance following radiometacarpal fusion.

wrist, the capitate and the hamate are already firmly bound by short, stout ligaments and motion between them is close to nil. Therefore, a fusion would do very little to change the behavior of the carpus. In effect, the *entire* distal carpal row migrates proximally in spite of the capitate-hamate

fusion, a displacement that is allowed by the scaphoid and triquetrum "getting out of the way" of the capitate, mainly by palmarflexion and foreshortening of the scaphoid on the radial side of the carpus (Fig. 8-18A), but also by distal migration of the triquetrum along the articular surface of the ha-

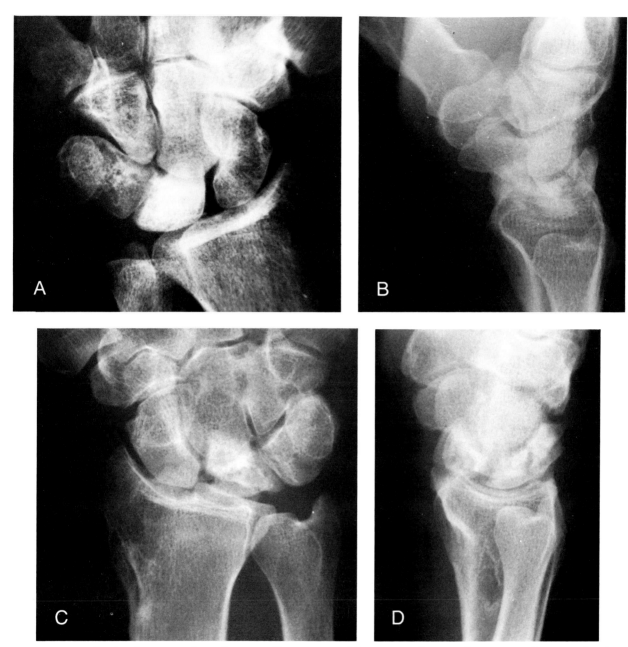

Fig. 8-17. Kienböck's disease without lunate collapse, treated by capitate-hamate fusion. *A* and *B*: Initial radiographs. *C* and *D*: Progressive fragmentation of the lunate three years later. (*A* from Taleisnik J: Fractures of the carpal bones. In Green DP (ed): Operative Hand Surgery. Vol. 1, Churchill Livingstone, New York, 1982.)

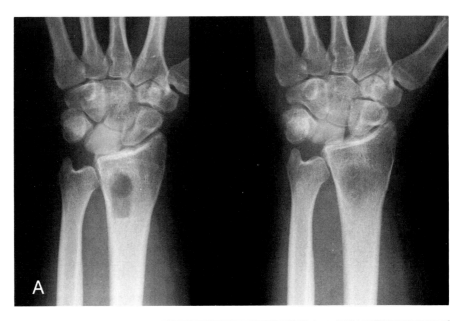

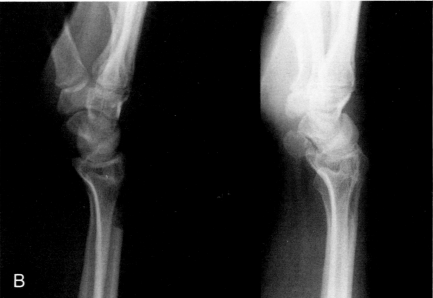

Fig. 8-18. Combined lunate implant arthoplasty and capitate-hamate fusion for the treatment of Kienböck's disease. *A*: Early (left) and late (right) anteroposterior radiographs. There is loss of carpal height allowed by scaphoid foreshortening (palmarflexion) on the radial side, and by distal migration of the triquetrum (dorsiflexion) on the ulnar side. *B*: Early (left) and late (right) lateral views show gradual palmar flexion of lunate implant. In spite of radiographic changes, this patient has remained free of symptoms.

mate on the medial side. An intercarpal arthrodesis that would eliminate midcarpal joint collapse should be more effective. The scaphoid can be fused to either the capitate or the trapezium in a near-longitudinal alignment,[117] thereby providing a load-bearing column for forces to be transmitted from the hand across the wrist into the forearm, bypassing the lunate implant (Fig. 8-19).

Technique of Capitate-Hamate Fusion (Chuinard and Zeman)

The capitate-hamate fusion is performed through a transverse incision. The joint is identified, and the overlying capsular periosteal layer is divided and reflected. The joint surfaces are curetted down to subchondral bone. Cancellous bone obtained from the distal radius through a separate incision is packed into the capitate-hamate space. Compression between the hamate and capitate is carefully avoided, to preserve the outside dimension of these carpal bones leaving the entire carpal relationship undisturbed. A cortical graft obtained from the radius is fitted across the fused joint. The wound is closed in layers. Internal fixation is not

necessary. A bulky dressing with plaster reinforcement is used postoperatively for the initial five to seven days and is replaced by a short arm circular plaster dressing for a total period of six weeks of immobilization.

Technique of Scaphoid-Trapezium Fusion

The technique of schaphoid-trapezium fusion is discussed in Chapter 11.

Summary

I believe that the treatment of Kienböck's disease must be correlated with the radiographic stages of the disease, as suggested by Lichtman.[62] One feature is common to all stages: the lunate has been rendered structurally weak by the lunatomalacia. There are three other factors that determine the staging of this disease and, consequently, its treatment (Fig. 8-20). These are (1) lunate collapse, (2) carpal collapse or instability, and (3) perilunar osteoarthritis. During stage I the weakened lunate is not fragmented or collapsed; carpal alignment is normal and there is no perilunar os-

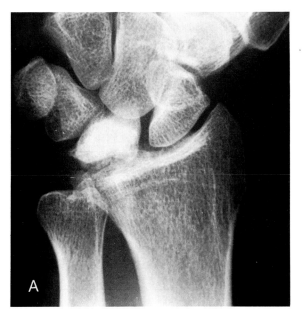 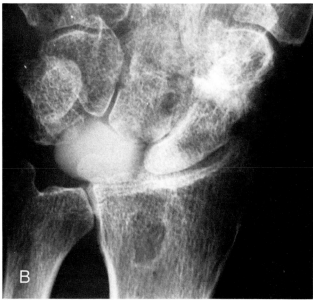

Fig. 8-19. Combined lunate implant arthroplasty and scaphotrapezium-trapezoid fusion for the treatment of Kienböck's disease. *A:* Preoperative radiograph. *B:* Radiographic appearance two years following scaphotrapezium-trapezoid fusion, and lunate implant arthroplasty. Carpal height and alignment are satisfactory. Patient is asymptomatic.

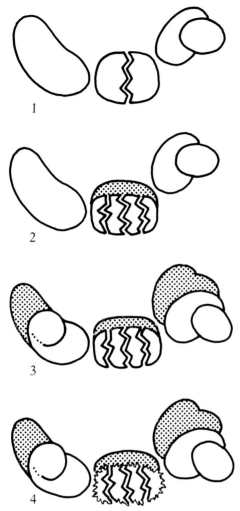

Fig. 8-20. Diagrammatic representation of stage of progression of lunatomalacia. *1*: Lunate is not collapsed. Carpal alignment is normal. There is no osteoarthritis. *2*: There is lunate fragmentation and initial collapse. Carpal height is normal. There is no osteoarthritis. *3*: There is lunate fragmentation and collapse, and carpal shortening and instability. There is no evidence of osteoarthritis. *4*: This is the last stage, when perilunate osteoarthritic changes are present.

mobilization, a review of the literature suggests that symptomatic improvement is actually accompanied by limitation of motion and decreased grip strength and increasing osteoarthritic changes. Immobilization in plaster or in a splint does not mechanically prevent the "nutcracker" effect on the weakened lunate. This can only be effectively blocked by a distraction of the carpus which could be secured by the use of external fixation. Theoretically, the addition to this of a pulsing electromagnetic stimulation device may in effect result in the best prognosis for reconstitution of the lunate. Surgical procedures could be performed at this stage if the patient's disability is severe or if successive roentgenograms suggest that lunate collapse is imminent. These procedures are likewise designed to "unload" the lunate, either by a fusion of the scaphoid to the trapezium or else by a joint leveling operation. For stage II lunates, when there is fragmentation with lunate shortening but without carpal collapse, excision of the lunate and its replacement with a silicone implant is the procedure of choice, particularly if the lunocapitate articular surface is involved. In stage III, there is lunate fragmentation and, in addition, evidence of carpal collapse and instability. The insertion of a lunate implant should be accompanied by the provision of a load bearing column preferably by a fusion across the midcarpal joint, easiest to accomplish by a limited arthrodesis between the scaphoid and the trapezium and trapezoid. For the stage IV, when there are perilunate osteoarthritic changes, the procedure of choice will have to be determined by the radiographic appearance of the carpus as well as by the findings during operation. The principle here is that if possible only those carpal joints that are involved should be treated either by the insertion of implants and/or by limited arthrodesis, leaving joints that are intact to provide stable, pain-free motion. If, however, the osteoarthritic changes are too advanced to consider a technique with salvage of some degree of wrist motion, then a full radiocarpal fusion is the procedure of choice.

teoarthritis. Lunate architecture is undisturbed, but there are linear fractures or sclerosis with minimal, if any, increase in lunate density. An attempt should be made to "unload" the lunate to allow healing and revascularization to proceed. Although this may be accomplished by prolonged im-

REFERENCES

1. Agerholm JC, Goodfellow JW: Avascular necrosis of the lunate bone treated by excision and pros-

thetic replacement. J Bone Joint Surg [Br] 45:110, 1963

2. Almquist EE, Burns JF: Radial shortening for the treatment of Kienböck's disease. A 5 to 10 year follow-up. J Hand Surg 7:348, 1982

3. Alnot JY, Badelon O, Sommariva L, et al: Revascularization d'un os nécrotique par implant d'un pédicule artério-veineux. Etude expérimentale chez la rat. Ann Chir Main 1:274, 1982

4. Antuña Zapico JM: Malacia del semilunar. Tesis doctoral. Universidad de Valladolid. Industrias y Editorial Sever Cuesta, Valladolid, 1966

5. Armistead RB, Linscheid RL, Dobyns JH, Beckenbaugh RD: Ulnar lengthening in the treatment of Kienbock's disease. J Bone Joint Surg [Am] 64:170, 1982

6. Axelsson R: Behandling av lunatomalaci. Elanders Boktryckeri Aktiebolag, Goteberg, 1971

7. Axhausen G: Nicht malacie sondern nekrose des os lunatum carpi. Arch Klin Chir 129:26, 1924

8. Bar P, Labourdette P: A clinical and radiological study of Kienböck's disease. Ann Chir Main 1:239, 1982

9. Barber HM, Goodfellow JW: Acrylic lunate prosthesis. A long term follow-up. J Bone Joint Surg [Br] 56:706, 1974

10. Beckenbaugh RD, Shives TC, Dobyns JH, Linscheid RL: Kienböck's disease: The natural history of Kienböck's disease and consideration of lunate fractures. Clin Orthop 149:98, 1980

11. Bellinghausen HW, Weeks PM, Young LV, Gilula LA: Roentgen Rounds #62. Orthop Rev 11:73, 1982

12. Blaine ES: Lunate osteomalacia. JAMA 96:492, 1931

13. Bolhofner B, Belsole RJ: Kienböck's disease: Current concepts in diagnosis and management. Contemp Orthop 3:713, 1981

14. Bowers WH: Distal radioulnar joint. In Green DP (ed): Operative Hand Surgery. Churchill Livingstone, New York, 1982

15. Braun RM: Pronator pedicle bone grafting in the forearm and proximal carpal row. Presented at the 38th Annual Meeting, American Society for Surgery of the Hand, Anaheim, CA, March 1983

16. Brolin I: Post-traumatic lesions of the lunate bone. Acta Orthop Scand 34:167, 1964

17. Buck-Gramcko D: Denervation of the wrist joint. J Hand Surg 2:54, 1977

18. Cave EF: Kienböck's disease of the lunate. J Bone Joint Surg 21:858, 1939

19. Chan KP, Huang P: Anatomic variations in radial and ulnar lengths in the wrists of Chinese. Clin Orthop 80:17, 1971

20. Chuinard RG, Zeman SC: Kienböck's disease: An analysis and rationale for treatment by capitate-hamate fusion. Orthop Transl 4:18, 1980

21. Codega G, Codega O, Kus H: Neurolysis of the median nerve in the carpal tunnel as a surgical treatment of Kienböck's disease. Int Surg 58:378, 1973

22. Cordes E: Über die Entstehung der subchondralen Osteonekrosen. Beitr Klin Chir 149:28, 1930

23. Crabbe WA: Excision of the proximal row of the carpus. J Bone Joint Surg. [Br] 46:708, 1964

24. Danis A: Ostéomalacie du semilunaire traitée par exérèse et prothèse acrylique; resultat après trois ans. Acta Chir Belg 50:120, 1951

26. Decoulx P, Marchand M, Minet P, Razemon JP: La maladie de Kienböck chez le mineur. Étude clinique et pathogénique (avec analyse de 1330 radios du poignet). Lille Chir 2:65, 1957

26. Desenfans G: A propos de la maladie du semi-lunaire. Opération de Persson. Acta Chir Belg 1:58, 1953

27. Dobyns JH, Linscheid RL: Fractures and dislocation of the wrist. In Rockwood CA Jr, Green DP (eds): Fractures. Lippincott, Philadelphia, 1975

28. Domotor E: Lunatum necrosis kezelese pisiform beuletessel. Magy Traumatol Orthop 17:192, 1974

29. Dornan A: The results of treatment in Kienböck's disease. J Bone Joint Surg [Br] 31:518, 1949

30. Dunn AW: Fractures and dislocations of the carpus. Surg Clin North Am 52:1513, 1972

31. Duparc J, Christel P: Traitement chrirurgical des nécroses du semi-lunaire par arthrodèse intercarpienne. Ann Chir 32:656, 1978

32. Durbin FC: The early changes of Kienböck's disease of the carpal lunate bone. Proc Soc Med 44:482, 1951

33. Eiken O, Niechajev I: Radius shortening in malacia of the lunate. Scand J Plast Reconstr Surg 14:191, 1980

34. Epner RA, Bowers WH, Guilford WB: Ulnar variance. The effect of wrist positioning and roentgen filming technique. J Hand Surg 7:298, 1982

35. Evrard H, Guillaume C, Hoet F, et al: La maladie du semi-lunaire. Ann Chir Main 1:280, 1982

36. Fabricius-Møller J: Den subcutane isolere de fraktur af os lunatum. Bibl Laeger 111:137, 1919

37. Fenollosa J, Valverde C: Résultats des arthrodèses intracarpiennes dans le traitement des nécroses du semilunaire. Rev Chir Orthop 56:745, 1970

38. Foucher G, Saffar PL: Revascularzation of the necrosed lunate, stages I and II, with a dorsal intermetacarpal arteriovenous pedicle. J Chir Main 1:259, 1982

39. Franck P: Die Pathogenese der Lunatum Necrose. Une ihre Bezielung zur Funktionellen. Belastung des Handgelenks. Beitr Z Klin Chir 164:200, 1936

40. Gelberman RH, Salamon PB, Jurist JM, Posch JL: Ulnar variance in Kienböck's disease. J Bone Joint Surg [Am] 57:674, 1975

41. Gelberman RH, Bauman TD, Menon J, Akeson WH: The vascularity of the lunate bone and Kienböck's disease. J Hand Surg 5:272, 1980

42. Geldmacher J, Legal HR, Brug E: Results of denervation of the wrist and wrist joint by Wilhem method. Hand 4:57, 1972

43. Gentaz R, Lespargot J, Levame J-H, Polis J-P: La maladie de Kienböck. Approche tomographique. Analyse de 5 cas. Nouv Presse Med 1:1207, 1972

44. Gillespie HS: Excision of the lunate bone in Kienböck's disease. J Bone Joint Surg [Br] 43:245, 1961

45. Goldsmith R: Kienböch's disease of the semilunar bone. Ann Surg 81:857, 1925

46. Gordon ME: Kienböck's disease. Aetiology. Br Med J 2:200, 1943

47. Graner O, Lopes EK, Costa Carvalho B, Atlas S: Arthrodesis of the carpal bones in the treatment of Kienböck's disease, painful ununited fractures of the navicular and lunate bones with avascular necrosis, and old fracture-dislocations of carpal bones. J Bone Joint Surg [Am] 48:767, 1966

48. Herndon JH, Acevedo M, Hecht O, et al: A long term evaluation of 607 cases of lunate and scaphoid arthroplasty. Orthop Trans 1:7, 1977

49. Hori Y, Tamai S, Okuda H, et al: Blood vessel transplantation to bone. J Hand Surg 4:23, 1979

50. Hultén O: Über anatomische Variationen den Hand. Gelenkknochen. Acta Radiol Scand 9:155, 1928

51. Inglis AE, Jones EC: Proximal-row carpectomy for diseases of the proximal row. J Bone Joint Surg [Am] 59:460, 1977

52. Iselin F: Role of decompression of the median nerve in the carpal tunnel in the treatment of Kienböck's disease. Ann Chir Main 1:273, 1982

53. Jorgensen EC: Proximal-row carpectomy: An end result study of 22 cases. J Bone Joint Surg [Am] 51:1104, 1969

54. Kapandji IA: A technique for shortening of the radius. Ann Chir Main 1:265, 1982

55. Kashiwagi D, Fukiwara A, Inoue T, et al: An experimental and clinical study on lunatomalacia. Orthop Trans 1:7, 1977

56. Kienböck R: Über traumatishe Malazie des Mondbeins, und ihre Folgezustände: Entartungsformen und Kompressions Frakturen. Fortschr Roengenstr 16:77, 1910

57. Konjetzny P: Welche Stellung nimmt die Lunatumnekrose in der Unfallchirurgie ein? Zentrbl Chir 3:929, 1931

58. Köstler J: Randständige Mondbeinsschädigungen. Z Orthop 75:111, 1944

59. Lee MLH: The intra-osseous arterial pattern of the carpal lunate bone and its relation to avascular necrosis. Acta Orthop Scand 33:43, 1963

60. Leriche R, Fontaine R: Contribution á l'étude de la maladie de Kienboeck; son traitement par la sympathectomie périhumérale. Strassbourg Med 89:581, 1929

61. Lesire MR, Allieu U: Étiologie traumatique de la maladie de Kienböck (luxations péri-lunariennes et nécrose du semi-lunaire). Ann Chir Main 1:242, 1982

62. Lichtman DM, Mack GR, MacDonald RI, et al: Kienböck's disease: The role of silicone replacement arthroplasty. J Bone Joint Surg [Am] 59:899, 1977

63. Lichtman DM, Alexander AH, Mack GR, Gunther SF: Kienböck's disease—Update on silicone replacement arthroplasty. J Hand Surg 7:343, 1982

64. Lippman EM, McDermott LJ: Vitallium replacement of lunate in Kienböck's disease. Milit Surg 105:482, 1949

65. MacConaill MA: The mechanical anatomy of the carpus and its bearings on some surgical problems. J Anat 75:166, 1941

66. Marek FM: Avascular necrosis of the carpal lunate. Clin Orthop 10:96, 1957

67. Merle M, Memeteau D, Michon J: Le remplacement prothétique du semi-lunaire. Ann Chir Main 1:253, 1982

68. Michon J: Lunarectomie avec remplacement prothétique. Rev Chir Orthop 39:180, 1973

69. Möberg E: Discussion. J Bone Joint Surg [Am] 52:251, 1970

70. Möberg E: Treatment of Kienböck's disease by shortening of the radius. Presented at the Joint Meeting of Japanese and American Hand Surgeons. Hiroshima, 1974

71. Mouat TB: Isolated fracture of the carpal semilunar and Kienböck's disease. Br J Surg 19:577, 1931

72. Müller W: Ueber die Erweichung und Verdichtung des Os Lunatum, eine typische Erkrankung des Handgelenks. Beitr Z Klin Chir 119:664, 1920

73. Nahigian SH, Li CS, Richey DG, Shaw DT: The dorsal flap arthroplasty in the treatment of Kienböck's disease. J Bone Joint Surg [Am] 52:245, 1970

74. Narakas A, Neff G: Results of surgical treatment of

15 cases of Kienböck's disease. Hand Chir 1:8, 1970

75. Nonnenmacher J, Naett R, Benabdid M: Arthrodése intracarpienne de revascularisation avec transposition du grand os (Graner type II). Ann Chir Main 1:256, 1982

76. Nordmann O: Die Behandlung der Lunatumnekrose und ähnlicher Erkrankungen mit der Gipsplombe. Zentralbl Chir 15:834, 1939

77. Ovesen J: Shortening of the radius in the treatment of lunatomalacia. J Bone Joint Surg [Br] 63:231, 1981

78. Palmer AK, Glisson RR, Werner FW: Ulnar variance determination. J Hand Surg 7:376, 1982

79. Persson M: Pathogenese und Behandlung der Kienböckshen Lunatummalazie. Acta Chir Scand 92: Suppl 98, 1945

80. Persson M: Causal treatment of lunatomalacia. Further experiences of operative ulna lengthening. Acta Chir Scand 100:531, 1950

81. Peste: Discussion. Bull Soc Anat Paris 18:169, 1843

82. Pfitzner W: Variations in the structure of the bones of the hand. Morphol Arb 4:349, 1895

83. Pfitzner W: Die morphologischen Elements des menschlichen Hand Skelets. Morphol Anthropol 2:76, 1895

84. Potma JN: Verlängerung Sosteotomie der Ulna Mittels einer A.A.—Halbrohrplatte als Distraktion Sosteosynthese bie der Behandlung der Lunatummalazie. Z Orthop 111:116, 1973

85. Ramakrishna B, D'Netto DC, Sethu AU: Long-term results of silicone rubber implants for Kienböck's disease. J Bone Joint Surg [Br] 64:361, 1982

86. Razemon JP: Étude pathogénique de la maladie de Kienböck. Ann Chir Main 1:240, 1982

87. Razemon JP: Les différentes méthodes thérapeutiques. Ann Chir Main 1:249, 1982

88. Razemon JP: Le Raccourcissement du radius. Ann Chir Main 1:261, 1982

89. Reichelt A, Seibold J: Die Therapie der Lunatummalacie II. Mitteilung: Die operative Behandlung. Arch Orthop Unfall Chir 84:299, 1976

90. Remijnse: Fractura carpi. Zentrbl Chir 41:378, 1914

91. Roca J, Beltran JE, Fairen MF, Alvarez A: Treatment of Kienböck's disease using a silicone rubber implant. J Bone Joint Surg [Am] 58:373, 1976

92. Rosemeyer B, Artmsnn M, Viernstein K: Lunatummalacie, Nachuntersuchungsergebnisse und therapeutische Erwägungen. Arch Orthop Unfallchir 85:119, 1976

93. Rossak K: Druckverhaltnisse am handgelenk unter besonderer berucksichtigung von fraktur-mechanismen. Z Orthop 103 (Suppl):296, 1967

94. Rostlund R, Somnier F, Axelsson R: Dennervation of the wrist joint. Acta Orthop Scand 51:609, 1980

95. Roth FB: Aseptic necrosis of the lunate bone. A case report with a study of the pathological changes. J Bone Joint Surg 25:683, 1943

96. Roullet J, Walch G: Technique d'allongement de l'ulna dans la maladie de Kienböck. Résultats av de la de dix ans. Ann Chir Main 1:268, 1982

97. Saffar Ph: Remplacement du semi-lunaire par le pisiforme. Description d'une nouvelle technique pour le traitement de la maladie de Kienböck. Ann Chir Main 1:276, 1982

98. Saffar Ph, Gentaz R: Comparaison entre le traitement médical et chirurgical de la maladie de Kienböck. Ann Chir Main 1:250, 1982

99. Seibold J, Reichelt A: Die therapie der lunatummalacie. I. Mittelung: Die konservative behandlung. Arch Orthop Unfall Chir 82:325, 1975

100. Simmons EH, Dommissee IG: The pathogenesis and treatment of Kienböck's disease. Clin Orthop 105:300, 1974

101. Simmons, EH, Dommissee, IG: An investigation into the pathogenesis and treatment of Kienbock's disease. Presented at the 35th Annual Meeting, American Society for Surgery of the Hand, Atlanta, GA. 1980

102. Simmons EH, Fu F: Kienböck's disease. Orthop Consult 2(11):1, 1981

103. Soeur R, Navarre M, DeRacker Ch: L'allongement du cubitus respectant l'articulation radio-cubitale inférieure dans la maladie de Kienböck. Ann Chir Main 1:261, 1982

104. Sommelet J, Hahn P, Schmitt D, et al: L'allongement du cubitus dans le traitement de la maladie de Kienböck. Rev Chri Orthop 56:731, 1970

105. Ståhl F: On lunatomalacia (Kienböck's disease): A clinical and roentgenological study, especially on its pathogenesis and the late results of immobilization treatment. Acta Chir Scand 95(Suppl 126):1, 1947

106. Stark HH, Zemel MP, Ashworth CR: Use of a hand-carved silicone-rubber spacer for advanced Kienböck's disease. J Bone Joint Surg [Am] 63:1359, 1981

107. Swanson AB: Silicone rubber implants for the replacement of the carpal scaphoid and lunate bones. Orthop Clin North Am 1:299, 1970

108. Swanson AB: Flexible Implant Resection Arthroplasty in the Hand and Extremities. Mosby, St. Louis, 1973

109. Taine GJ: Excision of the lunate in Kienböck's disease. J Bone Joint Surg [Br] 47:599, 1965

110. Tajima T: An investigation of the treatment of Kienböck's disease. J Bone Joint Surg [Am] 48:1649, 1966

111. Therkelsen F, Andersen K: Lunatomalcia. Acta Chir Scand 97:503, 1949

112. Tillberg B: Kienboeck's disease treated with osteotomy to lengthen ulna. Acta Orthop Scand 39:359, 1968

113. Ueba Y, Obara A, Fujikawa S, Matsumoto J: Kienböck disease treated by excision of the lunate and tendon transplantation. Orthop Surg (Japan) 23:1173, 1972

114. Verbrugge J, Verjans H: L'allongement du cubitus comme traitement de choix de la maladie de Kienböck. Rev Chir Orthop 49:563, 1963

115. Verdan CI: Les fractures ignorées du semi-lunaire. Ann Chir Main 1:248, 1982

116. Viernstein K, Weigert M: New methods for the treatment of lunatomalacia. Reconstr Surg Traumatol 11:154, 1969

117. Watson HK: Limited wrist arthrodeses. Clin Orthop 149:126, 1980

118. Wickenhauser J, Beck E: Die Kienbock'sche Erkrankung: diagnostic, therapie und postoperative Verlaufskontrolle. Fortschr Geb Roentgenstr Nuklearmed 132:303, 1975

119. Wilhelm A: Die gelenkdenervation und ihre anatomischen grundlagen. Ein nerves behandlungsprinzip in der hand chirurgie. Hefte Unfallheilkd 86:1, 1966

120. Youm Y, McMurtry RY, Flat AE, Gillespie TE: Kinematics of the wrist. I. An experimental study of radial-ulnar deviation and flexion extension. J Bone Joint Surg. [Am] 60:423, 1978

9 Dislocations and Fracture-Dislocations of the Carpus

This chapter is devoted to the discussion of those injuries that result in complete dislocation of one or more carpal bones, with or without simultaneous fractures of the carpus, radius or ulna. These injuries are complex, and an almost endless array of variations is possible. The earliest description of a volar dislocation of the lunate is found in Malgaigne's[63] treatise on fractures and dislocations, an enucleation of the lunate through a palmar wound. Malgaigne also described a case of Maisonneuve of what appears to be a dorsal transscaphoid, transtriquetral, perilunate fracture dislocation. Albertin[5] described a similar case, and originated the "cherry pit" theory to explain the mechanism of dislocation of the lunate. The earliest American publication on this subject was in 1866 by Hodges[48] on an open dislocation of the lunate, as a result of which the patient developed a massive infection of his arm leading to his death on the tenth day after the injury.

Following the discovery of the x-ray, reports of these injuries accumulated.[1,7,16,20,25,26,30,42,45,54,58–60,76,77,102,103,116] In 1902 Bialy[11] proposed to classify *volar dislocations of the lunate* into three stages, according to the degree of lunate rotation: in the first stage, the distal concavity of the lunate faces distally; in the second stage it faces palmarward, the lunate having rotated 90 degrees; in the third stage, it faces proximally, after a 180-degree rotation. *Volar perilunate dislocations* are considerably more infrequent. Goullioud and Arcelin[38] were probably the first to publish a report of a volar

transscaphoid perilunate fracture dislocation. Throughout the ensuing years, the terminology applied to these dislocations and fracture dislocations, although largely anatomic, became somewhat confusing. In effect, these injuries may be divided into two large groups, according to whether or not there are simultaneous fractures. When there is a major *carpal dislocation without fracture*, it is either a dislocation of the carpus around the lunate, with the lunate remaining in normal alignment with the radius (dorsal or volar perilunate dislocations) or a dislocation of the lunate, palmar or rarely dorsal to the radius. When there is a *fracture as well as a dislocation*, the terminology includes the fracture.[35] Therefore, when the fracture is of the scaphoid, the resulting entity is called transscaphoid perilunate or transscaphoid lunate fracture dislocation. If the capitate is also fractured, then the resulting injury should include transcapitate in its name. Therefore, the terminology in use at the present time attempts to describe not only the nature but also the path of the injury, as it progresses around and across the carpus, at times involving the radius and ulna. Most carpal fractures and dislocations are confined to the "vulnerable zone,"[55] an area comprising the scaphoid and trapezium and the bony surfaces that bound the midcarpal joint. The "vulnerable zone" is largely contained within a more proximal "lesser arc," that closely hugs the lunate, and a distal or "greater arc" that crosses the middle third of the scaphoid and continues in an ulnar direction, distal to the midcarpal joint (Fig. 9-1).[55] Based on these two arcs, carpal dislocations and fracture-dislocations may be classified into four main groups (Fig. 9-2):

I. *Dislocations and fracture-dislocations of the lesser arc:* These include the dorsal and volar perilunate dislocations and the dorsal and volar dislocations of the lunate.

II. *Dislocations and fracture-dislocations of the greater arc:* A complete example would be a transscaphoid, transcapitate, transhamate, transtriquetral perilunate fracture dislocation. Several variations are possible, depending on the number and location of the carpal fractures. The most frequent representative of this group is the dorsal transscaphoid perilunate fracture dislocation.

III. *Variants*[41]: These include fractures involving the radial styloid (transradial styloid perilunate fracture dislocations), the scaphocapitate syndrome, and isolated dislocations of one or more carpal bones.

IV. *Radiocarpal dislocations, volar and dorsal:* These include all complete volar or dorsal dislocations of the carpus on the radius. Excluded from this group are the more subtle, incomplete carpal subluxations and the radiocarpal injuries in which fractures of the distal radius are accompanied by dorsal or palmar carpal subluxations. These are discussed in the section on Carpal Instability.

MECHANISMS OF INJURY

It has been suggested that volar dislocations of the lunate result when the wedge-shaped lunate is squeezed forward "like the pit of a cherry pressed between two fingers,"[5] or as a "pea from a pod,"[110] or as a "watermelon seed,"[14] as the wrist is forcibly dorsiflexed. The actual mechanism of injury is, however, more complex and the damage that allows the lunate to subluxate is considerably more extensive. Carpal dislocations and fracture dislocations represent a continuum of progressive bony and ligamentous damage.[67] In 1906 Tavernier[99] had already pointed out that in all cases "only one displacement is constant; the lunate has lost its normal relationship with the head of the capitate." He stated that the mechanism which resulted in these injuries is unique and suggested that these are "the

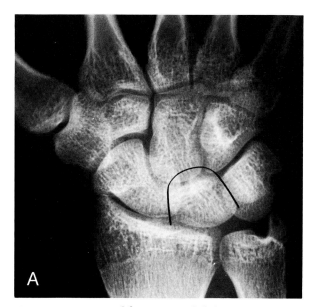
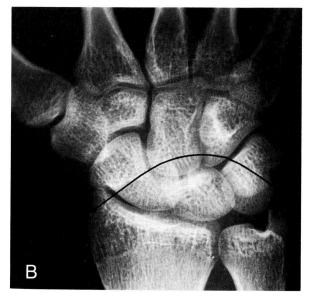

Fig. 9-1. Most carpal fractures and dislocations are confined to the "vulnerable zone," bound by a proximal "lesser arc" *(A)* and a distal "greater arc" *(B)* (see Fig. 7-1). (See Ref. 55.)

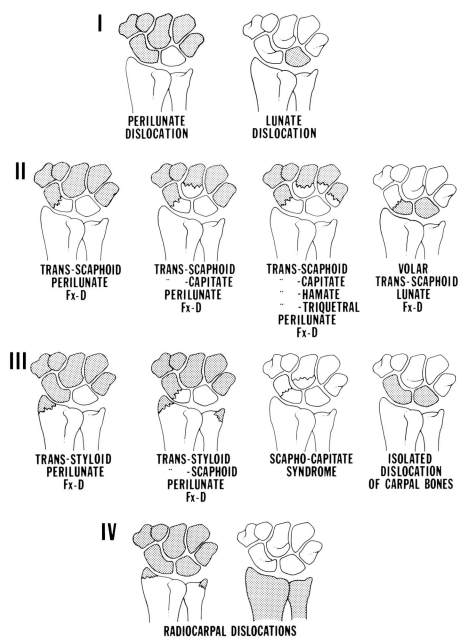

Fig. 9-2. Classification of common carpal dislocations and fracture-dislocations. I: Dislocations and fracture-dislocations of the lesser arc. II: Dislocations and fracture-dislocations of the greater arc. III: Variants. IV: Radiocarpal dislocations. (Modified from Watson-Jones R: Fractures and Joint Injuries. Vol. 2. 4th Ed. © 1960 Williams & Wilkins, Baltimore.)

stages and the varieties of one and the same lesion." Thus, he felt justified in grouping them under the single name of "traumatic displacements of the lunate."

The final outcome of a fall on the hand depends on (1) *the characteristics of the injuring force:* this includes its point of application, its magnitude, rate of loading and direction;[54,55] (2) *the position of the hand at impact*,[54,96] including the further angulatory and rotatory changes produced by the progression of the injury[54,98]; and (3) *the relative strength of carpal bones and ligaments.*[54,80,96] The same mechanism that results in a radiocarpal fracture-dislocation in a young adult, would produce a comminuted fracture of the distal radius in an elderly female or an epiphyseal injury in a child (although the exceptional occurrence of a transscaphoid perilunate fracture dislocation in a 10-year-old boy has been reported[80]). A force similar to that which causes a fracture of the scaphoid, if allowed to continue could end in a transcaphoid perilunate fracture dislocation. Thus, wrist injuries may progress from the minor sprain, to more significant ligament disruption, to tears or avulsions with varying degrees of carpal collapse and, finally, to the more severe dislocations and fracture-dislocations. Excessive dorsal mid carpal laxity may need to be present for these injuries to lead to carpal subluxations and dislocations.[96] In most dislocations it is the head of the capitate that is dislodged from the cup of the lunate. For this to occur, the scaphoid bridging across the lunocapitate space must either fracture or dissociate from the lunate.[19,26,107,108] The loss of the stabilizing influence of the scaphoid, either because of a fracture, or because of a scapholunate dissociation, effectively renders the carpus susceptible to further subluxation or dislocation, should the abnormal force persist. The position of the hand at the time of impact determines the point of application of the force at the wrist. Fractures of the scaphoid have been produced in the laboratory by forces applied to the radial half of the palm, with the wrist in dorsiflexion and slight radial deviation[111] (see Chapter 6). Conversely, a force applied to the hypothenar area while holding a cylindrical object in the hand (the handlebars of a motorcycle or the handle of a tennis racquet) is frequently recalled by patients who have sustained a rotatory subluxation of the scaphoid[8] (see Chap-

ter 11). There is also enough clinical evidence to suggest that loading on the ulnar side of the carpus, with carpal hyperpronation, results on triquetrolunate sprains, and dissociations (see Chapter 12).

The importance of rotation in the mechanism of production of these injuries was stressed at the turn of the century by Abadie,[1] in 1919 by Jeanne and Mouchet,[54] and was later emphasized by others[55,68,98,113] Tanz[98] believed that both lunate and perilunate dislocations resulted from longitudinal compression, dorsiflexion, and ulnar deviation of the wrist, with added hand pronation producing a dislocation of the lunate, and supination a perilunate dislocation. This was an important consideration, for manipulation for the reduction of these injuries should include rotation maneuvers in a direction opposite to that which produced a dislocation in the first place.

Mayfield and colleagues,[68] devised an experimental study designed to reproduce these carpal dislocations and fracture-dislocations. The mechanism of injury used for their experiments was extension, ulnar deviation and intercarpal supination. The ensuing sequence of dislocations was named progressive perilunar instability (PPI) and included four stages (Fig. 9-3). At the end of stage I, a scapholunate diastasis was produced, the least significant degree of perilunar instability. Progression of loading produced an additional dorsal dislocation of the capitate, the stage II. In stage III, the triquetrum was gradually peeled away from the lunate, resulting in a triquetrolunate diastasis, or an avulsion fracture of the triquetrum. Jeanne and Mouchet[54] had shown that forced carpal supination resulted in dislocation or erosion fractures of the triquetrum, and Destot had also suggested that a fracture of the triquetrum was an indication of a more severe type of carpal dislocation.[26] The presence of a triquetrolunate gap or malalignment and/or an avulsion fracture of the triquetrum are considered to be diagnostic of stage III injuries. Intercarpal supination was the significant factor in producing ligament damage at the level of the triquetrum. The end-stage IV was typified by a dislocation of the lunate, the highest degree of perilunate instability. This study supported previous clinical assumptions that dislocations of the lunate are preceded by perilunate dislocations and that both are in effect manifestations of the same jury,

Fig. 9-3. Schematic representation of Progressive Perilunar Instability. Stage I: scapholunate diastasis. Stage II: dorsal dislocation of the capitate. Stage III: triquetrolunate dissociation. Stage IV: dislocation of the lunate. (See Ref. 68.)

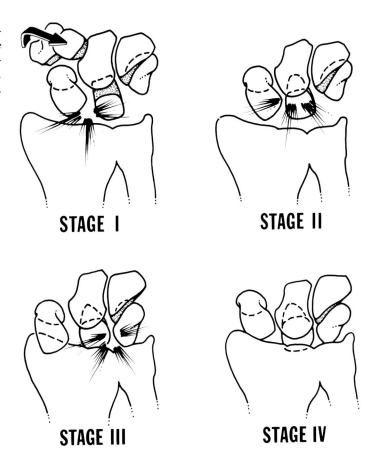

a concept first advanced, as we have seen, by Tavernier[99] in 1906, by Destot[26] in 1925, and by Farr[31] in 1926, and later adopted by many others.[2,4,9,17,18,29,40,57,62,91,98,107,108] It was with this unifying concept of dislocations about the lunate in mind that Destot proposed a classification of these injuries into two stages: first, when the capitate is displaced, but the lunate retains its relationship to the radius, and second, when the lunate has dislocated both from the radius and the head of the capitate,[26] stages that we have come to recognize as perilunate dislocations and dislocations of the lunate, respectively.

The mechanism of transscaphoid perilunate fracture dislocations may be somewhat different to that of the perilunate dislocations or dislocations of the lunate, in that a fracture through the scaphoid is the initial destabilizing factor.[108] The experimental mechanisms that may result in fractures of the scaphoid have already been reviewed (see Chapter 6). Once the scaphoid is fractured, the complex formed by the proximal fragment of the scaphoid and the lunate is subjected to the same loads that act on the lunate alone to produce a progressive perilunar instability. Weiss and coworkers[114] were able to produce a dorsal transscaphoid perilunate fracture dislocation when a hard blow was applied longitudinally to the palm of the hand with the wrist in full dorsiflexion and ulnar deviation.

Although initial destabilization requires a fracture of the scaphoid or its dissociation from the lunate,[19,26,108] further damage should occur to allow first the capitate, then the triquetrum, to dislocate from the lunate. Dislocation of the capitate is possible after a tear or failure of the volar radiocapitate ligament (see Chapter 2) or an avulsion fracture of the radial styloid, the displaced styloid fragment containing the origin of the radiocapitate ligament. If the capitate impinges against the dorsal margin of the radius, its head may be trapped

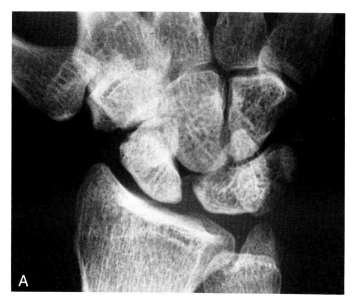

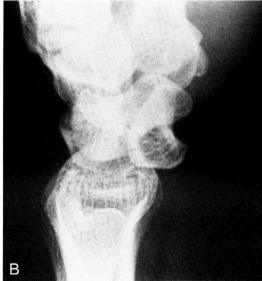

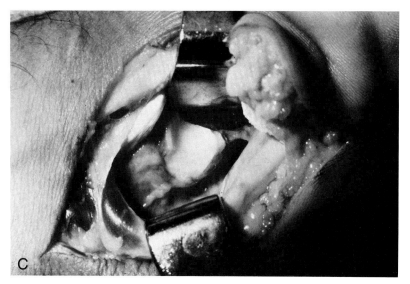

Fig. 9-4. Unrecognized, 6-months-old palmar dislocation of the lunate. *A:* Anteroposterior radiograph shows break in the continuity of Gilula's arcs (see Fig. 5-2), overlap of carpal rows across midcarpal joint space, palmar-flexed scaphoid and a triangular lunate. *B:* Lateral view shows palmar dislocation of the lunate (the "spilled teacup" sign) palmar flexion of the scaphoid and dorsal alignment of the capitate. *C:* Operative view of dislocated lunate.

and sheared off at the neck, or the neck itself may be fractured by the dorsal lip of the radius resulting in a scaphocapitate fracture syndrome[3,32,33,70,72,93,105] or in a transscaphoid transcapitate perilunate fracture dislocation. The location of the fracture of the capitate, and the further displacement of the head of the capitate may depend on the degree of dorsiflexion of the wrist at the time of impact.[54]

For the rare palmar perilunate dislocation, and its associated injury, the dorsal dislocation of the lunate, forced hyperflexion has been postulated as the mechanism of injury resulting from a load applied to the dorsum of the hand.[4,81,87,90] Pournaras and Kappas[81] suggested that a predisposing factor may be important in some of these injuries because of a preexisting abnormal alignment of the radiolunate axis with the lunate in a pre-position of palmar flexion. Saunier and Chamay[88] stated that hyperflexion of the wrist alone would actually be conducive to a Smith-type fracture of the radius, and that for a volar perilunate dislocation to occur,

Fig. 9-4 (cont.). D: Appearance after reduction. *E*: Postoperative radiographs.

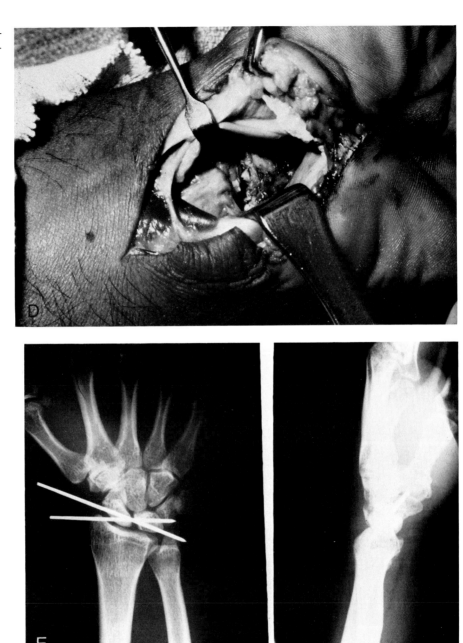

a component of ulnar deviation is necessary. Although in many of these case reports hyperflexion was clearly the mechanism of injury, other mechanisms may also be possible. Postmortem studies of a wrist with a volar perilunate dislocation in a patient who died two weeks later from associated injuries suggested that the likely mechanism of injury for this particular wrist was supination of the proximal carpal row (lunate) around the triquetrum, which behaves as the center of this abnormal rotation, while the distal carpal row (capitate) and the hand are fixed on the ground.[40] This interpretation agrees with Navarro's[76] observation published in 1935. Upon describing a palmar perilunate dislocation, Navarro noticed that in all seven cases which he had reviewed from the literature, the triquetrum had remained attached to the lunate. He further observed that there were only two cases of dorsal dislocations of the lunate and that in both the triquetrum had dissociated from the lunate, and suggested that it is the condition of the triquetrolunate ligaments which determines whether a palmar perilunate or a dorsal lunate dislocation will develop. He also stressed that the dorsal lunate displacement is never as total as that found in palmar dislocations of the lunate, a feature which he attributed to the longer dorsal overhang of the articular surface of the radius, and postulated that the prerequisite for a true dorsal lunate dislocation is a fracture of the dorsal rim of the radius. For palmar perilunate dislocations to take place, just as for the more common dorsal perilunate dislocations, a dissociation between the lunate and the distal carpal row is a prerequisite, occurring either at the scapholunate space, or through the body of the scaphoid.

Volar transscaphoid perilunate fracture dislocations frequently show associated radial carpal translocation.[118]

DIAGNOSIS

Considering the severity of these injuries and the major disruption of carpal anatomy that is present, it is surprising that a number of perilunate dislocations and dislocations of the lunate are not diagnosed, even in modern times, until very late (Fig. 9-4).[17,71] Jeanne and Mouchet[54] were distressed, in 1919, by the number of late unrecognized dislocations that were seen and wished that "a day will come, soon we hope, when unrecognized luxations will be the exception, and when one will have only to treat recent luxations." This wish has only been partially fulfilled. Dislocations diagnosed late comprise up to 40 percent of the total number of cases

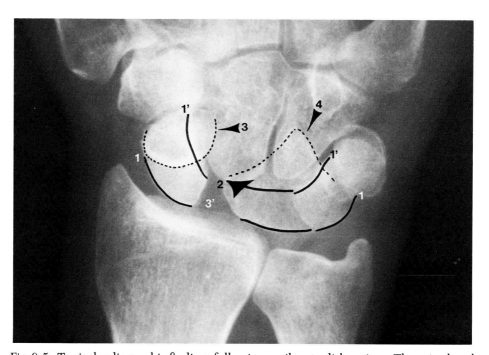

Fig. 9-5. Typical radiographic findings following perilunate dislocations. There is a break in the continuity of Gilula's lines (1 – 1 and 1' – 1'); arrow 2 points to an overlap of distal and proximal carpal rows, obscuring the midcarpal space. The shape of the scaphoid is abnormal. The distal pole is seen "end-on" (Ring-sign, arrow 3), and there is a scapholunate dissociation (3'). The lunate shape is triangular (4).

in some series.[17,71] Zolczer[119] recently reviewed 65 unreduced, chronic dislocations about the lunate that needed late treatment by open reduction. Lack of recognition is, therefore, the first complication arising from the handling of these injuries. The clinical findings are not diagnostic. Swelling of the wrist is diffuse, particularly in the early, acute cases. Tenderness is also poorly localized, although it may be more limited later on, as the acute initial reaction subsides. The range of motion is usually severely limited, and grip strength is very weak, if there is any grip at all. In volar dislocations of the lunate the fingers are usually semiflexed, and any attempt at passive finger extension or active finger flexion is very painful. There may be telltale skin marks and abrasions,[96] but these are not diagnostic. Open volar dislocations of the lunate are, for the most part, historical relics known to have led to amputation[15] or death[48] because of associated infection. Symptoms of median nerve compression, the "anaesthesia dolorosa" of Destot,[26] although not diagnostic, should strongly suggest a carpal dislocation when present in young patients, frequently male, after major injuries to the region of the carpus. Median neuropathies usually occur in the volar varieties of dislocations and fracture dislocations.[14,17,18,29–31,36,40,41,44,47,54,62,73,86,87,99,109] Elaborate palpation of bony landmarks was part of the exhaustive examination of these patients in the pre-Röntgen and early post-Röntgen eras.[1,20,25,26,30,42,49,50,54,58–60,74,76,77,99] Likewise, the presence of crepitus was considered necessary for the diagnosis of carpal fractures.[20,49,50] Such detailed examinations of the wrist however, are no longer justified. Although the diagnosis may be suspected, it is still the radiographic recognition of radiolunocapitate malalignment that provides the key to the injury. Gilula[35] proposed an analytic approach to the radiographic evaluation of carpal injuries. He pointed out that there are three major radiographic features that must be surveyed sequentially on the posteroanterior view: the carpal arcs (Fig. 5-2), the symmetry of joint spaces, and the correct shape of the individual bones, particularly scaphoid and lunate (see Chapter 5). Any breaks in the smooth outline of an arc, abnormal widening of a joint space, unusual bony overlap or bony shapes that do not correspond to a normal PA view in the neutral position should alert the physi-

cian to the presence of a carpal abnormality. Following are the essential radiographic features found in carpal dislocations and fracture dislocations.

Posteroanterior

See Figure 9-5.

1. Break in the continuity of Gilula's arcs.
2. Overlap of proximal and distal carpal rows, obscuring the mid carpal space.
3. Abnormal scaphoid shape; usually it is seen in palmar flexion and foreshortened. A wide scapholunate space may be present, although initial carpal distortion makes this difficult to recognize, at least until after reduction of the major dislocation is completed. Persistent or recurrent scapholunate dissociation, even while the wrist is immobilized in plaster, is a frequent sequela of reduced lesser arc dislocations (Fig. 9-6)[17,18,62,101,107,110] and should be of concern to the treating physician, requiring radiographic follow up at weekly intervals for the initial four to six weeks after reduction. The second reason for an abnormal scaphoid shape, other than that due to malrotation, is a fracture (Fig. 9-7). The proximal fragment usually remains with the lunate, while the distal fragment dislocates with the remainder of the carpus. Just like for "lesser arc" injuries, transscaphoid fracture-dislocations require careful post reduction scrutiny and follow up, for any loss of scaphoid alignment becomes an indication for open reduction and internal fixation. Posteroanterior and routine oblique views are most helpful to study scaphoid alignment and should be obtained at weekly intervals for at least four to six weeks post reduction. Particular attention must be paid to the concave outline of the scaphoid opposite the capitate, where early malalignment may be easier to detect. Loss of scaphoid alignment, whether due to scaphoid subluxation or fracture, will lead to a permanently unstable carpus unless corrected early.
4. The lunate is triangular in shape.
5. Associated fractures may be present, involving the radial styloid, the scaphoid as already mentioned, the capitate, hamate, or triquetrum.

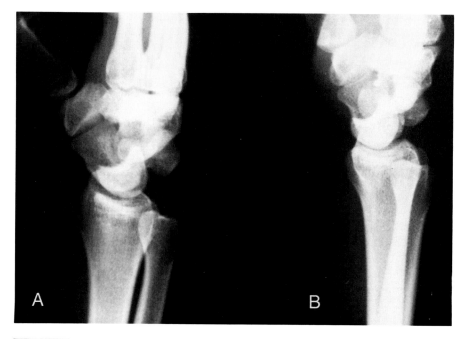

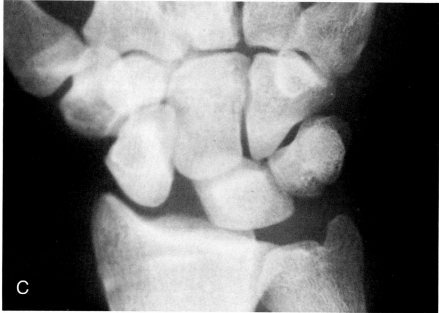

Fig. 9-6. Perilunate dislocation (*A* and *B*) shows persistent scapholunate dissociation after reduction *(C)*.

Lateral View

1. The lunate is not in line with the radius, or else it has remained distal to the dome of the radius but tipped into palmarflexion (the "spilled teacup sign") (Fig. 9-8).[40,41] The lunate is also palmar-flexed, but translated dorsally in the less frequent volar perilunate dislocations.

2. The scaphoid is usually palmarflexed (Fig. 9-8A), its long axis perpendicular to that of the radius; its proximal pole maybe dorsal to the dorsal rim of the radius. It is exceptional for the

Fig. 9-7. Posteroanterior radiograph of transcaphoid-perilunate fracture dislocation. PS, proximal scaphoid fragment is outlined; DS, distal scaphoid fragment.

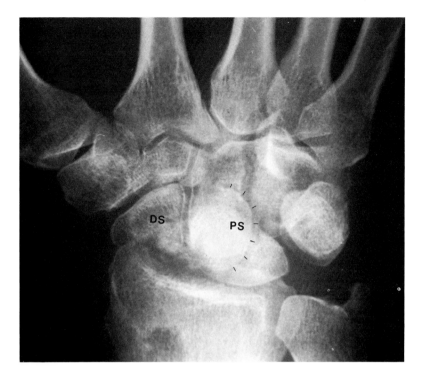

scaphoid to remain in a longitudinal alignment (Fig. 9-8B). If the injury includes a transscaphoid fracture, then the outline of a single scaphoid is missing, and two major fragments may be made out in the lateral views, the proximal having remained with the lunate, the distal displaced with the capitate and the rest of the carpus (Fig. 9-9).

3. The capitate is not aligned with the radius, or if it is, there is no colinearity of radius, lunate and capitate (Figs. 9-8, 9-9). The diagnosis between a perilunate dislocation and a dislocation of the lunate is often a matter of radiologic interpretation, and may depend on the position of the wrist at the time the radiograph was obtained. These very unstable wrists may easily and readily shift from the alignment of a perilunate dislocation to that of a dislocation of the lunate. The distinction is, to a great extent, largely academic, for both are just stages of the same injury and their treatment is identical.[41] The lunate may rarely dislocate dorsally.

"Exploded" views obtained in traction with the fingers suspended in finger traps are excellent for the assessment of the actual extent of the bony and articular disruption (Fig. 9-10).[39,41] Special studies are rarely necessary. Although arthrograms may help to delineate the severity of the capsular and ligamentous damage,[34] they add very little information to that which should be simply surmised from the evaluation of plain films and from a knowledge of the mechanism of injury.

TREATMENT

In general it must be understood that there are two stages to the treatment of these injuries. The initial goal is the restoration of the alignment between radius, lunate, and capitate. Late treatment may need to be directed to the correction of the mechanism that allowed the dislocation to occur in the first place, namely, the scapholunate dissociation (Fig. 9-6C) or the fracture through the scaphoid, both of which may remain as the telltale signs of the reduced major injuries. Therefore, most if not all of these injuries are first treated by manipulation. Indications for open reduction become apparent either immediately following an attempt at manipulation or shortly thereafter. These indications are as follows[18]:

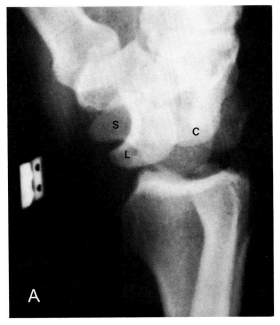

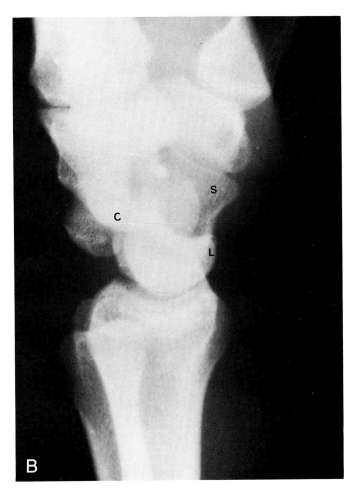

Fig. 9-8. Lateral views of perilunate and lunate dislocations. *A*: The capitate (C) is almost colinear with the radius. The scaphoid (S) is palmarflexed. The lunate (L) *is* tipped palmarward, the "spilled teacup" sign. *B*: The lunate (L) has remained aligned with the radius. The capitate (C) is aligned dorsally and the scaphoid (S) remains in a longitudinal alignment.

1. Irreducible dislocations of the lunate
2. Persistent displacement of carpal fracture fragments
3. Persistent rotatory subluxation of the scaphoid

TREATMENT OF LESSER ARC INJURIES

DORSAL PERILUNATE DISLOCATIONS

Dorsal perilunate dislocations are easier to reduce if seen while fresh, before swelling obscures anatomic landmarks and makes manipulation more difficult. A satisfactory anesthesia and complete muscle relaxation[39,41] are essential. The hand is suspended, usually with wire finger traps, or with a Weinberger apparatus. Counterweights are then hung from the arm near the elbow flexure, with the elbow at 90 degrees of flexion. Usually 10 lb are sufficient, although for the larger, more muscular arms greater weights may be required. Uninterrupted traction is continued for five to ten minutes.[40] Preliminary radiographs are now obtained. These will assist in demonstrating what traction alone has accomplished, and will provide a more accurate rendition of the extent and nature of the injury (Fig. 9-10B). Small fractures that may be difficult to visualize in routine films are better seen in the traction views. Manipulation may now be attempted, following the guidelines proposed by Codman and Chase[20] in 1905 and by Tavernier[99] in 1906, and later modified by Sir Watson Jones.[109] There is no need to use hard objects applied to the volar side of the wrist to exert a lever action

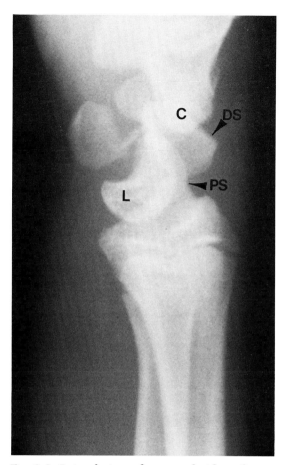

Fig. 9-9. Lateral view of transcaphoid perilunate fracture-dislocation. C, capitate, aligned dorsal to the radius. DS and PS, distal and proximal fragments of the scaphoid. The lunate (L) is minimally tilted into palmarflexion.

to facilitate reductionof the lunate, the so-called "broomstick"[6,24] or "wrench"[94] methods. Conwell had originally used the Davis broomstick method[21] but later stressed the advantage of utilizing thumb pressure only.[22] In effect, all maneuvers should be gentle; in general, manipulation results in surprisingly easy reduction[26,41,47,54]. The surgeon holds the patient's hand as the finger traps are removed (Fig. 9-11). The patient's wrist is dorsiflexed; the thumb opposite to the side of injury is used to apply pressure against the palmar projection of the lunate, the aim being to stabilize the lunate as manipulation proceeds rather than to physically push it back under the radius, as interpreted by Destot.[26]

The patient's hand is now gradually palmar flexed, until the distinct snap of capitolunate reduction is felt. Rotation of the hand on the forearm may be required for this maneuver to succeed. Jeanne and Mouchet[54] implied this when they advocated that palmarflexion be accompanied by ulnar deviation, in effect imparting a pronation effect to the hand. Tanz[98] also advocated pronation for the reduction of perilunate dislocations. Radiographs are now obtained. Requisites for a satisfactory reduction are restoration of a normal capitolunate relationship and reduction of the scaphoid without evidence of residual rotatory subluxation. If this has been accomplished, a long arm plaster fixation is applied, with the wrist in just as much volarflexion as needed for a stable reduction, and the forearm and hand in pronation to lessen the tendency of the scaphoid to malrotate in supination. The maintenance of a satisfactory reduction should be assessed by radiographs obtained weekly for the first four to six weeks. If reduction is maintained, the long arm immobilization is discontinued at the end of six weeks and a short arm thumb spica cast is applied for an additional four-week period.

Indications for Surgical Treatment

1. *Perilunate dislocations past the acute stage*, either because the nature of the injury was not recognized initially or because the initial manipulation was unsuccessful. In these cases an attempt should be made by surgical means to correct the persistent carpal displacement. The actual choice of treatment may have to be made at the time of operation. With the carpus exposed, two factors are assessed: the feasibility of reduction, and the condition of the articular surfaces involved. A dorsal approach is used first; a second palmar approach may be required if reduction appears possible but difficult from the dorsal approach only. When reduction is no longer possible, or when the articular surfaces are damaged, a proximal row carpectomy may be performed.[47] However, a fusion across the mid carpal joint is an attractive alternative to proximal row carpectomy, particularly for these usually young and active patients, permitting preservation of pain-free, but limited motion,

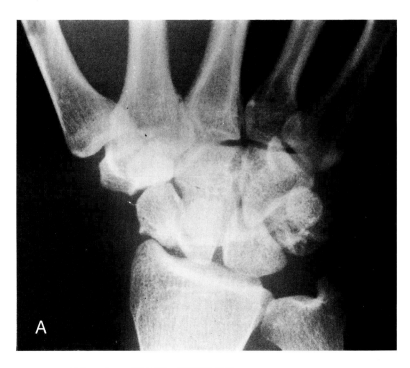

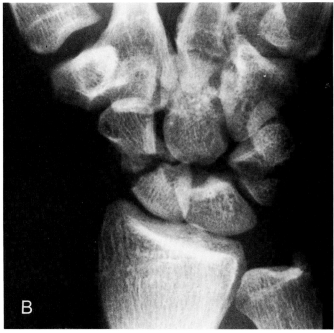

Fig. 9-10. Transcaphoid transtriquetral perilunate fracture dislocation. Carpal relationship
(A) is better appreciated in an "exploded" view
obtained with the hand in traction *(B)*.

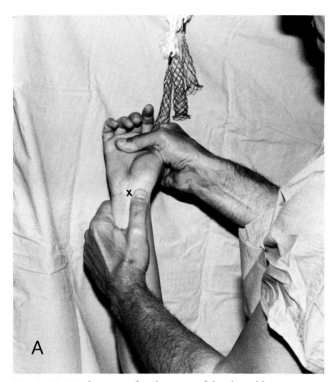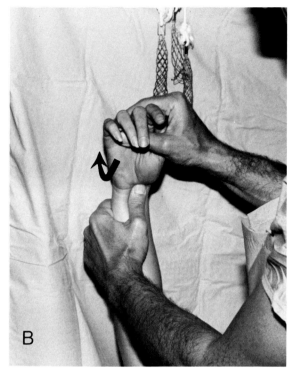

Fig. 9-11. Technique of reduction of displaced lesser arc injuries. *A:* After 5 to 10 minutes of uninterrupted traction, and following preliminary "exploded" radiographic views (see Fig. 9-10B), the surgeon supports the patient's hand as fingerstraps are removed. The injured wrist is dorsiflexed. The surgeon's thumb applies pressure against the palmar projection of the lunate (**X**). *B:* The patient's hand is gradually palmarflexed. Capitolunate reduction is felt as a distinct snap.

and maintenance of carpal height. Panarthrodesis is reserved for osteoarthritic wrists or for failed carpectomies and partial fusions.

2. *Persistent subluxation of the scaphoid,* either as a residual from the initial manipulation, or present at any time after an early satisfactory reduction (Fig. 9-12). The surgical treatment of rotatory subluxation is discussed in Chapter 11. Within the first three weeks following the injury, pinning of the reduced scaphoid to the lunate and the capitate under cineradiographic control may be attempted.[40] In my experience, although pure primary rotatory subluxations of the scaphoid may be successfully managed by manipulation and pinning under cineradiographic control, the scaphoid subluxation that is the residual of the reduced perilunate dislocation necessitates an open reduction, for it is considerably more unstable and difficult to treat. Therefore, in most

cases, an open reduction is preferred. In these early stages, a dorsal approach alone may suffice,[2] and ligament reconstructions or partial arthrodeses are not needed. If subluxation of the scaphoid recurs after immobilization is discontinued, or after the Kirschner wires are removed, or when residual secondary rotatory subluxation is not diagnosed or is treated more than three weeks after the initial injury, the surgical reduction of the malrotated scaphoid must be completed by a ligament reconstruction,[79] or preferably by a limited arthrodesis (see Chapter 11).

3. *Large unreduced bone fragments,* frequently from the radial styloid or the triquetrum, which are not reduced anatomically after manipulation, or interfere with reduction. In most cases, internal fixation of these fragments is required, using small smooth Kirschner wires, for an acceptable stabilization of the carpus.

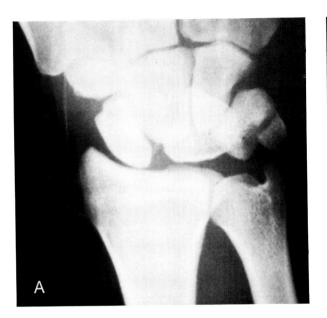

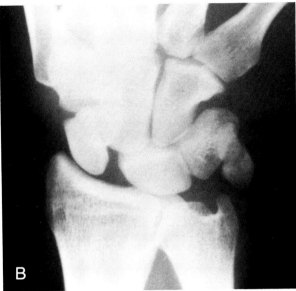

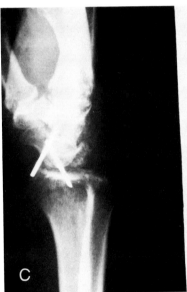

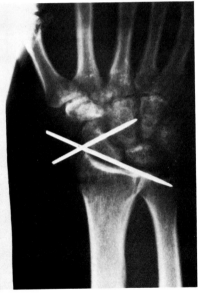

Fig. 9-12. Perilunate dislocation. *A:* Initial posteroanterior radiograph. *B:* Appearance following manipulative reduction; there is a persistent gap between scaphoid and lunate. *C:* Open reduction and internal fixation are required to correct residual scapholunate dissociation.

Surgical Technique

The initial approach is routinely dorsal. A transverse[2] or longitudinal skin incision can be used. Dorsal longitudinal veins and superficial nerves are protected. It is my preference in these wrists to enter the joint through the floor of the tunnel for the extensor pollicis longus tendon (Figs. 6-23, 6-25). This tendon is unroofed, retracted and the underlying floor is incised longitudinally to expose the joint. Both medial and lateral composite flaps are elevated subperiosteally and subcapsularly, preserving the integrity of the dorsal extensor compartments, particularly that containing the tendons of the extensor digitorum communis and the extensor indicis proprius. The exposure should be wide enough to visualize the scaphoid, lunate, the head of the capitate, and, if needed, the lunotriquetral joint. Reduction of residual dislocations, subluxations or fracture fragments is now per-

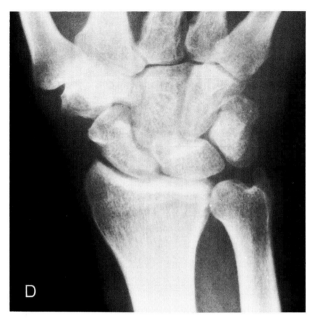

Fig. 9-12 (cont.) D: Final radiograph.

formed. Attention should be paid to actual reduction of the lunocapitate joint, with correction of any residual lunate tilt, and to restoration of the normal scapholunate relationship. Normally, the articular surface of the head of the capitate is completely covered by the lunate.[2] Any degree of exposure of this head is, therefore, abnormal. Manipulation of the lunate and scaphoid is facilitated by the insertion of short sturdy Kirschner wires from the dorsal toward the palmar side, to be used as handles for the control of angulation, and, particularly, of rotation (Fig. 9-13). The scapholunate joint is reduced first and immobilized with two 0.045 Kirschner wires introduced from just distal to the tip of the radial styloid, along the scaphoid and into the lunate. Any dorsiflexion tilt of the now fixed scapholunate complex is corrected, until the head of the capitate is covered; two additional Kirschner wires may now be needed, inserted usually from the scaphoid into the capitate. Closure is performed in layers. The extensor pollicis longus tendon may be left outside of its tunnel and dorsal to the repaired retinaculum without deleterious effect. A long arm thumb plaster spica is applied and worn for six weeks, followed by a short arm thumb plaster spica for four weeks. The Kirschner wires are usually removed at this time.

VOLAR DISLOCATION OF THE LUNATE

In the series of Campbell and coauthors[17] anterior dislocation of the lunate was the most frequent of the three common perilunate dislocations or fracture-dislocations. The treatment by manipulation of the acute injury is identical to that described for dorsal perilunate dislocations; dorsiflexion of the wrist prior to reduction should be accompanied by dorsal translation of the hand, in an attempt to "regress" one step in this cycle of progressive perilunate instability, changing a volar dislocation of the lunate into a dorsal perilunate dislocation. Stabilization of the lunate by thumb pressure is most important, as the capitate is brought over the lunate to the reduced position. As volarflexion proceeds, the hand should be rotated to facilitate reduction (Fig. 9-11B). Although Tanz[98] advocated supination of the hand on the forearm for the volar dislocations of the lunate, I find pronation usually just as effective and feel more comfortable with a postoperative immobilization with the hand in pronation to maintain scaphoid position more effectively. Avascular necrosis of the lunate is not usually a complication of this type of injury.

Indications for Surgical Treatment

1. *Chronic unreduced volar dislocations of the lunate.* Unreduced or unrecognized volar dislocations are not infrequent. In these cases, up to two or three weeks following the injury, a closed reduction may be attempted. Destot[26] had been able to reduce neglected dislocations that were two months old, but stated that he could not recommend this procedure. If manipulation fails, or if several months have elapsed since the original injury, an attempt should be made to reduce the lunate surgically (Fig. 9-4).[14] The lunate remains viable even in its dislocated position because blood supply may still reach it through its remaining attachment to the palmar radiolunate ligament. Surgical reduction of the lunate, attempted as early as 1897 by Vallas[104] is preferable to excision.[110] In most patients, a routine carpal tunnel incision is used first to carefully free up the lunate taking care not to damage the pal-

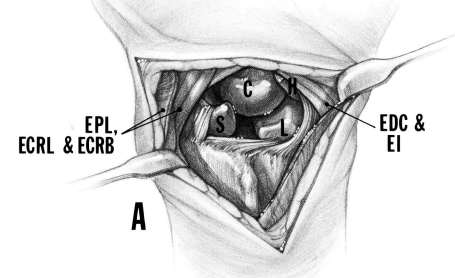

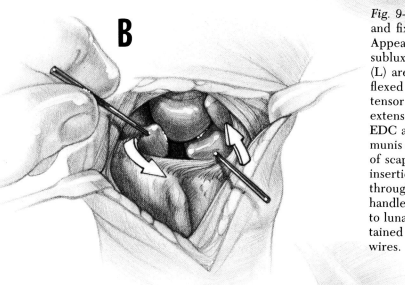

EPL,
ECRL & ECRB

C H

S L

EDC &
EI

A

B

Fig. 9-13. Surgical technique for reduction and fixation of scapholunate instability. *A*: Appearance of carpus. The capitate (C) is subluxed dorsally. Scaphoid (S) and lunate (L) are dissociated and the lunate is dorsiflexed and displaced palmarward. **EPL** is extensor pollicis longus. **ECR** and **ECRB** are extensor carpi radialis longus and brevis. **EDC** and **EIP** are extensor digitorum communis and indicis proprius. *B*: Manipulation of scaphoid and lunate is facilitated by the insertion of short, sturdy Kirschner wires through nonarticular surfaces to be used as handles. Arrows indicate motions imparted to lunate and scaphoid. *C*: Reduction is obtained and secured with multiple Kirschner wires.

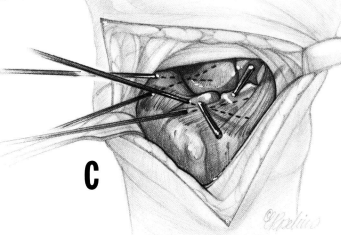

C

mar radiolunate ligament. In many cases, this approach is enough. A dorsal incision may be required to recreate the original space occupied by the lunate and facilitate its reduction. These may be difficult and laborious procedures. For those chronic dislocations, when reduction is not possible by surgical means, excision of the lunate and its replacement with a silastic implant has been proposed.[82] If this procedure is attempted, it would seem reasonable to reconstruct the palmar capsule using a tendon graft for an adequate reinforcement of the palmar wall, together with a scaphotrapezium-trapezoid or scaphocapitate fusion with the scaphoid in a neutral, noncollapsed alignment; this would restore carpal height and provide these patients with a load-bearing column from the hand to the radius. Proximal row carpectomy has also been suggested for these late injuries.[47] In most cases, however, particularly in the presence of isolated or generalized osteoarthritic changes, limited intracarpal arthrodeses, or radiocarpal fusions are the procedures of choice.

2. *Rotatory subluxation of the scaphoid.* Once capitolunate alignment is restored, attention must be directed to the scaphoid and its tendency to rotate into subluxation. Should this occur, the correction is identical to that following perilunate dislocations.

3. *Median neuropathy.* Open surgical treatment is indicated following reduced dislocations of the lunate when there is persistent, severe or progressive, or even delayed symptoms of median nerve compression at the level of the carpal tunnel. If these symptoms are not relieved by a change in the position of the wrist in plaster, the nerve should be explored and decompressed. This affords the opportunity to evaluate the extent of the volar capsular damage and to repair it.[27] The carpus is internally fixed at the same time, using an additional dorsal approach if needed, thus avoiding postoperative positioning of the wrist in extreme palmar flexion. Avascular necrosis of the lunate, even after open reductions, is extremely rare,[18,27,62,73,86] as long as the important source of blood supply through the intact palmar radiolunate ligament is undisturbed (see Chapter 4).

4. *Flexor tendon ruptures.* These have been described following an old unreduced dislocation of the lunate.[94] These are also indications for the surgical treatment of these injuries.

Fig. 9-14. Dorsal transcaphoid perilunate fracture-dislocation. L, lunate; C, capitate; DS and PS, distal and proximal fragments of the scaphoid; T, triquetrum.

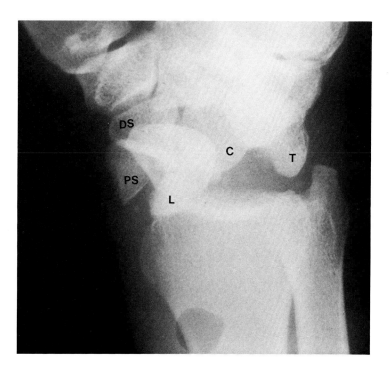

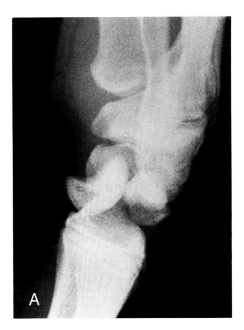

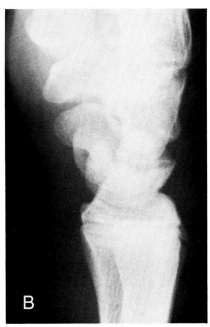

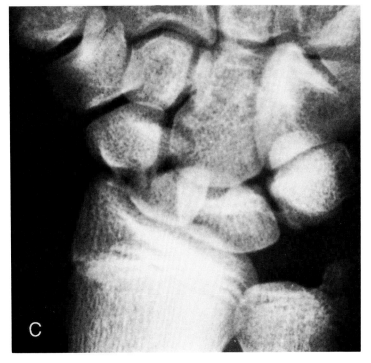

Fig. 9-15. *A*: Transcaphoid perilunate fracture-dislocation. *B*: Lateral view after closed reduction. *C*: Posteroanterior radiograph after closed reduction.

VOLAR PERILUNATE DISLOCATIONS/ DORSAL DISLOCATION OF THE LUNATE

In 1905 Codman and Chase[20] deplored the increased confusion created within the already confusing spectrum of carpal injuries by the introduction of "posterior (dorsal) dislocation of the semilunar, the occurrence of which we have good reason to doubt." They were right, because the earliest report of a dorsal dislocation of the lunate proven by radiographic examination was published in the following year, 1906, by Thebault.[100] These

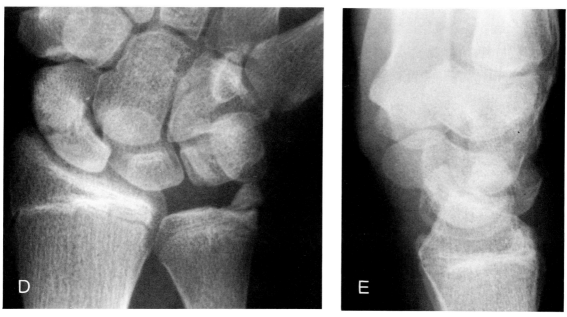

Fig. 9-15 (cont.) D and E: Radiographic appearance after 8 weeks of immobilization. (Courtesy of Dr. Glenn G. Almquist, Orange, CA.)

are indeed, very unusual injuries; single reports are rarely found in even large series[92] and case reports are exceedingly rare.[12,89] Volar perilunate dislocations are somewhat more frequent.[23,28,29,62,66,71,74,75,90,112,117] The overall approach to the treatment of these injuries is similar to that proposed for the more common forms of fracture dislocations and dislocations of the carpus. Acute injuries are managed by gentle finger-trap traction, allowed to continue for several minutes before manipulation is tried under satisfactory anesthesia and muscle relaxation. Reduction of the dorsally shifted lunate

Fig. 9-16. Internal fixation for the scaphoid fragments following closed reduction for transcaphoid-perilunate fracture-dislocation.

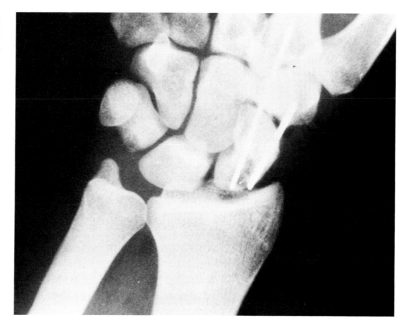

is attempted by direct pressure from the dorsum (the lunate is more readily palpable than in volar dislocations), while at the same time the hand is palmarflexed and rotated into supination around an imaginary pivot point passing through the triquetrum. Volar perilunate dislocations are more difficult to reduce than the dorsal variety, and when reduced are more likely to recur.[90] Open reduction and internal fixation with smooth Kirschner wires is indicated in these cases, after failure of manipulative reduction, or because of residual carpal instability, and for the neglected cases. The same surgical technique used for dorsal perilunate dislocation is applicable to these injuries. For volar perilunate dislocations, the general plan of postoperative care suggested for the more common injuries is also pertinent, except that usually immobilization is more effective with the wrist in neutral or slight dorsiflexion.

TREATMENT OF GREATER ARC INJURIES

DORSAL TRANSSCAPHOID PERILUNATE DISLOCATION

In 1902 De Quervain[84] described a combination of dislocation of the semilunar bone and fracture of the scaphoid. This is one of the three most frequent dislocations or fracture-dislocations of the carpus, together with the volar dislocations of the lunate and the dorsal perilunate dislocations. A review of the literature shows some controversy as to the treatment of this injury during the acute stages. While some authors[86] report satisfactory results with manipulative reductions, others propose immediate wrist arthrodeses[108] or excision of the lunate and the proximal fragment of the scaphoid[62] should initial reduction be less than anatomic. There is, however, no reason to resort to these more drastic procedures when treating fresh transscaphoid perilunate fracture-dislocations. Actually, the only difference between these injuries and the dorsal perilunate dislocations is the location of the main destabilizing injury, across the scaphoid rather than between the scaphoid and the lunate (Figs. 9-7, 9-9, 9-14). Therefore, the *initial* treatment is directed to reduction by manipulation, using a technique identical to that described for perilunate dislocations and volar dislocations of the lunate (Fig. 9-15). Jahna[53] had suggested slight supination of the forearm to facilitate reduction. Careful postmanipulation radiographic follow up is required at weekly intervals until stability is apparent, usually no sooner than four to six weeks later (Fig. 9-15D,E).

Indication for Surgery

Indications for surgical treatment are similar to those discussed for the lesser arc injuries, namely, initial reductions that are not entirely anatomic, recurrence of subluxation or instability, or the treatment of the older unrecognized chronic dislocations. In transscaphoid injuries, the emphasis is placed on the reduction and fixation of the fracture fragments of the scaphoid (Fig. 9-16), and on the restoration or correction of secondary or recurrent carpal collapse alignments. An open reduction becomes indicated as soon as reduction of the scaphoid appears less than anatomic. Alignment of the scaphoid fragments is best evaluated by studying the concave outline of the scaphoid in posteroanterior, anteroposterior, and oblique views. Internal fixation may be secured with two 0.045 Kirschner wires, or with a screw.[46,51,52] Bone grafting is usually not necessary if this treatment is provided within the first three weeks following the injury, unless the fracture of the scaphoid is comminuted. Loss of reduction of the scaphoid fragments, if these were not stabilized, is the rule rather than the exception following these highly unstable injuries. Failure to fix the fracture fragments results in a distressingly high number of nonunions[67,73] and on an increased incidence of avascular necrosis.[108] In the late stages, treatment is directed toward correcting residual nonunions of the scaphoid (see Chapter 6). An uncommon mistake is to attempt stabilization by bone grafting *alone* (Fig. 9-17). This will inexorably fail.

In summary, the surgical approach, the selection of the internal fixation technique, and the indications for bone grafting vary with the characteristics of the fracture and the time elapsed since injury. In general, an anterior, Russe type of approach is preferred (see Chapter 6). In my hands, internal fixation with smooth Kirschner wires is easier to accomplish and just as effective as fixation with screws. Green[41] advocated the temporary place-

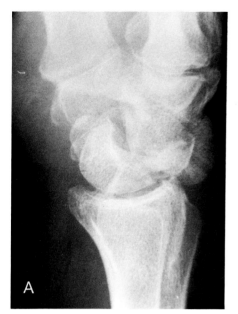

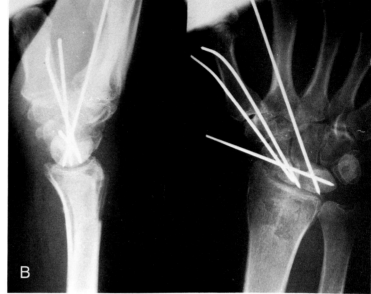

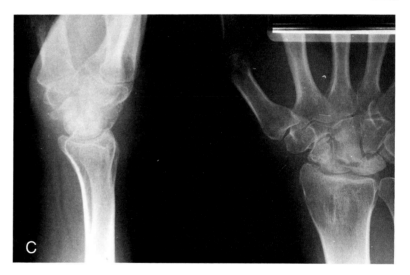

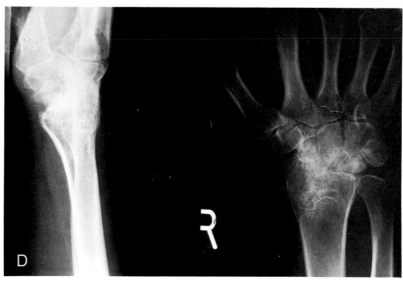

Fig. 9-17. Transcaphoid perilunate fracture-dislocation. A: Radiographic appearance after failed reduction and Russe's bone graft as only initial treatment. There is a complete recurrence of carpal dislocation. B: Postoperative radiographs following open reduction, internal fixation and insertion of a bone graft for the scaphoid fracture. This procedure failed (C). D: Final appearance 4 months after radiocarpal fusion.

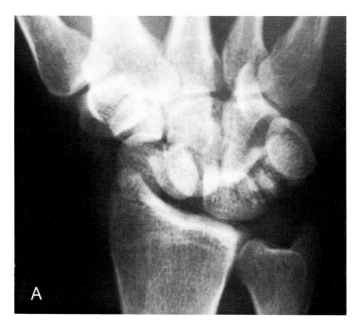
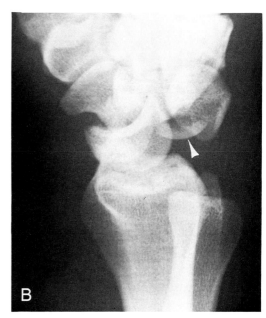

Fig. 9-18. Transcaphoid transcapitate perilunate fracture-dislocation. *A:* Posteroanterior radiograph. *B:* Lateral view shows head of capitate (arrow).

ment of a threaded 0.045 Kirschner wire into each of the two scaphoid fragments, to be used as "handles" for manipulation and reduction. Bone grafts, as we have seen, are not recommended for fractures under three weeks, and rarely for fractures under six weeks, unless there is radiographic and operative evidence of early bony sclerosis at the fracture site. Radiographic proof of scaphoid reduction, adequate insertion of pins or screws, and satisfactory restoration of carpal alignment must be obtained intraoperatively. Persistence of instability as evidenced by an abnormal lunate tilt, usually into dorsiflexion, may require an additional dorsal exposure and reduction and fixation of the lunocapitate joint.[41] Postoperatively these wrists are immobilized in a compression dressing incorporated into a long arm circular plaster dressing. This is followed by a long arm plaster that includes the thumb in opposition and the index and long fingers in an intrinsic-plus position. At three weeks, a routine long arm thumb plaster spica is applied and worn for an additional three weeks. At the end of six weeks it is replaced with a short arm thumb plaster spica, which is worn until twelve weeks have elapsed. If the Kirschner wires used for inter-

nal fixation were parallel to each other, they may be left in place until the twelfth postoperative week. If the Kirschner wires crossed each other on either plane, then one of the wires should be removed no later than six weeks postoperatively to prevent persistent distraction. For the treatment of persistent nonunion or avascular necrosis of the scaphoid, consult Chapter 6.

VOLAR TRANSSCAPHOID PERILUNATE FRACTURE-DISLOCATIONS

Volar transscaphoid perilunate fracture-dislocations are lesions similar to the volar perilunate dislocations, except that destabilization of the carpus occurs through the scaphoid rather than at the level of the scapholunate joint. Goullioud and Arcelin[38] were most likely the first to publish a proven case of volar transscaphoid perilunate fracture-dislocation. Five years later, on March 1, 1913, in a report to the Surgical Society at Lyon, France, Destot (quoted by Auvray[10]) stated that he knew of only two authentic cases of this type of midcarpal forward dislocation, that of Goullioud and Arcelin,

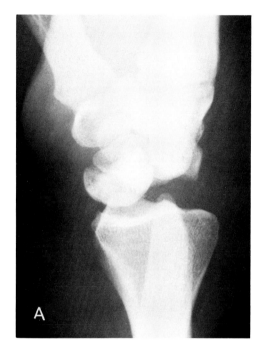

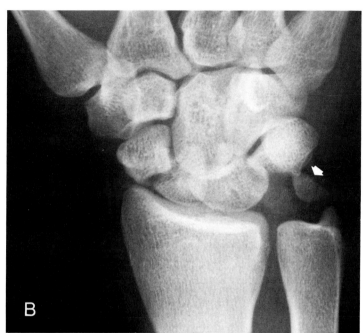

Fig. 9-19. Transcaphoid transtriquetral perilunate fracture-dislocation. *A:* Lateral view. *B:* Posteroanterior view shows fracture of the scaphoid and triquetrum (arrow). *C:* Both fractures are well visualized in postreduction view (arrows).

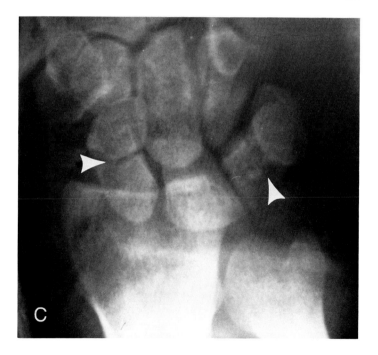

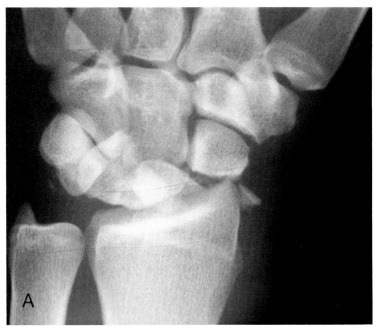

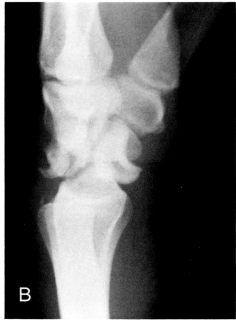

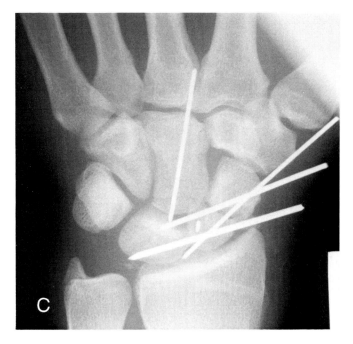

Fig. 9-20. Transcaphoid transcapitate perilunate fracture-dislocation. *A:* Initial posteroanterior radiograph. *B:* Lateral radiograph. *C:* Immediate postoperative appearance.

and a case that he had observed at Val de Grâce. This patient (who was also the subject of a communication by Mouchet and Vennin[75]) had been presented by Vennin to Destot during the latter's visit to Val de Grâce. Since these early reports, only isolated cases have been published.[4,90,97,118] Most large series mention only dorsal transscaphoid perilunate fracture dislocations.[17,29] Rarely, a few cases of a similar volar fracture-dislocation are included.[62,92,117]

The care of this injury is identical to that proposed for the more frequent dorsal transscaphoid

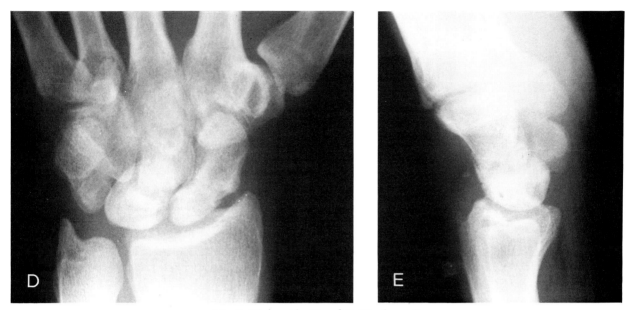

Fig. 9-20 (cont.)   D and E: Final result.

perilunate fracture-dislocation, except that the position of immobilization should be that which proves more stable, frequently with the wrist in dorsiflexion.[4] Attention should again be directed to restoration of radiolunocapitate alignment, and to a stable accurate reduction of the scaphoid frag-

ments. Persistence of a fracture malalignment is usually the reason for an operative intervention, for an anatomic reduction of the scaphoid by closed means is highly unlikely and, furthermore, maintenance of reduction without internal fixation is near-impossible. The treatment of this injury is

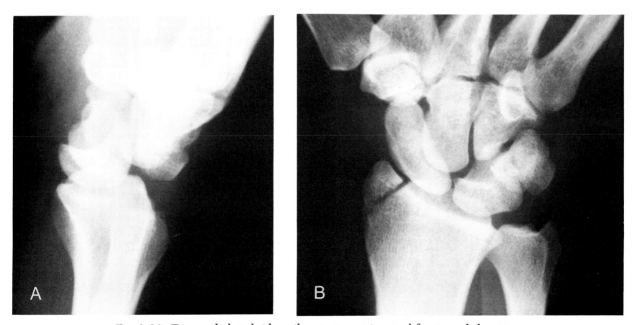

Fig. 9-21. Transradial-styloid perilunate transtriquetral fracture-dislocation.

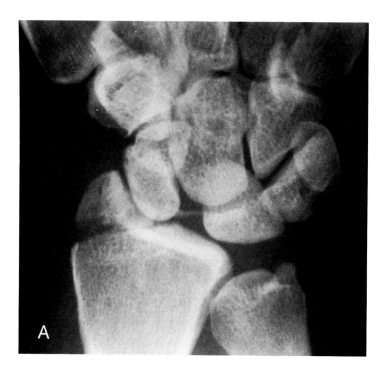

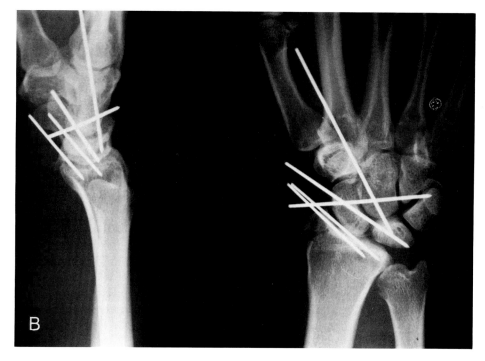

Fig. 9-22. Transradial-styloid perilunate fracture-dislocation. *A:* After closed reduction. There is residual scapholunate dissociation. The radial styloid fragment is tilted. *B:* Appearance after open reduction and internal fixation with multiple Kirschner wires.

best accomplished through a volar, Russe-type surgical approach[29,40,41] that may be supplemented by a dorsal approach, usually when intraoperative radiographs show unsatisfactory reduction.

OTHER "GREATER ARC" FRACTURE-DISLOCATIONS

There are some more unstable variations of the frequent dorsal transscaphoid perilunate fracture-dislocations, in which additional carpal fractures have occurred, involving the capitate (Fig. 9-18), the capitate and hamate, the capitate and triquetrum (Fig. 9-10), or the triquetrum alone (Fig. 9-19). In my experience, these rare injuries require initial manipulation to restore gross radiolunocapitate alignment, followed immediately or within a few days by an open reduction with internal fixation of the carpal fractures (Fig. 9-20). The postoperative care is thereafter dictated by the progress of the fractures, particularly those of the scaphoid and capitate (see previous discussions of the treatment of dorsal transscaphoid perilunate fracture-dislocations and Chapters 6 and 7).

VARIANTS

The most common variant is the transradial styloid fracture accompanying a perilunate or transscaphoid perilunate fracture-dislocation (Fig. 9-21). Noble and Lamb[78] published an exceptional case of transradial styloid-transscaphoid-translunate fracture-dislocation, in which a horizontal fracture line cut across the base of the radial styloid, the proximal scaphoid, and the body of the lunate. In this same category are the more extensive fracture-dislocations of the "greater arc," typically the transscaphoid-transcapitate-transtriquetral perilunate fracture-dislocations when radial and ulnar styloids are also involved.[115] Other var-

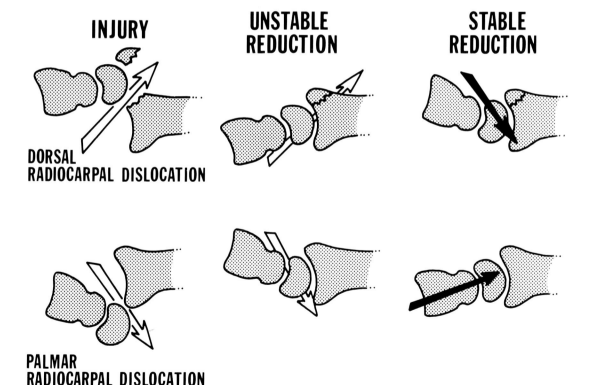

Fig. 9-23. Radiocarpal dislocations and fracture-dislocations are very unstable. When the carpal dislocation is dorsal, stable reduction is possible with the wrist in dorsiflexion. Palmar carpal dislocations are more stable after reduction if immobilized with the wrist in palmarflexion.

iants include the scaphocapitate fracture syndrome, isolated dislocations of one or more carpal bones (see Chapter 7) and some very rare, very bizarre injuries.[61] Most, if not all, of these variants, should be treated by open reduction and internal fixation of the displaced fracture fragments and a reduction and fixation of the dislocated carpal bones (Fig. 9-22).

RADIOCARPAL DISLOCATIONS

In 1838 Malle[64] presented a patient with a volar radiocarpal dislocation without evidence of fracture, in all probability the first such a case to be found in the medical literature. The earliest descriptions of *dorsal* radiocarpal dislocations are attributed to Marjolin[65] and to Voillemier,[106] both published in 1839. In all these cases, an initial clinical assumption of the presence of a radiocarpal dislocation was proven by postmortem examination of the wrists. Abadie[1] and Tavernier[99] present an exhaustive listing of these as well as other carpal injuries, and agree that, reviewing the literature, proven dorsal radiocarpal dislocations were considerably more frequent than volar radiocarpal dis-

locations. Abadie could gather only 18 case reports of volar radiocarpal dislocations in a review of the literature published until 1901, compared to 52 dorsal radiocarpal dislocations. Abadie quotes Jarjavay[1] who described a dry specimen that he found in a medical school laboratory dedicated to surgical practice, of a volar (forward) carpal dislocation with a small fracture fragment, still movable, attached to the volar lip of the radius. Goodall[37] also described an autopsy specimen of the wrist with a volar carpal dislocation, except that in his case, the triquetrum had remained in its normal location, while the remaining carpus dislocated. In 1919 Henry Judet[56] presented a case to the 28th French Congress of Surgery, following Jeanne and Mouchet's encyclopedic discussion or wrist injuries. His report was the first instance of recurrent voluntary palmar radiocarpal dislocation, eight days following an injury. This displacement pattern was proven by radiographs and was successfully treated by plaster immobilization. Gui[43] states that the incidence of radiocarpal dislocations with or without fractures of the styloid process of the radius is about 0.2 percent of all dislocations. These are all highly unstable injuries which may need external skeletal fixation to maintain reduction,[29,69] al-

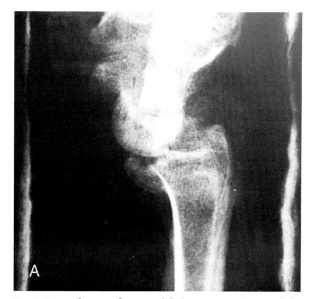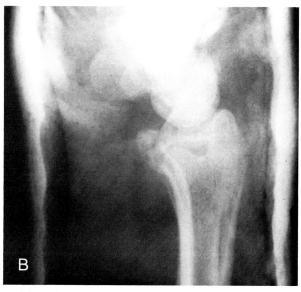

Fig. 9-24. Palmar radiocarpal dislocation with a small fracture of the palmar rim of the radius. *A:* Recurrence of carpal displacement with the wrist in dorsiflexion. *B:* Satisfactory, stable reduction obtained three weeks later with the wrist in slight palmarflexion.

though in general, stability after manipulation may be achieved by immobilization in some dorsiflexion for the dorsal dislocations[13,29,85] or by immobilization in neutral[83] or slight palmarflexion[29] for the treatment of volar dislocations (Figs. 9-23, 9-24).

REFERENCES

1. Abadie J: Des luxations radio-carpiennes traumatiques. Thèse Montpellier, 1901
2. Adkinson JW, Chapman MW: Treatment of acute lunate and perilunate dislocations. Clin Orthop 164:199, 1982
3. Adler JB, Shaftan GW: Fractures of the capitate J Bone Joint Surg [Am] 44:1357, 1962
4. Aitken AP, Nalebuff EA: Volar transnavicular perilunar dislocation of the carpus. J Bone Joint Surg [Am] 42:1051, 1960
5. Albertin: Note sur un cas de luxation traumatique de l'os semilunaire sur la face palmaire du poignet gauche. Province Med 27:420, 1887
6. Andrews FT: A dislocation of the carpal bones. The scaphoid and semi-lunar: Report of a case. Mich St Med Soc J 31:269, 1932
7. Apelt F: Zur Casuistik der Luxation des Os Lunatum Carpi. Monatschr Unfallheilk (Leipzig) 10:213, 1903
8. Armstrong GWD: Rotational subluxation of the scaphoid. Can J Surg 11:306, 1968
9. Aufranc OE, Jones WN, Harris WH: Transnavicular retrolunar dislocation of the wrist. JAMA 181:131, 1982
10. Auvray N: Rapport de luxation médio-carpienne en avant du poignet droit, par Mouchet A et Vennin H. Bull Mem Soc Chir 32:1376, 1913
11. Bialy F: Über die luxation des os lunatum. Julius Klinkhardt, Leipzig, 1902
12. Bilos ZJ, Hui PW: Dorsal dislocation of the lunate with carpal collapse. J Bone Joint Surg [Am] 63:1484, 1981
13. Bounds TB: Bilateral radiocarpal dislocation: A case report. Orthopedics 5:42, 1982
14. Boyes JH: Bunnell's Surgery of the Hand. 5th Ed. Lippincott, Philadelphia, 1970
15. Buchanan G: Case of compound dislocation of the semilunar bone of the carpus. Med Times Gaz (London) 1:113, 1885
16. Buzby BF: Perinavicular-lunar dorsal dislocation of the wrist with comminuted fracture of the navicular. Ann Surg 100:557, 1934
17. Campbell RD Jr, Lance EM, Yeoh CB: Lunate and perilunar dislocation. J Bone Joint Surg [Br] 46:55, 1964
18. Campbell RD Jr, Thompson TC, Lance EM, Adler JB: Indications for open reduction of lunate and perilunate dislocation of the carpal bones. J Bone Joint Surg [Am] 47:915, 1965
19. Cave EF: Retrolunar dislocation of the capitate with fracture or subluxation of the navicular bone. J Bone Joint Surg 23:830, 1941
20. Codman EA, Chase HM: The diagnosis and treatment of fracture of the carpal scaphoid and dislocation of the semilunar bone, with a report of thirty cases. Part II. Ann Surg 41:863, 1905
21. Conwell HE: Closed reduction of acute dislocation of the semilunar carpal bone. Ann Surg 92:289, 1925
22. Conwell HE: Closed reduction of recent dislocation of the semilunar (lunate) bone with results and discussion regarding necrosis (malacia). Report of eleven cases. Ann Surg 103:978, 1936
23. Cotte G: Luxation du grand os en avant. Bull Soc Chir 45:1252, 1919
24. Davis GG: Treatment of dislocated semilunar carpal bones. Surg Gynecol Obstet 37:225, 1923
25. Delbet P: Luxation du poignet avec fracture du scaphoïde. Bull Soc Chir, 30:949, 1904
26. Destot E: Traumatismes du poignet et rayons X. Masson, Paris, 1923
27. Dobyns JH, Linscheid RL: Complication of treatment of fractures and dislocations of the wrist. In Epps CH Jr (ed): Complications in Orthopaedic Surgery. Vol. 2. Lippincott, Philadelphia, 1978
28. Douarre M: Luxation du grand os en avant. Bull Soc Chir 47:185, 1921
29. Dunn AW: Fractures and dislocations of the carpus. Surg Clin North Am 52:1513, 1972
30. Eigenbrodt: Ueber isolierte luxationen der carpal knochen, speziell des mondbeins. Beitr Klin Chir 30:805, 1901
31. Farr CE: Dislocation of the carpi semilunar bone. Ann Surg 84:112, 1926
32. Fenton RL, Rosen H: Fracture of the capitate bone: Report of two cases. Bull Hosp Joint Dis 11:134, 1950.
33. Fenton RL: The naviculo-capitate fracture syndrome. J Bone Joint Surg [Am] 38:681, 1956
34. Ganel A, Engel J, Ditzian R, et al: Arthrography as a method of diagnosing soft tissue injuries of the wrist. J Trauma 19:376, 1979
35. Gilula LA: Carpal injuries: Analytic approach and case exercises. Am J Roentgenol 133:503, 1979
36. Golden WW: Dislocation of the semilunar bone:

report of case in which reduction was successful. JAMA 76:446, 1921

37. Goodall WP: Forward dislocation of the wrist. Death. Dissection of the articulation. Lancet 1:937, 1878

38. Goullioud and Arcelin: Luxation en avant de la tête du grand os. Lyon Med 2:550, 1908

39. Green DP, O'Brien ET: Open reduction of carpal dislocations: Indications and operative techniques. J Hand Surg 32:250, 1978

40. Green DP, O'Brien ET: Classification and management of carpal dislocations. Clin Orthop 149:55, 1980

41. Green DP: Carpal dislocations. In Green DP (ed): Operative Hand Surgery. Vol. I. Churchill Livingstone, New York, 1982

42. Gross H: Der Mechanismus der Luxatio Ossis Lunati, nebst Bemerkungen über die Enstehung der Fraktur desselben knochen. Archiv Klin Chir 70:793, 1903

43. Gui L: Fratture e lussazioni. Firenze Edizioni Scientifiche Istituto Ortopedico Toscano, 1957

44. Hamill RC: Forward dislocation of semilunar bone, undiagnosed. Int Clin 3:124, 1920

45. Hémery GEJ: Contribution a l'etude des luxations du semi-lunaire. Thèse, Lille, 1902

46. Herbert TJ: Management of the fractured scaphoid bone using a new surgical technique. Orthop Trans 6:464, 1982

47. Hill NA: Fractures and dislocations of the carpus. Orthop Clin North Am 1:275, 1970

48. Hodges RM: Compound dislocation of the semilunar bone of the carpus. Boston Med Surg J 73:261, 1866

49. Höfliger (of Zurich): Ueber Frakturen und Luxationen der Carpalknochen. Korrespondenzblatt Schweiz Aerzte 10:297, 1901

50. Höfliger (of Zurich): Ueber Frakturen und Luxationen der Carpalknochen. Korrespondenzblatt Schweiz Aerzte 10:338, 1901

51. Huene DR: An alignment instrument for pin fixation of small bone fractures. Orthop Rev 6:93, 1977

52. Huene DR: Primary internal fixation of carpal navicular fractures in the athlete. Am J Sports Med 7:175, 1979

53. Jahna H: Erfahrungen und Nachuntersuchungsergebnisse von 47 de Quervainschen Verrenkungsbrüchen. Arch Orthop Unfallchir 57:51, 1965

54. Jeanne LA and Mouchet A: Les lesions traumatiques fermeés du poignet. 28th Congrès Français de Chirurgie, 1919

55. Johnson RP: The acutely injured wrist and its residuals. Clin Orthop 149:33, 1980

56. Judet H: Lésions traumatiques fermeés du poignet. p. 204. Presented at the 28th Congrès Français de Chirurgie, 1919

57. Key JA, Conwell HE: The management of fractures, dislocations and sprains. 3rd Ed. p. 781. Mosby, St. Louis, 1942

58. Lesser LF von: Über die Luxationen der Mondbeins. Dtsche Z Chir 67:408, 1902

59. Lilienfeld A: Die luxatio ossis lunati volaris. Eine luxatio ossis capitati dorsalis. Arch Klin Chir 76:644, 1903

60. Lilienfeld A: Luxatio ossis lunati volaris. Munch Med Wochenschr 5:234, 1904

61. Lourie JA: An unusual dislocation of the lunate and the wrist. J Trauma 22:966, 1982

62. MacAusland WR: Perilunar dislocation of the carpal bones and dislocation of the lunate bone. Surg Gynecol Obstet 79:256, 1944

63. Malgaigne JF: Traité des fractures et luxations. Vol. 2. Baillière, Paris, 1855

64. Malle PNF: Lúxation du poignet en avant. Autopsie Rec Mem Méd Chir Milit 44:25, 1838

65. Marjolin N-R: Observation de luxation du poignet en arrière sans fracture du radius. Thèse, Paris, 1839

66. Maróttoli O: Luxación antelunar del carpo. Bol Soc Cir Rosario (Argent) 17:341, 1943

67. Mayfield JK: Mechanism of carpal injuries. Clin Orthop 149:45, 1980

68. Mayfield JK, Johnson RP, Kilcoyne RK: Carpal dislocations: Pathomechanics and progressive perilunar instability. J Hand Surg 5:226, 1980

69. McLaughlin HL: Trauma. p 168. Saunders, Philadelphia, 1959

70. Meyers MN, Wells R, Harvey JP: Naviculocapitate fracture syndrome. Review of the literature and a case report. J Bone Joint Surg [Am] 53:1383, 1971

71. Mikic Z, Somer T, Ercegan G: Perilunarne luksacije. Lijec Vjesn 104:405, 1982

72. Monahan PRW, Galasko CSB: The scaphocapitate fracture syndrome. A mechanism of injury. J Bone Joint Surg [Br] 54:122, 1972

73. Morawa LG, Ross PM, Schock CC: Fractures and dislocations involving the navicular-lunate axis. Clin Orthop 118:48, 1976

74. Mouchet A: Deux cas de luxation medio-carpienne en avant. Bull Soc Chir 44:1736, 1918

75. Mouchet A, Vennin H: Luxation medio-carpienne en avant du poignet droit. Bull Mem Soc Chir 32:176, 1913

76. Navarro A: Las luxaciones del carpo, pre o retrolunares. Pp. 233 in Anatomía y Fisiología del carpo, Anales del Instituto de Clinica Quirurgica y Cirugia Experimental. Imprenta Artistica de Dornaleche Hnos., Montevideo, 1935

77. Née L: De la luxation du semi-lunaire. Thèse, Paris, 1905

78. Noble J, Lamb DW: Translunate scapho-radial fracture. A case report. Hand 11:47, 1979

79. Palmer AK, Dobyns JH, Linschied RL: Management of post-traumatic instability of the wrist secondary to ligament rupture. J Hand Surg 3:507, 1978

80. Peiró A, Martos F, Mut T, Aracil J: Transscaphoid perilunate dislocation in a child. A case report. Acta Orthop Scand 52:31, 1981

81. Pournaras J, Kappas A: Volar perilunate dislocation. A case report. J Bone Joint Surg [Am] 61:625, 1979

82. Prinzivalli A: Lussazione inveterata del semilunare trattata mediante endoprotesi. Riv Chir Mano 16:33, 1979

83. Puig Rosado A: A possible relationship of radiocarpal dislocation and dislocation of the lunate bone. J Bone Joint Surg [Br] 48:504, 1966

84. Quervain F de: Beitrag zur Kenntnis der combinirten fracturen und luxationen der Handwurzelknochen. Monatsschr Unfallheilk Invalidenwesen (Leipzig) 9:3, 1902

85. Reynolds ISR: Dorsal radiocarpal dislocations. Injury 12:48, 1980/81

86. Russell TB: Intracarpal dislocation and fracture dislocation. A review of fifty-nine cases. J Bone Joint Surg [Br] 31:524, 1949

87. Sandzén SC Jr: Atlas of wrist and hand fractures. PSG Publishing, Littleton, MA, 1979

88. Saunier J, Chamay A: Volar perilunar dislocation of the wrist. Clin Orthop 157:139, 1981

89. Seidenstein H: Two unusual dislocations at the wrist. J Bone Joint Surg [Am] 38:1137, 1956

90. Sgrosso JA: Traumatismos del carpo: Tratamiento (Fracturas y luxaciones). 16th Congreso Argentino de Cirugia. Buenos Aires, 1944

91. Spar I: Bilateral perilunate dislocation: Case report with review of literature and anatomic study. J Trauma 18:64, 1978

92. Speed K: Traumatic injuries of the carpus. Including Colles' fracture. Appleton Century Crofts, New York, 1925

93. Stein F, Siegel MW: Naviculocapitate fracture syndrome: A case report. J Bone Joint Surg [Am] 51:391, 1969

94. Stern PJ: Multiple flexor tendon ruptures following an old anterior dislocation of the lunate. A case report. J Bone Joint Surg [Am] 63:489, 1981

95. Stern WG: Dislocation of carpal semilunar bone. JAMA 75:1389, 1920

96. Taleisnik J: Wrist: Anatomy, function and injury. Am Acad Orthop Surgeons Instruct Course Lect 27:61, 1978

97. Tanton J: A propos de qelques traumatismes du carpe. Bull Soc Chir 41:2131, 1915

98. Tanz SS: Rotation effect in lunar and perilunar dislocations. Clin Orthop 57:147, 1968

99. Tavernier L: Les déplacements traumatiques du semilunaire. Thèse, Lyon, 1906

100. Thebault V: A propos d'une luxation dorsale du semilunaire chez un accidenté du travail. Arch Gen Méd 83:1473, 1906

101. Thompson TC, Campbell RD Jr, Arnold WD: Primary and secondary dislocation of the scaphoid bone. J Bone Joint Surg [Br] 46:73, 1964

102. Tilmann: Beitrag zur lehre der luxation der handwurzelknochen. Dtsch Z Chir 49:98, 1898

103. Urban K: Ein fall von isolierte luxation des mondbeines. Wien Med Wochenschr 8:357, 1903

104. Vallas: Traitement de la luxation médio-carpiennne ancienne. Lyon Med 102:478, 1904

105. Vance RM, Gelberman RH, Evans ET: Scaphocapitate fractures: Patterns of dislocation, mechanisms of injury, and preliminary results of treatment. J Bone Joint Surg [Am] 62:271, 1980

106. Voillemier L-C: Histoire d'une luxation complète et récente du poignet en arrière, suivie de réflexions sur le mécanisme de cette luxation et sur son diagnostic différentiel. Arch Gen Med 6:404, 1839

107. Wagner CJ: Perilunar dislocations. J Bone Joint Surg [Am] 38:1198, 1956

108. Wagner CJ: Fracture-dislocations of the wrist. Clin Orthop 15:181, 1959

109. Watson-Jones R: Carpal semilunar dislocations of the carpal bones and dislocation of the lunate bone. Proc R Soc Med 22:1071, 1929

110. Watson-Jones R: Fractures and Joint Injuries. Wilson JN (ed): Vol II. 5th ed. Churchill Livingstone, London, 1976

111. Weber ER, Chao EY: An experimental approach to the mechanism of scaphoid waist fractures. J Hand Surg 3:142, 1978

112. Weeks PM: Acute bone and joint injuries of the hand and wrist. A clinical guide to management. Mosby, St. Louis, 1981

113. Weiss C, Laskin RS, Spinner M: Irreducible radiocarpal dislocation. A case report. J Bone Joint Surg [Am] 52:562, 1970

114. Weiss C, Laskin RS, Spinner M: Irreducible trans-scaphoid perilunate dislocation. A case report. J Bone Joint Surg [Am] 52:565, 1970

115. Weseley MS, Barenfeld PA: Trans-scaphoid trans-capitate, transtriquetral perilunate fracture-dislocation of the wrist. A case report. J Bone Joint Surg [Am] 54:1073, 1972

116. Wittek A: Ueber verletzungen der handwurzel (os lunatum). Beitr Z Klin Chir 42:578, 1904

117. Witwoët J, Allieu Y: Lésions traumatiques fraiches du semilunaire. Rev Chir Orthop 59:98, 1973

118. Woodward AH, Neviaser RJ, Nisenfeld F: Radial and volar perilunate transcaphoid fracture-dislocations. South Med J 68:926, 1975

119. Zolczer L, Nemes J, Nyári T, Gyárfás F: A nem friss és idösült perilunaris ficamok mütéti kezelése Magy Traumatol 23:81, 1980

10 Classification of Carpal Instability

The recognition of carpal instability as a clinical entity is relatively recent.[8,20] Until 1783, when Pouteau's description of a fracture of the distal radius was published posthumously, all injuries resulting in wrist deformity were thought to be radiocarpal dislocations.[6] The discovery of x-rays by Röntgen in 1895 provided clinicians and investigators with a sophisticated tool for the study of the normal wrist, and for the evaluation of the many wrist injuries which had previously been considered extremely rare.[4-6,9,17,18,22-24] In 1913 Chaput and Vaillant[4] published radiographic studies of carpal injuries, and stated that in some "there are abnormal separations between the bones of the carpus, separations about which it is difficult to say whether they correspond to diastasis, subluxations or dislocations." At least one of their cases showed a loss of the colinear alignment of the radius, lunate, and capitate, without frank dislocation or associated fracture. Of the early reports of carpal injuries that appeared in the European literature, particularly in the French literature, few qualified as true descriptions of carpal instability; perhaps the case of Chaput and Vaillant[4] and a patient of Mayersbach.[22] Auvray, discussing a case reported by Mouchet and Vennin[23] proposed a classification of "midcarpal luxations," into *total* or *partial*, depending on the number of carpal bones involved, and *complete* or *incomplete*, according to their relative degree of displacement. Jeanne and Mouchet[17] were aware of dorsal carpal subluxations following malunions of fractures of the distal radius, and dis-

cussed this potential complication in their extensive report of wrist injuries to the 28th French Congress of Surgery. In 1934 Mouchet and Belot[25] first called attention to midcarpal subluxations. In 1940 Marcelino Reyes (quoted by Bindi[3]), and in 1949 Vaughan-Jackson[37] reported on subluxation of the scaphoid, an injury that had been recognized and described by Destot[6] several years previously. This particular injury was called "Rotational dislocation of the scaphoid" by Fitton[13] and was more extensively described by Armstrong[2] in 1968. Prior to the publication of the landmark paper by Linscheid and coauthors[20] in 1972, instability of the scaphoid was the subject of most reports dealing with carpal instability.[3,7,10,28] Occasional references are found to subluxation of the medial side of the carpus[14] and to traumatic[1] and nontraumatic[16] radiocarpal dislocations not associated with fractures of the radius.

Gilford et al.[15] discussed the potential for instability present in the carpus. They compared the wrist to a link joint, stable under tension, but likely to crumple under compression loads, unless stabilized by a stop mechanism, represented in the wrist by the scaphoid. Fisk[11] first used the term "carpal instability" in reference to fractures of the scaphoid, in the title of his Hunterian Lecture, delivered to the Royal College of Surgeons of England on May 7, 1968. He described the zigzag alignment of the radius and carpus that may result from fractures of the scaphoid, and called it a "concertina deformity."

229

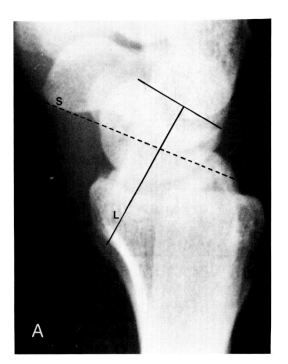

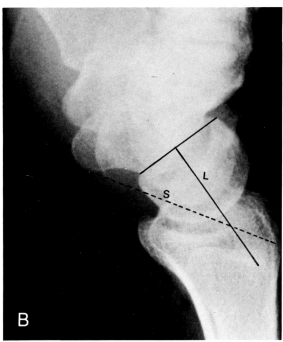

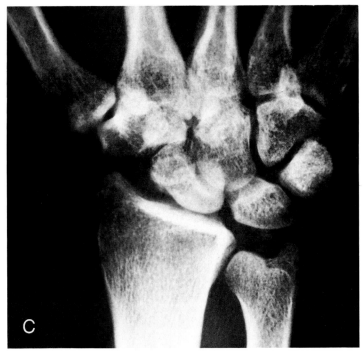

Fig. 10-1. Four major types of carpal instability. *A*: Dorsal instability (DISI). L, lunate axis; S, scaphoid's tangential axis. SL angle is 84 degrees. *B*: Volar instability. L, lunate axis; S, scaphoid's tangential axis. Both lunate and scaphoid are palmarflexed. The capitate is not colinear with the radius, but palmar to it. *C*: Ulnar translocation. The entire carpus has shifted in an ulnar direction. There is widening of the radial styloid-scaphoid space. The carpal-ulnar distance is decreased (see Fig. 5-5).

Fig. 10-1 (cont.) D: dorsal carpal sub-luxation following healed, malunited fracture of the distal radius.

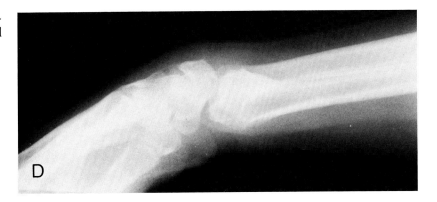

In 1972 and 1975 Dobyns, Linscheid, and collaborators,[8,20] proposed to group all these forms of carpal injuries under the name "traumatic instability of the wrist," which was defined as "a carpal injury in which loss of normal alignment of the carpal bones develops early or late." They also proposed to group carpal instabilities into four major types (Fig. 10-1):

1. Dorsiflexion instability
2. Palmarflexion instability
3. Ulnar translocation
4. Dorsal subluxation

The most frequent type, *dorsiflexion instability* (Fig. 10-1A), is present when the lunate is rotated into dorsiflexion in lateral roentgenograms. The normal colinear alignment of radius, lunate, and capitate is lost, the long axis of the capitate now dorsal to that of the radius. The term "dorsal intercalated segment instability," or DISI, was used to identify this condition, the "intercalated segment" being the lunate in lateral radiographs. The opposite pattern of *volar instability* or VISI (volar intercalated segment instability) is characterized by palmarflexion of the lunate (Fig. 10-1B). There is a zigzag alignment of the radiolunocapitate link, the capitate in these cases aligned palmar to the radius. Ulnar translocation occurs when the carpus shifts ulnar to its normal position (Fig. 10-1C). Dobyns et al.[8] stressed that the critical point in making this diagnosis is the presence of an increased space between scaphoid and radial styloid. This feature, however, is not always present in ulnar translocations. *Dorsal carpal subluxation* is an instability

pattern in which the carpus has subluxed dorsal to its normal alignment in relationship to the radius as seen in lateral radiographs (Fig. 10-1D).

These four basic types of instability were expanded in 1980.[33] Two primary instability patterns were recognized: static and dynamic (see Table 10-1). Further subdivisions were based on Navarro's concept of the columnar carpus (see Chapter 1).

STATIC AND DYNAMIC CARPAL INSTABILITY

Watson[38] has stated that the carpal joints are "a little like a 'Jack-in-the-box'" as if they were spring-loaded but kept under control by ligamentous restraints. A ligament tear is akin to releasing the spring in the Jack-in-the-box, allowing it to assume a different, paradoxically more stable, but abnormally aligned position. In effect, the Jack-in-

Table 10-1. Classification of Carpal Instability

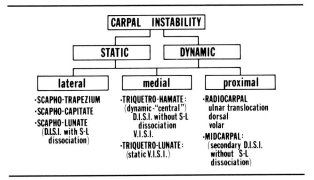

CARPAL INSTABILITY		
STATIC	DYNAMIC	
lateral	medial	proximal
·SCAPHO-TRAPEZIUM ·SCAPHO-CAPITATE ·SCAPHO-LUNATE (D.I.S.I. with S-L dissociation)	·TRIQUETRO-HAMATE: (dynamic-"central") D.I.S.I. without S-L dissociation V.I.S.I. ·TRIQUETRO-LUNATE: (static V.I.S.I.)	·RADIOCARPAL ulnar translocation dorsal volar ·MIDCARPAL: (secondary D.I.S.I. without S-L dissociation)

the-box in the carpus is represented by the lunate, held in a state of potentially unstable equilibrium by (1) its own shape, and position as an intercalated segment between the forearm and the hand; (2) the shape of the surrounding articular surfaces (particularly that of the distal radius); (3) pressures exerted by neighboring carpal bones; and (4) the guiding and restraining support of carpal ligaments. Changes of any of these characteristics can potentially lead to unstable alignments: (1) when the lunate collapses, such as in Kienböck's disease; (2) when the radiolunate relationship is reversed after malunion of fractures of the distal radius; (3) when scaphoid action on the lunate becomes abnormal after unstable scaphoid fractures; and (4) after various types of ligamentous tears. The resulting changes in carpal alignment, usually represented by dorsiflexion or palmar flexion of the lunate, or by its ulnar migration, cannot be actively reversed by the patient, nor can they be modified by manipulation or casting. These types of collapse, which may be recognized clinically and are readily seen in routine radiographs, are *static* forms of carpal instability (Fig. 10-1).[33,34] There is a group of patients, however, who do not fall into this category. Routine radiographic studies of their wrists are usually entirely within normal limits (Fig. 10-2A). These patients can change radiocarpal alignment almost at will, usually by bringing their hands into ulnar deviation with the forearm in pronation and by simultaneous longitudinal loading of their wrists, produced by the contraction of the extrinsic muscles that cross this joint. These patients exhibit a *dynamic* form of carpal instability,[33,34] which becomes apparent only when radiographs are obtained after the patient has actively assumed the position of collapse (Fig. 10-2B). These instabilities can be reversed to a normal alignment either by the patient or by the examining physician and can in turn be recognized in cineradiographic studies. The differentiation between static and dynamic types has diagnostic and therapeutic implications. Most dynamic forms are secondary to destabilization of the midcarpal joint and

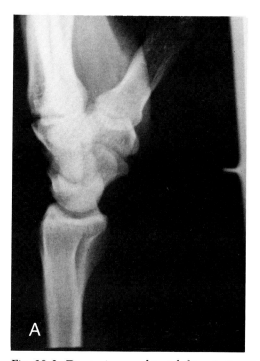
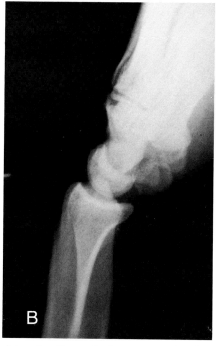

Fig. 10-2. Dynamic carpal instability. *A:* Routine lateral radiograph shows normal radiocarpal alignment. *B:* VISI is apparent only after patient assumes position of instability. This radiograph is obtained with the beam directed to the radial aspect of the wrist, and the plate vertical against the ulnar aspect (see Fig. 5-14A).

are treated by ligament repair or reconstruction or by limited intracarpal arthrodesis performed across the midcarpal joint.

ANATOMIC BASIS FOR A CLASSIFICATION OF CARPAL INSTABILITY

According to Navarro[26] the carpus should not be viewed as two horizontal carpal rows of four bones each, but rather as three vertical columns. Navarro's concept was modified in 1976[31] (Fig. 3-2). Based on this columnar concept, both dynamic and static instabilities may be further classified as *lateral,* occurring between the lateral column (scaphoid) and the central column (lunate-capitate-trapezium and trapezoid); *medial,* between the medial column (triquetrum) and the central column (lunate or hamate); and *proximal,* taking place between the entire carpus as a unit and the proximal radioulnar articular surface, frequently as a consequence of morphologic changes of the distal radius.

CLASSIFICATION OF CARPAL INSTABILITY

LATERAL CARPAL INSTABILITY

Scapholunate Dissociation

Scapholunate dissociation (rotatory subluxation of the scaphoid) is the most common form of carpal instability. It is secondary to the loss of support to the proximal pole of the scaphoid following trau-

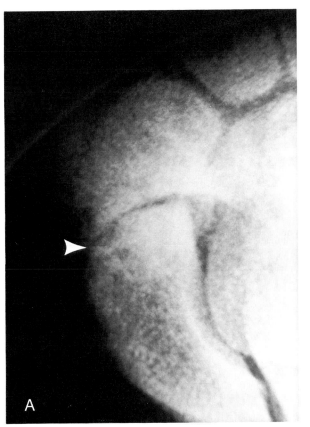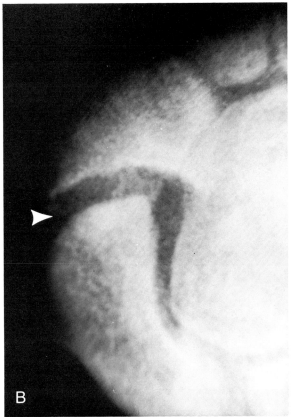

Fig. 10-3. *A* and *B*: Cineradiographs of patient showing voluntary scaphotrapezium-trapezoid instability (arrows). (Courtesy of Dr. Brian A. Ewald, Orange, CA.) (From Taleisnik J: Post-traumatic carpal instability. Clin Orthop 149:73, 1980.)

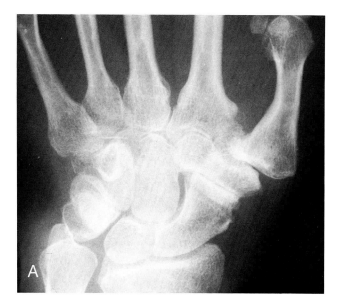

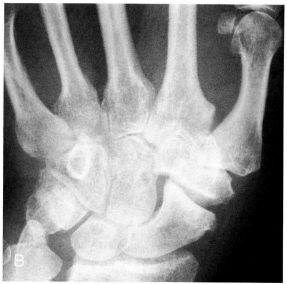

Fig. 10-4. Osteoarthritis in unstable scaphotrapezium-trapezoid joint. *A* and *B* show dynamic instability. *C*: Appearance one year following trapezium replacement arthroplasty.

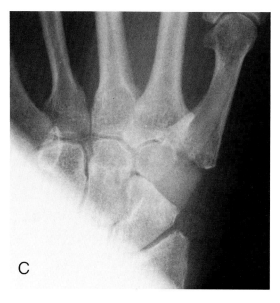

matic or inflammatory conditions (rheumatoid arthritis). Frequently, patients are young adults with excessive midcarpal laxity in the uninjured wrist.[8,32] Scaphoid malrotation may occur as a primary condition or be the residual manifestation of a reduced perilunate dislocation.[36] In this type of carpal collapse, the scaphoid is palmarflexed, its longitudinal axis perpendicular to that of the radius. Simultaneously, the lunate is dorsiflexed, a DISI pattern. The scapholunate angle is increased

(Fig. 10-1A). Since both the lunate and the scaphoid have rotated in opposite directions, this is a form of DISI *with* scapholunate dissociation. As we will see, there are other forms of DISI that are not accompanied by a scapholunate dissociation.

Scaphocapitate Diastasis

The os centrale has been described as an embryonic cartilaginous nodule in the primitive carpus,[19,29] located between the scaphoid and the capitate (Fig. 1-4). It usually disappears in the adult, but it may persist as a separate ossicle[39] or as an interosseous ligament.[19] Its presence should be suspected when radiographs show a notch of the capitate opposite the scaphoid (Fig. 1-5). In 1949 Sacks[29] reported a patient with bilateral occasional painful clicking in the wrist joints. Roentgenograms showed an unusually large gap between the scaphoid and the capitate. This was attributed to the persistence of an unossified os centrale. More recently, this structure was mentioned in relationship to a scaphocapitate diastasis[12] allowed by a tear of this interosseous ligament.

Scaphotrapezium-Trapezoid (STT) Instability

A review of the literature discloses only two reported cases of traumatic STT dissociation, one in a 13-year-old boy who had sustained a forced abduction injury to his left thumb, resulting in radiographic widening of the STT space,[30] and the second in a 36-year-old male who developed a "catching" or "locking" sensation of his wrist following a twisting injury.[33] Roentgenographic examination disclosed some narrowing of the STT joint compatible with early minimal osteoarthritis. Cineradiographs clearly demonstrated a recurring, longitudinal subluxation of the STT joint (Fig. 10-3). In addition to these posttraumatic forms it is my belief that the development of osteoarthritis of the scaphotrapezium-trapezoid joint may, in many patients, be the result of an unstable articulation. In some cases, residual STT instability can still be proven in osteoarthritic STT joints, by radiographs obtained in radial and ulnar deviation (Fig. 10-4).

MEDIAL CARPAL INSTABILITY

Triquetrolunate Dissociation

The loss of triquetral control on the lunate following ligamentous dissociation, places the lunate under the now uncontested influence of the palmarflexing scaphoid (Fig. 1-8). The result is a pro-

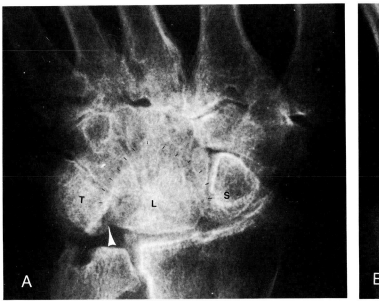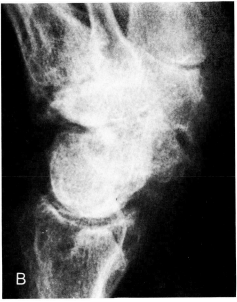

Fig. 10-5. Triquetrolunate dissociation (static VISI) in patient with rheumatoid arthritis of the wrist. A: Posteroanterior radiograph. Arrow points to triquetrolunate dissociation. S (scaphoid) is foreshortened (palmarflexed). L (lunate) is triangular (palmarflexed). T (triquetrum) is distal (dorsiflexed) in relation to the hamate. (See Fig. 3-4C,D.) B: Lateral radiograph. The lunate is palmarflexed. The capitate is aligned palmar to the center of the articular surface of the radius.

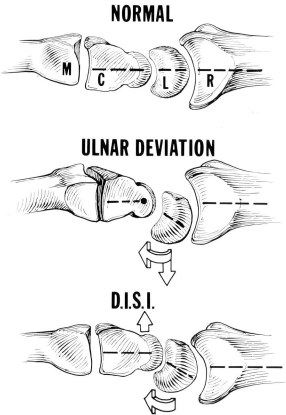

NORMAL

ULNAR DEVIATION

D.I.S.I.

Fig. 10-6. Schematic representation of normal and abnormal radiocarpal alignment. In neutral deviation, radius, lunate, and capitate are aligned. Normally, in ulnar deviation, the lunate dorsiflexes and shifts in a palmar direction, to allow radius and capitate to remain colinear. In dynamic dorsal instability, the lunate fails to shift in a palmar direction, resulting in the capitate aligned dorsal to the radius.

gressive, fixed palmarflexion of the lunate, a static **VISI** deformity (Fig. 10-1B). This type of instability is more frequent in the rheumatoid wrist. Both scaphoid and lunate appear palmarflexed in posteroanterior radiographs, the scaphoid foreshortened and the lunate triangular in shape, coexisting with a dorsiflexed triquetrum in a "low" or distal position in relationship to the hamate (Fig. 10-5A). There is uniform loss of radial and ulnar carpal height. The dissociated triquetrum shifts proximal to the scaphoid and lunate and closer to the ulnar head[22] due to the greater compliance of the cartilaginous ulnocarpal complex, resulting in a loss of

continuity of the smooth convex outline of the proximal carpal condyle (called the "Shenton line of the wrist" by Linscheid).[27] On the lateral view, the lunate is palmarflexed and so is the scaphoid (Fig. 10-5B). This is a static type of deformity which the patient is unable to reverse voluntarily, and is not correctible by passive manipulation of the wrist.

Triquetrohamate Dissociation

Midcarpal joint support depends on the scaphoid laterally, and on the integrity of the ulnar limb of the palmar intercarpal or V ligament medially.[31] Lichtman et al.[21] demonstrated that only after this ligament is divided can midcarpal joint subluxation be reproduced in the cadaver wrist during ulnar deviation. Patients who exhibit midcarpal instability can shift the distal carpal row dorsal or palmar to the axis of the radius, during ulnar or radial deviation. This is frequently painful and may be disabling. These are dynamic forms of instability, both

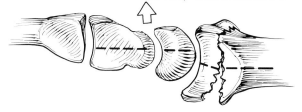

PROX.(RADIOCARPAL) INSTABILITY

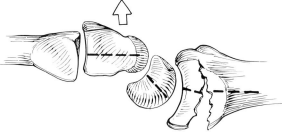

PROX.(MIDCARPAL) INSTABILITY

Fig. 10-7 Radiocarpal and midcarpal instability secondary to malunited fracture of the radius. The abnormal dorsal tilt of the articular surface of the radius caused the carpus to align in a potentially unstable position. This proximal carpal instability may occur at the radiocarpal or at the midcarpal joint level.

dorsal (dynamic DISI) (Fig. 10-6) and volar (dynamic VISI) and occur without any dissociation between scaphoid and lunate (see Chapter 12).

PROXIMAL CARPAL INSTABILITY

Proximal carpal instability occurs without actual primary intracarpal pathologic changes consequent to disruption of radiocarpal ligaments or to changes of alignment of the distal radioulnar joint surfaces. The carpus as a whole may migrate ulnarly (ulnar translocation (Fig. 10-1C)), dorsally (Fig. 10-1D) or volarly (dorsal and volar subluxations) to the articular surface of the radius, or else a midcarpal collapse deformity may develop secondary to the change of alignment of the distal radius.[35] There are, therefore, two main types of proximal carpal instability: (1) radiocarpal (ulnar translocation, dorsal radiocarpal subluxation, volar radiocarpal subluxation), and (2) midcarpal, a dynamic dorsal instability pattern occurring during ulnar deviation, in patients with healed fractures of the distal radius with residual malunion and a reversal of the normal palmar angulation of the distal radius (Fig. 10-7). These are dynamic DISI deformities without scapholunate dissociation, secondary to malunion of fractures of the distal radius (see Chapter 13).

REFERENCES

1. Abadie J: Des luxations radio-carpiennes traumatiques. Thèse de Montpellier, 1901
2. Armstrong GWD: Rotational subluxation of the scaphoid. Can J Surg 11:306, 1968
3. Bindi R: La luxación del escafoides carpiano. Bol Trab Soc Argent Ortop Traumatol 29:194, 1964
4. Chaput and Vaillant: Étude radiographique sur les traumatismes du carpe. Rev Orthop 4:227, 1913
5. Cotte G: Luxation du grand os en avant. Bull Soc Chir 45:1252, 1919
6. Destot E: Traumatismes du poignet et rayons X. Paris, Masson, 1923
7. Dobyns JH, Perkins JC: Instability of the carpal navicular (abstract). J Bone Joint Surg [Am]49:1014, 1967
8. Dobyns JH, Linscheid RL, Chao EYS, et al: Traumatic instability of the wrist. Am Acad Orthop Surgeons Instruct Course Lect 24:182, 1975
9. Douarre M: Luxation du grand os en avant. Bull Soc Chir 47:185, 1921
10. England JPS: Subluxation of the carpal scaphoid. Proc R Soc Med 63:581, 1970
11. Fisk GR: Carpal instability and the fractured scaphoid. Ann R Coll Surg Eng 46:63, 1970
12. Fisk GR: Personal communication. 1979
13. Fitton JM: Rotational dislocation of the scaphoid. In Stack GH, Bolton H (eds): Procedings of the Second Hand Club, British Society for Surgery of the Hand. Westway Press, Brentwood, Essex, 1962
14. Fitton JM: Subluxation on the medial side of the midcarpal joint. In Stack GH, Bolton H (eds): Proceedings of the Second Hand Club, British Society for Surgery of the Hand. Westway Press, Brentwood, Essex, 1962
15. Gilford W, Bolton R, Lambrinudi C: The mechanism of the wrist joint. Guy's Hosp Rep 92:52, 1943
16. Horwitz T: An anatomic and roentgenologic study of the wrist joint. Observations on a case of recurrent radiocarpal dislocation complicating Madelung's deformity and its surgical correction. Surgery 1:773, 1940
17. Jeanne LA, and Mouchet A: Les lésions traumatiques fermées du poignet. 28th Congres Français de Chirurgie, 1919
18. Johnston MB: Varying positions of the carpal bones in the different movements at the wrist. J Anat Physiol 41:109, 1907
19. Jones FW: The principles of anatomy as seen in the hand. 2nd ed. Baillier, Tindall and Cox, London, 1949
20. Linscheid RL, Dobyns JH, Beabout JW, Bryan RS: Traumatic instability of the wrist. Diagnosis, classification and pathomechanics. J Bone Joint Surg 54:1612, 1972
21. Lichtman DM, Swafford AR, Mack GR: Ulnar midcarpal instability — clinical and laboratory analysis. J Hand Surg 6:515, 1981
22. Mayersbach L von: Ein seltener Fall von Luxatio Intercarpea. Dtsch Z Chir 123:179, 1913
23. Mouchet A, Vennin H: Luxation médio-carpienne en avant du poignet droit. Bull Mem Soc Chir 32:1376, 1913
24. Mouchet A: Deux cas de luxation médio-carpienne en avant. Bull Soc Chir 44:1736, 1918
25. Mouchet A, Belot J: Poignet à ressaut (subluxation médio-carpienne en avant). Bull Mem Soc Nat Chir 60:1243, 1934
26. Navarro A: Luxaciones del carpo. An Fac Med (Montevideo, Uruguay) 6:113, 1921

27. Reagan DS, Linscheid RL, Dobyns JH: The lunotri-quetral sprain. Presented at the 36th Annual Meeting. The American Society for Surgery of the Hand. Las Vegas, Nevada, 1981

28. Rettig H: Zur gewohnheitsmäbigen Subluxation des Kahnbeines der Hand. Arch Orthop Unfallchir 53:498, 1961

29. Sacks S: Painful clicking wrists associated with os centrale. S Afr Med J 23:766, 1949

30. Tachakra SS: A case of trapezio-scaphoid subluxation. Br J Clin Pract 31:162, 1977

31. Taleisnik J: The ligaments of the wrist. J Hand Surg 1:110, 1976

32. Taleisnik J: Wrist: Anatomy, function and injury. Am Acad Orthop Surgeons Instruct Course Lect 27:61,1978

33. Taleisnik J: Post-traumatic carpal instability. Clin Orthop 149:73, 1980

34. Taleisnik J: Carpal instability. Symposium. Contemp Orthop 4:107, 1982

35. Taleisnik J, Watson HK: Midcarpal instability secondary to malunited fractures of the distal radius. J Hand Surg 8:612, 1983

36. Thompson TC, Campbell RD, Arnold WD: Primary and secondary dislocation of the scaphoid bone. J Bone Joint Surg [Br] 46:73, 1964

37. Vaughn-Jackson OJ: A case of recurrent subluxation of the carpal scaphoid. J Bone Joint Surg [Br] 31:532, 1949

38. Watson HK: Carpal instability. Symposium. Contemp Orthop 4:107, 1982

39. Watson-Jones R: Fractures and Joint Injuries. Vol. 2. Williams and Wilkins, Baltimore, 1960

11 Scapholunate Dissociation

The functional dissociation between scaphoid and lunate secondary to rotatory subluxation of the scaphoid is a frequent form of carpal instability. Jeanne and Mouchet[35] and Destot[17] recognized and described its typical radiographic features. Since the early references to scaphoid participation in carpal instability by MacConnaill[46] and by Gilford and associates[23] and reports by Cave,[12] Russell[59] and Vaughan-Jackson,[75] considerable progress has been made toward the understanding of the pathogenesis of this form of carpal collapse deformity, as well as toward the treatment of the chronic subluxations. The most persistent problem continues to be the lack of recognition of this entity in its early stages, since rotatory subluxation of the scaphoid diagnosed in the acute phase offers the best opportunity for successful correction.

MECHANISM OF INJURY

MacConnaill[46] and Gilford and associates[23] first stressed the role the scaphoid plays as a connecting rod between the proximal and distal carpal rows, protecting the wrist against the imbalance that is inherently built into the intercalated segment of a three-link system.[40] The loss of scaphoid support through fracture or ligamentous injury allows the carpus to collapse under compression loads and to assume a stance variously described as "crumpling,"[23] "zig-zag,"[40] or "concertina"[20] deformity. The scaphoid is stabilized at its proximal pole by

the deep palmar radioscapholunate and both volar and dorsal scapholunate interosseous ligaments[48,63,70] (see Chapter 2). Rotation of the proximal pole is also supported by the weak scaphoid attachment of the radiocapitate[41] or "sling" ligament.[63] The distal pole is controlled by the radial collateral and lateral arm of the V or deltoid ligaments and by the support provided by the scaphotrapezium ligaments. Considerable motion of the scaphoid is allowed by these ligaments: it dorsiflexes during full ulnar deviation and dorsiflexion of the wrist, and palmarflexes at the extreme of radial deviation or palmarflexion of the wrist (Figs. 1-10, 2-21, 3-4). For the scaphoid to become unstable, there must be attenuation, relaxation, tear, or destruction of the scaphoid components of the palmar deep radioscapholunate ligament, and the "sling" or radiocapitate ligament[66] (Fig. 11-1). Although unstable, it may fail to actually sublux (unless subjected to severe loading, or under manipulation) when the scaphotrapezium capsular and ligamentous support remains strong and the more proximal ligaments are not totally torn. Patients who can recall the mechanism of their injury, describe it as a force applied to the palm of their hands, particularly at the hypothenar area, with the wrist in dorsiflexion and ulnar deviation. Not infrequently a cylindrical object (racquet handle, motorcycle handlebar) was held in the hand at the time of the injury.[4,5] Isolated subluxation of the scaphoid may be considered the initial result of an injury that, if allowed to progress, would result in a

239

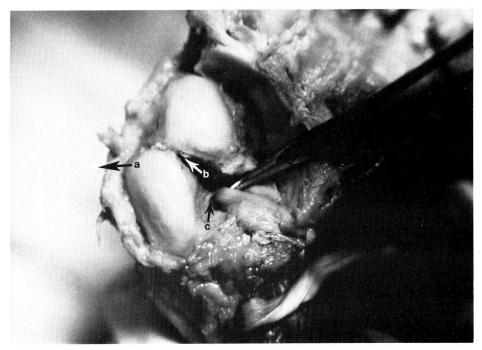

Fig. 11-1. For the scaphoid to become unstable and sublux dorsally *(a)*, there must be attenuation, relaxation, tear, or destruction of the scaphoid components of the deep radioscapholunate *(b)*, and radioscaphocapitate ligaments *(c)*.

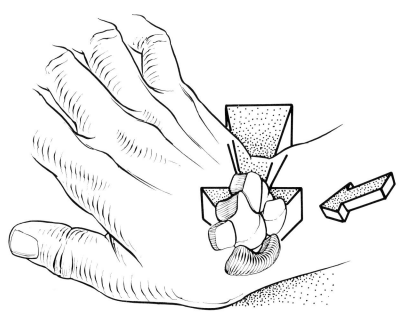

Fig. 11-2. Typically, scapholunate dissociations occur with the wrist in dorsiflexion and ulnar deviation, and the hand pronated in relation to the forearm. The initial load is applied to the base of the hypothenar area, and is directed against the scaphoid (large arrow) driving it away from the lunate (small arrow).

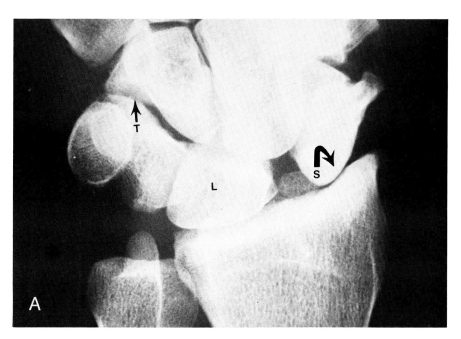

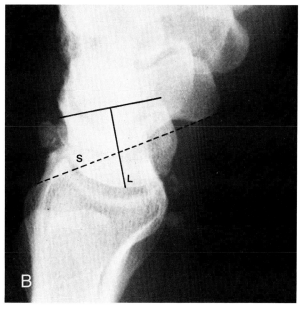

Fig. 11-3. Isolated primary scapholunate dissociation. *A:* Anteroposterior radiograph. The scaphoid is palmar flexed (arrow S). The triquetrum is distal (dorsiflexed) in relation to the hamate (arrow T). L, lunate. *B:* lateral projection, the scapholunate (SL) angle is 100 degrees.

perilunate carpal dislocation, just as a fracture of the scaphoid, if subjected to continuation of the injury force, could lead to a transscaphoid-perilunate-fracture dislocation.[9] Isolated dislocation of the scaphoid, after scapholunate connections are disrupted, although possible, is exceedingly infrequent.[10,14,31,39,47,51,52,61,69,71,76] Fitton[21] suggested

in 1962 that rotatory subluxation of the scaphoid is associated with a pronation-subluxation of the midcarpal joint. A case described by Fitton required supination of the hand in order to stabilize the scaphoid after reduction. England[19] believed that a forced pronation and palmar flexion injury was the mechanism of injury. Conversely, Mayfield and

Johnson[49] loaded to failure cadaver wrists into dorsiflexion, ulnar deviation, and midcarpal supination. In this manner they could reproduce a sequential, progressive pattern of ligamentous disruption which they classified into several stages. The fourth or highest degree of carpal instability, according to these authors, was the dislocation of the lunate (Fig. 9-3). Stage I included those specimens with scapholunate diastasis, the least severe of the carpal instability patterns. I believe that most frequently the initial impact loading takes place against the base of the hypothenar region with the hand in dorsiflexion, ulnar deviation and pronated in relationship to the forearm (Fig. 11-2). The direction of the floor-reaction force causes the scaphoid to dissociate from the lunate. After this initial destabilization, midcarpal supination would ensue, leading to the remaining three stages of Mayfield, Johnson and Kilcoyne's progressive perilunate instability: Stage II of partial perilunate dislocation (scaphoid and capitate are dislocated), Stage III of complete perilunate dislocation (the triquetrum is also dislocated), and Stage IV of dislocation of the lunate. In the anatomic specimen, division of the interosseous scapholunate ligaments alone fails to produce a subluxation; it is not until the palmar support from the radiocarpal ligaments is divided that a rotatory subluxation of the scaphoid can be obtained.[64] Because of its dissociation from the lunate, the scaphoid is no longer capable of counteracting a dorsiflexion influence of the triquetrum on the lunate, or the lunate's own, built-in dorsiflexion bias (Figs. 1-8, 1-10).[36] Therefore, in anteroposterior radiographs the volarflexed scaphoid is seen separated from the lunate by a gap, and coexisting with a dorsiflexed, quadrilateral lunate and a dorsiflexed triquetrum in a distal position in relation to the hamate. There is a **DISI** deformity *with* scapholunate dissociation. For these instability patterns to develop, excessive midcarpal laxity may need to be present, secondary to either a systemic hypermobility involving multiple joints,[62] or to a local carpal anatomical weakness.[63] Fisk's[20] assumption that deficient volar capitate-lunate support may facilitate intercarpal dislocation correlates well with the frequent anatomical absence of a capitolunate ligament and the dorsal-stress instability that is present in the uninjured wrists of patients who have sustained scapholunate dissociations.

DIAGNOSIS

Scapholunate dissociations may be *primary, secondary* (to a more extensive injury or disease), or *associated* (with extracarpal injuries). *Primary dissociations* occur when the scaphoid malrotation is the only end-result of the wrist injury (Fig. 11-3). Primary dissociations may also be idiopathic, without any clear preceding injury, or with a history of minor, insignificant, repetitive trauma (i.e., crutch walking).[30,32,43,74] *Secondary dissociations* are the residual findings of reduced, major carpal injuries

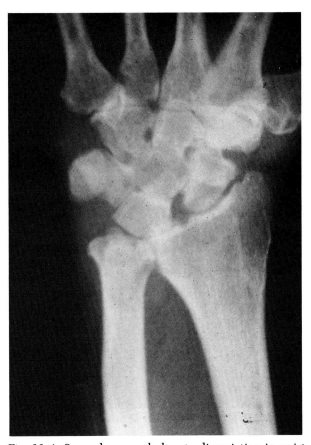

Fig. 11-4. Secondary scapholunate dissociation in wrist of patient with rheumatoid arthritis. There is some ulnar translocation of the carpus.

Fig. 11-5. Scapholunate dissociation associated with intraarticular fracture of the distal radius.

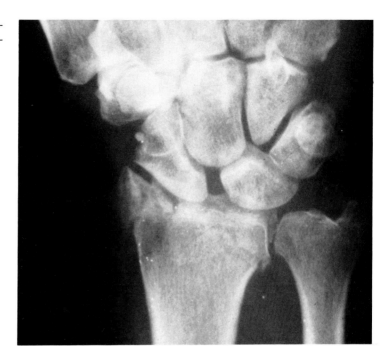

(perilunate dislocations and dislocations of the lunate) (Fig. 9-12). The scapholunate gap remains as the telltale sign of a severe carpal dislocation that has been reduced.[1,2,4,68,72] Secondary scapholunate dissociations may also be found consequent to ligament damage produced by synovitis, as seen in some patients with rheumatoid arthritis of the wrist[13,29,42,65,67] (Fig. 11-4). The third category of scapholunate dissociations are *associated* with extracarpal injuries, most frequently with fractures of the distal radius (Figs. 11-5, 11-6)[6,58] or with fractures of other bones of the same extremity (Fig. 11-7).

The early recognition of scapholunate dissociation is important for it improves the chances of obtaining a successful result. Posttraumatic *secondary* rotatory subluxations follow major carpal injuries (Fig. 9-12). For this reason, these patients are usually under medical care or supervision at the time the diagnosis of scapholunate dissociation becomes apparent. Malrotation of the scaphoid may take place even while the wrist is adequately immobilized in plaster. Acute lunate and perilunate dislocations are inherently unstable. In a study by Adkison and Chapman[1] only 41 percent of 32

wrists that were restored to anatomic position by closed reduction maintained a satisfactory alignment. Patients with *primary* scapholunate dissociation frequently seek medical help days or weeks following their injury, partly because the original accident is rather trivial, partly because symptoms may remain surprisingly minimal for several weeks. Frequently, these patients are adults with excessive carpal laxity of the uninjured wrist. Because the primary form of rotatory subluxation frequently follows a deceivingly minor injury,[16,19] the true nature of the carpal instability is not recognized by the physician, or else both the patient and his doctor dismiss the injury as "just a sprain." Progressive pain and weakness with loading of the wrist is the most consistent presenting complaint. At times a painful, loud snap can be reproduced, usually during palmarflexion of the wrist. Howard et al.[33] attributed this snap to the penetration of the head of the capitate into the scapholunate space. In my opinion, this clinical finding is secondary to the displacement of the proximal pole of the scaphoid as it subluxes past the dorsal rim of the radius (Fig. 11-8). Severe limitation of motion is rarely encountered early. Because of the disturbed me-

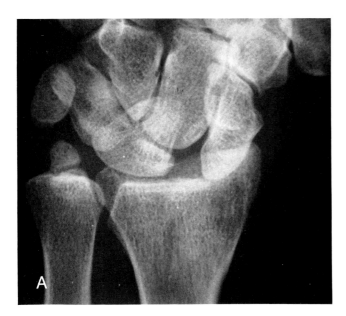

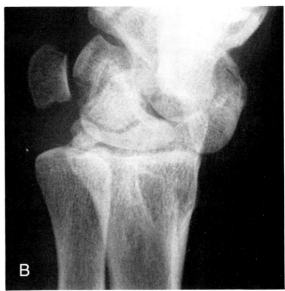

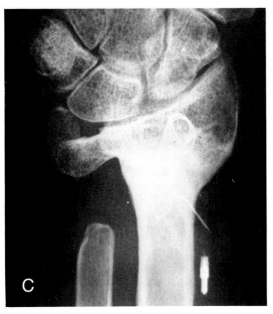

Fig. 11-6. Scapholunate dissociation occurring in young male patient with healed malunited fracture of the radius. *A:* Anteroposterior radiograph. There is an abnormal, dorsal tilt of the radius and ununited fracture through the base of the ulnar styloid. *B:* Reverse oblique view shows fixed dorsal subluxation of the proximal pole of the scaphoid. *C:* Late (one year) appearance following osteotomy of the radius, distal radioulnar fusion and surgical pseudarthrosis of the ulna, and reduction and tenodesis of subluxed scaphoid.

chanics of radiocarpal motion, these patients' wrists are very susceptible to the rapid onset of degenerative changes, particularly between the radial styloid and the subluxated scaphoid. As arthrosis develops, limitation of motion and pain become more constant and disabling.[66]

On examination, the diagnosis may be suspected by the patient's description of his accident, and by the presence of pain or tenderness on the radial aspect of the wrist, aggravated by loading. Strength may be near normal, although in many cases patients need to support the wrist with the opposite hand when gripping. In some cases scapholunate instability may exist even when radiographs are normal. For these patients, Watson[79] described a useful test. The patient's elbow rests on his or her lap, and the forearm is pronated. The examiner uses his opposite hand to take the patient's wrist

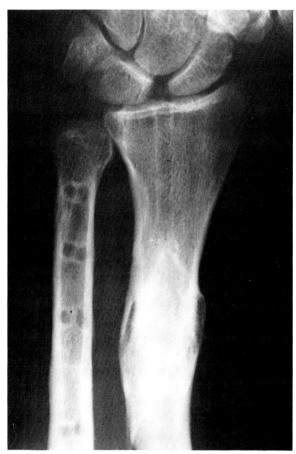

Fig. 11-7. Scapholunate dissociation associated with fractures of both bones of the forearm.

using these projections alone, special views should be obtained.

Frontal Radiographs

The importance of obtaining a proper *frontal projection* was stressed by Hudson and associates[34]: a projection was considered ideal when the distal ulna and radius did not overlap. Increasing overlap suggested unwanted obliquity, at times enough to obscure the presence of a scapholunate dissociation. Findings suggestive of scapholunate dissociation seen in frontal projections are as follows:

1. *A scapholunate gap.* This is the classic radiographic sign of malrotation of the scaphoid. The gap should be wider than that in the opposite uninjured wrist (the Terry-Thomas sign)[22]; this is usually more noticeable in the anteroposterior (supinated) view, rather than in the more usual posteroanterior (pronated) projection[72] (Fig. 11-10). Moneim[50] described a tangential posterior anterior view (see Chapter 5) for a better visualization of the scapholunate gap (Fig. 11-11). He observed that in routine posteroanterior radiographs scaphoid and lunate normally overlap. When the ulnar border of the hand is elevated 20 degrees off the table, the x-ray beam, directed vertically, aligns with the scapholunate articulation. Normally, the width of this space should not exceed 2 mm, or be greater than any other intercarpal space.
2. *The cortical "ring" sign* (Figs. 11-10, 11-11, 11-12). This is due to the end-on projection of the distal pole of the palmarflexed perpendicular scaphoid.[6,15,16,18]
3. *Foreshortening of the scaphoid* (Figs. 11-10, 11-11, 11-12).
4. *Loss of the normal scapholunotriquetral correlation* (Figs. 11-10, 11-11, 11-12). A foreshortened (palmarflexed) scaphoid coexists with a quadrilateral (dorsiflexed) lunate and a triquetrum in a distal position in relation to the hamate (dorsiflexed).
5. *Decrease in the scaphoid ring proximal pole distance* to less than 7 mm[37,56] (Fig. 11-12).

Additional posteroanterior views in ulnar deviation and radial deviation and longitudinal compres-

into full ulnar deviation (Fig. 11-9). In this position, the scaphoid is longitudinal. Next, the patient's hand is radially deviated, while the examiner uses his thumb against the distal pole of the scaphoid, in an attempt to prevent its normal palmarflexion. When the scapholunate joint is unstable, this maneuver will force the dorsal pole to sublux. Although the scaphoid in the uninjured wrist may also be somewhat unstable to this type of manipulation, the test will be painful only in the injured side.

The diagnosis is established by appropriate radiologic studies.[4,15,18,24,33,34,72] Roentgenograms should routinely include a lateral view with the wrist in neutral flexion, and an anteroposterior projection with the forearm and hand in full supination.[11,72] When a scapholunate dissociation is strongly suspected, but cannot be demonstrated

(Text continues on page 248.)

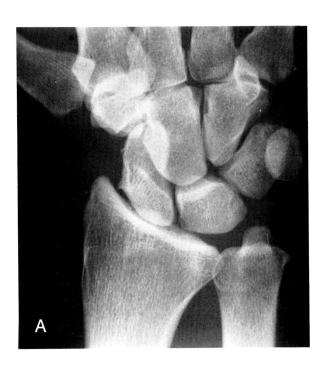

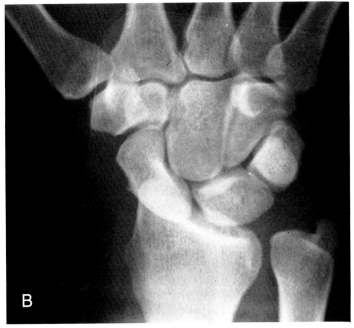

Fig. 11-8. Dynamic subluxation of the scaphoid. *A:* Anteroposterior radiograph shows normal alignment. *B:* Subluxation is accompanied by a loud, painful "snap."

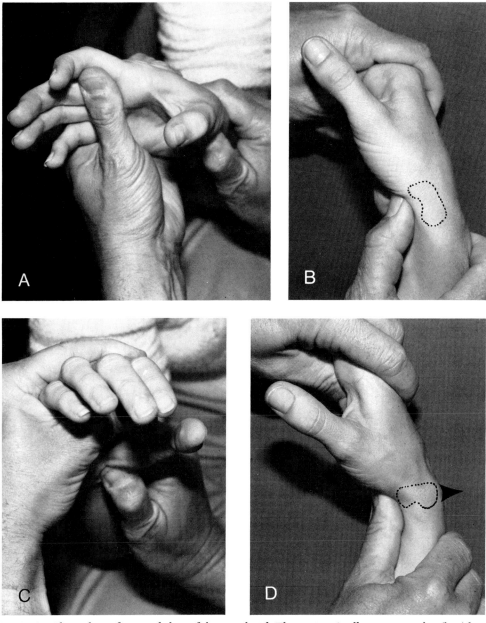

Fig. 11-9. Clinical test for instability of the scaphoid. The patient's elbow rests on his (her) lap. Forearm is pronated. The hand is brought into ulnar deviation and pressure is applied to the distal pole of the scaphoid (*A* and *B*). Next the hand is radially deviated while pressure is maintained on the distal pole of the scaphoid, in an attempt to prevent its normal palmarflexion (*C* and *D*). When the scaphoid is unstable, its proximal pole is forced to sublux dorsally, a maneuver that is accompanied by pain. (From Watson HK: Personal communication, 1982.)

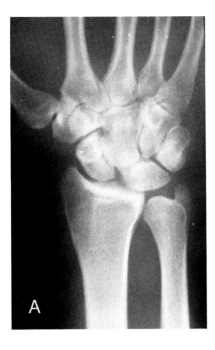

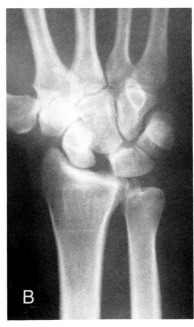

Fig. 11-10. Posteroanterior and anteroposterior radiographs of the same wrist show an abnormal scapholunate relationship which is less apparent in posteroanterior radiograph in pronation *(A).* The scapholunate gap becomes wider in the anteroposterior projection with the forearm in supination *(B).*

sion-load views[18] created by having the patient make a tight fist may also assist to widen the scapholunate gap. Gilula and Weeks[24] proposed a "ligamentous instability series" for the survey of all carpal bones and their relationships. The series includes posteroanterior views in neutral, ulnar, and radial deviation, anteroposterior views with the fist tightly clenched, routine oblique, a 30 degree off lateral (semisupination) oblique, and lateral views in neutral, full palmarflexion, full dorsiflexion, and with the fist tightly clenched. Usually, these many views are not necessary when a scapholunate dissociation is suspected.

Lateral Radiograph

The *lateral projection* must also be true; the long axis of radius and third metacarpal must be colinear in a properly aligned lateral view of the wrist. Lateral radiographs show the scaphoid with its long axis perpendicular to that of the radius,[19] and the lunate in dorsiflexion (DISI) (Figs. 5-8, 5-9, 10-1).[43,44] In some patients, the proximal pole of the scaphoid is clearly subluxated dorsal to the dorsal rim of the radius (Fig. 11-13). The normal

values of the angles between the axis of all the components of the radiocarpal link have been thoroughly discussed by Linscheid, Dobyns and associates[18,43] and by Sarrafian et al.[60] (see Chapter 5). The scapholunate angle ranges from 30 to 60 degrees with an average of 46 degrees (Fig. 5-7). Angles greater than 70 degrees are a clear indication of scapholunate dissociation. The average normal radioscaphoid angle is 58 degrees with the scaphoid palmarflexed (33–73 degrees). Normally, the long axis of the scaphoid and a line drawn tangential to the volar flare of the distal radius are closely parallel to each other. In the abnormally palmarflexed scaphoid, these lines converge at an acute angle.[64] For the same reason, the volar cortical outlines of the scaphoid and the radial styloid, which normally create a wide C bracket design open anteriorly, change into a sharp V when the scaphoid is subluxated[28,64] (Figs. 5-9, 11-13).

Cineradiographs

Cineradiographs (Fig. 11-14) may help to demonstrate the mechanical disturbance created by the scapholunate dissociation.[3] During ulnar and radial

Fig. 11-11. Moneim's view. *A:* Anteroposterior view is suggestive of malrotation of the scaphoid. Scapholunate gap is abnormal, but not very wide. *B:* Tangential posteroanterior view clearly demonstrates scapholunate dissociation (see Chap. 5). (See Ref. 50.)

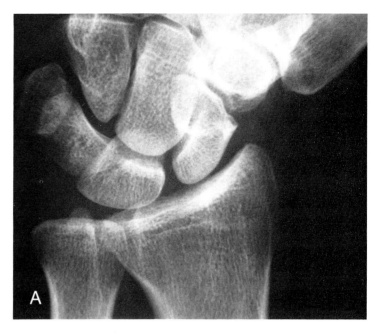

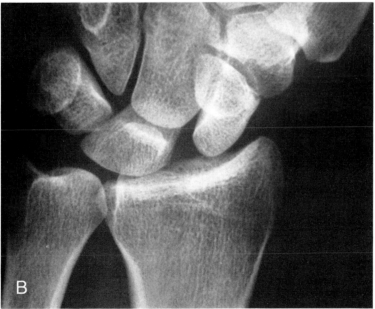

deviation there is a loss of the synchronous motions of the scaphoid and lunate. The abnormal widening of the scapholunate space, as well as the dorsal subluxation of the scaphoid can usually be documented. In the lateral projection, cineradiographs show the relative immobility of the lunate, which remains dorsiflexed throughout dorsal and palmar-flexion movements. The evaluation of cineradiographic studies requires a thorough knowledge of the normal mechanics of wrist motion, and a familiarity with the other types of dynamic carpal instability that may be present. An error in evaluating a

(Text continues on page 254.)

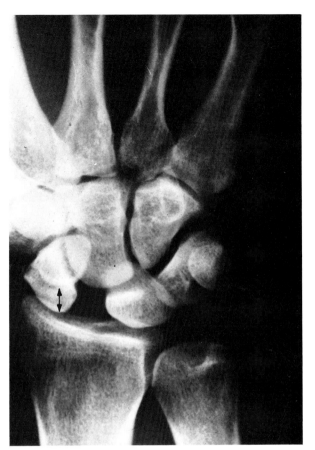

Fig. 11-12. Typical radiograph of wrist with scapholunate dissociation. The scaphoid is palmarflexed, its distal
pole seen end-on ("ring sign"). There is shortening of
the scaphoid ring-proximal pole distance (arrow).

Fig. 11-13. Different degrees of perpendicularization of
the scaphoid in scapholunate dissociation. *A:* Tangential
axes of scaphoid (S) and palmar flare of distal radius (RS)
meet at an acute angle A. Normally, both lines are almost
parallel. Palmar cortical outlines of scaphoid and radial
styloid delineate a sharp V (angle B) instead of the more
normal C or bracket (see Fig. 5-9). *B:* More severe subluxations create sharper angles. The proximal pole of this
scaphoid is dorsal to the dorsal rim of the radius.

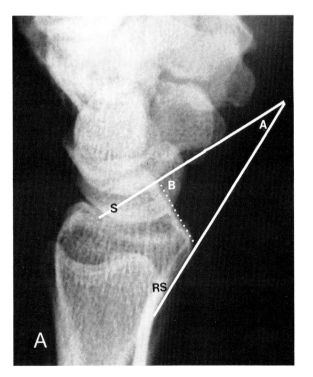

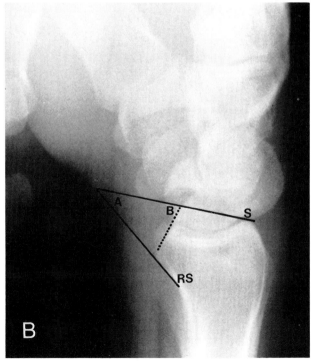

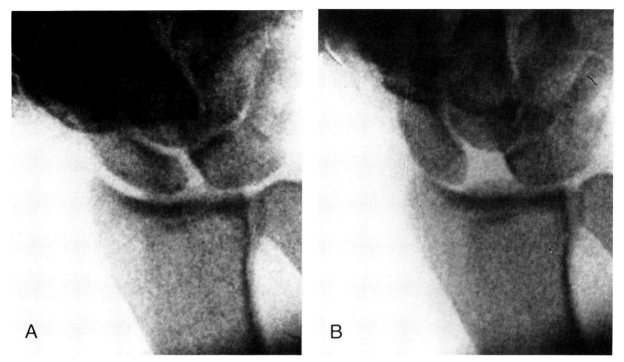

Fig. 11-14. Cineradiographic study of wrist with voluntary recurrent (dynamic) scapholunate dissociation. Successive frames *A* and *B* show sudden subluxation of the scaphoid and widening of the space between scaphoid and lunate. (Reproduced by permission from Taleisnik J: Wrist: Anatomy, function and injury. Am Acad Orthop Surgeons Instruct Course Lect 27:61, St. Louis, 1978, The C.V. Mosby Co.)

Fig. 11-15. Bone scan of abnormally unstable scaphoid (arrow).

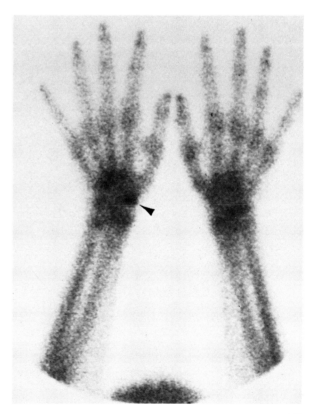

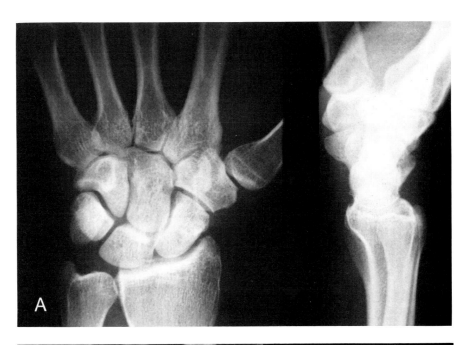

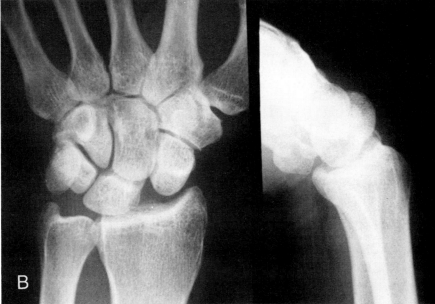

Fig. 11-16. Radiographic sequence of wrist following excision of a dorsal carpal ganglion. *A:* Posteroanterior projection three days following surgery suggests satisfactory alignment. *B:* At 16 weeks, and 10 days after manipulation of the wrist for postoperative stiffness, radiographs show a scapholunate dissociation.

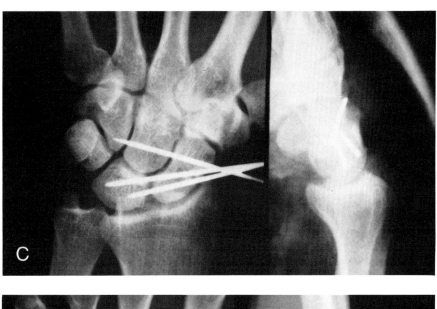

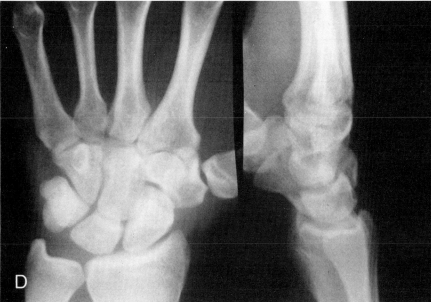

Fig. 11.16 (cont.) C: Appearance of carpus after reduction of scaphoid and fixation with multiple Kirschner wires under cineradiographic control, and further immobilization in a plaster cast with the wrist palmarflexed. *D:* 20 months later, there is satisfactory alignment. (From Crawford GP, Taleisnik J: Rotatory subluxation of the scaphoid after excision of dorsal carpal ganglion and wrist manipulation — case report. J Hand Surg 8:921, 1983.)

cineradiograph properly may lead to the wrong diagnosis and treatment.

Arthrography

Arthrography is rarely indicated for the diagnosis of rotatory subluxation of the scaphoid. It may, however, be of help in cases when radiographs or cineradiographs fail to establish a diagnosis, by delineating abnormal communications between radiocarpal and midcarpal joints along the scapholunate space.[34,44,54]

Bone Scans

Bone scans (Fig. 11-15) may be useful to further document an unstable scapholunate relationship in those patients with a positive clinical test (Fig. 11-9) and a negative radiograph.

TREATMENT

The best treatment for scapholunate dissociation is early, performed within the initial three to five weeks from injury.[8,45] Following is a discussion of the management of primary, secondary, and asso-

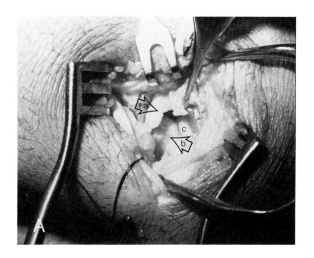

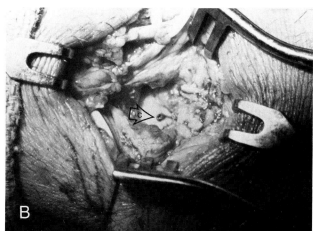

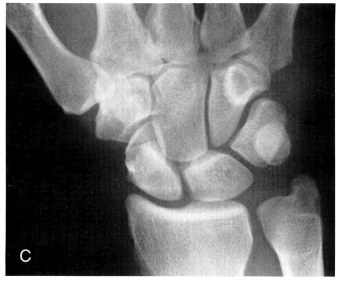

Fig. 11-17. Operative findings during exploration of recent scapholunate dissociation. *A:* Large cartilaginous fragment (a) elevated from underlying scaphoid (b). The head of the capitate (c) is sublexed dorsally. *B:* After reduction and fixation with multiple Kirschner wires, the cartilaginous fragment is sutured back in place (c). *C:* Radiograph obtained two years postoperatively.

ciated scapholunate dissociations, and of chronic dissociations after the onset of osteoarthritis.

The primary rotatory subluxation of the scaphoid may be successfully treated by closed pinning under cineradiographic control (Fig. 11-16), followed by prolonged immobilization.[57,64] Although reduction by manipulation of the scaphoid alone, followed by immobilization in plaster may be successful,[38,55] it is usually insufficient due to the "paradox" of closed reduction,[49] namely, when the wrist is palmarflexed in order to relax the torn palmar radiocarpal ligaments and facilitate their approximation and healing, the scaphoid is placed in the undesirable, unstable palmarflexed position of presubluxaton. If the scaphoid is reduced with the wrist in dorsiflexion, a gap is produced between the torn palmar ligaments, and their healing is either prevented or delayed. A satisfactory solution to the paradox consists of reducing the scaphoid with the wrist in dorsiflexion and, under cineradiographic control, securing this reduction by appropriate fixation with 0.045 Kirschner wires, from the scaphoid to the capitate and lunate, utilizing at least three pins. With scaphoid rotation under control, the radiocarpal joint, which should remain undisturbed by the Kirschner wires, is palmarflexed (Fig. 11-16C). This will afford relaxation to the torn palmar ligaments.

Loeb et al.[45] suggested that, in most cases, closed reduction fails, and an open reduction is indicated. Both palmar and dorsal approaches are used and ligaments are reconstructed "if possible." Actually, the volar capsular rent that is always present should be closed using interrupted nonabsorbable sutures. The technique for the insertion of the Kirschner wires remains unchanged, using at least three K-wires directed from the scaphoid to the capitate and lunate. There is no need to engage in complex ligament reconstructions in these acute injuries, for, although reduction may not remain anatomical, these patients' symptoms and function are not significantly different from those having undergone ligament reconstruction. Dorsal scapholunate interosseous ligament repair should be attempted. At times, the ligament has remained attached to an avulsed osteochondral fragment, which should be replaced when possible and stabilized with sutures or fine Kirschner wires (Fig. 11-17). After satisfactory reduction is obtained and

immobilization is secured with the Kirschner wires, a long arm thumb spica in comfortable palmarflexion is applied with the forearm in pronation. After six weeks this is replaced with a short arm plaster or with a splint that will allow removal for gentle, protected, daily radiocarpal motions. At the end of eight to ten weeks, all Kirschner wires are removed and exercises are increased.

Secondary rotatory subluxation of the scaphoid becomes usually apparent immediately following a successful reduction of a perilunate dislocation or a dislocation of the lunate, or at most a few days following their treatment. Because of the magnitude of the initial injury, as soon as the scaphoid becomes malrotated, and swelling has decreased, an open reduction is performed, using dorsal and palmar approaches. The latter will allow visualization and repair of what is, in most instances, a major ligament tear.[27] The dorsal exposure allows inspection of the proximal pole of the scaphoid, not infrequently the site of otherwise undetected cartilaginous fractures (Fig. 11-18). When the dorsal scapholunate ligament is avulsed together with a substantial piece of cartilage (usually from the scaphoid), this may be reapplied and sutured or pinned to the scaphoid (Fig. 11-17). This approach also permits adequate visualization of the scaphoid,

(Text continues on page 258.)

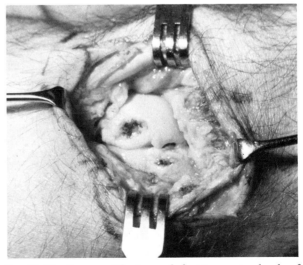

Fig. 11-18. Osteocartilaginous defect in proximal pole of scaphoid in patient with chronic scapholunate dissociation.

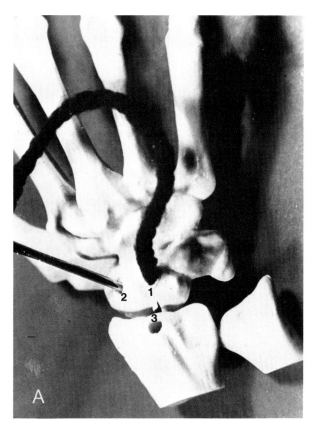

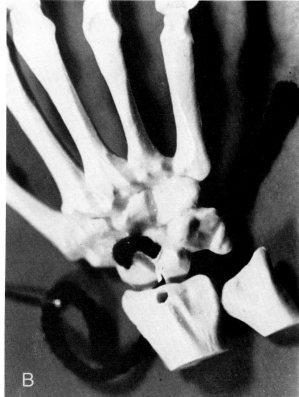

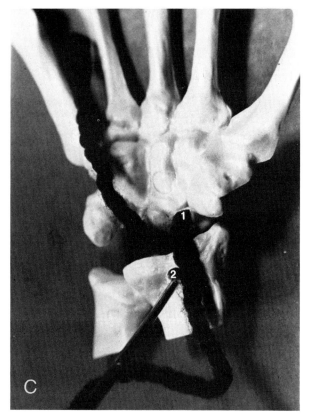

Fig. 11-19. Surgical reconstruction of torn radioscapho-lunate ligament. *A:* Dorsal view of radiocarpal joint. A tendon is threaded from palmar to dorsal through lunate (drill-hole 1) and is about to be introduced into scaphoid tunnel (2). A third tunnel (3) is needed. *B:* Dorsal scapho-lunate ligament completed. *C:* Palmar aspect shows ends of tendon graft from lunate and out through the scaphoid (1); it is next introduced into drill-hole in the radius (2).

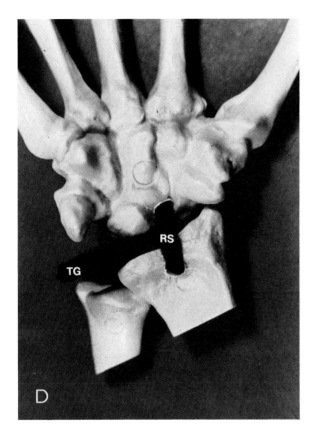

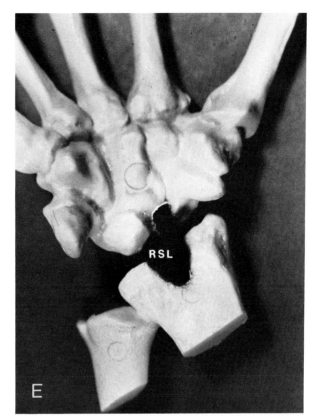

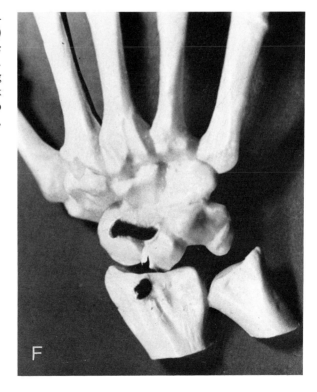

Fig. 11-19 (cont.) D: Palmar aspect after scaphoid is secured to distal radius (RS). Free end of tendon graft (TG) is then introduced through drill-hole in the radius. *E:* The deep radioscapholunate ligament is now completed. *F:* Dorsal view shows tendon sutured to the local, strong periosteum. (Reproduced by permission from Taleisnik J: Wrist: Anatomy, function and injury. Am Acad Orthop Surgeons Instruct Course Lect 27:61, St. Louis, 1978, The C.V. Mosby Co.)

lunate and capitate, useful when attempting to restore their anatomic alignment. Thus the scapholunate joint is reduced under direct vision, and pinning and postoperative immobilization are carried out thereafter as discussed for the postoperative care of primary subluxations.

Chronic scapholunate dissociations (without osteoarthritis): England stated in 1970 that "these chronic patients are best treated either by explanation and reassurance or by wearing a wrist strap."[19] These are, however, disabling injuries in many cases, more difficult to correct after the onset of osteoarthritis. Stabilization of the scaphoid is possible by ligament reconstruction using tendon grafts. This is a difficult procedure because of the considerable amount of force that is required to reduce and maintain the scaphoid as it tends to return to its subluxated alignment (which it may do in spite of plaster immobilization and internal fixation). The placement of the reconstructed ligamentous attachments on the carpus is crucial, if one is to restore the exquisite interplay between the intercarpal ligaments. Different techniques of ligament reconstruction have been described.[18,33,53,64] All share a common goal: to create a scapholunate ligament and restore a more normal scapholunate relationship. In some cases, an attempt is made to further reproduce the normal anatomy by reconstructing a palmar radioscaphoid "suspensory" ligament as well, in order to tether the proximal pole of the scaphoid and keep it from subluxating dorsally (Fig. 11-19).[64] Although good results may be obtained (Fig. 11-20) and have been reported with ligament reconstruction techniques,[33,53] these procedures are difficult, unreliable as to to the objective correction that is obtained and the degree of patient satisfaction and frequently disappointing because of late complications after prolonged follow up.[25,53] The modulous of elasticity of the actual ligaments at the wrist is much greater than that of tendon grafts used for ligament reconstruction. Therefore, a reconstructed ligament that is snug enough to restore the scapholunate relationship, will interfere with any attempts at regaining motion postoperatively. For the scaphoid to regain rotation on the lunate, either the new ligament will stretch or tear, becoming ineffective and allowing recurrence of the scapho-

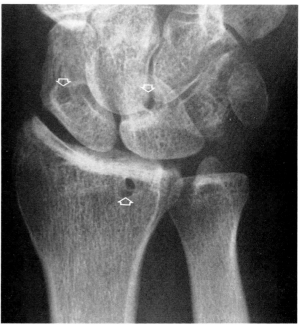

Fig. 11-20. Satisfactory restoration of carpal alignment following radioscapholunate tenodesis. Arrows indicate bone tunnels for the passage of a tendon graft. (Courtesy of Dr. Herbert H. Stark, Los Angeles, CA.)

lunate dissociation (Fig. 11-21); or the bony wall of the carpal tunnel through which the ligament was passed will fracture (Fig. 11-22); or slackening of the ligament reconstruction may indirectly occur because the joints that were spanned by the tendon graft become narrower, eventually leading to gradual osteoarthritis and pain (Fig. 11-23).

Blatt[7] has proposed to fashion a ligament from the dorsal capsule of the wrist, that is left attached to the radius proximally, and is inserted distally into a fresh groove on the reduced scaphoid (Fig. 11-24). By placing this dorsal capsular ligamentodesis insertion distal to the axis of rotation of the scaphoid, a proximal and dorsal check-rein effect is created on the distal pole. Scaphoid malrotation is thus corrected and, it is hoped, controlled. Although no attempt is made to reduce the persistent scapholunate dissociation, clinical results have been satisfactory (Fig. 11-25). I have successfully used this technique in three types of patients: (1) the very young with epiphysis still open, for whom the drilling of bone, or a limited arthrodesis would

(Text continues on page 262.)

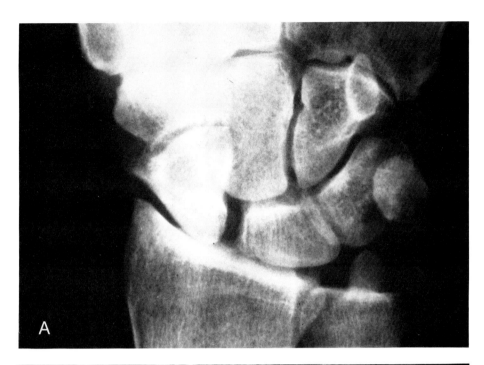

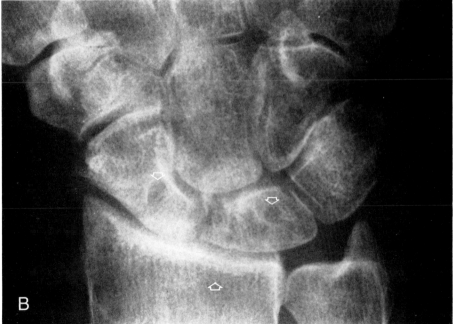

Fig. 11-21. Recurrent scapholunate dissociation following radioscapholunate tenodesis. *A:* Preoperative radiograph. *B:* Early (6 months) postoperative appearance is satisfactory. Arrows point to bone tunnels for the passage of a tendon graft.

(Fig. continues on next page.)

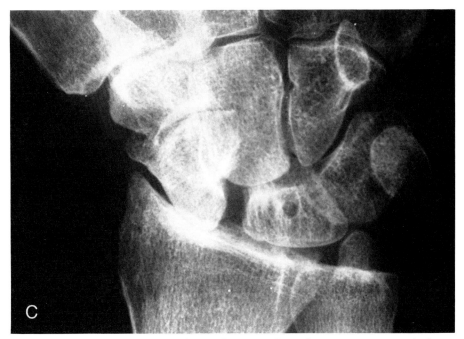

Fig. 11-21 (cont.) C: Radiograph obtained one year later shows recurrent scapholunate dissociation.

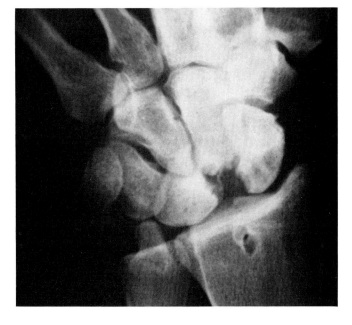

Fig. 11-22. Fractures through walls of osseous tunnels result in recurrence of instability.

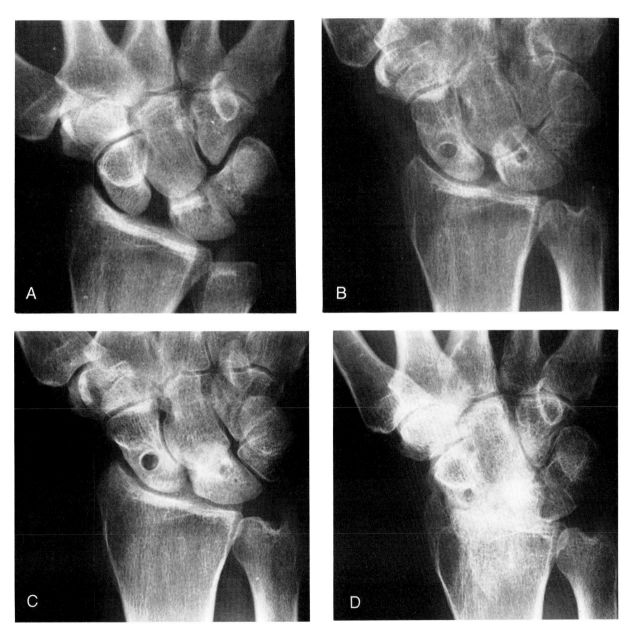

Fig. 11-23. *A:* Severe scapholunate dissociation. *B:* Incomplete but satisfactory correction at six months following radioscapholunate tenodesis. *C:* Recurrence of pain after onset of midcarpal joint (lunocapitate) narrowing; *D:* Final appearance after wrist fusion.

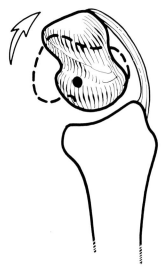

Fig. 11-24. Diagrammatic representation of the principle of dorsal capsuloligamentodesis. A capsular flap left attached proximally to the radius, is inserted into the scaphoid distal to its axis of rotation, to maintain scaphoid alignment after reduction. (From Blatt G: Personal Communication, 1981.)

either be contraindicated or too difficult to perform successfully; (2) the patient with scaphoid instability, but with minimal radiographic changes, in whom clinical examination suggests and surgical exploration demonstrates excessive scaphoid mobility, *provided* that normal preoperative grip strength is 80 lb or less using a standard Jamar dynamometer; and (3) scapholunate dissociations in wrists with rheumatoid arthritis.

Patients with frank scaphoid subluxations, and with stronger grip strength, require a more stable type of correction, only achieved, in my experience, through the use of limited arthrodesis. Although maximum mobility is a goal of the treatment of carpal instability many, if not all the procedures mentioned, result in some limitation of motion. I believe that a more accurate goal may be the preservation of the *maximum* amount of wrist mobility that is *compatible* with a pain-free, stable, and strong wrist.

In 1967 Peterson and Lipscomb[56] reported the successful use of arthrodesis between scaphoid, trapezium, and trapezoid for the treatment of rotatory subluxation of the scaphoid. In 1979 Uematsu[73] proposed to fuse scaphoid, lunate, and capitate for the treatment of this condition. Since 1980, limited arthrodeses of the scaphoid-trape-

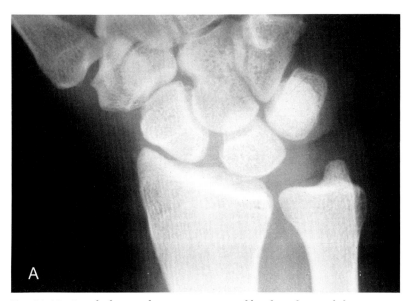

Fig. 11-25. Scapholunate dissociation treated by dorsal capsuloligamentodesis. A: Preoperative radiograph. B: Immediate postoperative radiograph.

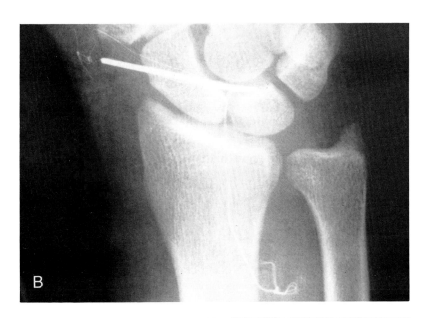

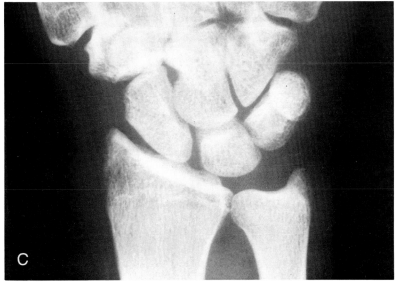

Fig. 11-25 (cont.) *C:* Final result (Courtesy of Dr. G. Blatt, Long Beach, CA.)

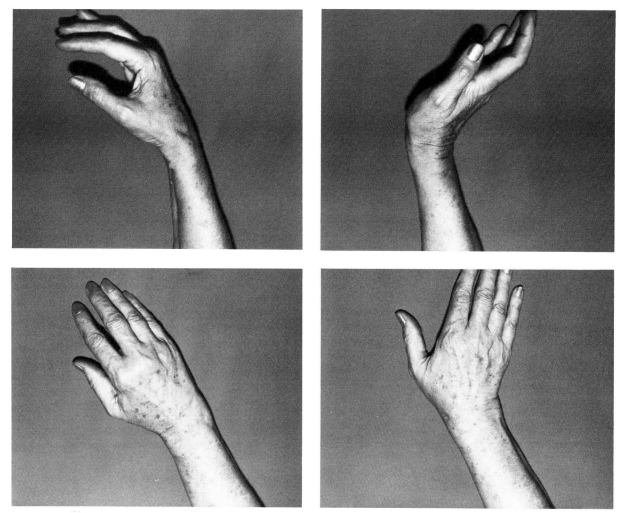

Fig. 11-26. Range of motion following scaphotrapezium-trapezoid fusion averages 80 percent of dorsal-palmar flexion, and 66 percent of radial-ulnar deviation.

zium-trapezoid (STT) joint, referred to as the "tri-scaphoid" joint by Watson and Hempton,[77] has been an accepted treatment for chronic scapholunate dissociations prior to the appearance of osteoarthritic changes. Although this procedure significantly alters normal wrist kinematics,[26,37] the placement of the proximal pole of the scaphoid under the dome of the distal articular surface of the radius restores the height of the radial carpus, and the patient's ability to load his wrist with stability and without pain. It also reduces the propensity for degenerative changes between radius and scaphoid.[37] Late osteoarthritis of other intercarpal joints has not been a problem.[56,77] An average of 80 per-

cent of dorsal-palmar flexion, and 66 percent of radial-ulnar deviation should be expected postoperatively (Fig. 11-26, 11-27). Kleinman et al.[37] described the cineradiographic changes occurring after successful STT fusions. They point out that in the normal wrist, the total arc of scaphoid motion from full dorsiflexion to full palmarflexion is 90 degrees, and that of the capitate 135 degrees. After STT fusions, both arcs average 90 degrees, suggesting that the capitate moves with the STT fusion mass (Fig. 11-28). In the anteroposterior plane, the loss of the scaphoid ability to foreshorten during radial deviation interferes with this motion (Fig. 11-27E). The more longitudinal the position of the

Fig. 11-27. Recurrent voluntary (dynamic) scapholunate dissociation. *A:* Anteroposterior radiograph is essentially within normal limits, although *B:* Lateral view shows a dorsiflexed lunate. *C:* Posteroanterior projection after the patient voluntarily subluxed his wrist. There is a clear scapholunate dissociation.

(Fig. continues on next page.)

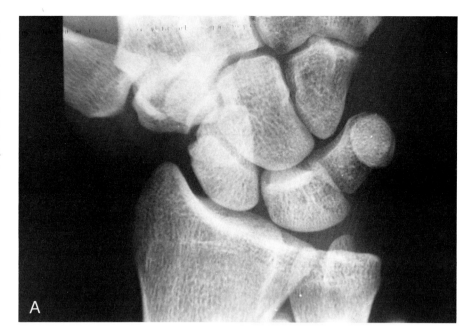

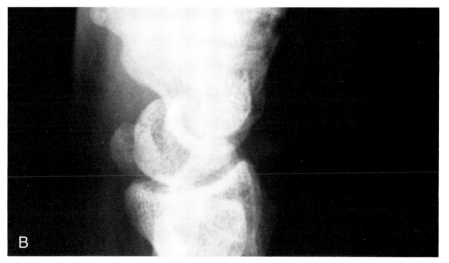

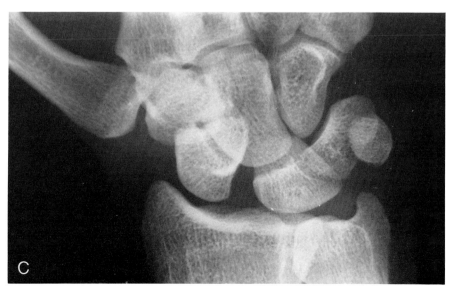

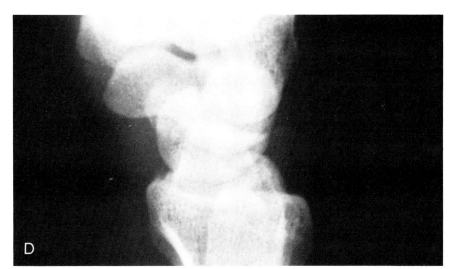

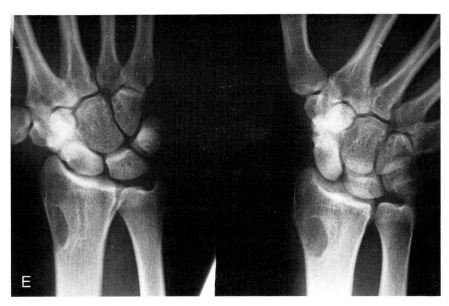

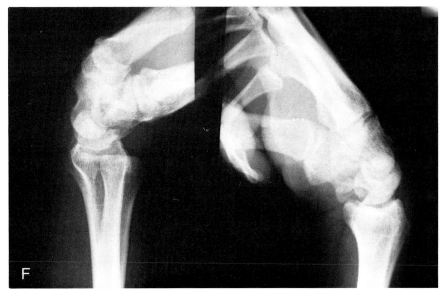

Fig. 11-27 (cont.) D: lateral view shows now a perpendicular, subluxed scaphoid. *E:* Postoperative radiographic range of radial and ulnar deviation following arthrodesis between scaphoid, trapezium and trapezoid. Bone graft was obtained from the distal radius. *F:* Postoperative radiographic range of dorsal-palmarflexion.

Fig. 11-27 (cont.) G, H, I, and J show clinical comparative range of motion.
(Fig. continues on next page.)

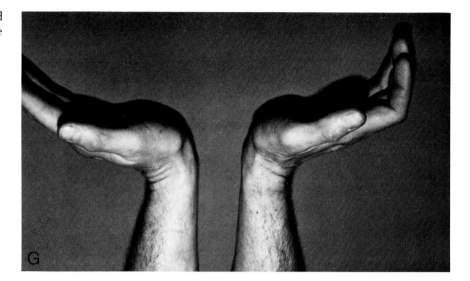

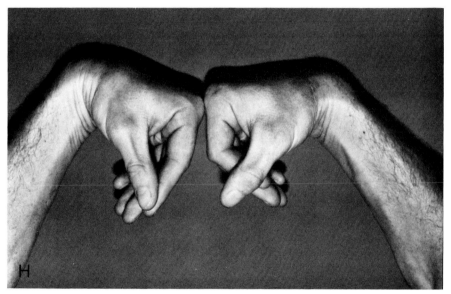

fused scaphoid, the more compromised will be the range of radial deviation. Some preservation of radial deviation is possible if the scaphoid is fused in a neutral alignment of approximately 45 degrees in relationship to the long axis of the radius (Fig. 11-27). During ulnar deviation, the scapolunate diastasis, which has remained untreated, opens widely, allowing substantial intercarpal motions (Fig. 11-29). The scaphoid clearly loses its influence to shift the lunate and triquetrum during lateral movements.[37] A new plane of motion, between scaphoid and lunate, is present in these wrists.

Technique of Scaphotrapezium Trapezoid Fusion (Watson)

A transverse incision is used to approach the STT joint, placed along the dorsoradial aspect of the carpus, 5 to 7 mm distal to the tip of the radial styloid[77] (Fig. 11-30). Care is taken to isolate and preserve the superficial branches of the radial nerve. The tunnel for the extensor pollicis longus is unroofed and the tendon is retracted. The radial artery may then be mobilized and kept out of the operating field. The dorsoradial wrist capsule is

Fig. 11-27 (cont.)

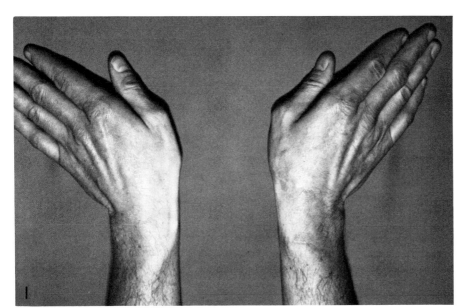

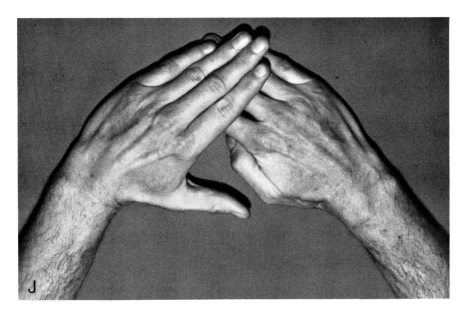

opened transversely. An additional vertical incision is used if needed. The scaphotrapeziotrapezoid articulation appears as a horizontal T. Retraction of the proximal capsule, or prolonging the capsular and skin incisions will allow examination of the proximal pole of the scaphoid. Usually, there is localized synovitis, not only at the scapholunate level, but also, surprisingly, at the scaphotrape-zium-trapezoid joint. A synovectomy is completed. The ability to reduce the scaphoid is tested at this point. The articular surfaces of the three joints (scaphotrapezium, scaphotrapezoid, trapezium trapezoid) are excised down to healthy cancellous bone. Fixation with several 0.045 Kirschner wires is required. Two wires are driven from distal to proximal until their tips become barely visible in

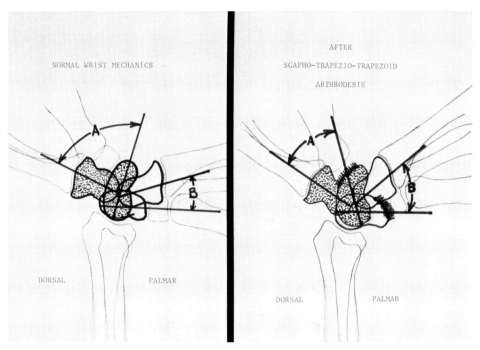

Fig. 11-28. Normal cineradiographs demonstrate that angle between scaphoid and capitate on lateral projection is quite variable through dorsiflexion/palmarflexion arc (compare angle "A" in dorsiflexion to angle "B" in palmarflexion). Following scaphotrapezium-trapezoid arthrodesis, this angle remains fixed through dorsiflexion/palmarflexion arc (angle "A" = angle "B"), suggesting that capitate moves with scaphotrapezium-trapezoid fusion mass. (From Kleinman WB, Steichen JB, Strickland JW: Management of chronic rotary subluxation of the scaphoid by scaphotrapezio-trapezoid arthrodesis. J Hand Surg 7:125, 1982.)

the center of the decorticated surfaces of the trapezium and trapezoid. This ensures correct pin placement before the bone graft is packed into place. A third wire is introduced from lateral to medial across the trapezium-trapezoid joint. The scaphoid is then manually reduced to neutral alignment, at roughly 45 degrees to the radius. Hyperextension of the scaphoid must be avoided for this may result in a fixed ulnar deviation position of the wrist, or in unnecessary loss of radial deviation. Reduction is maintained with two Kirschner wires driven from the scaphoid to the lunate and to the capitate. A second transverse incision is next placed proximal to the base of the radial styloid. Superficial branches of the radial nerve are retracted and the radius is exposed subperiosteally, usually between the tendons of the first and second compartments (extensor pollicis brevis and extensor carpi radialis longus). A small cortical window is elevated, and enough cancellous bone obtained to pack the interstices of the scaphotrapezium-trapezoid joint. Once this is completed, the two wires which were left prepositioned at the joint are driven across to engage the trapezium and trapezoid to the reduced scaphoid. Compression of the surfaces to be fused is avoided in order to preserve the entire form and dimensions of the scaphotrapezium-trapezoid unit (Fig. 6-27). The cortical bone graft obtained from the radius may next be used to bridge the fused joints. The wounds are closed in layers.

Immediately postoperatively, the wrist and hand are placed in a compression dressing, and immobilization secured in a long arm plaster dressing. This

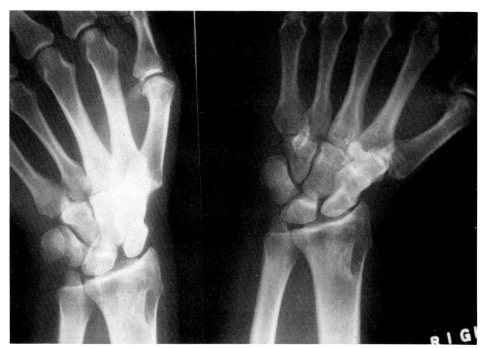

Fig. 11-29. Following scaphotrapezium-trapezoid arthrodesis, scapholunate diastasis opens widely as wrist rolls into ulnar deviation (left). Intercarpal motion occurs around axis formed by head of capitate, along plane beginning at triquetrohamate joint, coursing between capitate and lunate, and exiting at scapholunate diastasis and radioscaphoid joint. (From Kleinman WB, Steichen JB, Strickland JW: Management of chronic rotary subluxation of the scaphoid by scaphotrapezio-trapezoid arthrodesis. J Hand Surg 7:125, 1982.)

is removed at three to five days postoperatively and is replaced with a long arm plaster that includes the thumb and the index and long fingers in an intrinsic-plus position. At two weeks postoperatively, this cast is changed and replaced with a long arm thumb spica cast, worn until the end of the sixth week. At this point, the solidity of the fusion is radiographically determined. Usually, a short arm thumb spica cast is needed for an additional two to four week period, or until the fusion is solid. At eight to ten weeks, all pins can be removed and an exercise program commenced.

Chronic Scapholunate Dissocation with Osteoarthritis

When the malrotated scaphoid is allowed to remain outside of its normal relationship with the distal radius, degenerative changes, usually be-

tween radial styloid and scaphoid, are bound to occur. At times, radioscaphoid osteoarthritis appears very rapidly following scapholunate dissociation; narrowing and sclerosis of the radial styloid and the scaphoid may be seen as early as three months following the injury, and continue to progress at a fast pace (Fig. 11-31). Watson and Ballet[80] described a pattern of radiocarpal joint involvement, which they named scapholunate advanced collapse (SLAC wrist). They believed that the subluxated scaphoid fits poorly on the highly specific elliptical-shape scaphoid fossa of the radius, and that this is conducive to the rapid rate of wear of their articular cartilage. In comparison, the lunate facet of the radius and the proximal articular surface of the lunate are segments of a sphere and tolerate rotatory displacements without damage. When the proximal pole of the scaphoid is worn out, its stabilization by scaphotrapezium-trapezoid

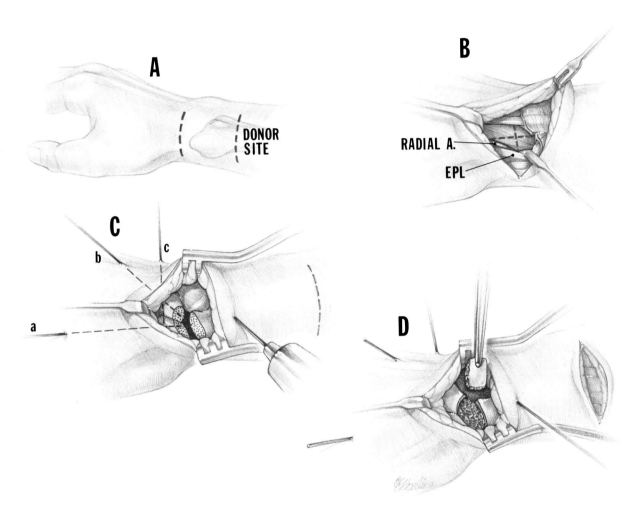

Fig. 11-30. Technique of scaphotrapezium trapezoid (STT) fusion. *A:* Transverse incisions used to expose STT joint and distal radius donor site. *B:* Capsule of STT joint exposed. Extensor pollicis longus tendon (EPL) retracted palmarward. A transverse capsular incision may be supplemented with a longitudinal incision if needed. *C:* Joint surfaces excised to underlying, healthy cancellous bone. Kirschner wires are prepositioned along the trapezium (a), the trapezoid (b) and across the trapeziotrapezoid joint (c). The scaphoid is reduced and pinned to the lunate and the capitate. Overreduction of the scaphoid (excessive "longitudinalization") must be avoided. *D:* Bone chips obtained from the distal radius are packed into the fusion site. The drawing shows a cortical window about to be inserted across the fusion. The Kirschner wires are advanced at this time, to secure fixation. (See Ref. 77.)

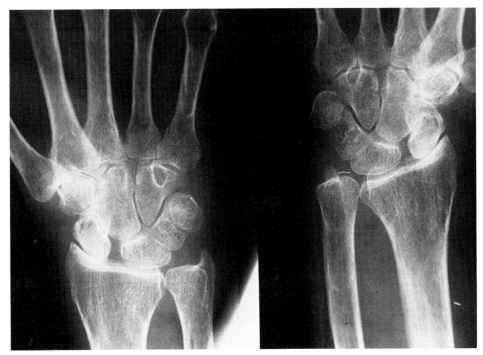

Fig. 11-31. Posteroanterior (left) and anteroposterior (right) radiographs three months following an acute scapholunate dissociation, show early osteoarthritic changes between radial styloid and scaphoid.

fusion will subject it to unyielding pressure against the radius. This will result in an accelerated process of progressive degenerative changes, and continuous pain (Fig. 11-32). In these cases, it it best to replace the scaphoid with an implant, with the addition of a lunocapitate arthrodesis to avoid further subluxation in an already unstable carpus (Fig. 11-33). Wrists with chronic unreduced scapholunate dissociations also develop progressive degenerative changes of the lunocapitate joint, subjected to abnormal stresses because of the dorsiflexion of the lunate and the dorsal subluxation of the head of the capitate (Fig. 11-34). Again, at this stage, any attempt at relocating and holding the scaphoid, either by ligament reconstruction or by limited arthrodesis, will fail in restoring pain free function, as worn out surfaces are brought to bear loads. For this type of wrist, the same procedure consisting of excision of the scaphoid, its replacement with a silicone implant, and a fusion across the degenerated lunocapitate joint is satisfactory. The removed scaphoid and additional bone from the distal radius provide the bone-graft for this fusion. The addition of the hamate and triquetrum to the lunocapitate arthrodesis does not significantly change the expected postoperative range of motion.[78] This procedure eliminates, by arthroplasty or by fusion, all abnormal joints, and leaves intact the usually excellent articulation between the radius and the lunate, for all motions of the wrist. It also provides a load-bearing column, from the hand, through the capitate and lunate, into the radius, bypassing the silicone implant that had replaced an already unstable scaphoid. This far, synovitis related to the presence of the silicone implant has not been seen in these patients with combined arthroplasties and limited arthrodesis. The technique for the insertion of a scaphoid implant has already been discussed (see Chapter 6). A transverse incision may be used instead of a longitudinal approach, placed overlying the midcarpal "four corner" joint between capitate, lunate, triquetrum, and hamate.

(Text continues on page 277.)

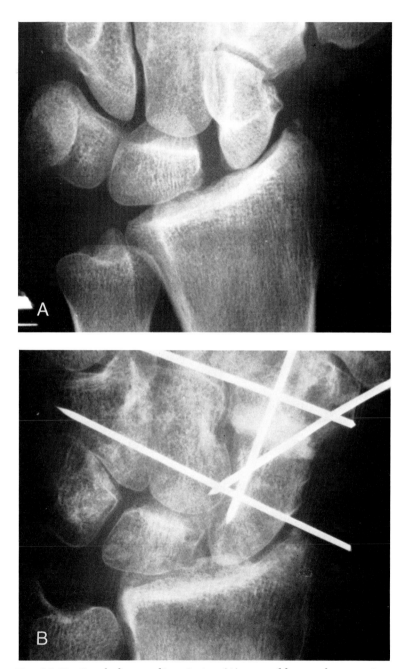

Fig. 11-32. Scapholunate dissociation *(A)* treated by scaphotrapezium trapezoid arthrodesis *(B).* Initial result was very satisfactory.

(Fig. continues on next page.)

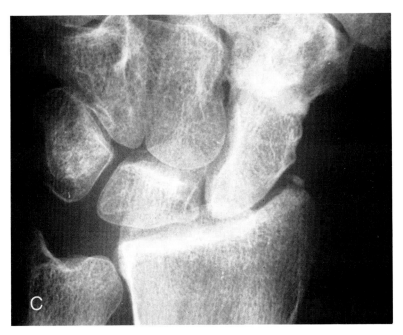

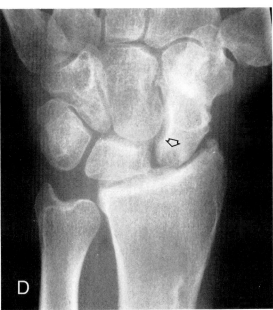

Fig. 11-32 (cont.) (C). At six months there was recurrence of pain and synovitis. Radiographs *(D)* show severe cystic erosion of the proximal pole of the scaphoid (arrow).

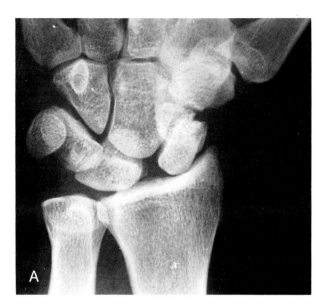

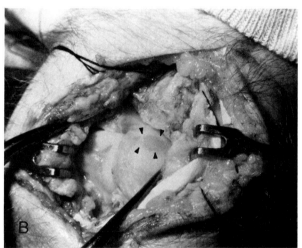

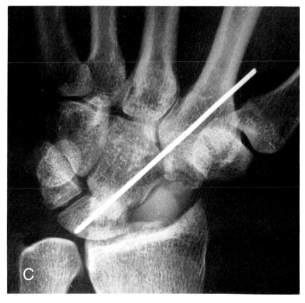

Fig. 11-33. Scapholunate dissociation *(A)* with degenerative posttraumatic changes of the proximal pole of the scaphoid *(B)* treated by excision of the scaphoid, insertion of scaphoid implant and carpal stabilization by lunocapitate arthrodesis *(C)*.

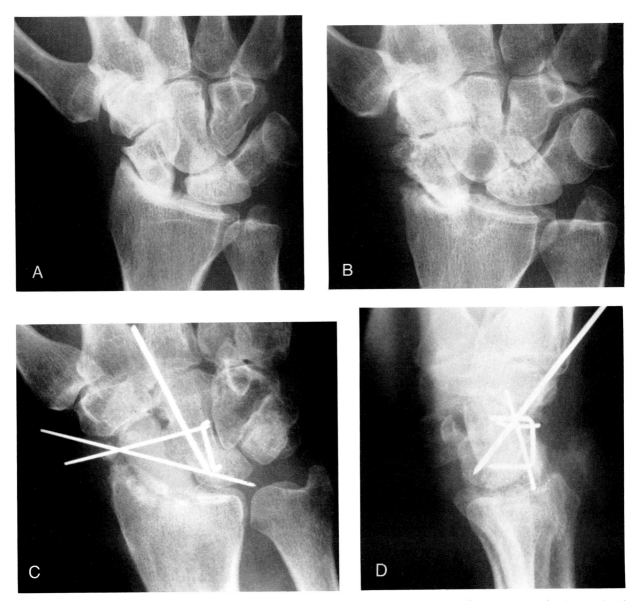

Fig. 11-34. Scapholunate advanced collapse deformity (SLAC wrist). *A* and *B* show different stages of radioscaphoid and lunocapitate osteoarthritis. *C* and *D* are postoperative radiographs following scaphoid implant arthroplasty and lunocapitate arthrodesis. (See Ref. 80.)

The fusion follows principles already discussed (Fig. 6-27):

1. The joint surfaces are excised until cancellous bone is exposed.
2. Kirschner wires are prepositioned, their tips at the site of the proposed fusion, but without crossing the joint space until bone has been packed. As many pins as needed may be used for a stable fixation.
3. Bone from the excised scaphoid and the distal radius is utilized as the graft.
4. The excised joints are packed with the bone grafts, without compression to avoid any change in the outside shape and dimensions of the arthrodesed unit.
5. The prepositioned pins are now driven across the joint. The radiocarpal space is left free of fixation. A staple between lunate and capitate may be needed for additional stabilization (Fig. 11-34).

The postoperative care is similar to that recommended following scaphotrapezium-trapezoid arthrodeses.

REFERENCES

1. Adkison JW, Chapman MW: Treatment of acute lunate and perilunate dislocations. Clin Orthop 164:199, 1982
2. Andrews FT: A dislocation of the carpal bones. The scaphoid and semilunar: Report of a case. Mich St Med Soc J 31:269 1932
3. Arkless R: Cineradiography in normal and abnormal wrists. Am J Roentgenol 96:837, 1966
4. Armstrong GWD: Rotational subluxation of the scaphoid. Can J Surg 11:306, 1968
5. Bindi R: La luxación del escafoides carpiano. Bol Trab Soc Argent Ortop Traumatol 29:194, 1964
6. Bjelland JC, Bush JC: Secondary rotational subluxation of the carpal navicular. Ariz Med 34:267, 1977
7. Blatt G: Personal communication, 1981
8. Boyes JG: Subluxation of the carpal navicular bone. South Med J 69:141, 1976
9. Boyes JH: Bunnell's Surgery of the Hand. 5th Ed. Lippincott, Philadelphia, 1970
10. Buzby BF: Isolated radial dislocation of carpal scaphoid. Ann Surg 100:553, 1934
11. Campbell RD Jr, Thompson TC, Lance EM, Adler

JB: Indications for open reduction of lurate and perilunate dislocations of the carpal bones. J Bone Joint Surg [Am] 47:915, 1965
12. Cave EF: Retrolunar dislocation of the capitate with fracture or subluxation of the navicular bone. J Bone Joint Surg 23:830, 1941
13. Collins LC, Lidsky MD, Sharp JT, Moreland J: Malposition of carpal bones in rheumatoid arthritis. Radiology 103:95, 1972
14. Connell MC, Dyson RP: Dislocation of the carpal scaphoid. Report of a case. J Bone Joint Surg [Br] 37:252, 1955
15. Crittenden JJ, Jones DM, Santerelli AG: Bilateral rotational dislocation of the carpal navicular: Case report. Radiology 94:629, 1970
16. Demos TC: Radiologic case study: Painful wrist. Orthopedics 1:151, 1978
17. Destot E: Traumatismes du poignet et rayons x. Masson, Paris, 1923
18. Dobyns JH, Linscheid RL, Chao EYS, et al: Traumatic instability of the wrist. Am Acad Orthop Surgeons Instruc Course Lect 24:182, 1975
19. England JPS: Subluxation of the carpal scaphoid. Proc R Soc Med 63:581, 1970
20. Fisk GR: Carpal instability and the fractured scaphoid. Ann R Coll Surg Engl 46:63, 1970
21. Fitton JM: Rotational dislocation of the scaphoid. In Stack GH, Bolton H (eds): Proceedings of the Second Hand Club, British Society of Surgery of the Hand. Brentwood, Essex. The Westway Press, 1962
22. Frankel VH: The Terry-Thomas sign. Clin Orthop 129:321, 1977
23. Gilford WW, Bolton RH, Lambrinudi C: The mechanism of the wrist joint; with special reference to fractures of the scaphoid. Guys Hosp Rep 92:52, 1943
24. Gilula LA, Weeks PM: Post-traumatic ligamentous instability of the wrist. Radiology 129:641, 1978
25. Glickel SZ, Millender L: Results of ligamentous reconstruction for chronic intercarpal instability. Ortho Trans 6:167, 1982
26. Goldner JL: Treatment of carpal instability without joint fusion—Current assessment. J Hand Surg 7:325, 1982
27. Green DP, O'Brien ET: Open reduction of carpal dislocations: Indications and operative techniques. J Hand Surg 3:250, 1978
28. Green DP: Carpal dislocation. In Green DP (ed): Operative Hand Surgery. Vol. I. Churchill Livingstone, New York, 1982
29. Hastings DE, Evans JA: Rheumatoid wrist deformities and their relationship to ulnar drift. J Bone Joint Surg [Am] 57:930, 1975

30. Hergenröeder PT, Penix AR: Bilateral scapholunate dissociation with degenerative arthritis. J Hand Surg 6:620, 1981

31. Higgs SL: Two cases of dislocation of carpal scaphoid. Proc R Soc Med 23:61, 1930

32. Hockley BJ: Carpal instability and carpal injuries. Aust Radiol 23:158, 1979

33. Howard FM, Fahey T, Wojcik E: Rotatory subluxation of the navicular. Clin Orthop 104:134, 1974

34. Hudson RM, Caragol WJ, Faye JJ: Isolated rotatory subluxation of the carpal navicular. Am J Roentgenol 126:601, 1976

35. Jeanne LA and Mouchet A: Les lésions traumatiques fermées du poignet. 28th Congrès Français de Chirurgie, 1919

36. Kauer JMG: Functional anatomy of the wrist. Clin Orthop 149:73, 1980

37. Kleinman WB, Steichen JB, Strickland JW: Management of chronic rotary subluxation of the scaphoid by scaphotrapezio-trapezoid arthrodesis. J Hand Surg 7:125, 1982

38. Kovalkovitz I, Ficzere O: Habituelle scapholunare Dissoziation. Chirurg 48:428, 1977

39. Kuth JR: Isolated dislocation of the carpal navicular. A case report. J Bone Joint Surg 21:479, 1939

40. Landsmeer JM: Studies in the anatomy of articulation. I. The equilibrium of the "intercalated" bone. Acta Morphol Neerl Scand 3:287, 1961

41. Lewis OJ, Hamshere RJ, Bucknill TM: The anatomy of the wrist joint. J. Anat 106:539, 1970

42. Linscheid RL: Mechanical forces affecting the deformity of the rheumatoid wrist. J Bone Joint Surg [Am] 51:790, 1969

43. Linscheid RL, Dobyns JH, Beabout JW, Bryan RS: Traumatic instability of the wrist. J Bone Joint Surg [Am] 54:1612, 1972

44. Linscheid RL, Dobyns JH, Beckenbaugh RD, et al: Instability patterns of the wrist. J Hand Surg 8:682, 1983

45. Loeb TM, Urbaniak JR, Goldner JL: Traumatic carpal instability: Putting the pieces together. Orthop Trans 1:163, 1977

46. MacConaill MD: Mechanical anatomy of the carpus and its bearing on some surgical problems. J Anat 75:166, 1941

47. Maki NJ, Chuinard RG, D'Ambrosia R: Isolated, complete radial dislocation of the scaphoid. A case report and review of the literature. J Bone Joint Surg [Am] 64:615, 1982

48. Mayfield JK, Johnson RP, Kilcoyne RF: The ligaments of the human wrist and their functional significance. Anat Rec 186:417, 1976

49. Mayfield JK, Johnson RP, Kilcoyne RF: Carpal dislocations: Pathomechanics and progressive perilunar instability. J Hand Surg 5:226, 1980

50. Moneim MS: The tangential posteroanterior radiograph to demonstrate scapholunate dissociation. J Bone Joint Surg [Am] 63:1324, 1981

51. Murakami Y: Dislocation of the carpal scaphoid. Hand 9:79, 1977

52. Nigst H: Luxations et subluxations du scaphoide. Ann Chir 27:519, 1973

53. Palmer AK, Dobyns JH, Linscheid RL: Management of post-traumatic instability of the wrist secondary to ligament rupture. J Hand Surg 3:507, 1978

54. Palmer AK, Levinsohn EM, Kuzma GR: Arthrography of the wrist. J Hand Surg 8:15, 1983

55. Parkes JC, Stovell PB: Dislocation of the carpal scaphoid: A report of two cases. J Trauma 13:384, 1973

56. Peterson HA, Lipscomb PR: Intercarpal arthrodesis. Arch Surg 95:127, 1967

57. Rask MR: Carponavicular subluxation: Report of a case treated with percutaneous pins. Orthopedics 2:134, 1979

58. Rosenthal DI, Schwartz M, Phillips WC, Jupiter J: Fracture of the radius with instability of the wrist. Am J Roentgenol 141:113, 1983

59. Russell TB: Intercarpal dislocations and fracture-dislocations: A review of fifty-nine cases. J Bone Joint Surg [Br] 31:524, 1949

60. Sarrafian SK, Melamed JL, Goshgarian GM: Study of wrist motion in flexion and extension. Clin Orthop 126:153, 1977

61. Schlossbach T: Dislocation of the carpal navicular bone not associated with fracture. J Med Soc NJ 51:533, 1954

62. Sutro CJ: Hypermobility of bones due to "over-lengthened" capsular and ligamentous tissues. Surgery 21:67, 1947

63. Taleisnik J: The ligaments of the wrist. J Hand Surg 1:110, 1976

64. Taleisnik J: Wrist: Anatomy, function and injury. Am Acad Orthop Surgeons Instruct Course Lect 27:61, 1978

65. Taleisnik J: Rheumatoid synovitis of the volar compartment of the wrist joint: Its radiological signs and its contribution to wrist and hand deformity. J Hand Surg 4:526, 1979

66. Taleisnik J: Scapholunate dissociation. In Strickland JW, Steichen JB (eds): Difficult Problems in Hand Surgery. Mosby, St. Louis, 1982

67. Taleisnik J: Rheumatoid arthritis of the wrist. In

Strickland JW, Steichen JB (eds): Difficult problems in hand surgery. Mosby, St. Louis, 1982

68. Tanz SS: Rotation effect in lunar and perilunar dislocations. Clin Orthop 57:147, 1968

69. Taylor AR: Dislocation of the scaphoid. Postgrad Med J 45:186, 1969

70. Testut L, Latarjet A: Tratado de anatomia humana. 9th Ed. Revised A. Latarjet. Vol. I. Salvat Editores, S.A., Buenos Aires, 1951

71. Thomas HO: Isolated dislocation of the carpal scaphoid. Acta Orthop Scand 48:369, 1977

72. Thompson TC, Campbell RD Jr, Arnold WD: Primary and secondary dislocation of the scaphoid bone. J Bone Joint Surg [Br] 46:73, 1964

73. Uematsu A: Intercarpal fusion for treatment of carpal instability: A preliminary report. Clin Orthop 144:159, 1979

74. Vance R, Gelberman R, Braun R: Chronic bilateral scapholunate dissociation without symptoms. J Hand Surg 4:178, 1979

75. Vaughan-Jackson OJ: A case of recurrent subluxation of the carpal scaphoid. J Bone Joint Surg [Br] 31:532, 1949

76. Walker GBW: Dislocation of the carpal scaphoid reduced by open operation. Br J Surg 30:380, 1943

77. Watson HK, Hempton RF: Limited wrist arthrodesis. I: The triscaphoid joint. J Hand Surg 5:320, 1980

78. Watson HK, Goodman ML, Johnson TR: Limited wrist arthrodesis. Part II: Intercarpal and radiocarpal combination. J Hand Surg 6:223, 1981

79. Watson HK: Personal communication, 1982

80. Watson HK, Ballet FL: The SLAC wrist: Scapholunate advanced collapse pattern of degenerative arthritis. J Hand Surg 9A:358, 1984

12 Medial Carpal Instability

Navarro[20] was the first to stress the functional importance of what he called the triquetropisiform system, at a time when Destot[4] had affirmed that "the scapho-lunary system is vital" and that "as far as the cuneiform is concerned, it is far from the ulna and its lesions are insignificant compared with those of the scaphoid and of the semilunar." It is true that injuries to the ulnar half of the carpus are infrequent compared to those involving the scaphoid. There is, however, a growing body of evidence indicating that these are important causes of pain along the ulnar side of the wrist. Medial carpal instability occurs because of ligamentous dissociation between the medial carpal column (triquetrum and pisiform) and either the lunate or the hamate.[27]

TRIQUETROLUNATE
INSTABILITY (STATIC VISI)

There are two types of triquetrolunate instability, which may be two stages in the progression of triquetrolunate instability, one without clinical or radiographic evidence of VISI, the other presenting a full-blown volar instability pattern. Historically, and until recently,[22] a review of the literature disclosed references to the latter type only. In 1913 Chaput and Vaillant[3] published a radiographic study of carpal injuries. One of their patients represents a classic example of what is now recognized as a VISI deformity.[5,15] During the same year, Mayersbach[18] reported a carpal injury in a 72-year-old man, whose lateral radiographs also showed a VISI deformity. Mayersbach noticed that "as a result of the injury, the cuneiform bone (triquetrum) is separated from the semilunar bone (lunate) but it is not substantially changed in its position. It *is only brought closer to the ulna in the direction of an ulnar abduction.*" In 1919, Jeanne and Mouchet[11] described partial "medial-carpal luxations," and shortly thereafter Navarro[20] described palmar subluxation of the capitate in a patient with abnormal displacements of triquetrum and scaphoid. He pointed out that the triquetrum had rotated "just like the scaphoid, but in the *opposite sense*" and showed a frontal radiograph with a loss of the normal convex outline of the carpal condyle, similar to that observed by Mayersbach.

The position of the lunate as the intercalated segment within the radiocarpal link, is influenced by its own shape[13] and by the scaphoid laterally and the triquetrum medially[12] (Fig. 1-10). In the normal wrist, during radial deviation, palmar flexion of the lunate and the triquetrum is determined by the need for the scaphoid to palmarflex to allow for radial carpal shortening. A posteroanterior radiograph obtained with the wrist in full radial deviation, therefore, will show a normal relationship between the three major carpal bones within the palmarflexed proximal carpal row, consisting of a foreshortened scaphoid, a triangular lunate and the triquetrum in a proximal position in relation to the hamate. In full ulnar deviation, ulnar carpal shortening is possible by a distal displacement of the triquetrum on the hamate (Fig. 3-4).[2] This is accompanied by triquetral dorsiflexion which augments the normal dorsiflexion bias of the lunate. This results in dorsiflexion of the entire proximal carpal row. The scaphoid appears now elongated, and coexists in the normal wrist with a quadrilateral lunate, and a triquetrum displaced distally in relation to the hamate. If the scaphoid is responsible for volarflexion of the lunate and the triquetrum for dorsiflexion of the lunate, a logical correlation is to expect a static dorsiflexion instability of the lunate (**DISI**) following a scapholunate dissociation, and a static volarflexion of the lunate (**VISI**) after a tri-

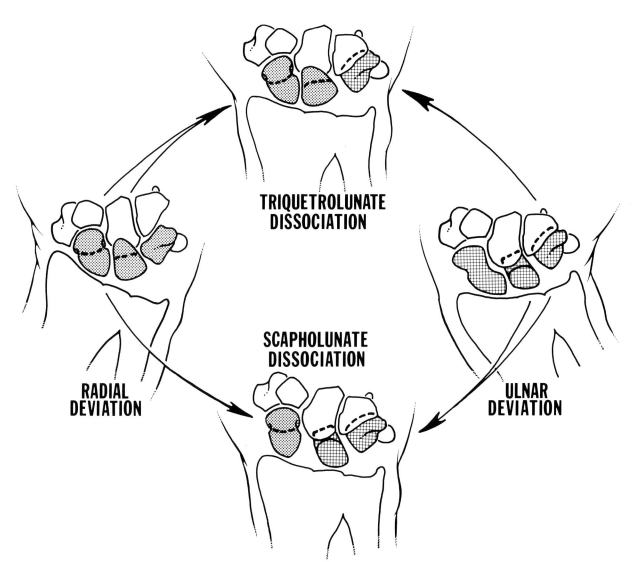

Fig. 12-1. Schematic representations of scapholunate and triquetrolunate dissociations show mixing carpal rotations normally found only in radial or in ulnar deviation. In *scapholunate dissociation* the scaphoid is palmarflexed (such as in normal radial deviation) while lunate and triquetrum are dorsiflexed (such as in normal ulnar deviation). In *triquetrolunate dissociation* scaphoid and lunate are palmarflexed (such as in normal radial deviation) while the triquetrum is dorsiflexed (such as in normal ulnar deviation). The net effect in both types of instability is a loss of carpal height, allowed by palmarflexion and foreshortening of the scaphoid (on the radial side) and by dorsiflexion and distal migration of the triquetrum (on the ulnar side).

quetrolunate dissociation (Fig. 12-1). The presence of such an injury within the proximal carpal row must be suspected when there is coexistence in frontal radiographs of a palmar flexed, foreshortened scaphoid (as seen in radial deviation) with a dorsiflexed triquetrum in a distal position in relation to the hamate (as occurs in ulnar deviation).[28,30] The actual location of the dissociation can be surmised by the shape of the lunate in the same frontal projection: if it is *quadrilateral*, it is dorsiflexed, and consequently, it has remained together with the triquetrum, but dissociated from the volarflexed scaphoid. This is the case in rotatory subluxations of the scaphoid, where the scapholunate dissociation is strikingly shown by the presence of a scapholunate gap (the Terry Thomas sign) (Fig. 12-2).[9] If the shape of the lunate is triangular in the frontal projection, it is because the lunate is palmar flexed, together with the scaphoid (Fig. 12-3). In these cases, the dissociation must have occurred at the interface with the dorsiflexed triquetrum, but is more difficult to see because, instead of a gap, there is a step-off between the triquetrum and lu-

nate (at times, almost imperceptible). A lateral radiograph will clearly show that both scaphoid and lunate are volarflexed together (Fig. 12-4). Clinical models in support of this concept of carpal behavior are rare; one such model was provided by a patient who had sustained a dislocation of scaphoid and lunate as a unit, without scapholunate dissociation (Fig. 12-5A,B).[28] Scaphotrapezium and scapholunate ligaments were preserved, but all lunotriquetral connections were torn. Following a successful closed reduction, a progressive VISI deformity developed (Fig. 12-5C). Linscheid and coauthors[15] reported two patients with static VISI deformities in their 1972 paper on traumatic instability of the wrist; one deformity accompanied a fracture of the scaphoid and the other was in a young man who had lost the triquetrum, the distal end of the ulna, and the extensor tendons of the fingers as a result of an electrical burn. Since excision of the distal ulna is not known to produce VISI deformities, it is safe to assume that in this patient it was the loss of the triquetrum, in effect an extreme form of triquetrolunate dissociation, which led to

Fig. 12-2. The "Terry Thomas sign" (gap between scaphoid and lunate) is a clear sign of scapholunate dissociation.

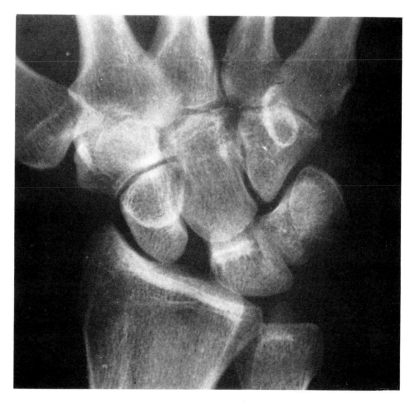

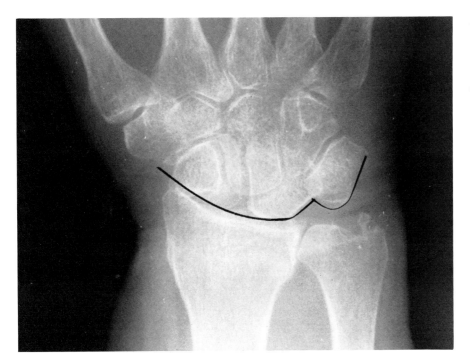

Fig. 12-3. Triquetrolunate dissociation. The posteroanterior view shows palmarflexion of the scaphoid. The lunate is triangular (palmarflexed). The triquetrum is distal in relation to the hamate (dorsiflexed). There is shortening of the distance between triquetrum and ulnar head (Mayersbach's sign). The convex outline of the proximal carpal condyle ("Shenton line of the wrist") is interrupted between lunate and triquetrum.

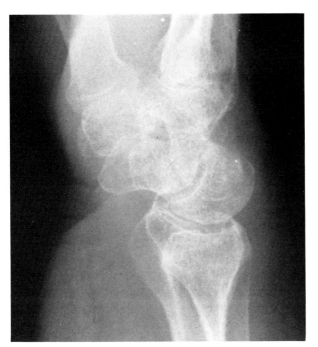

Fig. 12-4. Triquetrolunate dissociation. Lateral view shows palmarflexion of lunate and scaphoid. The radial styloid-scaphoid space has collapsed into a V.

the development of the **VISI** deformity. Static forms of **VISI** are more frequent in severe rheumatoid arthritis of the wrist. These rheumatoid patients show the same pattern of palmarflexion of scaphoid and lunate, coexistent with a dorsiflexed triquetrum displaced distally in relation to the hamate, and a step-off between lunate and triquetrum (Fig. 12-6).

Although attempts to reproduce this instability pattern in cadavers have been unsuccessful, based on the clinical experience just reviewed I believe that triquetrolunate dissociation is the mechanism responsible for the development of static **VISI** deformities.

Diagnosis

In 1981 Reagan et al.[22] reported on lunotriquetral sprains, and indicated that palmarflexion instability patterns represent a "more extensive continuation of this (sprain) injury" between lunate and triquetrum. Very early after injury, and in patients whose instability does not progress to a fully devel-

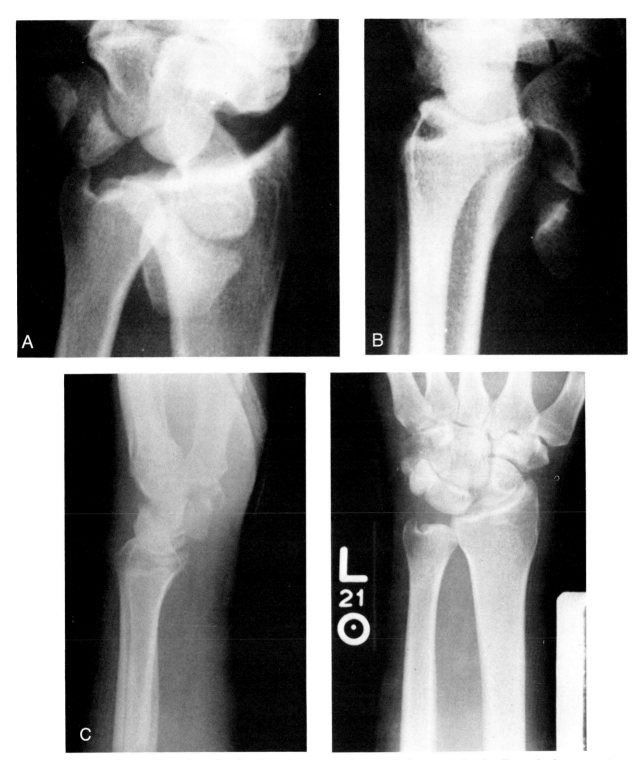

Fig. 12-5. Isolated dislocation of scaphoid and lunate. *A:* Initial PA view shows scaphoid still attached to trapezium and to lunate. *B:* Lateral radiograph shows the palmar dislocation of scaphoid and lunate without scapholunate dissociation. *C:* At six weeks following successful closed reduction, a VISI alignment is apparent in the lateral projection. The posteroanterior view shows the features of a palmar carpal instability; foreshortening of the scaphoid, a triangular lunate and a distal (dorsiflexed) triquetrum (see Fig. 12-1).

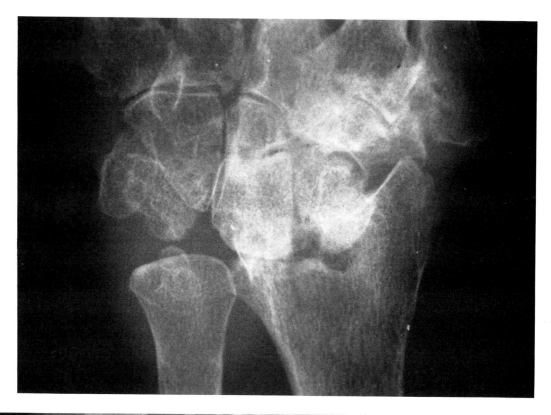

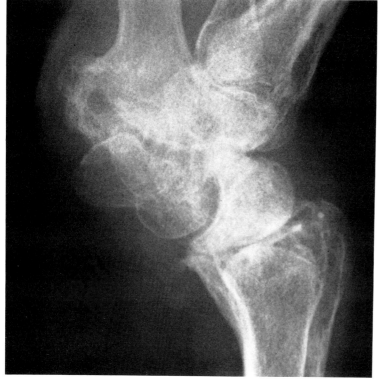

Fig. 12-6. Severe **VISI** deformity in wrist of patient with rheumatoid arthritis.

oped VISI, the diagnosis is difficult and is suggested only by the pain referred to the ulnar aspect of the carpus, and by tenderness localized to the triquetrolunate space. Radiographs are negative. A normal, bilateral alignment into some volarflexion of the lunate may be present (Fig. 12-7). A positive ulnar variance is not infrequent and, in some cases, an ulnolunate impingement exists. For the triquetrolunate dissociation following trauma, neither a knowledge of the mechanism of injury nor of the patient's complaints are helpful, in most cases, in arriving at a diagnosis. Although I believe that triquetrolunate dissociations are carpal hyperpronation injuries, this is difficult to prove from the patient's description of his accident, and could not be reproduced by impact loading of cadaver specimens. Rotation is an important factor in the production of this deformity. The importance of rotation was stressed as early as 1913 by Auvray[1] and is further supported by a relatively frequent mechanism of injury seen in these cases. Many patients describe a torque load applied to their wrists when using a power drill, as the drill bit gets stuck, causing a sudden reverse torsion of the hand at the wrist.[29] Examination of the wrist will disclose tenderness localized to the triquetrolunate space. In later stages, after a full VISI deformity is present, there is a subtle bayonet alignment of the hand on the forearm when seen in profile, the carpus slightly palmar to the distal radius (Fig. 12-8). This deformity may be corrected by applying pressure on the pisiform directed dorsally, a maneuver that is frequently accompanied by a feeling of increased stability and decreased pain.[16] Pain is frequently minimal or absent, except when attempting heavy lifting or gripping. Patients complain more of weakness and soreness than of pain. In many cases, these symptoms disappear after a period of splinting.

In the initial stages of triquetrolunate dissociation, when a VISI deformity is absent, an injection of an anesthetic agent precisely into the triquetrolunate space, under radiographic control, will assist in restoring painfree motion if the triquetrolunate space is, indeed, the source of pain. Radiographic motion studies into radial and ulnar deviation may demonstrate an abnormal displacement of the triquetrum on the lunate. Arthrograms are helpful when a leak of opaque material between triquetrum and lunate can be shown (Fig 12-9). When a complete VISI is present, frontal radiographs will show the following (Fig. 12-3):

1. The scaphoid is volarflexed and foreshortened. The ring sign is present and there is a decrease in the ring-proximal pole distance.
2. The lunate is volarflexed, and triangular in shape.

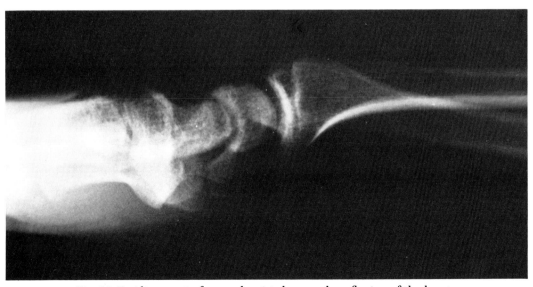

Fig. 12-7. Alignment of normal wrist shows palmarflexion of the lunate.

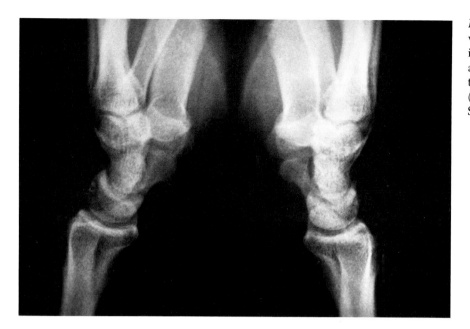

Fig. 12-8. Comparison lateral views of injured (left) and uninjured (right) wrists. There is a subtle bayonet alignment of the hand on the forearm. (Courtesy of Dr. Richard M. Salib, Carson City, Nevada.)

3. The triquetrum is dorsiflexed, in a distal position in relation to the hamate.
4. There is a shortening of the distance between the ulnar head and the triquetrum (Mayersbach's sign).
5. The convex outline from the proximal carpal condyle, called "Shenton line of the wrist" by Linscheid, is interrupted by a stepoff between lunate and triquetrum. Likewise, Gilula and Weeks[10] point out that the smooth arc, which can normally be drawn along the *distal* articular surfaces of the scaphoid, lunate, and triquetrum, is broken at the triquetrolunate joint.

Lateral radiographs (Fig. 12-4) show the lunate palmarflexed, the scaphoid also palmarflexed, its long axis perpendicular to that of the radius, and the styloid-scaphoid space collapsed into a V, a palmarflexed type of "concertina" deformity.[7] If triquetrum and lunate can be identified, a normal negative triquetrolunate angle of approximately 16 degrees is converted to a neutral or positive angle.[16]

TREATMENT

It is unusual to see a patient with a static type of VISI deformity soon after injury. At this early

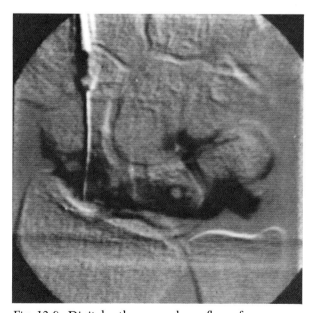

Fig. 12-9. Digital arthrogram shows flow of opaque material into midcarpal joint, through triquetrolunate dissociation.

stage, these patients show surprisingly minimal findings and, frequently, minimal disability. Treatment at this point consists of plaster immobilization of the wrist in ulnar deviation and dorsiflexion, the plaster molded to apply palmar pressure on the pisiform. Immobilization should include the elbow to prevent rotational stress on the carpus, and should be maintained for six weeks at least. When a VISI deformity is present, the position of immobilization should attempt to bring the scaphoid and lunate into enough dorsiflexion to match the position of the triquetrum, and at the same time to reverse the clinical deformity. Even though the deformity may recur after immobilization is discontinued, an essentially pain-free wrist may result. In my experience, it is infrequent for a patient to develop sufficient disability to justify a surgical correction. For the wrist with only arthrographic evidence of triquetrolunate dissociation, a triquetrolunate fusion is a reliable solution. When in ad-

Fig. 12-10. Tenodesis and capsulodesis techniques for VISI and DISI deformities.

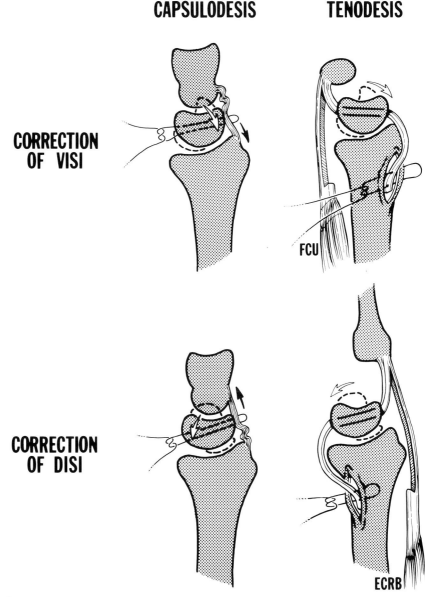

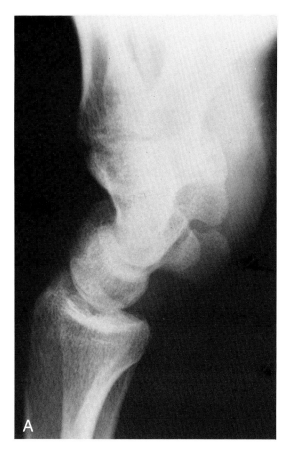

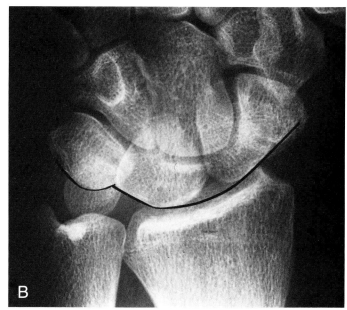

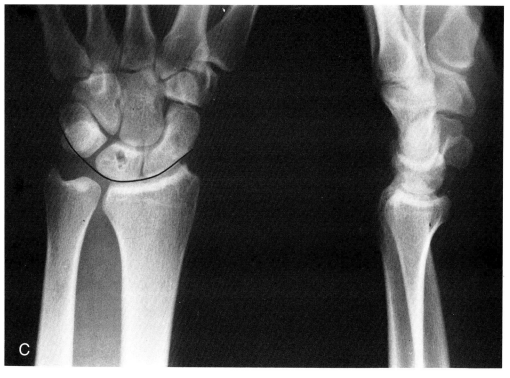

Fig. 12-11. VISI deformity. *A*: Preoperative lateral view. *B*: Preoperative PA view (the "Shenton line of the wrist" is interrupted). *C*: Postoperative radiographs two years following treatment by tenodesis using a slip from the flexor carpi ulnaris tendon (see Fig. 12-10).

dition to the triquetrolunate leak there is an ulna plus variant, shortening of the ulna must be considered. Ulnar recession will help to decompress the ulnocarpal space and will assist in stabilizing the ulnar carpus. For the fully developed VISI, stabilization of the lunate using one half of the flexor carpi ulnaris left attached distally has proven successful in my hands (Figs. 12-10 and 12-11). However, this procedure is technically demanding, and subjects the lunate to the danger of collapse and fragmentation. Recurrence is also possible. Indeed, an easier and more reliable correction is provided by a radiolunate arthrodesis, with the lunate in the correct, neutral rotation. Should radiolunate fixation intraoperatively be ineffective to maintain

scaphoid alignment, then the fusion should also include the scaphoid.

TRIQUETROHAMATE INSTABILITY (DYNAMIC VISI AND DISI DEFORMITY)

In 1934 Mouchet and Belot[19] reported a patient, a 58-year-old wife of a physician, with bilateral "forward mid-carpal subluxation" of the wrists, who had developed a "snapping" of the right wrist following an automobile accident. This trick motion was accompanied by a special sound, and could be reproduced with the slightest movement of dor-

Fig. 12-12. In the normal wrist (*A*), during ulnar deviation, the lunate dorsiflexes and at the same time shifts palmarward enough to allow capitate and radius to remain colinear. In patients exhibiting a **DISI** dynamic instability (*B*) the lunate pivots on its own center of rotation, forcing the capitate dorsal to the radius.

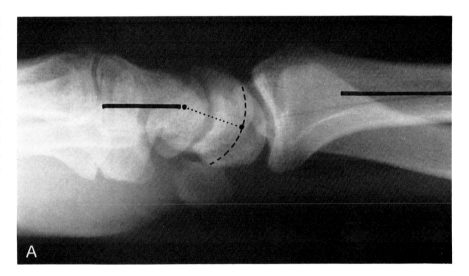

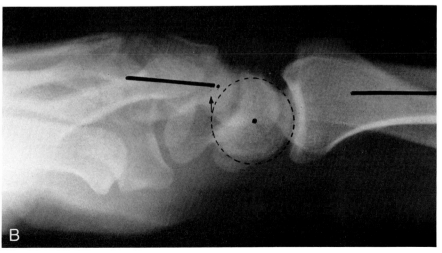

siflexion, and easily reduced in palmar flexion. The strength of her grip was diminished. On examination, she demonstrated a similar finding on the left wrist, although here it was less consistent, more fleeting, and free of discomfort. Radiographs taken after the subluxed position was assumed showed bilateral volar midcarpal subluxations. Mouchet and Belot were unable to find similar reports. They concluded that this phenomenon was due to a congenital malformation, aggravated on the right side by the accident sustained. Mauclaire[17] discussed this paper and recalled a similar patient whom he had seen in 1910. Two other cases were reported in 1946 by Sutro.[24] Both Sutro's patients showed bilateral findings without a history of trauma. One of these could reproduce a subluxation by strong active contraction of the fingers with the hand in radial deviation and palmarflexion. Both were successfully treated by a fusion between scaphoid, capitate, and lunate. These patients were representative of a group of individuals later grouped by Sutro under the name "hypermobility syndrome."[25]

In 1962 Fitton[8] presented a fifth case of recurrent carpal subluxation "on the medial side of the mid-carpal joint," that he had treated by placing a bone graft "between trapezium and lunate." Although Fitton did not specify whether the carpal subluxation occurred into VISI or DISI, his was the first clear mention of instability localized to the medial side of the midcarpal joint. Two other patients may be found in the group of *traumatic* car-

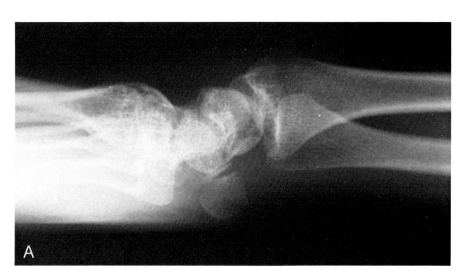

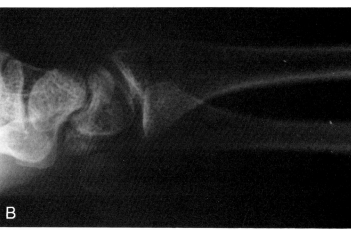

Fig. 12-13. Dynamic DISI. A: Normal alignment for this patient includes a slightly palmarflexed lunate and the capitate palmar to the radius. B: In ulnar deviation, this normal radiocapitate alignment is abruptly reversed.

Fig. 12-14. Dynamic VISI. *A* and *B*: Clinical and radiographic appearance show palmarflexion of the lunate, normal for this patient (whose opposite, uninjured wrist is shown in Fig. 12-7). *C* and *D* demonstrate clinical and radiographic alignment in VISI, after the patient actively assumes the subluxed position. (*B* and *D* from Taleisnik J: Current concepts of the anatomy of the wrist. In Spinner M (ed): Kaplan's Functional and Surgical Anatomy of the Hand. 3rd Ed. Lippincott, Philadelphia, 1984.)

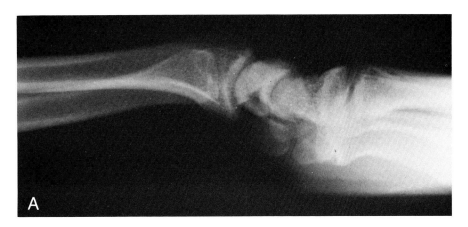

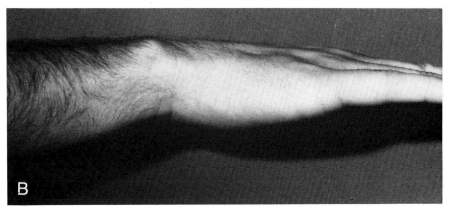

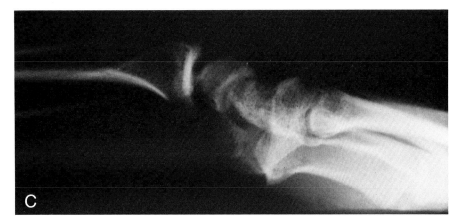

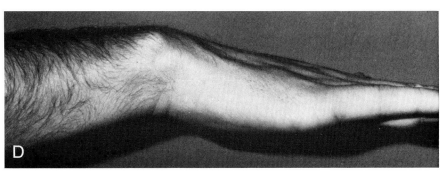

pal instabilites reported in 1972 by Linscheid and coauthors.[15] Both had voluntary recurrent volar subluxations without a previous history of injury.

According to Dobyns[6] "the topographically determined areas of the carpus . . . appear to dictate the volarflexed intercalated segment instability," once ligamentous restraints are no longer present, due to either congenital laxity, or attenuation and tear caused by disease or injury. In 1981 Lichtman et al.[14] presented a clinical laboratory analysis of ulnar (medial) midcarpal instability. These authors observed that the only important intrinsic ligament across the midcarpal joint is the palmar or V ligament, and that the ulnar limb of this ligament is the only structure to support the ulnar half of the midcarpal joint (see Chapter 2). It was only after this heavy fascicle was divided in cadaver wrists that the clinical syndrome could be reproduced by manipulation and ulnar deviation. These authors described ten patients, of whom seven showed a dynamic **DISI** collapse, reproducible in ulnar deviation. As we have seen, it is particularly in ulnar deviation that the wrist tends to assume a precollapse appearance (Fig. 10-6). In full ulnar deviation, dorsiflexion of the lunate is offset by an equal but opposite palmarflexion of the capitate. However, in order for the capitate and radius to remain colinear, the dorsiflexed lunate must shift in a palmar direction. During ulnar deviation, this shift is guided by the triquetrum which, as it dorsiflexes, descends along the *palmar* aspect of the hamate. In the lateral radiographs, lunate dorsiflexion takes place along the segment of a circle that is centered within the head of the capitate, the central axis of wrist rotation (Fig. 12-12A). It is the ulnar or capitotriquetral limb of the V ligament that controls and supports this motion. When this ligament is divided, dorsiflexion of the lunate is not accompanied by a concurrent palmar shift, and no longer takes place around a center within the head of the capitate. Instead, the lunate simply pivots on its own center of rotation, resulting in a displacement of the capitate *dorsal* to the radius (Fig. 12-12B) or dorsal to what is a normal radiocapitate alignment for that particular patient (Fig. 12-13). The wrist assumes a true zigzag or collapse alignment. The opposite pattern, dynamic VISI, is also possible, usually when the wrist is slightly palmar flexed and radially deviated (Fig. 12-14). I believe these patients have a preexisting alignment that prelocates the wrist in a slight dorsal or palmar flexed position (Figs. 12-13, 12-14A). Actually, the "normal" coaxial pattern of radius and lunate may be considerably less frequent than a pattern with some degree of lunate palmar flexion. Sarrafian and coauthors[23] found that 71 percent of *normal* wrists radiographed in a clinical neutral position presented an average of 12 degrees of radiolunate palmar flexion (1 to 31 degrees), and in 51 percent this palmar angulation of the lunate was not offset by an equal but opposite dorsiflexion of the capitate. Likewise, in 18 percent the lunate appeared dorsiflexed to an average of 9 degrees, and in 38 percent the capitate was extended anywhere from 1 to 43 degrees in relation to the radius. The presence of a predisposing loss of colinearity in individuals with

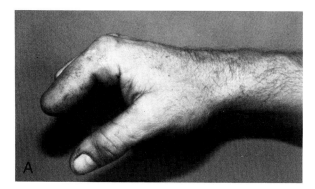 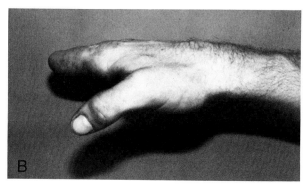

Fig. 12-15. Dynamic **DISI**. *A:* Neutral alignment. *B:* Prominence of head of capitate is apparent in ulnar deviation. Transition occurs abruptly, and is accompanied by a painful, loud, visible, and palpable snap.

Fig. 12-16. Midcarpal instability. *A* and *B* show manipulation of patient's wrist, reproducing the dynamic,
painful subluxation.
(Fig. continues on next page.)

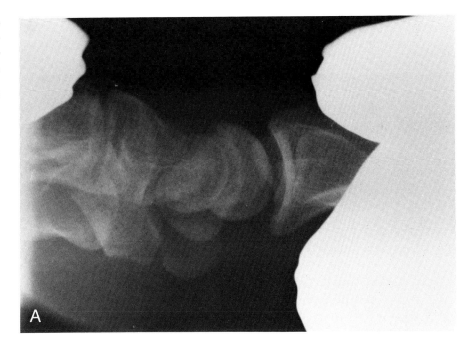

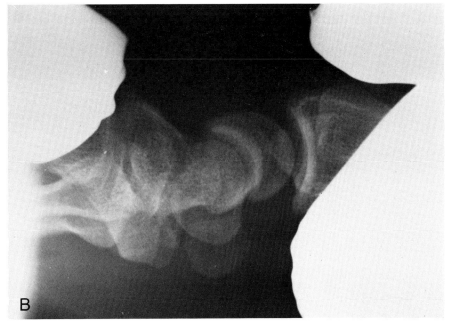

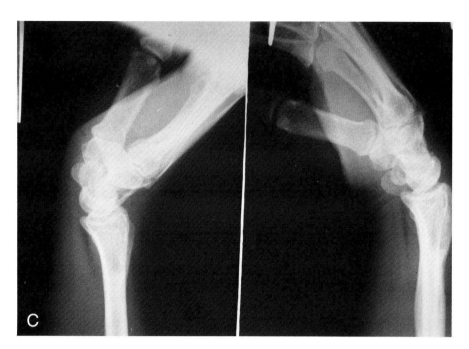

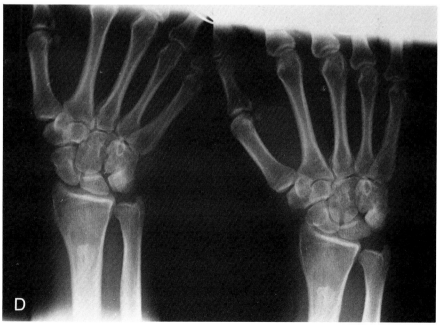

Fig. 12-16. (cont.) C and D show range of motion following triquetrohamate fusion. Patient is asymptomatic.

normally lax joints may, therefore, be the prerequisite to the development of these dynamic forms of carpal instability.

DIAGNOSIS

Patients are usually young adults who frequently conform to the hypermobility syndrome described by Sutro.[25] Routinely the uninjured wrist is lax and can be stressed with ease, producing a significant alteration of carpal alignment (Fig. 3-6E,F).[26] Not infrequently, although symptomatic in only one wrist, these patients present *bilateral* evidence of wrist instability.[19,21,25] A history of a specific traumatic episode may be absent. The presenting complaint is a painful snap, most consistently reproduced by bringing the hand into or out of ulnar deviation with the forearm in pronation while axial loading is either generated by the patient contracting his own muscles across the wrist (Fig. 12-15), or by the examiner.[14] This snap is often loud, and can be readily palpated between triquetrum and hamate, or between lunate and capitate. The midcarpal instability can be reproduced by manipulation of the ulnar half of the midcarpal joint, and al-though this phenomenon may be present bilaterally, it is only a meaningful finding when it reproduces the patient's pain (Fig. 12-16). The midcarpal joint is tender, particularly where it is most accessible to palpation: between lunate and capitate, and between triquetrum and hamate. The diagnosis should be strongly suspected in the presence of this history and the clinical findings described. Dynamic forms of **DISI** or **VISI** are secondary to loss of support across the ulnar half of the midcarpal joint.

Routine radiographs are usually considered normal, although the alignment of the radiocarpal link may show a clear palmar or dorsiflexion bias (Figs. 12-13, 12-14). Diagnostic radiographs are obtained with the patient's forearm and hand pronated against a vertically placed film, and with the x-ray beam directed from the side (Fig. 5-14). The patient is then asked to assume the position of collapse. Lateral radiographs obtained at this point will show a VISI or DISI deformity, *with loss of the alignment between capitate and radius which is normal for that particular patient.*

Cineradiography further demonstrates the sudden, abnormal displacement that occurs between the two carpal rows. Other diagnostic techniques,

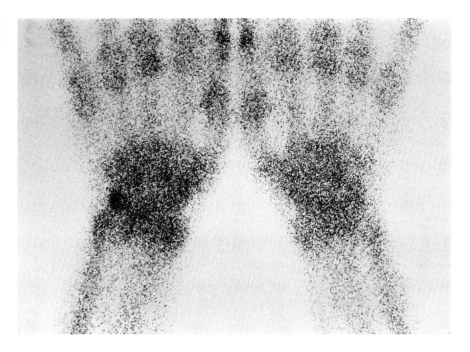

Fig. 12-17. Positive bone scan (left) shows increased uptake of the ulnar carpus.

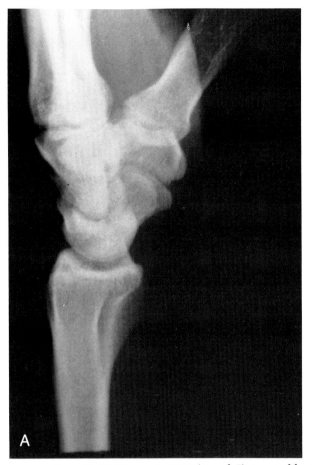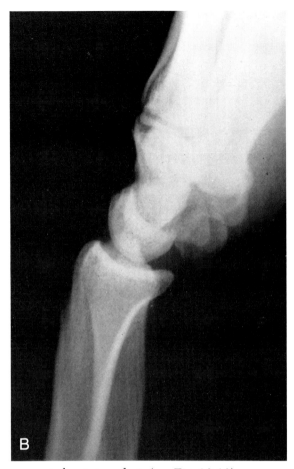

Fig. 12-18. Dynamic **VISI** (*A* and *B*), treated by Flexor carpi ulnaris tenodesis (see Fig. 12-10).

including arthrography, are usually not helpful. In some cases, a bone scan may show an increase in uptake in the lunocapitate, the triquetrohamate (Fig. 12-17) or both joint areas.

Treatment

A trial of nonsurgical management, antiinflammatory medications and local injections is justified for patients that are seen early after the onset of symptoms, and even if first examined late but without having received any previous treatment. Long-arm plaster immobilization with the forearm in supination and the wrist in neutral deviation for at least six weeks is frequently effective. In those pa-

tients with recurrent, persistent or disabling symptoms, unresponsive to nonsurgical measures, treatment should be directed to stabilization of the lunate, to prevent its uncontrolled abnormal dorsi- or palmarflexion, or to stabilization of the midcarpal joint. When demands on the wrist are not expected to be excessive, in females, for the minor wrist, when the patient's occupation does not involve excessive loading, and arbitrarily, when the grip strength of the normal hand is under 80 lb *capsulodesis or tenodesis* procedures are preferred (Fig. 12-10). *Limited arthrodeses* are used when the anticipated stress to be borne by the stabilization procedure is greater, in men, particularly when involved in heavy activities, for the major wrist, and when the grip strength exceeds 100 lb.

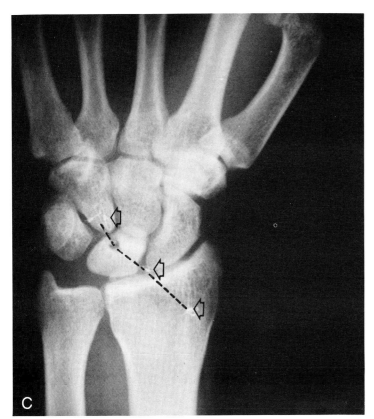 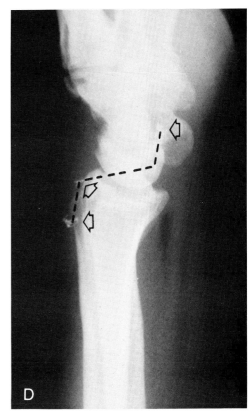

Fig. 12–18. (cont.) (C, D) Wire sutures (arrows) show path of new ligament. (From Taleisnik J: Post-traumatic carpal instability. Clin Orthop 149:73, 1980.)

Lunate Stabilization

Tenodeses and Capsulodesis. These procedures result in the creation of a sling or suspensory ligament which tends to counteract the abnormal rotation of the lunate (Figs. 12-18, 12-19). For dynamic **VISI** deformities, a strip fashioned from the lateral half of the flexor carpi ulnaris, left attached distally, is threaded from the palmar to the dorsal aspects of the lunate and attached to the dorsal aspect of the radius. For dynamic **DISI** deformities, the medial half of the extensor carpi radialis brevis is left attached distally and is similarly threaded through the lunate from dorsal to palmar, to be anchored under the pronator quadratus on the anterior surface of the distal radius (Fig. 12-10). Because of the concern arising from the drilling of the lunate, and the difficulty of the procedure, a capsulodesis may be used instead. The rationale for this

procedure is similar to that behind the stabilization of the scaphoid by capsulodesis (Fig. 11-24). A dorsal capsular flap based distally is used to tether the dorsal pole of the lunate distalward in cases of **DISI**. This capsular flap is secured to a small trap door on the dorsal pole of the reduced lunate, and is secured with a nonabsorbable suture passed through fine drill holes made with Kirschner wires, exiting on the palmar pole of the lunate, where the suture is tied. This requires a second, small palmar approach. For a **VISI** deformity, the dorsal capsular flap is left attached proximally (Fig. 12-10).

Radiolunate Fusion. Stabilization may also be provided by a radiolunate fusion, with the lunate held in neutral, colinear alignment in relation to the long axis of the radius. The radiolunate joint may be exposed using a longitudinal or a transverse skin approach along the dorsum of the wrist, and a

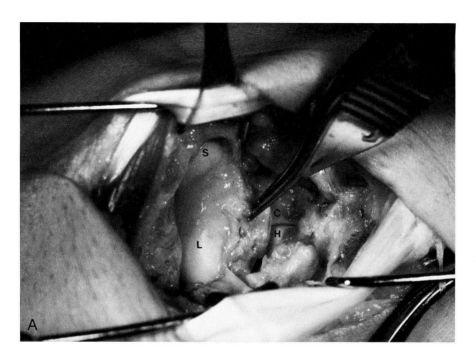

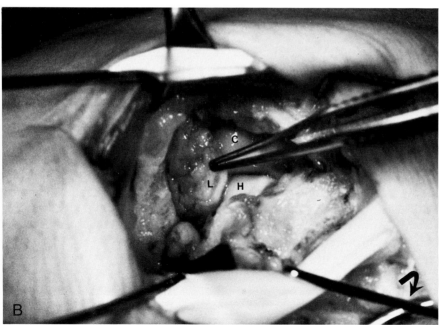

Fig. 12-19. Intraoperative views of wrist with dynamic DISI. *A*: in neutral alignment (note arms of self-retaining retractors), much of scaphoid (S) and lunate (L) can be seen. Capitate (C) and hamate (H) are partially hidden. The forceps points to the dorsal pole of the lunate. *B*: In ulnar deviation (arrow indicates change of alignment of distal self-retaining retractor), the lunate (L) dorsiflexes allowing capitate (C) and hamate (H) to sublux in a dorsal direction.

Fig. 12-19. (cont.) C: Radiographic alignment following tenodesis with one half of Extensor carpi radialis brevis tendon (see Fig. 12-10).

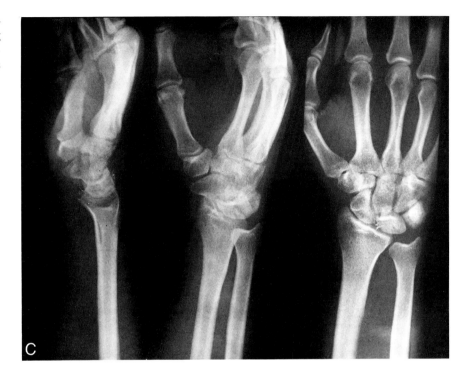

transverse capsular incision (Figs. 6-23, 6-25). The principles of this limited type of arthrodesis are common to all other limited fusions (Fig. 6-27), and include decortication of articular surfaces of lunate and radius down to healthy cancellous bone, the insertion of two or three Kirschner wires of suitable size (usually .054 or .045) through the radius, from its lateral cortex, in a medial and distal direction, until the tips of the wires show at the lunate surface of the radius. Cancellous bone is packed into the radiolunate space (the donor site is either the distal radius or the iliac crest) without applying any compression, and finally the Kirschner wires are driven across the fusion site to complete fixation. A small cortical bridge is then inset between the radius and the lunate to secure further fixation. The postoperative care includes an initial three-digit plaster immobilization cast for the first two weeks following the operation, replaced by a long arm thumb spica to be worn until the end of the sixth postoperative week. A short arm plaster cast is worn for the final four weeks or until healing is radiographically solid.

Midcarpal Stabilization

Restoration of stability across the midcarpal joint may also be achieved by one of several additional techniques: ligamentous reefing and/or interosseous tendon grafting[14] between triquetrum and hamate, or localized arthrodesis crossing the midcarpal joint, either medially (triquetrohamate or lunotriquetrohamate capitate) or laterally (scapholunocapitate) and conceivably between scaphoid, trapezium and trapezoid. Triquetrohamate fusions result in stable wrists, with minimal sacrifice of motion (Fig. 12-16C), but may create one of several postoperative problems, particularly pain over the hook of the now unyielding hamate, or accelerated degenerative changes of the pisotriquetral joint, or may allow a late recurrence of a painful snap that is usually localized to the unfused lunocapitate space. A fusion that includes the lunate, capitate, triquetrum, and hamate, the "four corners" of the carpus, although more extensive, may be more consistently successful, with minimal additional loss of wrist motion when compared with the more

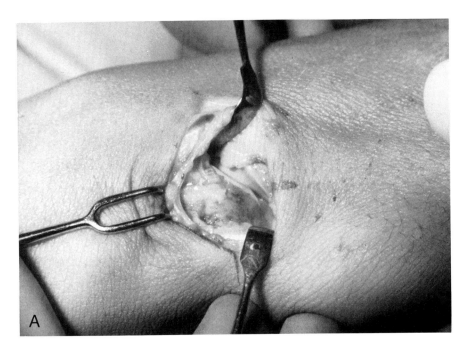

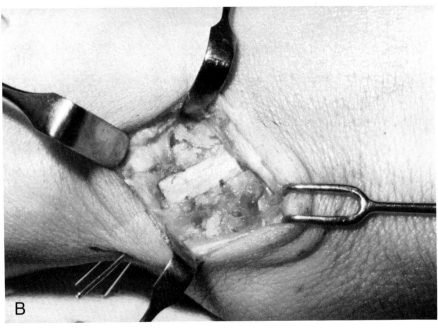

Fig. 12-20. Intraoperative photographs of wrist with midcarpal (dynamic) instability. *A:* Triquetrohamate joint. *B:* After fusion and internal fixation with multiple Kirschner wires.

limited triquetrohamate arthrodesis. The surgical technique follows the same guidelines that have already been mentioned for other types of limited arthrodesis (Figs. 6-27, 12-20).

REFERENCES

1. Auvray M: Discussion, in Mouchet, A, and Vennin, H: Luxation medio-carpienne en avant du poignet droit. Bull Mem Soc Chir 39:1376, 1913
2. Bryce TH: On certain points in the anatomy and mechanism of the wrist joint reviewed in the light of a series of roentgen ray photographs of the living hand. J Anat Physiol 31:59, 1896
3. Chaput and Vaillant: Étude radiographique sur les traumatismes du carpe. Rev Orthop 4:227, 1913
4. Destot E: Traumatismes du poignet et rayons X. Masson, Paris, 1923
5. Dobyns JH, Linscheid RL, Chao EYS, et al: Traumatic instability of the wrist. Am Acad Orthop Surgeons Instruct Course Lect 24:182, 1975
6. Dobyns JH: Personal communication, January 1979
7. Fisk G: Carpal instability and the fractured scaphoid. Ann R Coll Surg Engl 46:63, 1970
8. Fitton JM: Subluxation of the medial side of the midcarpal joint. In Stack GH, Bolton H (eds): Proceedings of the Second Hand Club, Leeds. Brentwood, Essex, The Westway Press, 1962
9. Frankel VH: The Terry-Thomas sign. Clin Orthop 129:321, 1977
10. Gilula LA, Weeks PM: Post-traumatic instabilities of the wrist. Radiology 129:641, 1978
11. Jeanne LA and Mouchet A: Les lésions traumatiques fermées du poignet. 28th Congres Français de Chirugie, 1919
12. Johnston MB: Varying positions of the carpal bones in the different movements at the wrist. J Anat Physiol 41:109, 1907
13. Kauer JMG: The interdependence of carpal articulation chains. Acta Anat 88:481, 1974
14. Lichtman DM, Schneider JR, Swafford AR, Mack GR: Ulnar midcarpal instability — Clinical and laboratory analysis. J Hand Surg 6:515, 1981
15. Linscheid RL, Dobyns JH, Beabout JW, Bryan RS: Traumatic instability of the wrist. Diagnosis, classification and pathomechanics. J Bone Joint Surg [Am] 54:1612, 1972
16. Linscheid RL, Dobyns JH, Beckenbaugh RD, et al: Instability patterns of the wrist. J Hand Surg 8:682, 1983
17. Mauclaire M: Discussion. In Mouchet A, Belot J: Poignet á ressáut (subluxation médio-carpienne en avant). Bull Mem Soc Nat Chir 31:1244, 1934
18. Mayersbach L von: Ein seltener Fall von Luxation Intercarpea. Dtsch Z Chir 123:179, 1913
19. Mouchet A, Belot J: Poignet á ressaut (subluxation medio-carpienne en avant). Bull Mem Soc Nat Chir 31:1243, 1934
20. Navarro A: Luxaciones del carpo. An Fac Med (Montevideo, Uruguay) 6:113, 1921
21. Pournaras J, Kappas A: Volar perilunar dislocation. J Bone Joint Surg [Am] 61:625, 1979
22. Reagan DS, Linscheid RL, Dobyns JH: Lunotriquetral sprain. (Abstract). J Hand Surg 6:296, 1981
23. Sarrafian S, Melamed J, Goshgarian G: Study of wrist motion in flexion and extension. Clin Orthop 126:153, 1977
24. Sutro CJ: Bilateral recurrent intercarpal subluxation. Am J Surg 72:110, 1946
25. Sutro CJ: Hypermobility of bones due to "overlengthened" capsular and ligamentous tissues. Surgery 21:67, 1947
26. Taleisnik J: The ligaments of the wrist. J Hand Surg 1:110, 1976
27. Taleisnik J: Post-traumatic carpal instability. Clin Orthop 149:73, 1980
28. Taleisnik J, Malerich M, Prietto M: Palmar carpal instability secondary to dislocation of scaphoid and lunate: Report of case and review of the literature. J Hand Surg 7:606, 1982
29. Watson HK: Carpal instability. Symposium. Contemp Orthop 4:107, 1982
30. Weber ER: Biomechanical implications of scaphoid waist fractures. Clin Orthop 149:83, 1980

13 Proximal Carpal Instability

The first reference to carpal instability secondary to malunion of fractures of the distal radius is found in Jeanne and Mouchet's study of closed injuries of the wrist.[12] These authors realized that a reversal of the normal palmar tilt of the articular surface of the distal radius could result in dorsal carpal subluxation. Fifty-three years elapsed before this entity was clearly incorporated as a form of post-traumatic instability of the wrist, by Linscheid and coauthors.[15] Proximal carpal instability follows major disruption of radiocarpal ligament support, or changes of alignment of the distal articular surface that radius, ulna, and ulnocarpal complex present for articulation with the carpus.[20] Primary intracarpal pathologic changes need not be present. There are two main types within this group (Fig. 10-7); in the first, or *radiocarpal*, symptoms, findings and radiographic features point to a disturbance of the relationship between the radius and ulna proximally and the carpus distally. Included within this category are instabilities resulting in ulnar, dorsal, or palmar translocation of the carpus. The second type, or *midcarpal*, includes patients who develop instability at the midcarpal joint level, a dynamic type of DISI without scapholunate dissociation, secondary to malunion of fractures of the distal radius with residual dorsiflexion of the distal fragment.[21]

ULNAR TRANSLOCATION

Ulnar translocation is rarely found as an isolated posttraumatic deformity. It is more frequent following attenuation of ligament support caused by chronic synovitis [rheumatoid arthritis (Fig. 13-1), psoriatic arthritis (Fig. 13-2)][8] when ulnar migration of the carpus is facilitated by an increased ulnar slope of the radius, and by the loss of ulnar stability secondary to the disease, and, at times, aggravated by the surgical excision of the distal ulna. A third cause of ulnar translocation is found in some developmental disturbances of skeletal growth, particularly hereditary multiple exostosis when there is severe and progressive shortening of the ulna relative to the radius (Fig. 13-3).[22]

DIAGNOSIS

The mechanism of injury is difficult to ascertain, although it must be significant to produce this major loss of alignment. There is massive swelling, at times present weeks following the original insult to the joint, in spite of protective splinting or casting. Loss of motion and weakness of grip are striking. There is pain even at rest, in spite of protective immobilization. When swelling is no longer present, the clinical alignment of the radius and carpus is patently abnormal, with the ulnar margin of the hand clearly medial to the ulnar margin of the forearm. The diagnosis, however, is established by radiographic examination, showing an abnormal translation of the lunate in an ulnar direction. McMurtry and coauthors[16] described a reproducible method for the measurement of what they called "carpal-ulnar distance," defined as that distance present between the center of rotation of the

305

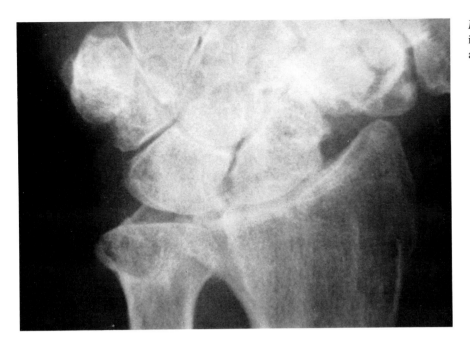

Fig. 13-1. Ulnar translocation in patient with rheumatoid arthritis.

carpus, within the head of the capitate, and a line prolonging distally the longitudinal axis of the ulna (Fig. 5-5). This distance, divided by the length of the third metacarpal, results in a consistent ratio which is 0.30 ± 0.03 in normal wrists. In ulnar translocation, this ratio is smaller, indicating that the capitate and the lunate are translocated in an ulnar direction. The behavior of the scaphoid determines a further subdivision of ulnar translocations into two types. In type I, the entire carpus is displaced, including the scaphoid (Fig. 13-4A). There is a widening of the radial styloid-scaphoid distance, a critical diagnostic feature.[8] In type II, the scaphoid is the only carpal bone that remains in a normal relation with the radius. Therefore, the radial styloid–scaphoid distance is unchanged. The migration of the rest of the carpus, however, results in volar flexion of the scaphoid, and in widening of the scapholunate space (Fig. 13-4C). The distinction between these two types is important, because the appearance of a wide scapholunate gap may lead to the erroneous diagnosis of scapholunate dissociation. In this case, any attempt at stabilization of what appears to be a rotatory subluxation of the scaphoid, by scapholunate ligament reconstruction or by scaphotrapezium-trapezoid fusion (Fig. 13-4D) or even by scapholunate arthrodesis (Fig. 13-4E,F), will fail to correct the underlying problem, which is the ulnar migration of the carpus. Ulnar translocation is frequently accompanied by a severe volar-flexion instability of the proximal carpus (Fig. 13-4G).

TREATMENT

There is no place in this injury for nonsurgical treatment, except for the initial protection of the wrist with splints or plaster. Although reduction may be achieved by manipulation (Fig. 13-4B), it is difficult to maintain and even if successful will result in recurrence of deformity after immobilization is discontinued. Likewise, attempts at surgical repair of the massively torn ligaments, with or without ligament reconstruction, are bound to fail in my experience (Fig. 13-5). Treatment should instead be directed, even early, to relocating and stabilizing the lunate, the carpal keystone, in its normal relationship to the radius, and to securing this reduction by a limited radiolunate arthrodesis (Fig. 13-6).[20,23] If this appears insufficient to provide stability, or in the presence of persistent palmar flexion of the scaphoid, or if radiocarpal osteoarthritis is present, a radioscapholunate fusion

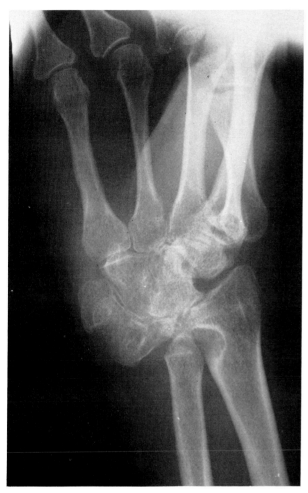

Fig. 13-2. Severe ulnar translocation in patient with psoriatic arthritis. Note "scallop sign" of distal radius opposite ulnar head. This patient had tears of multiple extensor tendons.

should be performed, leaving the uninjured midcarpal joint intact for motion.

Technique of Radiolunate and Radioscapholunate Fusion (Fig. 13-7)

The dorsal radiocarpal joint is approached using a longitudinal obliquely placed incision (Fig. 6-23). The extensor pollicis longus tendon is unroofed and retracted. The joint is exposed through an incision along the floor of the tunnel for this tendon and by subcapsular and subperiosteal dissection. The articular surfaces of the radius and lunate are excised

until healthy cancellous bone is exposed. The scaphoid surface and the corresponding facet of the radius are also excised if the scaphoid is to be included in the fusion mass. As for all types of limited arthrodesis, compression of the surfaces to be fused is carefully avoided. Large Kirschner wires (0.054 – 0.062) or small Steinman pins are then inserted obliquely from distally to proximally along the triquetrum and lunate, until the tips of the wires are visible at the level of the fusion surfaces. If the scaphoid is to be fused, additional wires are inserted for its fixation. Care is taken to avoid driving the wires across the midcarpal joint. The head of the capitate and its articulation with the lunate should be free of any fixation. At this point a sufficient amount of cancellous bone is obtained from the distal radius or from the ipsilateral iliac crest if a larger amount of bone is needed. The bone chips are tightly packed into the fusion site. A cortical graft may be slotted to cover the dorsal radiolunate or radioscapholunate areas for further fixation. The pins are then driven to engage the articular surface of the radius and the opposite cortices of the radius. Closure is performed in layers. Long arm immobilization is used for approximately 6 weeks, and is then replaced with a splint or a short arm plaster to be worn until the fusion appears to be solid. The pins are usually removed at eight to ten weeks postoperatively. If treatment of the distal radioulnar joint is required, this could be performed through the same incision immediately after the radioscapholunate fusion is completed.

DORSAL CARPAL TRANSLOCATION

A pure form of dorsal carpal subluxation may occur following a malunited extraarticular fracture of the distal radius. When the carpus slides along a dorsally directed radial articular slope, it ends in a precarious subluxated dorsal position, the lunate and capitate colinear but in a bayonet alignment in relation to the long axis of the radius (Fig. 13-8). A second type follows intraarticular fractures with dorsal angulation and displacement of the dorsal rim of the radius and the radial styloid; there is actually no radiocarpal subluxation: the carpus and a major dorsal fragment of the radius

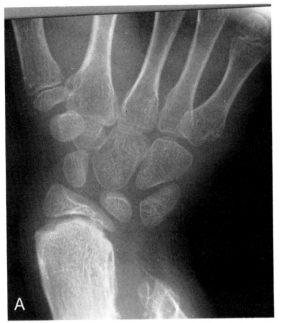
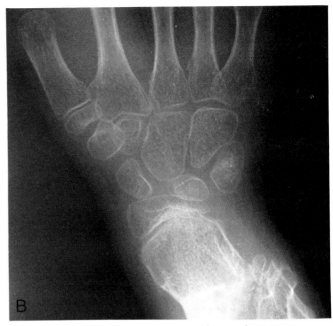

Fig. 13-3. Ulnar translocation in a child with hereditary multiple exostosis. *A:* Preoperative radiograph. *B:* Postoperative appearance following osteotomy of the radius and excision of fibrous ulnar anlage.

remain normally aligned with each other, but dorsally displaced in relation to the shaft of the radius. The clinical appearance and the functional limitations, including weakness and instability, are similar in both forms (Fig. 13-9).

DIAGNOSIS

These patients have had known extraarticular fractures of the distal radius, resulting in a loss or reversal of the normal palmar tilt of the articular surface of the distal radius or intraarticular fractures with dorsal displacement of a major articular fragment. The clinical appearance is typical, the wrist exhibiting a dorsal concavity, a smooth "silver-fork" type of alignment, frequently with swelling or tenderness at the level of the radiocarpal joint (Fig. 13-10). These patients complain of loss of strength and of an ill-defined, deep-seated feeling of instability, particularly if the wrist is subjected to compressive loads. They feel best when the hand is dorsiflexed to accommodate the dorsal angulation of the malunited distal radius. In these

cases, the carpus remains subluxated throughout the entire range of motion. Radiographic studies confirm the presence of a malunion of the radius, and the translocation of the lunocapitate complex dorsal to the long axis of the radius (Fig. 13-8A). The frontal views may show varying degrees of radial shortening, radioulnar discrepancy and, particularly in Barton's fractures, some element of malrotation.

TREATMENT

When dealing with extraarticular malunions, a dorsal open wedge osteotomy of the distal radius is performed, designed to rectify, if possible, all elements of deformity. At least the abnormal dorsal tilt of the distal radius must be corrected. Intraarticular fractures may be treated by an osteotomy along the plane of the fracture and the correction of the abnormal alignment, although in most cases the presence of degenerative, posttraumatic osteoarthritic changes of the radioscapholunate articulation dictates the need for a restoration of the

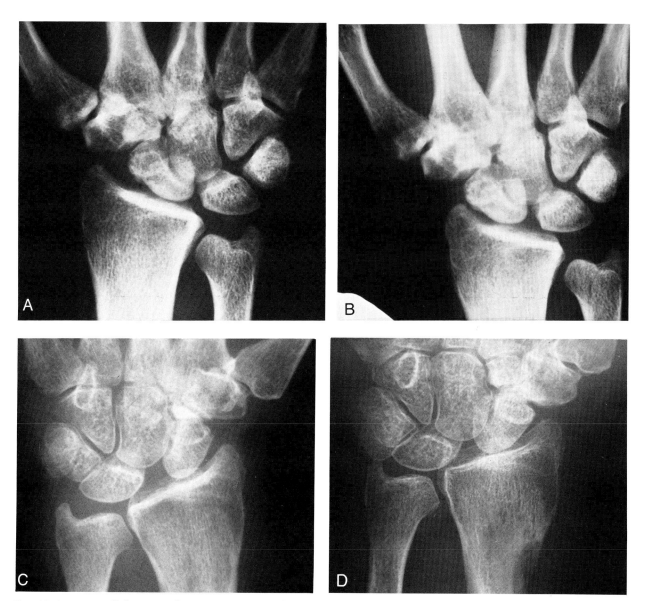

Fig. 13-4. Types of ulnar translocation. *A*: Type I shows ulnar translocation, increased styloid-scaphoid distance. *B*: The same after attempted manual reduction. *C*: Type II ulnar translocation. There is a wide scapholunate gap. The scaphoid is the only carpal bone in satisfactory alignment in relation to the radius. This was erroneously diagnosed as rotatory subluxation of the scaphoid, and (*D*) was unsuccessfully treated by scaphotrapezium-trapezoid fusion.

Fig. continues on next page.

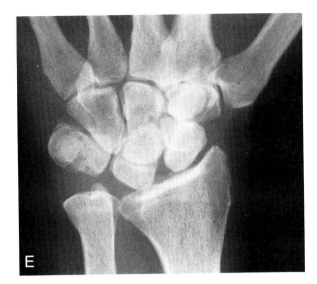

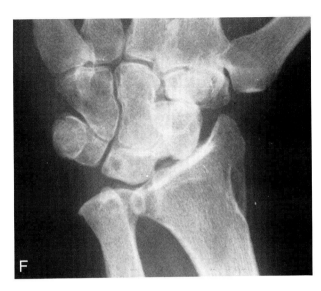

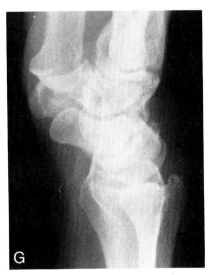

Fig. 13-4. (cont.)   E: Type II ulnar translocation with palmarflexion of the proximal carpal row (VISI). This was diagnosed as scapholunate dissociation. *F:* Unsuccessful treatment by scapholunate arthrodesis (there is persistent translocation and wider styloid-scaphoid space). *G:* Lateral view shows persistent VISI.

radiocarpal relationship, through a radioscapholunate fusion without inclusion of the midcarpal joint (Figs. 13-7, 13-9).

Dorsal Open Wedge Osteotomy of the Distal Radius (Fig. 13-11)

The distal radius is approached using a dorsal longitudinal incision, starting at the end of Lister's tubercle distally and extending proximally. The tendon of the extensor pollicis longus is identified distally and is retracted medially. The outcropping group of muscles (extensor pollicis brevis and abductor pollicis longus) is gently elevated and retracted proximally and radially. The distal radius is exposed subperiosteally, using a longitudinal incision between the extensor carpi radialis brevis and the extensor digitorum communis tendons. The plane of the osteotomy is parallel to the articular surface of the radius in both, anteroposterior and lateral planes.[9] Two Kirschner wires may be driven from dorsal to palmar to assist in manipulating the

Fig. 13-5. Recent posttraumatic type I ulnar translocation. *A:* Initial PA radiograph. *B:* Intraoperative photograph. Forceps is holding entire palmar radiocarpal capsule, avulsed from its origin from the radius. *C:* Multiple
sutures passed through drill holes in the distal radius will
be used to secure fixation of avulsed palmar radiocarpal
structures.   *(Figure continues on next page.)*

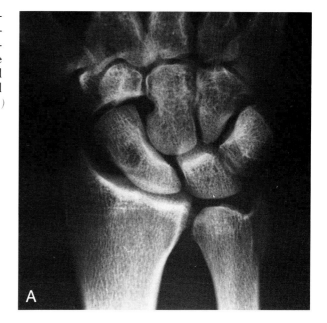

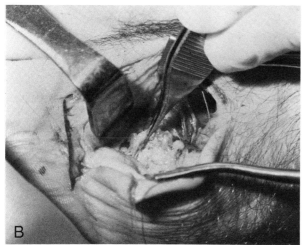

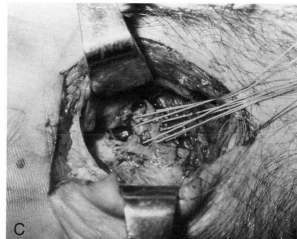

fragments and to assist in the determination of the
degree of tilt to be applied to the distal fragment.[9]
The proximal Kirschner wire is introduced perpendicular to the long axis of the radius, while the distal
wire is introduced parallel to the articular surface
of the radius. I find intraoperative radiographs
helpful at this point. The osteotomy is now performed, and the distal fragment is levered distally
to correct the palmar tilt of the distal radius. If at all
possible, the distal Kirschner wire should end approximately 5 degrees palmarflexed compared to

the proximal Kirschner wire. Ulnar tilt (and radial
length) may also be corrected by opening the radial
side of the osteotomy. A laminar spreader is useful
for this purpose. This maneuver will correct a radioulnar discrepancy that is no greater than 12
mm.[9] The position of the fragments is maintained
temporarily using a large Kirschner wire inserted
obliquely from the radial styloid into the proximal
fragment. This wire is placed as close as possible to
the anterior cortices, and serves to maintain palmar
cortex-to-cortex alignment while at the same time

(Text continues on page 317.)

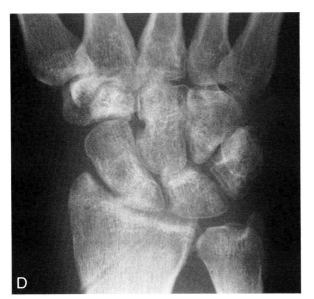

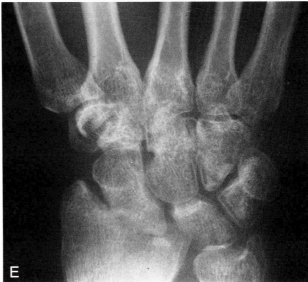

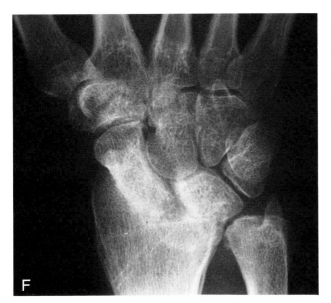

Fig. 13-5. (cont.) D: Radiograph 8 weeks later, immediately after Kirschner wires used for fixation were removed. Alignment is satisfactory. *E*: Radiographs one week later show recurrence of ulnar translocation. There is severe loss of radioscaphoid joint space. There was no evidence of infection during reoperation for a limited radioscapholunate fusion. *F*: Final radiographs. Patient is asymptomatic.

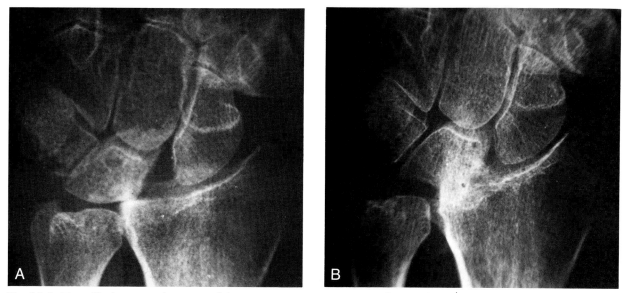

Fig. 13-6. Type II ulnar translocation of the carpus. *A*: Preoperative radiograph. *B*: Postoperative appearance after carpal relocation and radiolunate fusion. (From Taleisnik J: Subtotal arthrodesis of the wrist joint. Clin Orthop 187:81, 1984.)

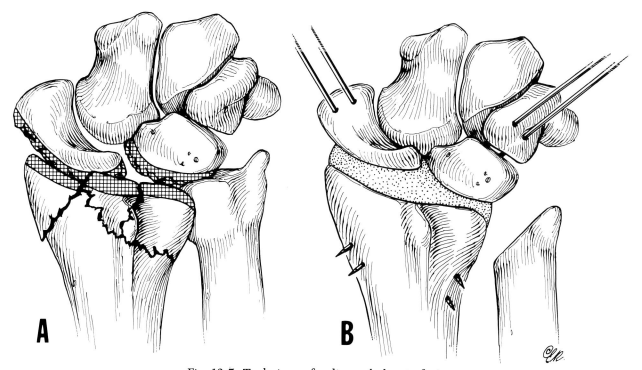

Fig. 13-7. Technique of radioscapholunate fusion.

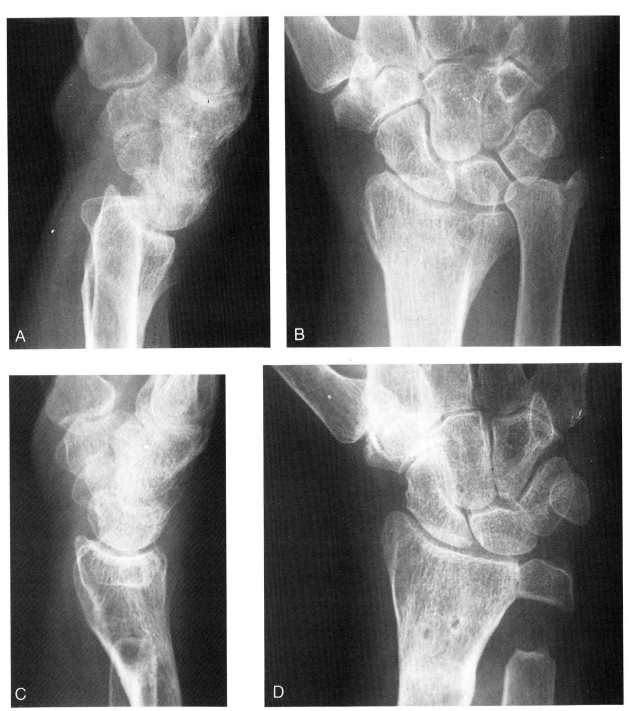

Fig. 13-8. Malunited fracture of distal radius with dorsal carpal translocation. *A:* Lateral view. There is a reversed tilt of the articular surface of the distal radius. The entire carpus is subluxed dorsally. *B:* Anteroposterior view shows loss of radial length and a secondary radioulnar dislocation. This patient was treated by corrective osteotomy of the distal radius, distal radioulnar relocation and fusion and surgical pseudarthrosis of the ulna. *C:* Final lateral radiograph. *D:* Final posteroanterior view.

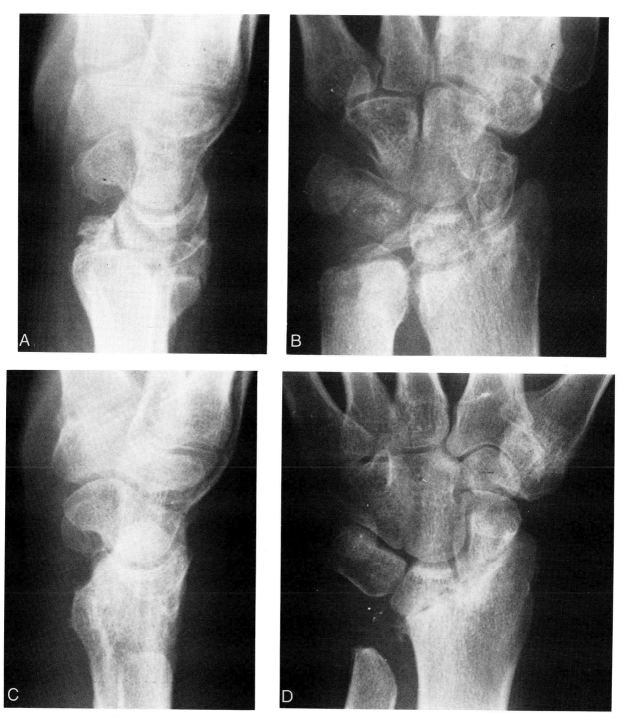

Fig. 13-9. Dorsal radiocarpal translocation secondary to intraarticular fracture of the distal radius. *A* and *B* are radiographs obtained several months following the original injury. *C* and *D* show final appearance following radio-scapholunate fusion.

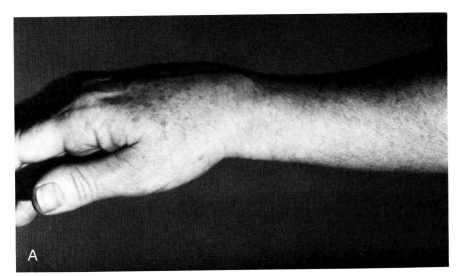

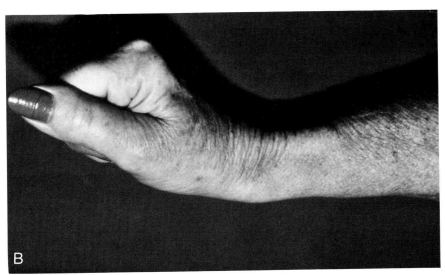

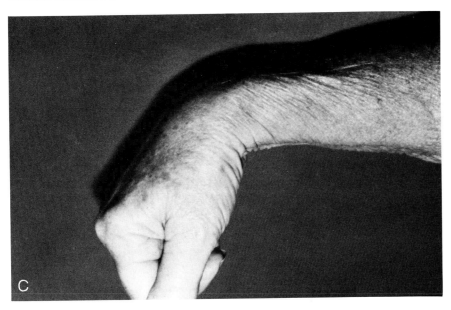

Fig. 13-10. Preoperative (*A*) and postoperative (*B,C*) clinical appearance of wrist with malunion of fracture of distal radius and radiocarpal instability, treated by osteotomy of the radius, radioulnar relocation, and fusion and surgical pseudarthrosis of the ulna.

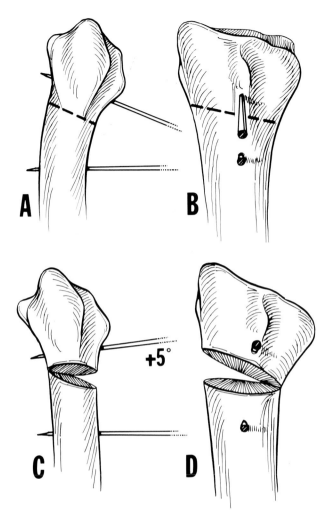

Fig. 13-11. Dorsal open wedge osteotomy of the distal radius. Restoration of palmar tilt (*A* and *C*) and radial inclination (*B* and *D*) should be attempted. Sturdy Kirschner wires are used as handles and as visual aids for the alignment of the distal fragment. The distal Kirschner wire is introduced parallel to the articular surface of the radius.

providing the surgeon with a fixed, stable palmar hinge on which to pry open the osteotomy site. A corticocancellous bone graft is obtained from the iliac crest, and is shaped to fit the defect. Internal fixation is secured with a T plate, contoured to match the surface of the radius. The prominence of Lister's tubercle may be flattened with an osteotome in order to further facilitate fit (Fig. 13-12). At this time, the need to correct any distal radioul-

nar joint incongruity must be assessed. If the radioulnar relationship appears restored, and passive pronation and supination are satisfactory, treatment may be postponed until the time when the plate is removed, giving the patient and the treating physician the opportunity to evaluate the range and freedom of forearm rotation. If the radioulnar congruency is obviously unsatisfactory, in the presence of degenerative changes of the distal radioulnar joint, or when pronation and supination remain clearly limited after the osteotomy is completed, then this problem must be solved, either by excision of the distal ulna[4-6,13] or by a distal radioulnar fusion with an ulnar osteotomy proximal to the fusion site (Fig. 13-8D).[10,18,19] Postoperatively, I prefer above-elbow immobilization for six weeks. At the end of this period removable splints are used, as the patient regains motion and strength. All immobilization is usually discontinued at eight to ten weeks following surgery. The plate and screws may be removed any time after the osteotomy site is healed and the bone graft appears to be fully incorporated, usually no sooner than six months postoperatively. The plate and screws may be removed earlier if the patient develops problems related to their presence, particularly a troublesome tendonitis of the extensor pollicis longus.[9]

Radioscapholunate Fusion

The technique of radioscapholunate fusion is discussed under Ulnar Translocation earlier in this chapter.

PALMAR CARPAL TRANSLOCATION

In their classification of carpal instability, Dobyns and coauthors[8] include dorsal carpal subluxation as an actual type of instability, but mention a similar palmar subluxation as only a theoretical possibility. Here, as in dorsal carpal translocation, there are two main types of palmar carpal subluxation, the most common accompanying intraarticular fractures of the distal articular surface of the radius, of the Barton's type, resulting in palmar displacement of the major articular fragment with the carpus still attached to it (Fig. 13-13).[20] A pure

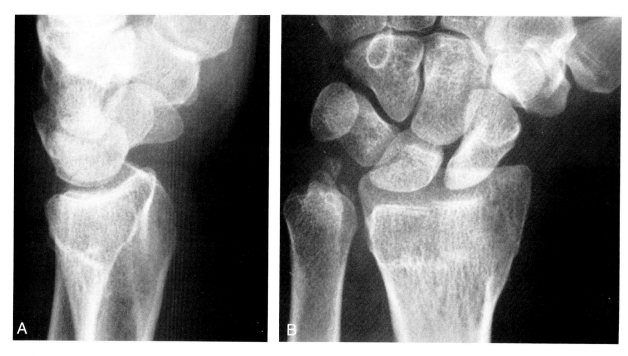

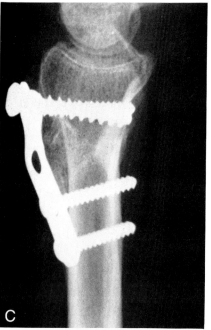

Fig. 13-12. Malunited fracture of distal radius with radiocarpal instability. *A* and *B*: Preoperative radiographs. *C*: after dorsal open wedge osteotomy and internal fixation with plate and screws.

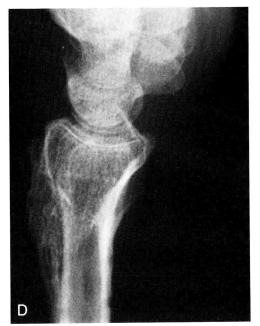
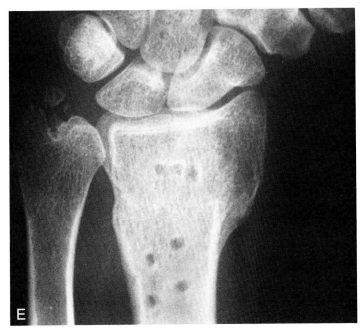

Fig. 13-12. (cont.) D and E: Final radiographs.

type of volar subluxation, taking place at the radiocarpal joint itself, is extremely rare (Fig. 13-14). Unlike the typical Colles fracture, the reversed Colles or Smith's fractures, although producing a palmar angulation of the distal radius, do not result in palmar carpal subluxation. A third example of palmar radiocarpal instability is found in inflammatory arthritides (Fig. 13-15). Horwitz[11] described a case of recurrent voluntary palmar subluxation of the entire carpus on an abnormal radius in a patient with a preexisting Madelung's deformity. Recently Bellinghausen and coauthors[2] reported two patients with pure, posttraumatic palmar carpal subluxations, the first two well-documented cases in the literature.

DIAGNOSIS

These patients' complaints are similar to those following the more frequent dorsal carpal translocations: there is limitation of motion, weakness, and a sense of instability on attempting to load the wrist. Pain may not be as severe as in dorsal subluxations. The alignment of the hand may be abnormal and the range of motion decreased, particularly for extension. Grip strength is usually diminished. The diagnosis is established by roentgenographic examination. Lateral radiographs show the lunate palmar to the center of the articular surface of the radius. In the case of a Barton's-type fracture, the lunate remains colinear with the capitate, and with the displaced volar radial fragment, all palmar to the long axis of the radius. In palmar radiocarpal subluxations the lunate subluxates volarward and also rotates into dorsiflexion. Ulnar translocation may accompany this type of deformity.[2] The mechanism of injury postulated for these posttraumatic palmar subluxations involves hyperextension with resulting tear of volar radiocarpal ligaments and a shear force directed ulnarward, which produces dorsal radiocarpal ligament avulsion or tear and results in an added ulnar translocation.[2]

TREATMENT

There is very limited experience in the treatment of this type of carpal instability. When a fracture of the distal radius is present, an osteotomy through

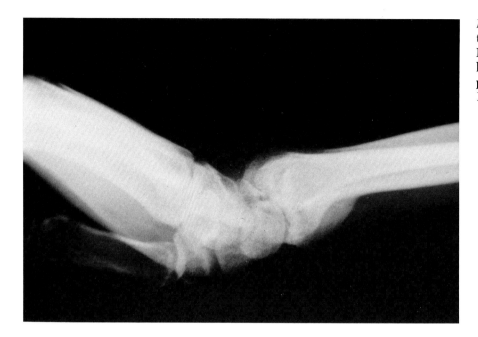

Fig. 13-13. Palmar carpal translocation in patient with a Barton's fracture. (From Taleisnik J: Post-traumatic carpal instability. Clin Orthop 149:73, 1980.)

the plane of fracture, relocation of the displaced fragment and internal fixation are indicated for as long as the radiocarpal articular surface between the displaced fragment proximally and the scaphoid and lunate distally remains satisfactory. When this procedure is not technically feasible, and in the presence of arthritic changes between radius and proximal carpal row, a fusion limited to the radius, scaphoid and lunate is indicated (Fig. 13-15). The surgical technique is similar to that employed for other types of limited carpal or radiocarpal fusions. For the pure palmar radiocarpal subluxation, with or without ulnar translocation, I believe that carpal relocation and stabilization by fusion is again the

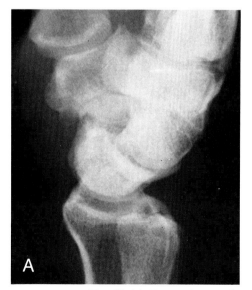
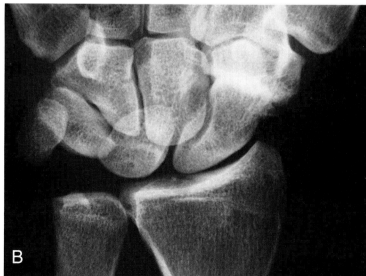

Fig. 13-14. Rare palmar radiocarpal subluxation. A and B: Preoperative radiographs.

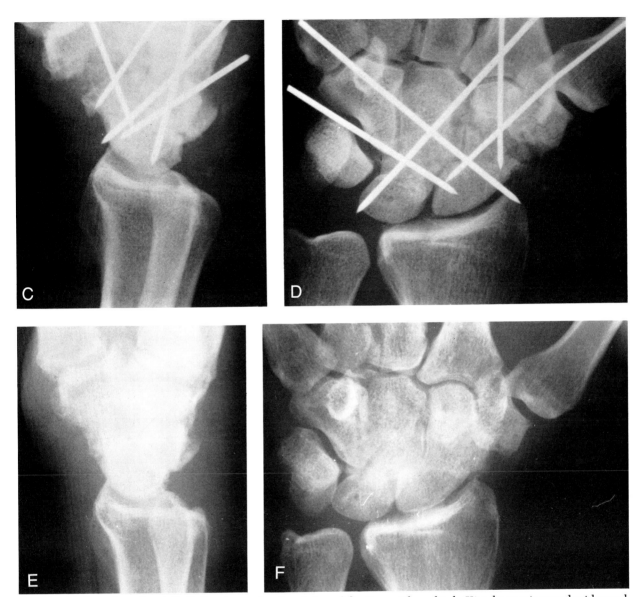

Fig. 13–14. (cont.) C and D: Following reduction, internal fixation with multiple Kirschner wires and midcarpal fusion. E and F: Final appearance.

procedure of choice. If this stability can be satisfactorily achieved intraoperatively by an arthrodesis limited to the radiolunate joint, then only this is needed. Otherwise, the fusion should be extended to encompass radius, scaphoid, and lunate in the reduced, neutral alignment, or an arthrodesis across the midcarpal joint may be done, after satisfactory lunocapitate alignment is restored (Fig. 13-14C,D).

MIDCARPAL INSTABILITY SECONDARY TO MALUNITED FRACTURES OF THE DISTAL RADIUS

Intracarpal instability associated with fractures of the distal radius is rare.[3,7,15,17] Scapholunate dissociations are probably the most frequent.[3,17] In 1972 Linscheid and coauthors[15] described loss of carpal alignment of proximal and distal carpal rows,

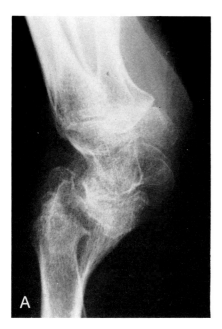

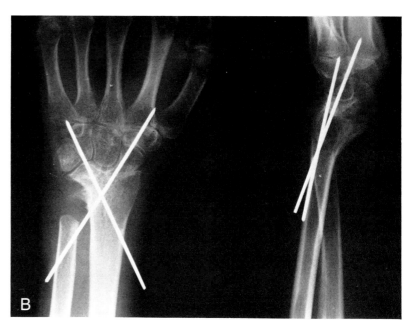

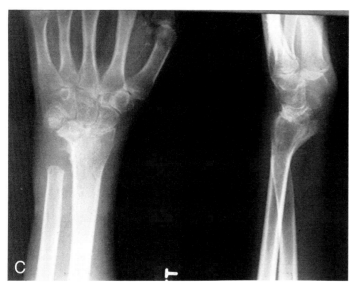

Fig. 13-15. Neglected palmar radiocarpal fracture-subluxation. *A*: Preoperative lateral view. *B*: Postoperative appearance following reduction, internal fixation with multiple Kirschner wires and radioscapholunate arthrodesis. *C*: Final radiographs.

specifically a dorsiflexion instability pattern, following fractures of the distal radius with residual loss of the normal articular palmar tilt. This loss of radiocarpal alignment was interpreted as a compensatory realignment through balancing of the articular components, rather than as a true form of instability, a concept shared by Allieu and coauthors.[1] There is, however, a dynamic form of carpal instability that may develop as a complication of malunion of fractures of the distal radius without involvement of the radiocarpal joint.[21] The instability is localized to the midcarpal area and results in painful synovitis, accompanied at times by a dynamic collapse deformity, similar to the dynamic DISI seen following triquetrohamate ligament tear, attenuation, or avulsion.[14]

Fig. 13-16. Midcarpal instability secondary to malunited fracture of the distal radius. *A:* Presubluxation appearance. *B:* In ulnar deviation there is a loud, painful snap. The head of the capitate (arrow) becomes prominent dorsally.

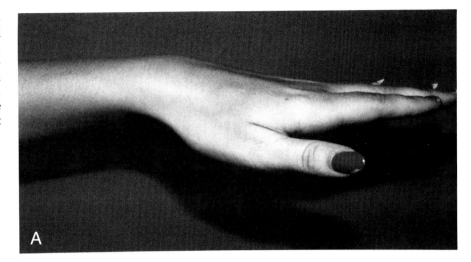

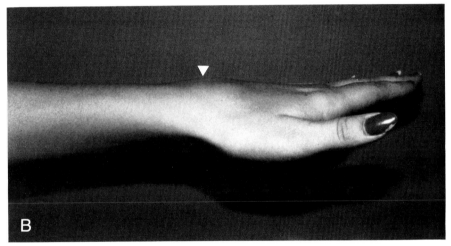

DIAGNOSIS

These patients are usually young and active and may show evidence of carpal laxity when the uninjured wrist is stressed. They seek medical advice several weeks or months after having sustained an extraarticular fracture of the distal radius, which went on to heal with a loss of the normal palmar tilt of the distal radius. Their presenting complaints are pain, localized to the ulnar half of the midcarpal joint, increased by lifting, pushing, and accompanied by swelling, which is most visible at the midcarpal level. There is weakness of grip, and a feeling of instability. Some patients gradually develop a painful, loud "snap," which can be seen and palpated with ease at the level of the triquetrohamate and lunocapitate joints, and is reproduced by bringing their hands into ulnar deviation with the forearm pronated (Fig. 13-16). This subluxation is very similar to that described by Lichtman et al.[14] in their patients with midcarpal instability (see Chapter 12). The range of motion of the wrist is modified in proportion to the severity of the dorsal angulation of the radius. In general, loss of palmarflexion is greater than that of dorsiflexion. Pronation and supination may be limited due to the involvement or incongruity of the distal radioulnar joint. Grip strength is severely weakened. Routine

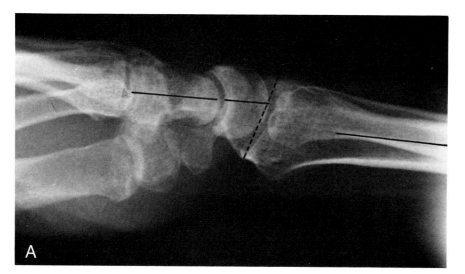

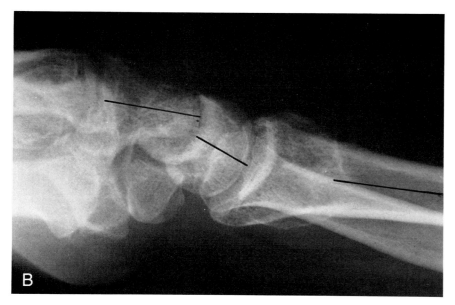

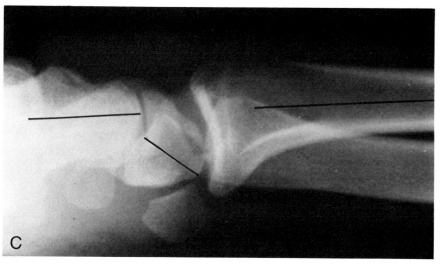

Fig. 13-17. Midcarpal instability secondary to malunited fracture of the distal radius. *A:* Abnormal dorsal tilt of distal radius. In neutral deviation, lunate and capitate are colinear but dorsal to axis of radius. *B:* In ulnar deviation, the lunate dorsiflexes but fails to shift palmarward against the reversed slope of the distal articular surface of the radius. The capitate subluxes with a sudden painful snap. *C:* Lateral view of normal wrist in ulnar deviation. Capitate-radius colinearity is preserved.

Fig. 13-17. (cont.) D: Lateral view of injured wrist in ulnar deviation, after successful dorsal open wedge osteotomy. Normal lunate rotation and palmar shift are restored.

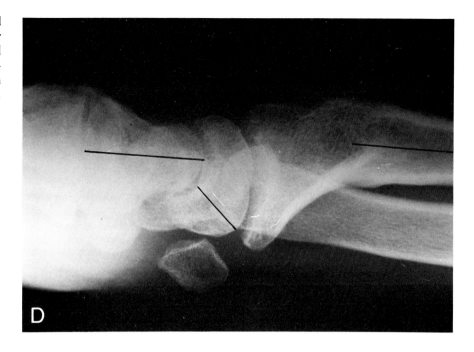

lateral and posteroanterior radiographs show a malunion of a fracture of the distal radius, usually extraarticular. The major architectural change of the radius is the reversal of the palmar tilt of its distal articular surface (Fig. 5-1D). Routine lateral radiographs show colinear lunate and capitate axes, both along a plane that is parallel, but dorsal, to the long axis of the shaft of the radius (Fig. 13-17A). Lateral radiographs obtained with the wrist in ulnar deviation, after the patient actively subluxates his carpus, show that the lunate dorsiflexes as in normal ulnar deviation (Fig. 13-17B), but unlike the normal wrist (Fig. 13-17C) it fails to shift simultaneously in a palmar sense. Consequent to this dorsiflexion of the lunate with reduced or absent palmar shift, and to the residual dorsal angulation of the distal radius, during ulnar deviation the capitate is pushed in a dorsal direction, and aligns in a position of dorsal subluxation in relation to the radius. It is in this position that these patients experience subluxation at the midcarpal joint level.

TREATMENT

The loss or reversal of the normal palmar tilt of the distal radius is responsible for two major changes: the transfer of loads to the dorsal ligaments, poorly prepared to handle this added stress, and prepositioning of the carpus in a dorsal-type collapse alignment. Commonly, after malunited fractures of the distal radius, compensatory angulation to realign the hand to the forearm takes place at the radiocarpal joint (Figs. 10-7, 13-8, 13-12). In these patients, however, the compensatory angulation occurs at the lunocapitate level. Restoration of radius alignment by a dorsal, open wedge osteotomy is the treatment of choice (Fig. 13-17D). Realignment of the palmar tilt of the distal radius restores normal carpal mechanics and allows the lunate to shift palmarward as it dorsiflexes during ulnar deviation, thereby restoring normal colinear alignment of capitate and radius as well. The operative technique and the postoperative care following osteotomies of the distal radius have already been discussed.

REFERENCES

1. Allieu Y, Brahin B, Asencio G: Les instabilités du carpe bilan et sémiologie radiologique. Ann Radiol 25:275, 1982
2. Bellinghausen H-W, Gilula L, Young LV, Weeks

PM: Post-traumatic palmar carpal subluxation. Report of two cases. J Bone Joint Surg [Am] 65:998, 1983

3. Cooney WP, Dobyns JH, Linscheid RL: Complications of Colles' fractures. J Bone Joint Surg [Am] 62:613, 1930

4. Darrach W: Anterior dislocation of the head of the ulna. Ann Surg 56:802, 1912

5. Darrach W: Partial excision of lower shaft of ulna for deformity following Colles's fracture. Ann Surg 57:764, 1913

6. Darrach W, Dwight K: Derangements of the inferior radio-ulnar articulation. Med Rec 87:708, 1915

7. Dobyns JH, Linscheid RL: Fractures and dislocations of the wrist. p 345. In Rockwood CA Jr, Green DP (eds): Fractures. Lippincott, Philadelphia, 1975

8. Dobyns JH, Linscheid RL, Chao EYS, et al: Traumatic instability of the wrist. Am Acad Orthop Surgeons Instruct Course Lect 24:182, 1975

9. Fernandez DL: Correction of post-traumatic wrist deformity in adults by osteotomy, bone-grafting and internal fixation. J Bone Joint Surg [Am] 64:1164, 1982

10. Gonçalves D: Correction of disorders of the distal radioulnar joint by artificial pseudoarthrosis of the ulna. J Bone Joint Surg [Br] 56:462, 1974

11. Horwitz T: An anatomic and roentgenologic study of the wrist joint. Observations on a case of recurrent radiocarpal dislocation complicating Madelung's deformity and its surgical correction. Surgery 1:773, 1939

12. Jeanne LA, Mouchet A: Les lésions traumatiques fermées du poignet. 28th Congrès Français de Chirurgie, 1919

13. Lauenstein C von: Zur Behandlung der nach Karpalen Vorderarmfraktur zurückbleibenden Störung der Pro- und Supinations Bewegung. Zentralbl Chir 23:433, 1887

14. Lichtman DM, Schneider JR, Swafford AR, Mack GR: Ulnar midcarpal instability. Clinical and laboratory analysis. J Hand Surg 6:515, 1981

15. Linscheid RL, Dobyns JH, Beabout JW, Bryan RS: Traumatic instability of the wrist: Diagnosis, classification and pathomechanics. J Bone Joint Surg [Am] 54:1612, 1972

16. McMurtry RY, Youm Y, Flatt AE, Gillespie TE: Kinematics of the wrist. II. Clinical applications. J Bone Joint Surg [Am] 60:955, 1978

17. Rosenthal DI, Schwartz M, Phillips WC, Jupiter J: Fracture of the radius with instability of the wrist. Am J Roentgenol 141:113, 1983

18. Steindler A, Marxer JL: The Traumatic Deformities and Disabilities of the Upper Extremity. Charles C Thomas, Springfield, IL, 1946

19. Steindler A: Orthopedic Operations. Indications, Technique and End Results. 4th Ed. Charles C Thomas, Springfield IL, 1947

20. Taleisnik J: Post-traumatic carpal instability. Clin Orthop 149:73, 1980

21. Taleisnik J, Watson HK: Midcarpal instability secondary to malunited fractures of the distal radius. J Hand Surg 9A:350, 1984

22. Taleisnik J: Classification of carpal instability. Bull Hosp Joint Dis 44:511, 1984

23. Watson HK, Goodman ML, Johnson TR: Limited arthrodesis. Part II: Intracarpal and radiocarpal combinations. J Hand Surg 6:223, 1981

14 Rheumatoid Arthritis of the Wrist

INTRODUCTION

The first reference to an arthritic process with the characteristics of rheumatoid arthritis is found in a thesis presented in 1800 by a French medical student, Augustin Jacob Laudre Beauvais, entitled "Should we recognize a new type of gout to be called primary asthenic gout?"[10] In 1859, the first edition of *The Nature and Treatment of Gout and Rheumatic Gout* was published by Sir Alfred Baring Garrod.[6] At the time, gout had become a well-defined disease, separate from a host of poorly understood, non gouty arthritides, that were grouped under the term "rheumatic gout." This nomenclature was confusing, and led Garrod to introduce for the first time the term rheumatoid arthritis, ". . . an inflammatory affection of the joints, not unlike rheumatism, in some of its characteristics, but differing materially from it." Thus, the initial definition of rheumatoid arthritis encompassed a large group of articular problems, whose only common characteristic was to be different from gout and from the better known rheumatic fever. Other investigators, including Garrod's youngest son, helped to separate osteoarthritis from within this group.[9] It was not, however, until the turn of the century that rheumatoid arthritis, degenerative joint disease, and the then prevalent tuberculous arthritis became distinct entities. This brief review suggests that rheumatoid arthritis is a relatively "young" disease, although according to some investigators it may have been in existence for at least 400 years. Indeed, Domen points out that there is enough paleopathologic evidence to suggest that rheumatoid arthritis was more prevalent in antiquity than is suspected.[5] Signs of joint involvement strongly reminiscent of rheumatoid arthritis have been found in an Egyptian mummy from the fifth dynasty (2750 to 2625 B.C.)[8] and in the skeleton of an American Indian from the Mississippi (700 to 1650 A.D.).[5] Five paintings by artists from the Flemish school (1400 to 1700) depicted deformities that resembled those found in rheumatoid arthritis.[4] A scholarly analysis of the hands in paintings attributed to Peter Paul Rubens[2] suggests that the artist had introduced his own "rheumatoid disease" in his work depicting progressive stages of deformity in paintings in successive years. Documents from Rubens contemporaries, however, tend to categorize his malady as gout, although it was not until much later that gout established its own distinct identity. There is no convincing evidence, however, nor descriptions of rheumatoid arthritis before the eighteenth or nineteenth centuries, unlike osteoarthritis, which was found in remains of dinosaurs and early man, or gout and ankylosing spondylitis, that were found in mummified remains several thousands of years old.[2,10] Furthermore, although several forms of arthritis are mentioned in the bible, nothing resembling rheumatoid arthritis was described.[10]

To explain the historical development of rheumatoid arthritis, unknown environmental factors that first made their appearance around the seventeenth century, or some infectious agent, have been implicated.[10] Until the 1930s, rheumatoid arthritis was believed to be produced by a focus of infection somewhere in the body, and was often called "chronic infectious arthritis." The orthopaedic care for this condition was largely nonoperative, and consisted of the use of rest in casts to prevent, and of serial casts to correct, joint deformities.[3] Since then, an unusual immune reaction, taking place predominantly within the synovial membranes of joints and tendon sheaths, has been implicated to explain the frequently devastating inflammatory response that is found in some of these patients. An infectious agent is still thought to be ultimately responsible for the onset of the disease.[1] Recently, an immune reactivity to collagen II (present in the hyaline cartilage of joints) has been shown to produce a rheumatoidlike synovitis in rats.[7,10–12] This reaction is largely controlled by immune response genes, that are responsible for the presence or absence of an immune response to a specific antigen. The understanding of these complex mechanisms has gradually translated into improvements in the overall medical treatment of the disease. Surgery, throughout the years, has been but one part of this total management of the rheumatoid patient, and has retained a fundamental role in the prevention and correction of disabilities. There are shortcomings to surgery that must be recognized, both by the surgeon and by the patient. Much of the emphasis of operative treatment is directed to relieving pain; although full restoration of normal function by surgical means alone is rarely achieved, a rewarding improvement in the patient's ability to cope with activities is frequently obtained.

REFERENCES

1. Alspaugh MA, Tan EM: Serum antibody in rheumatoid arthritis reactive with a cell-associated antigen. Demonstrated by precipitation and immunofluorescence. Arthritis Rheum 19:711, 1976
2. Appelboom T, Boelpaepe C de, Ehrlich GE, Famaey J-P: Rubens and the question of antiquity of rheumatoid arthritis. JAMA 245:483, 1981
3. Bayles TB: The history of the treatment of rheumatoid arthritis (1939–1975). Orthop Clin North Am 6:603, 1975
4. DeQueker J: Arthritis in Flemish paintings (1400–1700). Br Med J 1:1203, 1977
5. Domen RE: Paleopathological evidence of rheumatoid arthritis (letter). JAMA 246:1899, 1981
6. Garrod AB: The nature and treatment of gout and rheumatic gout. 1st Ed. Walton & Maberly, London, 1859
7. Griffiths MM, Eichwald, EJ, Martin JH, et al: Immunogenetic control of experimental type II collagen-induced arthritis. I. Susceptibility and resistance among inbred strains of rats. Arthritis Rheum 24:781, 1981
8. Karsch RS, McCarthy JD: Archeology and arthritis. Arch Intern Med 105:640, 1960
9. Rodnan GP, McEwen C, Wallace SL: Primer on the rheumatic diseases. JAMA 224, No. 5 (Suppl), 1973
10. Stobo JD: Rheumatoid arthritis—From Rubens to restriction maps. Medical Staff Conference, University of California, San Francisco. West J Med 137:109, 1982
11. Stuart JM, Cremer MA, Townes AS, et al: Type II collagen-induced arthritis in rats: Passive transfer with serum and evidence that IgG anticollagen antibodies can cause arthritis. J Exp Med 155:1, 1982
12. Trentham DE, Townes AS, Kang AH, et al: Humeral and cellular sensitivity to collagen in type II collagen-induced arthritis in rats. J Clin Invest 61:89, 1978

15 Surgery for the Rheumatoid Wrist: Indications and Timing

It is often difficult for the surgeon to decide whether or not a given surgical procedure will benefit the patient with rheumatoid arthritis, particularly during the early stages of the disease. Even later on, as the disease progresses, the mere existence of deformity is not necessarily an indication for surgery.[19] The wrist is the initial site of synovitis in only 2.7 percent of patients with rheumatoid arthritis, almost six times less frequently than the hand.[17] However, with persistence and progression of the disease, the wrist is eventually involved in close to 95 percent of cases.[10] The decision to operate should be shared by the patient, a rheumatologist, and the surgeon. The majority of patients do respond to a full and conscientious nonsurgical program that includes rest, antiinflammatory, immunosuppressive, and other medications, physical therapy, the use of splints and braces, and the judicious utilization of steroids, including local injections. Early in the disease, when symptoms are secondary to tissue distention and to increased intraarticular pressures produced by synovitis, these nonsurgical measures may restore comfortable function and delay the onset or progression of deformities and joint destruction. Surgical treatment is indicated when pain and disability have progressed or persist, and when instability and joint disorganization have already developed. It is not necessary, or indicated, to delay operative intervention until the rheumatoid process is quiescent.[1,2,6,11-13]

The surgeon and the patient must be prepared for the recurrence of synovitis following surgical synovectomy, either within the same compartments that were treated or from neighboring compartments. Recurrence is more likely in the very active, uncontrolled seropositive rheumatoid patient.[1]

Once a surgical course is elected, the next step is the selection, from the many procedures that have been described in the literature, of the one which is likely to benefit that particular patient. As stated by Millender et al,[15] "a cookbook approach" cannot be used. There are several factors that should be considered. These include the patient's age, sex, handedness, occupation, functional needs, and expectations. Signs and symptoms suggestive of digital arteritis, particularly in patients receiving large dosages of steroids with evidence of rheumatoid nodule formation, should alert the physician to the potential for vascular compromise postoperatively.[1,5,22] Additional tests may be required for these patients (Doppler, arteriography) before extensive surgery is recommended (Fig. 15-1).

The patient with juvenile arthritis is also deserving of individualized care. The course of the arthritis is milder in children, and the eventual disability less severe. Between 50 and 70 percent of children with juvenile rheumatoid arthritis (JRA) will go into remission.[9] Once past puberty, the characteristics of the active juvenile rheumatoid arthritis change to resemble adult-onset rheumatoid disease.[8] Early involvement of the wrist in juvenile rheumatoid arthritis is seen in 30 percent of pa-

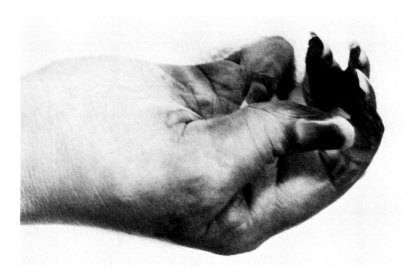

Fig. 15-1. Necrotizing vasculitis resulting in gangrene in patient with rheumatoid arthritis. (From Cummings JK, Taleisnik J: Peripheral gangrene as a complication of rheumatoid arthritis. Report of a case and review of the literature. J Bone Joint Surg [Am] 53:1001, 1971.)

tients and eventual involvement in at least 60 percent. In anywhere from 15 to 47 percent of these patients, when the disease process is severe it will culminate in stiffness and ankylosis.[7,8,14] This fact, and the frequent occurrence of subluxations, are arguments in favor of early, efficient, and prolonged splinting, alternating with a judicious exercise program dictated by the degree of activity of the disease and the severity of pain. The goal is a wrist that will eventually be stable, somewhat mobile, pain-free, and in satisfactory alignment. The wrists of children with juvenile rheumatoid arthritis show a frequent tendency toward ulnar deviation.[3] Chaplin et al.[3] found that 34 percent of over 400 patients with juvenile rheumatoid arthritis developed ulnar metacarpal shift (Fig. 15-2), as opposed to the more frequent radial metacarpal shift seen in adults. These authors believed that ulnar deviation of the wrist was allowed by ulnar shortening, attributed by them to damage of the distal ulnar epiphysis caused by the rheumatoid process. In Granberry and Mangum's[8] study of 100 patients, a clinically significant ulnar deviation was found in only 10 percent of wrists. Conversely, 79 of 93 wrists with radiographic documentation demonstrated an average of 13 degrees of ulnar deviation (4–25 degrees). This suggests that in many cases radiographic evidence of ulnar deviation may be due to positioning rather than to an actual deformity. Altogether, there was clinical or radiographic involvement of the wrist in 24.5 percent of their patients. In Granberry and Mangum's experience, loss of extension (dorsiflexion) of the wrist was a more meaningful finding, while in general, palmar flexion was comparatively well preserved. Loss of complete dorsiflexion was not only frequent but was also found to be an early sign of juvenile rheu-

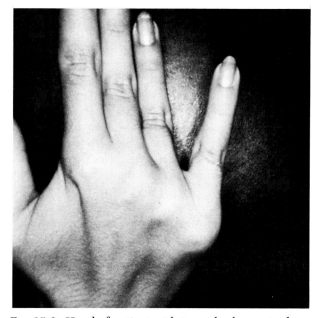

Fig. 15-2. Hand of patient with juvenile rheumatoid arthritis shows ulnar metacarpal shift and radial drift of the fingers.

Fig. 15-3. Stiff subtype of rheumatoid arthritis, resulting in ankylosis of the wrist.

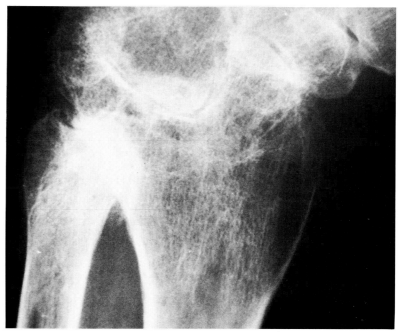

matoid arthritis, detectable prior to the presence of clinically apparent synovitis or of any other findings suggestive of juvenile rheumatoid arthritis. Granberry and Mangum[8] point out that loss of extension "serves as a barometer of the disease and usually precedes roentgenographic changes by several months." In their experience, ulnar metacarpal angulation was not necessarily associated with radial deviation of the fingers.

Established contractures and deformities of the wrist in juvenile rheumatoid arthritis must be individually evaluated. Serial casting or wedging casts, followed by progressive, static splinting, and alternating with dynamic splints are all helpful. Surgery in the patient with juvenile rheumatoid arthritis is a relatively small part of the overall management program. In general, major surgical procedures are rarely indicated or justified. Tenosynovitis is rarely if ever severe enough in children to justify tenosynovectomy.[8] In the few patients reported to have undergone joint synovectomy, postoperative loss of motion was significant. In the late phase of the disease, surgical treatment is reserved for those patients in whom pain and functional loss interfere with daily activities. The procedures that may be

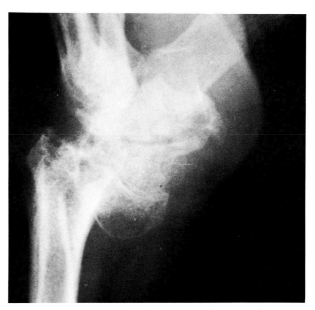

Fig. 15-4. Radiocarpal dislocation of wrist of patient with rheumatoid arthritis.

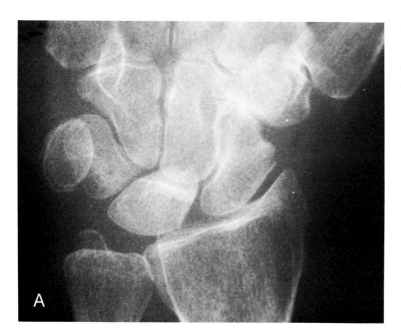

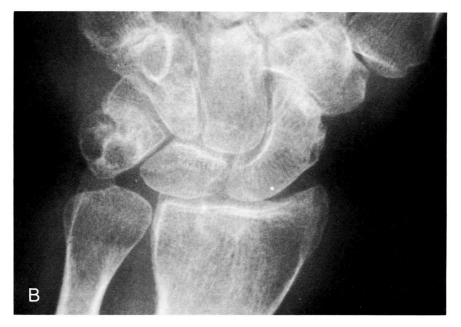

Fig. 15-5. Stages of radiographic changes in rheumatoid arthritis. *A*: Stage I: minimal changes. *B*: Stage II: erosive changes with satisfactory preservation of joint architecture.

used during this stage are similar to those suggested for rheumatoid arthritis of adult onset.

Rheumatoid disease follows one of three basic patterns[18]: *polycyclic*, when periods of activity alternate with periods of complete or partial remission; *monocyclic*, in the rare patient in whom a single episode of rheumatoid arthritis is followed by a seemingly permanent arrest of the disease, and *progressive*, when the ever-present inflammatory process becomes gradually worse, although with peaks and valleys due to periodic flare-ups and partial transient remissions. Within each pattern, there are two clinical subtypes[4]: *stiff*, which involves mainly the articular synovium; there is acute

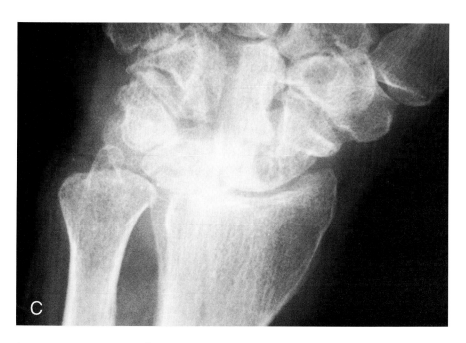

Fig. 15.5. (cont.) C: Stage III: increased bone destruction, dislocations and subluxations. *D:* Stage IV shows bony and fibrous ankylosis in addition to findings in stage III.

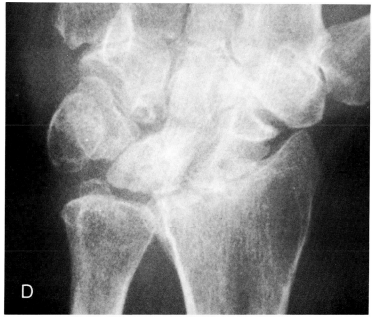

inflammation, progressive stiffness, and frequent ankylosis (Fig. 15-3); and *loose,* in which joint surfaces are eroded, destroyed, and rendered unstable (Fig. 15-4). It may be more important to assign the patient to one of four stages, based on clinical and radiologic findings.[16] In *stage I (early)* there is persistent synovitis; there are no radiographic changes and osteoporosis may be present. In *stage II (moderate),* there may be limitation of motion, adjacent muscle atrophy and continuous evidence of synovitis, although without clinical or radiographic deformity; there is, however, radiologic evidence of erosive changes and cartilage destruction, with satisfactory preservation of joint architecture. During *stage III (severe)* there are progressive deformities, and extensive muscle atrophy. Radiographic bone destruction, dislocations and subluxations are present. The stage IV (terminal) includes bony and fibrous ankylosis in addition to the findings present in stage III (Fig. 15-5).

Initial involvement of the wrist is, as we have seen, not as frequent as involvement of the hand and finger joints. The wrist is, however, a key joint in formulating a plan of treatment for hand and finger deformity and loss of function. Although there is a genuine question as to the importance of the wrist in initiating the typical subluxations and dislocations of the rheumatoid digits, it is clear that, when present, wrist collapse will facilitate the progression of finger deformity. More importantly, it will interfere with the successful correction of ulnar drift of the digits, unless the wrist itself is treated first.[20,21] In summary, surgery for the rheumatoid wrist is indicated for those patients who present pain, or disability, or progression of the disease in spite of adequate medical management. Special considerations should be given to the juvenile rheumatoid, and to each patient according to individual needs, and considering the progression pattern, the stage of the disease, and the rheumatoid subtype.

REFERENCES

1. Backhouse KM, Harrison SH, Hutchings RT: Color Atlas of Rheumatoid Hand Surgery. Yearbook Medical Publishers, Chicago, 1981
2. Campbell RD Jr, Straub LR: Surgical considerations for rheumatoid disease in the forearm and wrist. Am J Surg 109:361, 1965
3. Chaplin D, Pulkki T, Saarima A, Vainio K: Wrist and finger deformities in juvenile rheumatoid arthritis. Acta Rheumatol Scand 15:206, 1969
4. Clayton ML: Surgical treatment at the wrist in rheumatoid arthritis. A review of thirty-seven patients. J Bone Joint Surg [Am] 47:741, 1965
5. Cummings JK, Taleisnik J: Peripheral gangrene as a complication of rheumatoid arthritis. Report of a case and review of the literature. J Bone Joint Surg [Am] 53:1001, 1971
6. Flatt AE: Care of the arthritic hand. 4th. Ed. Mosby, St. Louis, 1983
7. Findley TW, Halpern D, Easton JKM: Wrist subluxation in juvenile rheumatoid arthritis: Pathophysiology and management. Arch Phys Med Rehabil 64:69, 1983
8. Granberry WM, Mangum GL: The hand in the child with juvenile rheumatoid arthritis. J Hand Surg 5:105, 1980
9. Hanson V, Konreich H, Bernstein B, et al: Prognosis of juvenile rheumatoid arthritis. Proceedings of the first ARA conference on the rheumatic disease of childhood. Arthritis Rheum (Suppl 2) 20:279, 1976
10. Hooper J: The surgery of the wrist in rheumatoid arthritis. Aust NZ J Surg 42:135, 1972
11. Lipscomb PR: Surgery of the arthritic hand: Sterling Bunnell Memorial Lecture. Mayo Clin Proc 40:132, 1965
12. Lipscomb PR: Synovectomy of the wrist for rheumatoid arthritis. JAMA 194:655, 1965
13. Lipscomb PR: Surgery for rheumatoid arthritis—timing and techniques: Summary. J Bone Joint Surg [Am] 50:614, 1968
14. Maldonado-Cocco JA, García-Morteo O, Spindler AJ, et al: Carpal ankylosis in juvenile rheumatoid arthritis. Arthritis Rheum 23:1251, 1980
15. Millender LH, Nalebuff EA, Feldon PG: Rheumatoid arthritis. In Green DP (ed): Operative Hand Surgery. Churchill Livingstone, New York, 1982
16. Rodnan GP, McEwen C, Wallace SL: Primer on the rheumatic diseases. JAMA 224(5)(Suppl), 1973
17. Short CL, Bauer E, Reynolds WE: Rheumatoid Arthritis. A Definition of the Disease and a Clinical Description Based on a Numerical Study of 293 Patients and Controls. Harvard University Press, Cambridge, MA, 1957
18. Sones DA: Surgery for rheumatoid arthritis—timing and techniques: General and medical aspects. J Bone Joint Surg [Am] 50:576, 1968
19. Souter WA: Planning treatment of the rheumatoid hand. Hand 11:3, 1979
20. Taleisnik J: Rheumatoid synovitis of the volar compartment of the wrist joint: Its radiological signs and its contribution to wrist and hand deformity. J Hand Surg 4:526, 1979
21. Taleisnik J: Rheumatoid arthritis of the wrist. In Strickland JW, Steichen JB: Difficult Problems in Hand Surgery. Mosby, St. Louis, 1982
22. Williams HB: Current status of the role of surgery in the rheumatoid hand. Orthop 9:29, 1980.

16 Evaluation of the Rheumatoid Wrist

CLINICAL EVALUATION

Synovitis

Swelling, pain, limitation of motion, and weakness are the complaints that bring the patient to a surgical consultation. Swelling, due to edema and synovitis, may be paradoxically less painful and disabling the more prominent it appears. Synovitis is easier to detect on the dorsum of the wrist, simply because structures that are lined with synovium are closer to the dorsal surface, and are covered by thinner, less constrictive ligaments and capsules. Dorsal swelling is usually secondary to tenosynovitis of the dorsal extensor tendons. The ulnar three compartments are more frequently and severely involved than the radial three (Fig. 16-1). Tenosynovitis surrounding the extensor indicis proprius, the extensor digitorum communis, and the extensor digiti quinti produces a typical hourglass deformity, the central constriction caused by the dorsal retinaculum (Fig. 16-2). Tenosynovitis within the extensor carpi ulnaris compartment produces an ovoid, elongated area of swelling on the dorsoulnar aspect of the wrist (Fig. 16-1A). The swelling may be cystic in the early cases, when actual synovial sacs are filled with a yellowish, thin fluid. Later on the fluid becomes thicker, and "rice bodies" may be present as well. Because the dorsal retinaculum accomodates to a considerable extent to the increased pressures produced by the space-occupying synovium, pain may remain relatively minimal. Conversely, synovitis within the radio-carpal and intercarpal joints, where increased local pressures are less well tolerated, results in a uniformly tense, warm wrist, with comparatively less swelling but considerably more pain and limitation of motion (Fig. 16-3).

Tendon Ruptures

Pain that is elicited by finger extension against resistance, and is referred to the distal margin of the dorsal retinaculum may indicate a serious tendon involvement, and impending rupture,[40] due to synovial invasion and attrition of tendons against bony spicules. Gradual and successive tear of the digital extensor tendons may be seen, usually starting by a painless, seemingly sudden loss of extension of the little finger, rapidly followed by the loss of extension of the ring and long fingers (Fig. 16-4). The single loss of the extensor digiti quinti or of the extensors of a central digit may cause minimal disability. The lack of full extension is masked by the associated pull through the junctura tendinum from the neighboring finger extensors and only the patient's subjective feel of a loss provides a clue to the existence of a tendon tear.[28,30]

Attrition and rupture of the extensor pollicis longus may also occur (Fig. 16-5). Although in many cases this rupture is localized to an area of bone roughness, or to a bony spicule, this complication is most likely secondary to the particular characteristics of the blood supply to the extensor pollicis longus tendon as it winds around Lister's

(Text continues on page 338.)

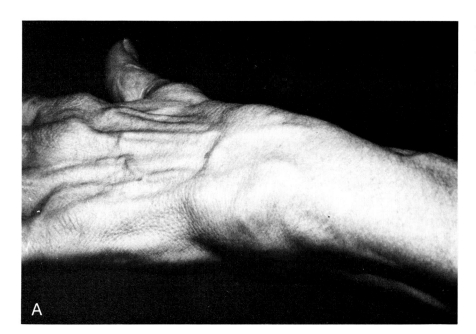

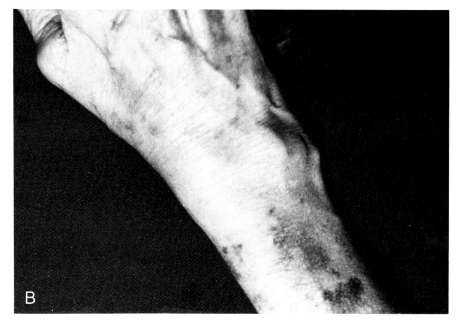

Fig. 16-1. A and B: the ulnar dorsal compartments are involved more frequently and severely than the radial three compartments.

Fig. 16-2. Hourglassing of dorsal tenosynovitis caused by fibers of the dorsal retinaculum (arrows). *A* and *B*: Clinical appearance. *C*: Intraoperative appearance.

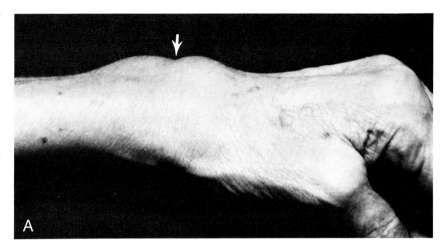

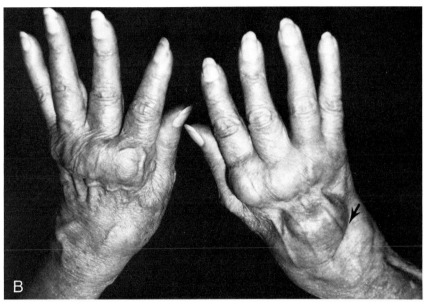

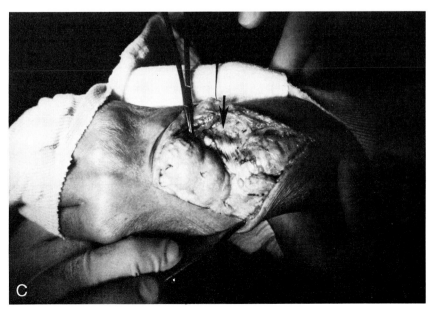

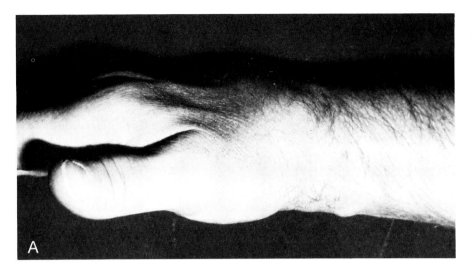

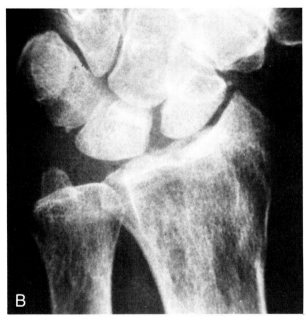

Fig. 16-3. Synovitis predominantly involving the radio-carpal and intercarpal joints. *A:* Clinical appearance. The wrist is tense, warm. There is considerable pain and limitation of motion. *B:* Radiograph of same wrist.

tubercle. Engkvist and Lundborg[9] suggested that increased pressure within the intact sheath of this tendon further restricts blood flow to a portion of the extensor pollicis longus that is already poorly vascularized under normal conditions. Ruptures of the extensor carpi ulnaris and of the radial wrist extensors are possible but not as frequent, and may be related to bony and articular changes (radiocarpal dislocation) rather than to tenosynovitis. Occasionally, a DeQuervain's tendinitis is seen,[18,20,21] either because of tenosynovitis, or caused by a bony roughness along the floor of the first dorsal extensor wrist compartment. Involvement of this compartment is, however, infrequent in rheumatoid patients. Tenosynovitis of the flexor compartment within the carpal tunnel is more difficult to detect clinically, unless compression of the median nerve develops,[13,14,40] or flexor tendon ruptures occur. Nocturnal paresthesias are common even if a clear-cut carpal tunnel syndrome is not present.

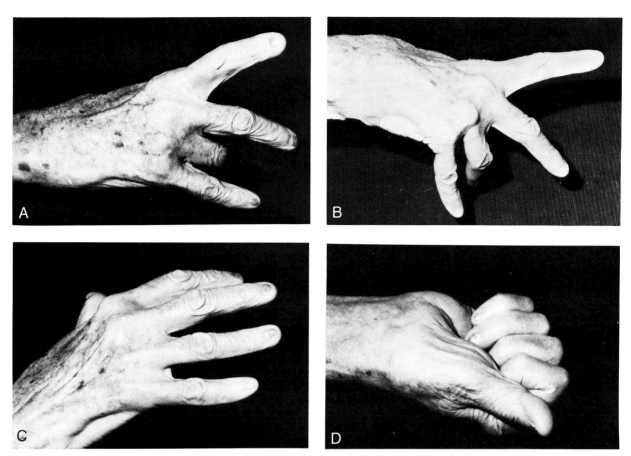

Fig. 16-4. Loss of extension to long, ring and little fingers. *A* and *B*: Preoperative appearance. *C*: Range of extension following tendon transfers. *D*: Flexion should be preserved.

At times, these patients exhibit triggering of flexion at the wrist, the "trigger wrist" phenomenon.[2,4,5,7] This may be secondary to nodular involvement of the flexor profundus or superficialis tendons. A "sublimis test" (a single finger flexion is examined while the flexor digitorum profundus is kept tenodesed distally by keeping all other fingers passively extended) (Fig. 16-6) may elicit pain which, in the case of flexor tenosynovitis within the carpal tunnel, is referred to the anterior surface of the wrist.[2] Limitation of finger flexion may be associated with carpal tunnel synovitis (Fig. 16-7) and is at times accompanied by a tense swelling of the palmar aspect of the wrist, and a palpable crepitation that can be felt during finger motion.[10] The presence of carpal tunnel symptoms, with greater passive than

active finger flexion, is strongly suggestive of flexor tenosynovitis.[28,41] Ruptures of flexor tendons may be due to synovial invasion or more frequently to attrition against bony spicules penetrating through the floor of the carpal canal, usually arising from the distal pole of the palmarflexed scaphoid (Fig. 16-8A,B), or from the tubercle of the trapezium (Fig. 16-8C).[15,19,22,29,31] The flexor tendons to the thumb and index are most commonly involved. Both extensor or flexor motor loss from tendon ruptures must be differentiated from other conditions that may produce the same appearance and disability. Loss of long flexion to the thumb and index finger may be the result of an anterior interosseous nerve syndrome; it may also be secondary to rupture of the tendon distal to the wrist, in the

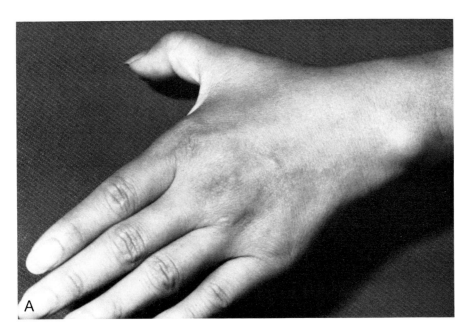

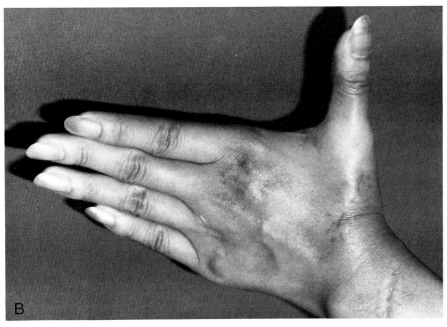

Fig. 16-5. Loss of extensor pollicis longus. *A*: Preoperative appearance. *B*: Postoperative range of extension, after tendon transfer.

Fig. 16–5. (cont.). C: Flexion and adduction are preserved.

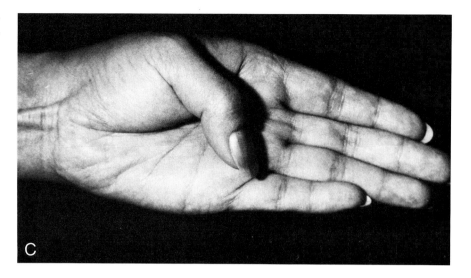

palm or within the digital sheath.[29] At times, the exact site of injury can be determined only during surgical exploration. Extensor tendon ruptures may be mimicked by dorsal interosseous nerve compressions,[24] or loss of extension of the fingers due to dislocations of the metacarpophalangeal joints, and/or dislocation of the extensor tendons themselves.[27,28,42] A careful examination of the hand should assist the surgeon in arriving at a proper diagnosis (Fig. 16-9). Active tensing of the tendon, palpable and visible, is indicative of tendon integrity and of an active muscle, even though this motor activity may be unsuccessful in producing finger extension. In many cases, only after the fingers are aligned by the examiner in full extension, can the patient actively maintain this position.[10,40] The dorsal interosseous nerve syndrome is more difficult to diagnose; it requires a greater degree of awareness to disregard the obvious, that is, a tendon rupture, in favor of a less frequent diagnosis. At times the diagnosis is not suspected until exploration of the extensor tendons shows them to be intact.[24,27] The history of painless, usually abrupt, loss of extension successively involving neighboring digits favors the diagnosis of ruptures. Soft tissue swelling or fullness about the elbow, a history of pain from the elbow preceding the paralysis by days or weeks, and palsy of muscles other than those to the fingers (extensor carpi ulnaris) favor a diagnosis of dorsal interosseous nerve syndrome.[27,29] A "tenodesis effect" test has been de-

scribed in paralysis due to dorsal interosseous nerve compression. Finger extension is produced by passive wrist flexion, a synchronous tenodesis effect which is absent when the tendons have been ruptured.[27,29] Enough palmarflexion of the wrist, however, should be present in these patients for the test to be meaningful. Tear of the extensor pollicis longus may be masked by residual extension of the thumb due to intrinsic action only; however,

(Text continues on page 344.)

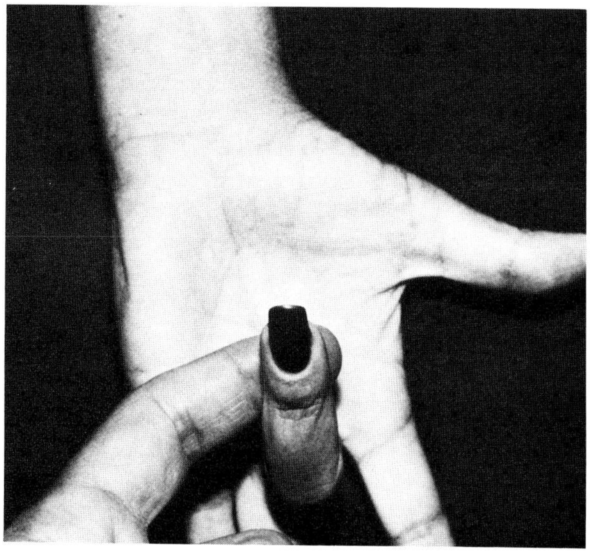

Fig. 16-6. "Sublimis test" may elicit pain on the palmar aspect of the wrist, in patients with flexor tenosynovitis within the carpal tunnel.

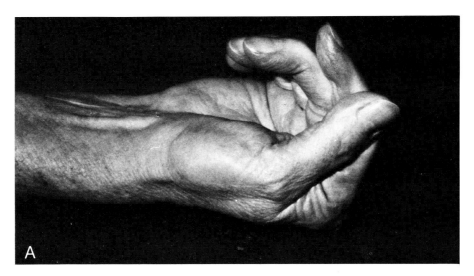

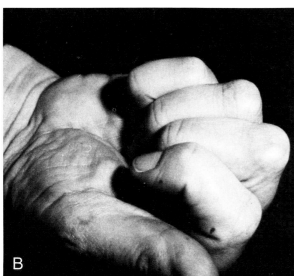

Fig. 16-7. Flexor tenosynovitis. *A:* Preoperative loss of flexion. *B:* Postoperative range of flexion after flexor tenosynovectomy within the carpal tunnel.

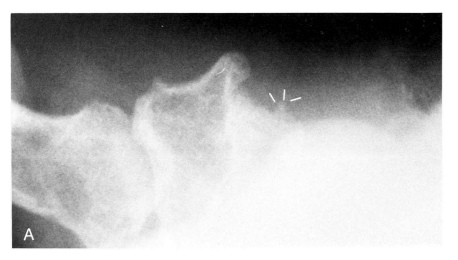

Fig. 16-8. Rupture of flexor tendons by attrition against bony spicules in the floor of the carpal tunnel. *A:* Carpal tunnel view shows a bony prominence arising from the scaphoid, in patient with loss of flexor pollicis longus.

Fig. 16–8. (cont.)   *B*: Same patient, intraoperative view. Instrument (arrow) points to bone spicule. Torn tendon ends are shown (a–a′). *C*: Instruments (*A* and *B*) hold torn tendon ends in wrist of a different patient. Arrow points to abnormal, rough prominence arising from the trapezium.

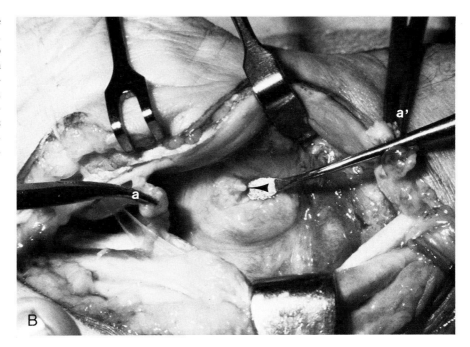

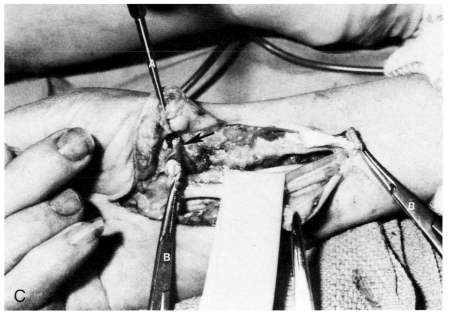

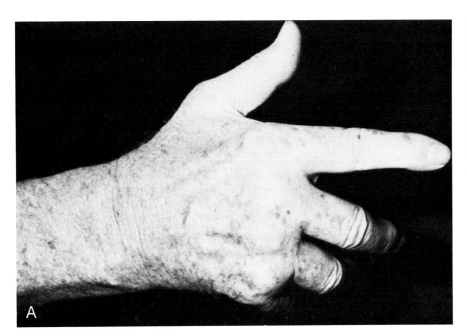

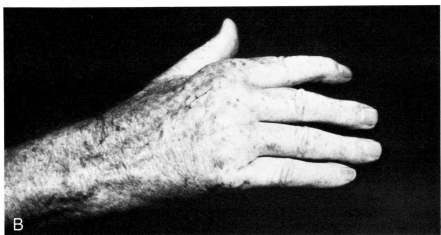

Fig. 16-9. Extensor tendon ruptures may be mimicked by loss of extension secondary to metacarpophalangeal joint dislocations. *A:* Preoperative appearance. *B:* Restoration of finger extension by replacement arthroplasties and relocation of dislocated extensor tendons at the level of the metacarpophalangeal joints.

this extension is not complete, and is *decreased* by thumb adduction. Conversely, thumb adduction would result in enhancement of extension in the presence of an intact extensor pollicis longus tendon. A more important finding after extensor pollicis longus tendon tears is the loss of retropulsion of the thumb, dorsal to the dorsal plane of the hand (Fig. 16-5).

Deformity

In the absence of acute synovitis, the surgeon must accurately assess the presence and degree of chronic deformities, of stiffness and crepitation of the wrist. Chronic rheumatoid arthritis of the wrist must be evaluated in relation to the patient's age, sex, and occupation. The degree of interference of wrist pain, limitation of motion and deformity with the activities of daily living must be noted. The potential for continuous destruction and collapse or damage to surrounding structures (i.e., tendons) should also be kept in mind. Some patterns of deformity are very typical and include a dorsal subluxation of the ulna, which, as will be discussed later, may be more apparent than real and represent instead a palmar subluxation of the radius and

Fig. 16-10. A: Palmar subluxation of radius and carpus in relation to ulnar head. FCU, flexor carpi ulnaris approaches the hand palmar to the ulnar head. *B*: Alignment improved by dorsal translation of the ulnar carpus.

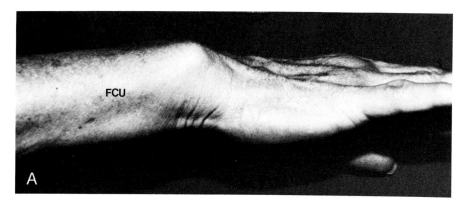

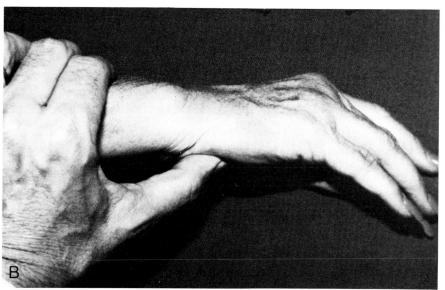

the carpus in relation to the ulnar head (Fig. 16-10). The ulnar half of the carpus is particularly prone to "drop" in a palmar direction (Fig. 16-11), while at the same time the metacarpals shift into radial angulation. The net effect is one of supination of the carpus and metacarpals in relation to the forearm (Fig. 16-12).[38,39] A second frequent pattern of deformity occurs when the carpus dislocates palmar to the radius (Fig. 16-13), and a third pattern is ulnar translocation of the carpus, resulting in a clinically recognizable deformity, in which the radial styloid is more prominent and the ulnar side of the hand is medial to the ulnar styloid (Fig. 16-14). Radial metacarpal shift is more apt to be associated with ulnar drift of the fingers (Fig. 16-15A). Conversely, the typical ulnar dislocation of the fingers is less prevalent in cases of wrist col-

lapse without radial metacarpal shift. Metacarpal angulation does not occur when the carpus collapses evenly, both radial and ulnar halves migrating proximally and equally (Fig. 16-15B); ulnar carpal translocations may also show preservation of radiometacarpal alignment, at least during earlier stages (Fig. 16-15C).

RADIOGRAPHIC EVALUATION

The radiologic features of advanced rheumatoid involvement of the wrist are well known. Less known are those early changes produced by synovitis at a stage when synovectomy could be most beneficial. These changes are not haphazard but develop in direct proportion to the concentration

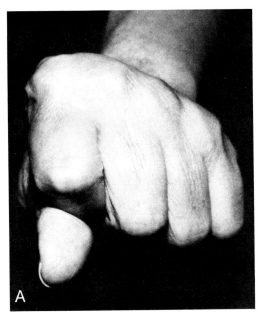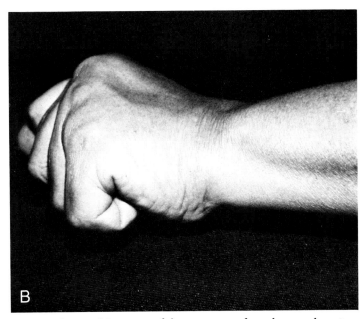

Fig. 16-11. *A:* Abnormal metacarpal descent. *B:* There is palmar subluxation of the carpus, and an abnormal supination of the wrist in relation to the forearm.

of synovium, the presence of synovial sacs and pouches in close relation to the supporting wrist ligaments, and the mechanical characteristics of the area involved.[3,25,26,33–37,43–45] Bywaters[3] described two sites where erosions are frequently seen: the ulnar head and its styloid and the most lateral portion of the scaphotrapezial joint. Likewise, Martel, Hayes, and Duff[26] found that the ulnar styloid was involved in 46 percent of radiographs they reviewed and that the radial aspect of the scaphoid was the next most frequent location of involvement. Ranawat and associates,[33] in a report on arthrographic changes in the rheumatoid wrist, reviewed 76 wrist radiographs. The earliest bone lesions were marginal erosions of the ulnar styloid in 41, of the scaphoid and lunate in 40, and of the radial styloid in 38. Pseudocysts of the distal portion of the radius were present in 22 wrists. Abnormalities noted in arthrograms included, in addition, communictions between the different wrist joint compartments; this correlated well with the surgical findings in 15 wrists, all of which showed, for instance, destruction of the scapholunate interosseous ligament. Resnick and Gmelich[36] also found fragmentation predominant at the level of

the ulnar aspect of the distal radius and "adjacent to the body of the scaphoid." All reports describe a pattern of involvement of the ulnar head and styloid, and, less frequently, of the midportion of the scaphoid. Conspicuously absent, however, is any mention of similar early erosive changes involving the midcarpal joint, particularly the head of the capitate, which may remain structurally intact in the midst of a complete dissociation of the carpal architecture (Figs. 15-4, 18-8). This feature is helpful in planning the treatment for the severely destroyed and unstable wrist. A review of the anatomy of the wrist ligaments[16,43] suggests that synovitis of the prestyloid recess is the cause of erosive changes of the ulnar styloid and that the scaphoid erosions occur deep to the radiocapitate or "sling" ligament, which runs across the concavity of the scaphoid, spanning the distance between the radial styloid and the neck of the capitate. Other areas where a close anatomic correlation can be found with radiographic changes in the rheumatoid wrist are the radioscapholunate junction, the dorsalulnar corner of the radius, and the triquetrum[44,45] (refer to Chapter 2 for a description of the ligamentous structures).

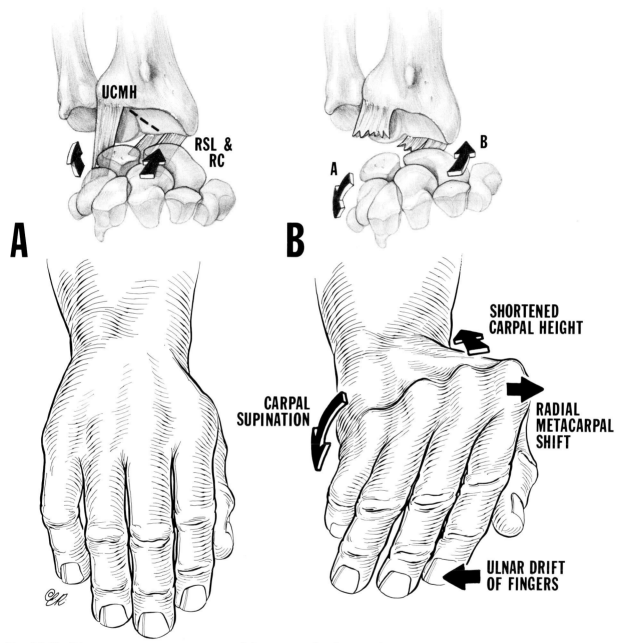

Fig. 16-12. Diagrammatic representation of factors involved in producing the typical deformity of the wrist in patients with rheumatoid arthritis. *A*: Normally, the ulocarpal complex suspends the ulnar carpus from the dorsal-ulnar corner of the radius (UCMH, ulnocarpal meniscus homologue). The palmar radiocarpal ligaments tether the proximal pole of the scaphoid to the palmar rim of the radius. RSL, radioscapholunate ligament. RC: radiocapite (radioscaphocapitate) ligament. *B*: In rheumatoid arthritis, typical elements of deformity of the wrist are carpal supination (allowed by the loss of the ulnocarpal complex), and shortening of radial carpal height (through palmar-flexion of the scaphoid after loss of its palmar ligamentous support).

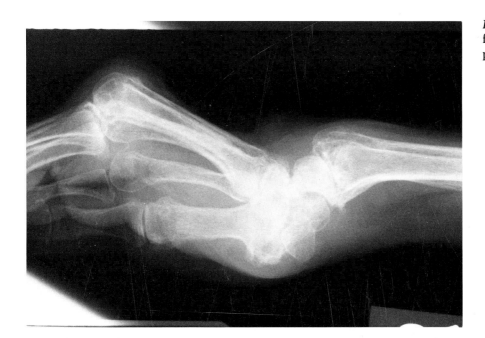

Fig. 16-13. Severe VISI deformity results in palmar carpal subluxation.

Scaphoid-Grooving: The Sling (Radiocapitate) Ligament

In 1964 Martel[25] called attention to an area of erosion of the radial aspect of the scaphoid. In very early synovitis all that may be seen is a band of decreased bony density across the waist of the scaphoid. This corresponds to the location of the radiocapitate ligament, which is weakly attached to the concave volar waist of the scaphoid, and on which it rotates as a gymnast does on a horizontal bar while executing a hip circle. Synovitis in this area is responsible for the appearance and progression of scaphoid grooving or notching (Fig. 16-16). It is one factor leading toward destabilization of the proximal pole of the scaphoid. The scaphoid subluxates into palmar flexion,[20,32] its longitudinal axis perpendicular to that of the radius. It appears foreshortened in posteroanterior radiographs. There is eventual loss of radial carpal height, and rotation of the carpus into supination (Fig. 16-12).

Pseudocysts of the Radius and Scapholunate Dissociation: The Deep Radioscapholunate Ligament

Pseudocysts of the radius in rheumatoid wrists have previously been reported.[6,12,19,20,23,33] The subchondral margin of the radius shows, in line with the scapholunate junction, a pseudocystic area of variable diameter (Fig. 16-17). This corresponds to the origin of the deep radioscapholunate ligament.[23,43] Opposite the pseudocyst of the radius, there are frequent erosions of the scaphoid and lunate, and eventually a progressive scapholunate dissociation similar to that seen after traumatic ligament tears or avulsions.[17,20] This, together with a detachment of the scaphoid from the radiocapitate ligament, completes the destabilization of the proximal pole of the scaphoid, allowing it to sublux into a position perpendicular to the long axis of the radius.

Ulnar Translocation

Ulnar migration of the carpus as seen in radiographs of the rheumatoid wrist, is very likely related to a gradual loss of all radiocarpal support, particularly the very strong volar radiolunate and dorsal radiocarpal ligaments (Fig. 16-18). Because of their size and orientation, these structures are principally responsible for maintaining the lunate (and consequently the carpus) in its proper relationship to the radius. Both ligament groups originate from the radius and progress in an almost hori-

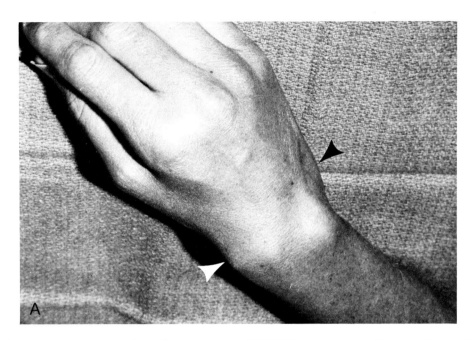

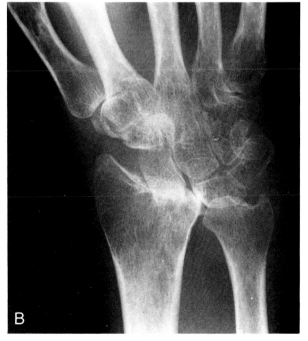

Fig. 16-14. Ulnar translocation. *A*: Clinical appearance. Arrows point to abnormal prominence of radial styloid laterally, and of carpus medially. *B*: Radiograph shows a type I ulnar translocation.

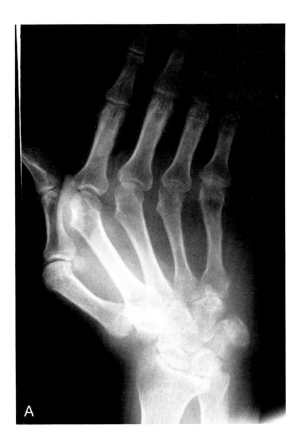

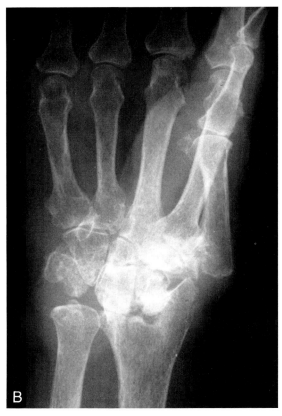

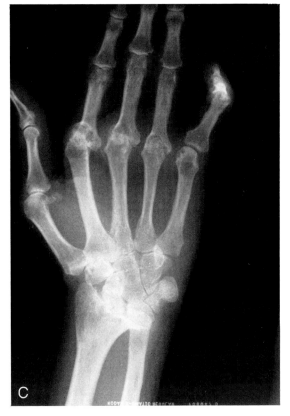

Fig. 16-15. Typical patterns of deformity of the wrist in rheumatoid arthritis. *A*: Zigzag deformity in the frontal plane. Carpal supination and radial shift of the metacarpals are frequently associated with ulnar deviation of the fingers. *B*: Even collapse of radial and ulnar carpus. There is no metacarpal angulation in the frontal plane, but a zigzag VISI deformity is present in the lateral projection (see Fig. 16-13). *C*: Ulnar translocation without metacarpal angulation. Metacarpodigital alignment is satisfactory.

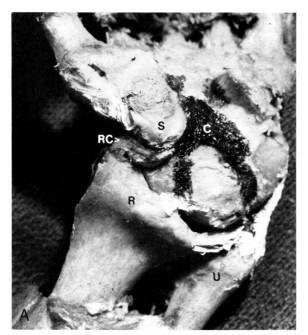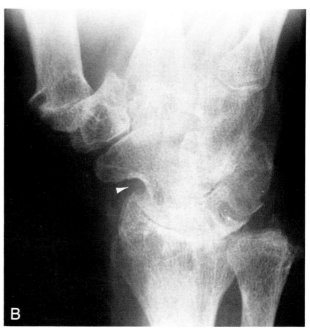

Fig. 16-16. Scaphoid-grooving and the radiocapitate ("sling") ligament. *A:* Shows the radiocapitate (RC) ligament. R, radius; U, ulna; S, scaphoid; C, capitate. *B:* Groove or notch (arrow) in midscaphoid. (*A* from Taleisnik J: The ligaments of the wrist. J Hand Surg 1:110, 1976.)

zontal direction medially and somewhat distally. They strongly tether the carpus laterally, preventing its ulnar migration along the inclined plane of the distal radius.

Erosions of the Ulnar Corner of the Radius and the Triquetrum: The Ulnocarpal Ligament Complex

Erosive and cystic changes at the level of the origin and insertion of the ulnocarpal complex are frequent in rheumatoid wrists (Figs. 2-12, 16-19). Erosions of the triquetrum are predominant along the ulnar confines of the midcarpal and radiocarpal joints. Arthrograms may show abnormal pooling of contrast material in these sites.[37] Loss of dorsoradial support, normally provided by the ulnocarpal complex, is a factor in the palmar subluxation of the ulnar carpus that is seen in these patients (Fig. 16-12). It may also be present in those wrists exhibiting ulnar translocation (Fig. 16-19D).

The Ulnar Styloid and the Prestyloid Recess (Fig. 2-13)

Resnick[35] distinguishes three areas of distal ulnar erosions: *lateral*, related to the inferior radioulnar joint compartment, and leading to the "scallop sign" described by Freiberg and Weinstein (Fig. 16-19D);[11] *distal*, corresponding to involvement of the synovial villi within the prestyloid recess, and *medial*, in connection with synovitis of the extensor carpi ulnaris tendon sheath, and attributed to subjacent bone resorption and periostitis beneath the inflamed sheath.[37] Early synovitis within the synovium-filled prestyloid recess is a cause of erosive changes of the ulnar styloid and an additional factor of destabilization of the ulnar carpus.

The Distal Radioulnar Joint

The distal radioulnar joint is surrounded by a synovial sac, and supported by the triangular fibrocartilage, the palmar and dorsal radioulnar liga-

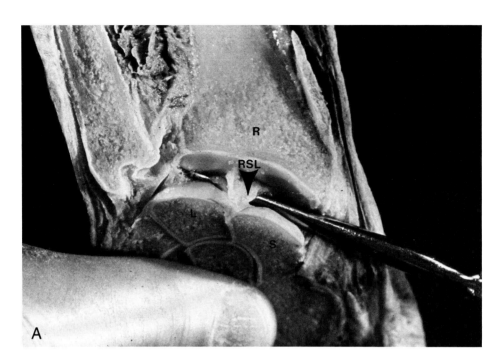

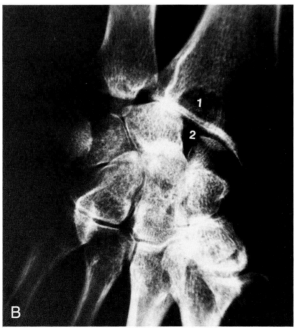

Fig. 16-17. Pseudocyst of the radius, scapholunate dissociation and radioscapholunate ligament. *A*: Coronal section of wrist; palmar half as seen from within the joint. R, radius; RSC, radioscapholunate ligament. *B*: Pseudocyst (1) and scapholunate dissociation (2) secondary to synovitis at origin and insertion of radioscapholunate ligament. Destabilized scaphoid is palmarflexed and foreshortened (*A* from Taleisnik J: The ligaments of the wrist J Hand Surg 1:110, 1976, *B* from Taleisnik J: Rheumatoid synovitis of the volar compartment of the wrist joint: Its radiological signs and its contribution to wrist and hand deformity. J Hand Surg 4:526, 1979.)

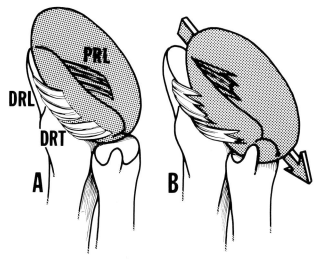

Fig. 16-18. A: Radiocarpal ligamentous apparatus keeps carpus against ulnar slope of distal radius. PRL, palmar radiolunate ligament; DRL, dorsal radiolunate ligament; DRT, dorsal radiotriquetral ligament. B: Without this support, the carpus tends to slide in an ulnar direction, down the incline of the articular surface of the distal radius.

ments, and the ulnocarpal complex (including the extensor carpi ulnaris and its retinacular tunnel). Distension by radioulnar synovitis, bony erosions, and loss of support from the triangular fibrocartilage and extensor carpi ulnaris contribute to the derangement of the distal radioulnar joint. The result is an apparent dorsal subluxation of the ulnar head (Figs. 16-10, 16-11). This is part of what Bäckdahl[1] named the "caput ulnae syndrome," which also consists of a fluctuant dorsal swelling (dorsal tenosynovitis), radioulnar instability and pain and weakness of the wrist, particularly during pronation and supination. In 1777, upon reporting a traumatic dislocation of the distal radioulnar joint found in a cadaver, Desault[8] pointed out that it is not the ulna which dislocates from the radius but the radius, together with the carpus and hand, which dislocate from the ulna. The net result is a deformity with a prominent ulnar head, which is accentuated by forearm pronation. Attenuation of all structures dorsal to the ulnar head, as well as the palmar pull exerted by radius and carpus, contribute further to the deformities found in the rheumatoid patient.

The VISI Deformity

Lateral roentgenographs may show a fixed palmarflexion of the lunate, resulting in a palmar displacement of capitate and metacarpals in relation to the long axis of the radius.[19,20] The deformity is similar to that seen in posttraumatic carpal instabilities and has been called VISI, (volarflexed intercalated segment instability; see Chapter 12) (Fig. 16-13). Progression of this deformity has been reported as a potential cause of palmar dislocation of the carpus;[20] in most patients with rheumatoid arthritis, it produces a zigzag alignment as seen in profile, that eventually becomes fixed by ankylosis and remains strangely symptom-free and functional in many patients. A true palmar dislocation of the carpus is somewhat different, and is due to changes at the radiolunate rather than at the lunocapitate levels, leading to a palmar drop of both, lunate and capitate together (Fig. 15-4). In these cases, there are extensive erosive changes of the palmar rim of the radius resulting in an abnormal increase of the palmar tilt of its articular surface. This, together with a destruction by synovitis of all palmar radiocarpal support, allows progressive palmar dislocation of the carpus.

Arteriography

The value of arthrography of the rheumatoid wrist joint has been investigated by Ranawat and coauthors.[33,34] Arthrographic abnormalities due to villous proliferation and infolding of the synovial lining consisted of a corrugated pattern of the synovial cavity, abnormal communications between radiocarpal and midcarpal joints, and of the radiocarpal and distal radioulnar joints, and between the wrist joint itself and the extensor or flexor tendon sheaths. These abnormalities can exist in many cases before erosive changes are visible in plain roentgenographs. This emphasizes the advantages of earlier surgical exploration of these patients' joints, even if preoperative radiographs have been inconclusive. During dorsal synovectomies, radiocarpal and midcarpal joints should be visualized, and the need for a joint synovectomy determined by direct inspection. When there is doubt as to the degree of joint involvement, in a patient with proven rheumatoid arthritis, but with normal ra-

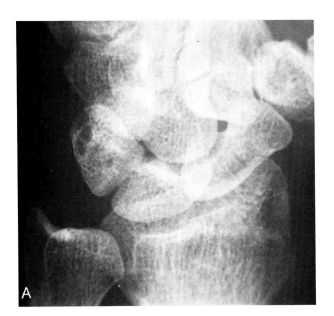

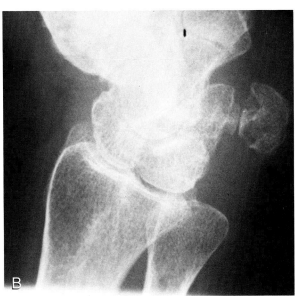

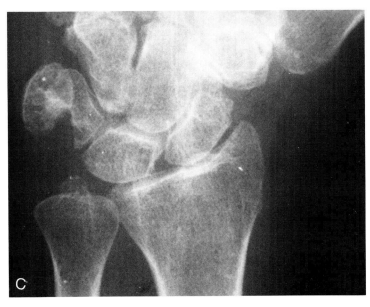

Fig. 16-19. Ulnar cysts of radius and triquetrum and the ulnocarpal ligament complex. *A*: Early cysts of the triquetrum. *B*: Triquetropisiform cysts. *C*: Erosive loss of triquetrum.

Fig. 16–19. (cont.). D: Severe distal radioulnar and triquetral erosions in ulnar translocated carpus.

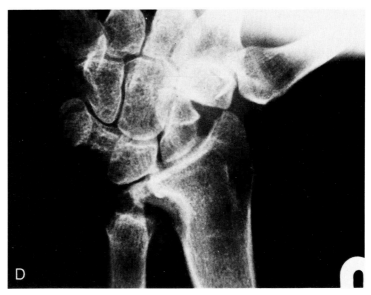

diographs and who has not as yet fulfilled the indications for surgical exploration, an arthrogram may provide a clue as to the extent and severity of the intraarticular synovitis.[34] Wu and coworkers[46] point out that, in addition to outlining the joint, delineation of lymphatic vessels is a frequent finding in arthrograms done for rheumatoid arthritis. They have used this technique to demonstrate that peripheral edema in rheumatoid arthritis is associated with lymphatic obstruction and to postulate that this edema is, in effect, secondary to the lymphatic obstruction itself.

REFERENCES

1. Bäckdahl M: The caput ulnae syndrome in rheumatoid arthritis: A study of the morphology, abnormal anatomy and clinical picture. Acta Rheumatol Scand [Suppl 5] 1–75, 1963
2. Brewerton DA: The rheumatoid hand. President's address. Section of Physical Medicine. Proc R Soc Med 59:225, 1966
3. Bywaters EGL: The early radiological signs of rheumatoid arthritis. Bull Rheum Dis 11:231, 1960
4. Carvell JE, Mowat AG, Fuller DJ: Trigger wrist phenomenon in rheumatoid arthritis. Hand 15:77, 1983
5. Clayton ML: Surgical treatment at the wrist in rheumatoid arthritis. A review of thirty-seven patients. J Bone Surg [Am] 47:741, 1965
6. Collins LC, Lidsky MD, Sharp JT, Moreland J: Malposition of carpal bones in rheumatoid arthritis. Radiology 103:95, 1972
7. Davalbhakta VV, Bailey BN: Trigger wrist: Report of two cases. Br J Plast Surg 25:376, 1972
8. Desault M: Extrait d'un mémoire de M. Desault sur la luxation de l'extrêmité inferieure du radius. J Chir 1:78, 1791
9. Engkvist O, Lundborg G: Rupture of the extensor pollicis longus tendon after fracture of the lower end of the radius. A clinical and microangiographic study. Hand 11:76, 1979
10. Flatt AE: Care of the Arthritic Hand. 4th Ed. Mosby, St. Louis, 1983
11. Freiberg RA, Weinstein A: The scallop sign and spontaneous rupture of finger extensor tendons in rheumatoid arthritis. Clin Orthop 83:128, 1972
12. Hastings DE, Evans JA: Rheumatoid wrist deformities and their relation to ulnar drift. J Bone Joint Surg [Am] 57:930, 1975
13. Henderson ED, Lipscomb PR: Surgical treatment of the rheumatoid hand. JAMA 175:431, 1961
14. Henderson ED, Lipscomb PR: Rehabilitation of the rheumatoid hand by surgical means. Arch Phys Med Rehab 42:58, 1961
15. Kleinert HE, Frykman G: The wrist and thumb in rheumatoid arthritis. Orthop Clin North Am 4:1085, 1973
16. Lewis OJ, Hamshere RJ, Bucknill TM: The anatomy of the wrist joint. J Anat 106:539, 1970
17. Lidsky MD, Collins L, Moreland J: Abnormal navic-

ular-lunate separation in rheumatoid arthritis. (Abstract). Arthritis Rheum 13:332, 1970

18. Linscheid RL: Surgery for rheumatoid arthritis — Timing and techniques: The upper extremity. J Bone Joint Surg [Am] 50:605, 1968

19. Linscheid RL: Mechanical forces affecting the deformity of the rheumatoid wrist. Presented at the meeting of the American Society for Surgery of the Hand, New York, 1969

20. Linscheid RL, Dobyns JH: Rheumatoid arthritis of the wrist. Orthop Clin North Am 2:649, 1971

21. Lipscomb PR: Surgery of the arthritic hand: Sterling Bunnell Memorial Lecture. Mayo Clin Proc 40:132, 1965

22. Mannerfelt L, Norman O: Attrition ruptures of flexor tendons in rheumatoid arthritis caused by bony spurs in the carpal tunnel. J Bone Joint Surg [Br] 51:270, 1969

23. Mannerfelt L, Raven MV: Die Ätiologie und Bedeutung der Radiuskrypte im rheumatischen Handgelenk. Verh Dtsch Ges Rheumatol 5:94, 1978

24. Marmor L, Lawrence JF, Dubois EL: Posterior interosseous nerve palsy due to rheumatoid arthritis. J Bone Joint Surg [Am] 49:381, 1967

25. Martel W: The pattern of rheumatoid arthritis in the hand and wrist. Radiol Clin North Am 2:221, 1964

26. Martel W, Hayes JT, Duff IF: The pattern of bone erosion in the hand and wrist in rheumatoid arthritis. Radiology 84:204, 1965

27. Millender LH, Nalebuff EA, Holdsworth DE: Posterior interosseous-nerve syndrome secondary to rheumatoid synovitis. J Bone Joint Surg [Am] 55:753, 1973

28. Millender LH, Nalebuff EA: Preventive surgery. Tenosynovectomy and synovectomy. Orthop Clin North Am 6:765, 1975

29. Millender LH, Nalebuff EA, Feldon PG: Rheumatoid arthritis. In Green DP (ed): Operative Hand Surgery. Churchill Livingstone, New York, 1982

30. Nalebuff EA, Potter TA: Rheumatoid involvement of tendons and tendon sheaths in the hand. Clin Orthop 59:147, 1968

31. Palmieri TJ: Rheumatoid arthritis in the volar aspect of the wrist. Bull Hosp Joint Dis 35:103, 1974

32. Pekin TJ Jr, Zvaifler NJ: Navicular displacement in rheumatoid arthritis: Its recognition and significance. (Abstract). Arthritis Rheum 6:292, 1963

33. Ranawat CS, Freiberg RH, Jordan LR, Straub LR: Arthrography in the rheumatoid wrist joint. J Bone Joint Surg [Am] 51:1269, 1969

34. Ranawat CS, Harrison MD, Jordan LR: Arthrography of the wrist joint. Clin Orthop 83:6, 1972

35. Resnick D: Rheumatoid arthritis of the wrist: Why the ulnar styloid? Radiology 112:29, 1974

36. Resnick D, Gmelich JR: Bone fragmentation in the rheumatoid wrist: Radiographic and pathologic considerations. Radiology 114:315, 1975

37. Resnick D: Rheumatoid arthritis of the wrist. Med Radiogr Photogr 52:50, 1976

38. Shapiro JS: Ulnar drift — Report of a related finding. Acta Orthop Scand 39:346, 1968

39. Shapiro JS, Heijna W, Nasatir S, Ray RD: The relationship of wrist motion to ulnar phalangeal drift in the rheumatoid patient. Hand 3:68, 1971

40. Souter WA: The hand in rheumatoid disease. In Lamb DW, Kuczynski K (eds): The Practice of Hand Surgery. Blackwell Scientific Publications, Boston, 1981

41. Straub LR, Ranawat CS: The wrist in rheumatoid arthritis. Surgical treatment and results. J Bone Joint Surg [Am] 51:1, 1969

42. Swanson AB: Implant arthroplasty in the hand and upper extremity and its future. Surg Clin North Am 61:369, 1981

43. Taleisnik J: The ligaments of the wrist. J Hand Surg 1:110, 1976

44. Taleisnik J: Rheumatoid synovitis of the volar compartment of the wrist joint: Its radiologic signs and its contribution to wrist and hand deformity. J Hand Surg 4:526, 1979

45. Taleisnik J: Rheumatoid synovitis of the wrist. In Strickland JW, Steichen JB (eds): Difficult Problems in Hand Surgery. Mosby, St. Louis, 1982

46. Wu G, Whitehouse GH, Littler TR: The demonstration of lymphatic channels on wrist arthrography in rheumatoid disease with particular reference to associated lymphoedema. Rheumatol Rehabil 21:65, 1982

17 Mechanism of Wrist Deformity in Rheumatoid Arthritis

There are three stages of the disease, similar in the wrist to those described by Zancolli for the hand of patients with rheumatoid arthritis: the initial inflammatory period of *synovitis*, a second stage leading to *joint disorganization*, and a final stage of *joint destruction*:[34] Throughout these stages several factors combine to produce a typical rheumatoid deformity of the wrist and hand. Some are normal *anatomic and functional* characteristics of the hand and wrist that become pathological after arthritic disruption has taken place.[25] Among these are the asymmetry of the metacarpal heads and metacarpophalangeal ligaments,[8,15] and of intrinsic muscles on each side of the fingers,[3,33] the location of synovial recesses and bursae,[33] the tendency of flexor tendons and metacarpophalangeal joints to deviate ulnarward in flexion,[6,25] augmented by the force of gravity and the pressures that are exerted against the radial side of the fingers.[30] Other factors of deformity are *pathologic*, entirely due to the disease process itself.[25] These include loss of bone and joint stability secondary to synovitis, subluxation of extensor and flexor tendons,[12,13,26] malalignment of the long finger,[10] and the contractures of the intrinsic muscles, clinically more significant for the ulnar wings because of their more direct relationship with the extensor mechanism. This characteristic permits full finger flexion only if the digits are, at the same time, brought into ulnar deviation to relax the ulnar wings (Fig. 17-1).[4,5]

Loss of bone and joint stability and increased tissue laxity secondary to rheumatoid synovitis, as well as to the elevation of the intraarticular pressures,[9,32] are also factors in causing deformity. In 1966 Millroy,[18] almost casually, mentioned that for the treatment of ulnar drift of the fingers it is important to correct the radial deviation of the wrist. In 1968 Shapiro[21] emphasized that radial deviation of the metacarpals, and radial rotation of the wrist, are deformities frequently associated with ulnar deviation of the fingers. In measuring radiographs, Shapiro utilized two coordinates. The first was drawn along the radial cortex of the shaft of the second metacarpal, the second from the tip of the radial styloid to the ulnar-palmar corner of the distal articular surface of the radius. The intersection of the lines makes an obtuse angle that measures an average of 112 degrees (average range 92 to 127 degrees) in the normal wrist.[21] A greater value indicates a radial shift of the metacarpals (Fig. 17-2). In Shapiro's study[22] those patients who eventually developed drift progressed from an an initial mean value of 117 degrees to a final mean value of 128 degrees. In those that never developed ulnar drift this angle remained consistently between normal limits (108 to 112 degrees). In 1971 Shapiro and associates[23] stated that "the individual who exhibits this set of variant findings (a normal tendency toward radial deviation during power grip) will be the one individual who may develop ulnar phalangeal drift should rheumatoid involvement occur." Linscheid[16] suggested that the corollary to this statement may also be true, in that correction of ulnar drift of the fingers may improve radial meta-

357

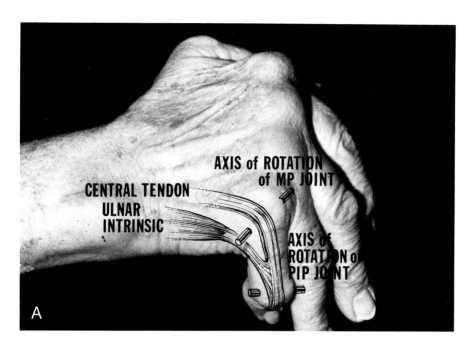

Fig. 17-1. Intrinsic ulnar wing contracture in rheumatoid arthritis permits full finger flexion if the finger is simultaneously brought into ulnar deviation.

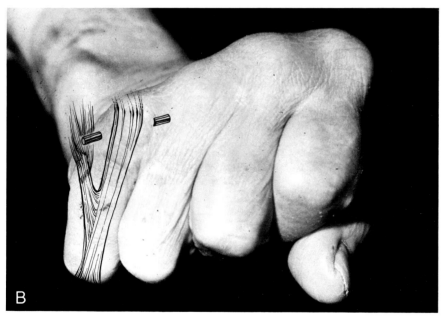

carpal alignment without direct intervention at the wrist level. This concept of a zigzag alignment tending to collapse under longitudinal loading (Fig. 17-2) was presented by Landsmeer[15] as part of his studies on the anatomy of joint function. Landsmeer stated that, in a biarticular system, a third element is necessary as a link between the opposing sides of the system to prevent its collapse under the longitudinal load that is produced by equal but opposite forces. In the wrist this function is provided by the scaphoid. Loss of its stabilizing influence allows zigzag deformities to develop, not only in the frontal plane[21] but also in the sagittal plane (VISI).[16,17] In an explanation of this pattern of

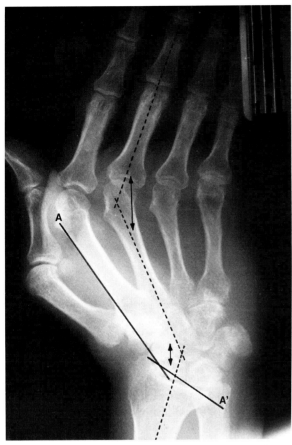

Fig. 17-2. Coordinates proposed by Shapiro[21] for radiographic measurements of metacarpal and finger deviations in rheumatoid arthritis. A is drawn along the radial cortex of the shaft of the second metacarpal. A' is traced from the tip of the styloid process of the radius to the ulnar-palmar corner of the distal articular surface of the radius. The normal A–A' angle averages 112 degrees. A greater value in this radiograph indicates a radial metacarpal shift. The interrupted lines depict the zigzag radiometacarpal-digital alignment in this patient with rheumatoid arthritis.

mits them to initiate digital flexion at the proximal interphalangeal (PIP) joint level. Already in 1960 Vaughan Jackson[31] had pointed out that the cause of the flexor-extensor imbalance which results in swan neck deformities may be found at the wrist, and that surgical reduction of the carpal malalignment was accompanied by a reversal of the swan neck deformity, the fingers seen thereafter to assume "the normal flexed position in the relaxed hand."

Shapiro and collaborators,[21] as well as others,[2,17,27] believe that the initial factor of wrist deformity is the loss of the stabilizing power of the extensor carpi ulnaris, a result of extensor carpi ulnaris tendon damage, rupture, subluxation, or muscle inhibition. Bäckdahl[2] demonstrated that the extensor carpi ulnaris is a true dorsiflexor with the forearm in supination, when it occupies a position dorsal to the center of rotation of the wrist. In supination, the extensor carpi ulnaris tendon is electromyographically active both in dorsiflexion and in palmarflexion. In pronation the extensor carpi ulnaris translates ulnarly and functions poorly as a dorsiflexor. In rheumatoid disease, electromyographic recordings show that the extensor carpi ulnaris is no longer active in dorsiflexion. Subluxation from its normal position further decreases its ability to influence dorsiflexion. When dislocated palmar to the transverse axis of wrist rotation, this tendon does, in effect, become a palmar flexor (Fig. 16-10). Without the extensor carpi ulnaris support, the ulnar carpus shows a progressive tendency toward volar subluxation (Fig. 16-12). During power grip, radial rotation of the carpus is increased, allowing the long digital flexors to exert an abnormal ulnar pull on already weakened finger joints. This inhibition of extensor carpi ulnaris activity was found, however, in those patients with already established ulnar digital drift. Whether this inhibition was primary and preceded the onset of ulnar drift, as proposed by Shapiro and associates,[21] or secondary to an established ulnar drift was not clearly demonstrated. This correlation of wrist and finger deformities was further suggested by Pahle and Raunio's investigation of wrist-hand alignment following wrist fusions.[19] Their findings confirmed Shapiro's concept that radiometacarpal shift frequently would lead to ulnar digital drift. Conversely, ulnar metacarpal

collapse, Shapiro[24] has suggested another hypothesis, that is, that the loss of carpal height effectively decreases the efficiency of the long extrinsic muscle-tendon units crossing the wrist, initiating an "extrinsic-minus" or, comparatively, an "intrinsic-plus" attitude of the fingers (Fig. 17-3). This may lead to the development of swan neck deformities. In these patients, distraction of the wrist allows them to improve their prehension ability, and per-

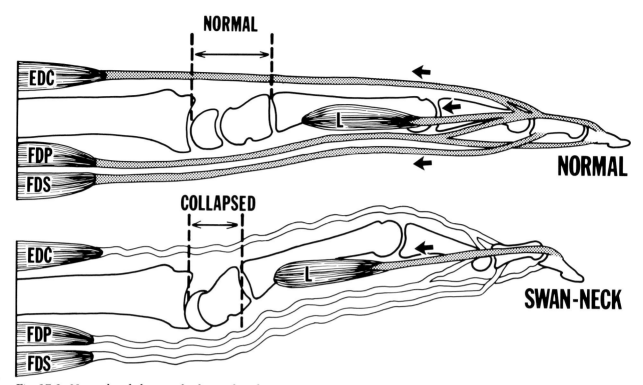

NORMAL

EDC

FDP

FDS

L

NORMAL

COLLAPSED

EDC

FDP

FDS

L

SWAN-NECK

Fig. 17-3. Normal and abnormal relationships between extrinsic and intrinsic musculotendinous units. In the normal skeleton (top) there is a balance between both groups of motors. In the presence of carpal collapse and proximal migration of the carpal-hand unit, long extrinsic motors no longer function at their optimal length while the intrinsics, distal to the collapsed carpus, still do. The resulting imbalance results in an "extrinsic minus" or, conversely, an "intrinsic plus" deformity. (Modified from Shapiro JS: Wrist involvement in rheumatoid swan neck deformity. J Hand Surg 7:484, 1982.)

shift may be conducive to radial deviation of the fingers as is more frequently seen in juvenile rheumatoid arthritis (Fig. 15-2). In patients whose wrists had undergone arthrodesis, it was clearly the position of fusion that determined the phalangeal deviation, and not the dynamic influence of the wrist motors which were no longer operative. Clinical experience indicates that patients deprived of the extensor carpi ulnaris through injury or transfer do not develop carpal malrotation, provided all other supportive structures are intact. Therefore, it must be assumed that in the wrist joint, just as in other joints with rheumatoid involvement, disorganization is initiated by intraarticular synovitis and the consequent loss of ligament support. Once articular malrotation and imbalance are present, then extensor carpi ulnaris inhibition or tear becomes a factor of deformity,

contributing to the development of the radial metacarpal shift. In addition, any support function of the extensor carpi ulnaris as a dynamic ulnar collateral ligament system is lost (Fig. 2-33).[14]

Arkless[1] showed that changes in carpal function *do* occur in the early stages of rheumatoid involvement. Forty-five of 110 wrists examined under cineradiography showed decreased or absent rotation of the distal pole of the scaphoid during radial and ulnar deviation. Over half of these had clear scapholunate joint widening. Fifty-eight of the wrists exhibited an abnormal lunate motion: the lunate failed to return to its normal position under the radius during ulnar deviation. In some, the lunate motion was described as "sticky." Linscheid[16] mentioned two predominant patterns of wrist involvement: ulnar translocation and radial metacarpal shift secondary to palmar flexion of the scaphoid (see Chapter 16). In all instances an apparent collapse of the radial half of the carpus was shown. Hastings and Evans[11] confirmed this in measurements of normal wrists and in wrists with rheumatoid arthritis. They attributed wrist collapse to loss of cartilage, with or without bone erosions, to proximal migration of the capitate through an abnormal scapholunate separation, and to rotation of the scaphoid itself. They also showed that, even though volarflexion of the scaphoid was preserved, dorsiflexion was lost. In the ulnar half of the wrist, volar subluxation and relative supination of the carpus, together with distal radioulnar and extensor carpi ulnaris synovitis, allowed the ulnar head to become prominent dorsally (see Chapter 16). Recently, Tubiana and coworkers[29] incorporated the kinematic concept of the columnar carpus to the understanding of the development of rheuma-

toid wrist deformities in rheumatoid disease. These deformities were classified as ulnar, central, and radial. This corresponds to the three longitudinal carpal columns and to what they describe as the vascular "axis of penetration" of rheumatoid synovitis. Propagation of this process would take place along one vascular axis per column, entering the corresponding carpal bones at the ligamentous attachments.

The combination of the altered *normal* characteristics of the wrist and hand, and the *pathologic* changes that are induced by the disease, result in the typical deformities that are seen in these patients. The carpus is normally "suspended" from the radius by a ligamentous sling that originates predominantly from the palmar radial and dorsal ulnar corners of the distal radius (Figs. 2-16, 16-12).[28] The radial half of this sling contributes to

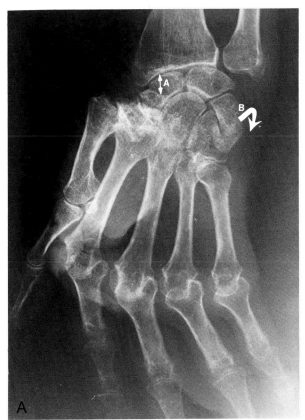

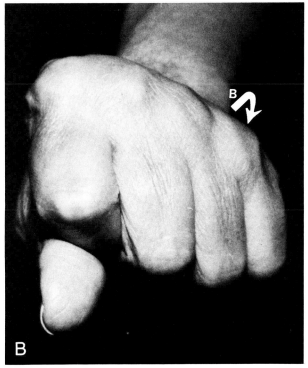

Fig. 17-4. *A*: Radiograph of typical deformity of the hand and wrist in rheumatoid arthritis. There is shortening of the radial carpal height (arrow **A**) and palmar subluxation of the ulnar carpus with carpal supination (arrow **B**). *B*: increased metacarpal descent and carpal supination (arrow **B**).

the stability of the lateral or "mobile" carpal column (scaphoid) and the ulnar half to the stability of the medial, or "rotation," column (triquetrum) (Fig. 16-12). On the radial side attenuation or destruction of the deep radioscapholunate and radiocapitate ligaments effectively destabilizes the proximal pole of the scaphoid, which gradually assumes a palmarflexed position, its longitudinal axis perpendicular to that of the radius (Fig. 17-4A). The scaphoid appears foreshortened in the frontal roentgenogram, leading to a proportional loss of radial carpal height. On the ulnar side of the carpus the ulnar half of the radiocarpal sling is no longer capable of providing dorsal support. The entire medial column gradually sinks in a palmar direction, appearing clinically as an increased metacarpal descent angle (Fig. 17-4A,B).[34] Therefore, this deformity may be secondary to the more proximal radiocarpal changes rather than to synovitis and loss of stability of the fourth and fifth carpometacarpal joints alone. The ulnar head becomes prominent dorsally, which is further accentuated by synovitis of the distal radioulnar joint, allowing dorsal subluxation of the ulna, or rather palmar subluxation of the radius. The combination of shortening of the radial carpus, palmar subluxation of the ulnar carpus, and dorsal subluxation of the ulnar head (or palmar subluxation of the radius) produce a relative carpal malrotation into supination, in relation to the distal forearm (Fig. 16-12). This gives those tendons that lie radial to the center of wrist rotation an advantage over those tendons ulnar to the center of rotation.[17] Every time the patient makes a fist or attempts to grasp, this abnormal alignment is dynamically accentuated, because the function of the extensor carpi radialis longus is facilitated and, on the opposite side, the extensor carpi ulnaris fails to act as a dorsiflexor as it gradually subluxates palmar to the prominent ulnar head, in fact carried palmarward by the drop of the ulnar carpus. Reversal of this dynamic malrotation by the transfer of the extensor carpi radialis longus from its insertion on the base of the second metacarpal to join the extensor carpi ulnaris at its insertion in the fifth metacarpal has proven valuable in correcting wrist deformity and as a prerequisite to correcting ulnar deviation of the fingers.[7]

REFERENCES

1. Arkless R: Rheumatoid wrists: Cineradiography. Radiology 88:543, 1967
2. Bäckdahl M: The caput ulnae syndrome in rheumatoid arthritis: A study of the morphology, abnormal anatomy and clinical picture. Acta Rheumatol Scand Suppl 5:1–75, 1963
3. Backhouse KM: The mechanics of normal digital control in the hand and an analysis of the ulnar drift of rheumatoid arthritis. Ann R Coll Surg Engl 43:154, 1968
4. Boyes JH: Bunnell's Surgery of the Hand. 5th Ed. Lippincott, Philadelphia, 1970
5. Brewerton DA: Hand deformities in rheumatoid disease. Ann Rheum Dis 16:183, 1957
6. Fearnley GR: Ulnar deviation of the fingers. Ann Rheum Dis 10:126, 1951
7. Ferlic DC, Clayton ML: Tendon transfer for radial rotation in the rheumatoid wrist. J Bone Joint Surg [Am] 55:880, 1973
8. Hakstian RW, Tubiana R: Ulnar deviation of the fingers. The role of joint structure and function. J Bone Joint Surg [Am] 49:299, 1967
9. Harris RW: The pathophysiology of rheumatoid hand deformities. Orthop Rev 10:33, 1981
10. Harrison SH: The importance of middle or long finger realignment in ulnar drift. J Hand Surg 1:87, 1976
11. Hastings DE, Evans JA: Rheumatoid wrist deformities and their relation to ulnar drift. J Bone Joint Surg [Am] 57:930, 1975
12. Henderson ED, Lipscomb PR: Surgical treatment of the rheumatoid hand. JAMA 175:431, 1961
13. Henderson ED, Lipscomb PR: Rehabilitation of the rheumatoid hand by surgical means. Arch Phys Med Rehabil 42:58, 1961
14. Kauer JMG: The collateral ligament function in the wrist joint. Acta Morphol Neerl Scand 17:252, 1979
15. Landsmeer JMF: Anatomical and functional investigations on the articulations of the human fingers. Acta Anat (Basel) (Suppl. 24) 25:169, 1955
16. Linscheid RL: Mechanical forces affecting the deformity of the rheumatoid wrist. Presented at the meeting of the American Society for Surgery of the Hand, New York, 1969
17. Linscheid RL, Dobyns JH: Rheumatoid arthritis of the wrist. Orthop Clin North Am 2:649, 1971
18. Milroy P: Surgery of the rheumatoid hand. J Bone Joint Surg [Br] 48:593, 1966
19. Pahle JA, Raunio P: The influence of wrist position on finger deviation in the rheumatoid hand: A clini-

cal and radiological study. J Bone Joint Surg [Br] 51:664, 1969

20. Resnick D: Rheumatoid arthritis of the wrist. Med Radiogr Photogr 52:50, 1976
21. Shapiro JS: Ulnar drift — Report of a related finding. Acta Orthop Scand 39:346, 1968
22. Shapiro JS: A new factor in the etiology of ulnar drift. Clin Orthop 68:32, 1970
23. Shapiro JS, Heijna W, Nasatir S, Ray RD: The relationship of wrist motion to ulnar phalangeal drift in the rheumatoid patient. Hand 3:68, 1971
24. Shapiro JS: Wrist involvement in rheumatoid swan-neck deformity. J Hand Surg 7:484, 1982
25. Smith RJ, Kaplan ER: Rheumatoid deformities at the metacarpophalangeal joints of the fingers. A correlative study of anatomy and pathology. J Bone Joint Surg [Am] 49:31, 1967
26. Snorrason E: The problem of ulnar deviation of the fingers in rheumatoid arthritis. Acta Med Scand 140:359, 1951
27. Stack HG, Vaughan-Jackson OJ: The zig-zag deformity in the rheumatoid hand. Hand 3:62, 1971
28. Taleisnik J: The ligaments of the wrist. J Hand Surg 1:110, 1976
29. Tubiana R, Kuhlmann N, Fahrer M, and Lisfranc R: Étude du poignet normal et ses déformations au cour de la polyarthrite rhumatoïde. Chirurgie 106:257, 1980
30. Vainio K, Oka M: Ulnar deviation of the fingers. Ann Rheum Dis 12:122, 1953
31. Vaughan-Jackson OJ: Swan neck deformity in rheumatoid arthritis. In Stack HG, Bolton H: The Proceedings of the Second Hand Club (10th meeting, London, 1960). The British Society for Surgery of the Hand. London, 1975
32. Williams HB: Current status of the role of surgery in the rheumatoid hand. Orthop Rev 9:29, 1980
33. Wise KS: The anatomy of the metacarpophalangeal joints with observations of the aetiology of ulnar drift. J Bone Joint Surg [Br] 57:485, 1975
34. Zancolli E: Structural and Dynamic Bases of Hand Surgery. 2nd Ed. Lippincott, Philadelphia, 1979

18 Treatment: Soft Tissue Procedures

The surgical plan of treatment of the rheumatoid wrist is based on clinical and radiographic evaluations. Nonsurgical measures may at times suffice to preserve function and prevent deformity. Local steroid injections, rest, and splinting are helpful. Tendon compartments should be injected sparingly, however, for the risk of tendon rupture is always present and may be accentuated by the increased function that is artificially allowed by the relief of pain that follows local steroid injections, and by the introduction of the medication within the tendon sheath.

Changes of joint and tendons go through three stages, similar to those described by Zancolli[50] for the hand: the initial inflammatory period of *synovitis*, a second stage leading to joint *disorganization*, and a final stage of *joint destruction*. The treatment of the wrist with rheumatoid arthritis may include one or more of the following procedures: synovectomy, capsular or ligament repair or reconstruction, tendon transfer, tendon relocation or repair, partial or total arthrodesis, with or without the simultaneous use of implants, and different types of wrist arthroplasties. Only the soft tissue procedures are reviewed in this chapter.

SYNOVECTOMY

Tenosynovitis was recognized as a clinical entity much earlier than joint synovitis. In 1827 Scudamore[38] first recorded involvement in patients suffering from "rheumatism." Helweg[17] specifically mentioned "snapping tendons" in rheumatoid arthritis, and Kahlmeter[20] described tendon nodules in rheumatoid patients. One of the earliest comprehensive studies of tendon lesions in rheumatoid arthritis was published in 1950.[21] Fifty-two percent of 100 patients presented tendon lesions.

The first joint synovectomies were performed for tuberculosis. It was not until much later that reports of synovectomies for rheumatoid arthritis began to appear in the literature. This relatively late application of this procedure was attributed by Steiger and Morscher[42] to the preoccupation of orthopedists of that time with other more prevalent problems (i.e., tuberculosis, osteomyelitis) and to the reluctance to proceed with operative treatment in the face of acute inflammatory changes. Furthermore, synovectomies for rheumatoid arthritis fell into disfavor, largely because of their indiscriminate use, especially in larger joints in advanced stages of destruction. It was later on resurrected[48] after it became apparent that bone and tendon damage in rheumatoid arthritis began, and remained confined for long periods of time, to areas in close contact with diseased synovium. It was natural to wonder what would happen if the synovium were removed.[49] Synovectomies were initially performed in the larger joints, and only infrequently in the wrist. As late as 1967 Arden reported the results of 35 synovectomies. These were good or excellent in 60 percent of knees and in 80 percent of shoulders. Only one was performed in the wrist, and it was unsuccessful.

There are no absolute indications for synovectomies. *Tendon synovectomies* are indicated for persistent disease after at least six months of adequate nonsurgical treatment, and also after extensor tendons rupture or following recurrence of synovitis.[25,26] *Synovectomies* of the wrist *joint* are reserved for patients with persistent, uncontrolled, slowly progressive synovitis after six months of adequate medical treatment,[8,22,25,26,40] particularly if radiologic changes are either absent or minimal. In the absence of radiologic abnormalities, and with meager clinical findings, arthrograms may help to demonstrate synovitis. According to Mitchell and Shepard,[28] even in early rheumatoid arthritis, when the disease appears to be confined entirely to the synovium, there may already be a profound change in the underlying cartilage. Early synovectomy in these cases is helpful. It decreases capsular and ligament stretching, thereby delaying joint instability. It may prevent erosions, progression of damage to the joint surface, and destruction of the underlying subchondral bone. Most important, however, is the excellent relief of pain that is obtained and the improvement of functional capability that follows synovectomies, as well as the chance that is afforded for systemic medications to act on the joints without the encumbrance of large masses of involved synovium. In a retrospective evaluation of synovectomies in rheumatoid arthritis, Mongan[30] found that 67 percent of their patients showed progressive roentgenographic changes postoperatively. In a review of the results of 314 wrist operations in 227 patients, Eiken and collaborators[11] agreed, and they concluded that the hope that synovectomy might arrest or prevent skeletal destruction was not realized. Progression of skeletal changes was found in 74 percent. These authors also observed that the main benefits to be derived from synovectomies are relief of pain and prevention of tendon ruptures. An interesting observation was that the main preoperative problem was pain, but the main complaint following operation was weakness, in spite of what appeared to be increased working capacity. In the opinion of Eiken and coauthors[11] the preoperative pain may actually mask underlying weakness. When pain is relieved, there is a potential increase in activity, which then reveals the preexisting weakness. Namba[33] reviewed 36 patients who had symmetrical wrist findings, but who underwent synovectomies in only one side. Although radiographic evidence of destruction was seen to increase bilaterally, synovectomized wrists exhibited less pain and greater range of motion in 80 percent of patients after an eight-year follow-up. My own experience also suggests that synovectomy is effective for the relief of pain and for the maintenance of function, in spite of postoperative progressive radiographic changes. It is also my belief that when left to its own progress, the wrist with rheumatoid arthritis will undergo more instability and greater destruction than it would have developed had a synovectomy been performed. Recurrence of synovitis is not infrequent. However, the new synovium is less likely to show severe inflammatory changes, since regenerated synovium contains fewer cells and is less vascular.[42]

Dorsal synovectomies are performed more frequently. These may be done for dorsal *tenosynovitis*, a most frequent manifestation of rheumatoid disease, at times present well in advance of joint involvement or for dorsal *wrist joint synovitis*, although customarily all tendon and joint compartments should be examined at the time of operation. Synovectomy of the palmar compartments of the radiocarpal and midcarpal joints has been proposed for those patients who exhibit radiographic evidence of palmar articular synovitis, and in whom the overall joint architecture is still well preserved.[45] Not all patients, however, have a satisfactory result from synovectomy. This appears to be related to the ultrastructure of synovium. Patients who maintain good clinical results are likely to develop joint lining cells with many of the features of normal synovial cells. Most important, these cells are supported, in the good cases, by an envelope of dense collagenous tissue which may be a barrier against aggressive infiltration by rheumatoid inflammatory cells.

In some patients, a thorough clinical, radiographic, and intraoperative evaluation may indicate the need for an "all compartment" synovectomy, which includes both palmar and dorsal tendon spaces, palmar and dorsal radiocarpal and intercarpal, and distal radioulnar and ulnocarpal joints.

SURGICAL TECHNIQUE

Although a skin incision over the area of most significant synovitis may be used, my experience and that of others indicates that the involvement found intraoperatively is usually more extensive than suspected clinically and radiographically, justifying a wider exposure, now standard for most procedures in the dorsum of the wrist (Fig. 18-1). A straight dorsal incision is preferred, obliquely placed from the proximal one third of the second metacarpal, proximally and ulnarward to a point 5 cm proximal to the projection of the distal radioulnar joint (Fig. 18-1A). The incision should be long enough to afford satisfactory exposure without excessive skin retraction.[10] An area of frequent postoperative skin necrosis and dehiscence, immediately distal and ulnar to Lister's tubercle, directly over the extensor tendon to the long finger, should not be crossed by the incision. The surgical approach should be ulnar to this area, keeping this tendon under the intact radial skin flap. The skin must be handled with utmost care in these patients, avoiding rough retraction and unnecessary dissection; necrosis of the skin edges exposes the tendons beneath, and may require extensive plastic maneuvers for closure (Fig. 18-2). The skin flaps are kept full thickness by dissecting immediately on the plane of the dorsal retinaculum. As many as possible of perforating and longitudinal vessels and, of course, all superficial nerve branches are kept intact within these skin flaps. Only those vessels that cross the operative field are sacrificed when necessary. When a synovectomy of the extensor tendon compartments is not anticipated, dissection and elevation of the skin flaps should be kept to a minimum. In these cases, the extensor pollicis longus tendon is unroofed and retracted, and the wrist joint is entered using a longitudinal subcapsular incision through the floor of its tunnel (Figs. 18-1B,C). In most patients, however, when a tenosynovectomy is needed, the entire expanse of the attenuated but always present dorsal retinaculum must be exposed. The compartment for the extensor carpi ulnaris tendon is opened first, using a step-cut retinacular incision (Fig. 18-1D). This incision creates a longer distal retinacular flap, based radially, which will be used to retain the extensor

carpi ulnaris in a more dorsal position at the completion of the procedure.[23,41] Proximal and distal transverse incisions are then used to delineate the width of the retinacular flap that will be elevated. Care is taken to preserve the deep antebrachial fascia proximal to the retinaculum and the pretendinous fascia distal to the retinaculum. An exception is the forearm fascia over the extensor carpi ulnaris which may need to be incised longitudinally to free this muscle enough to allow its mobilization and its replacement dorsal to the ulnar head during closure. In most cases, preservation of the forearm and hand fascia will prevent postoperative tenting of the extensor tendons. When the range of dorsiflexion of the wrist is near-normal, the danger of bowstringing is increased. In these cases a very narrow proximal retinacular strip may be preserved. All involved tendon synovium is then excised by sharp dissection and by the selective use of rongeurs. Savill[37] suggested that it is the mechanical decompression of the tendons by relocation over the retinaculum that is important, rather than the synovectomy itself. Abernethy and Dennyson[1] presented a similar clinical experience. Even in the presence of florid synovitis, they did not do an active synovectomy. This placement of tendons in the more favorable environment superficial to the relocated retinaculum, was sufficient to produce a gradual disappearance of the synovitis. Clayton agrees that meticulous removal is not necessary, as long as the tendons are replaced over the retinaculum and under the fat: "rheumatoid synovium does not proliferate and invade tendons in healthy fat."[10]

Rheumatoid nodules within tendons may be evacuated by short longitudinal incisions on the tendon surface, later repaired with very fine sutures (Fig. 18-1E). Likewise, frayed-out areas of tendon may be reinforced or repaired when present. Once this step is completed, the extensor tendons are retracted both medially and laterally to expose the underlying wrist capsule and the infratendinous retinaculum. The radiocarpal joint is exposed by a transverse incision a few millimeters distal to the dorsal rim of the radius, leaving a proximal apron that can be used for later capsular repair (Fig. 18-1F). The distal capsular flap is elevated from the scaphoid and lunate, and then from the

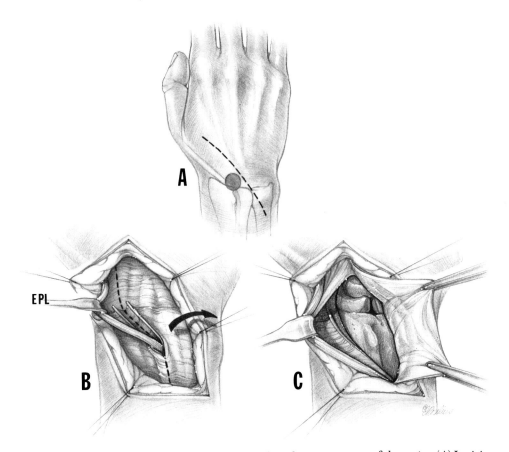

Fig. 18-1. Surgical approach recommended for dorsal synovectomy of the wrist. (*A*) Incision. Circle indicates intersection of dorsal wrist crease and extensor tendon to the long finger, frequent site of postoperative necrosis and dehiscence of wound margins. (*B*) When the extensor tendons do not need to be exposed, the extensor pollicis longus tendon (EPL) is unroofed, and (*C*) the joint is entered by a longitudinal division of the dorsal capsule and periosteum. When work needs to be done within the tendon compartments, the entire expanse of the supratendinous retinaculum is first exposed.

capitate, exposing both radiocarpal and midcarpal joints. A synovectomy of the radiocarpal and midcarpal joints may then be performed (Fig. 18-1G). The distal radioulnar joint can also be exposed through a longitudinal incision that connects with the first to complete a L shape capsular incision (Fig. 18-1F). The dorsal interosseous neurovascular bundle is identified at this point, ligated or coagulated and divided proximal to the capsular incision. A synovectomy of the distal radioulnar and ulnocarpal compartments can now be completed. The distal ulna is either left intact, relocated against the radius, or treated according to the pre-

operative clinical and radiographic evaluation. Soft tissue stabilization of the distal ulna depends on whether or not there is a radioulnar subluxation (with ulna dorsal) or a destruction of the distal radioulnar joint requiring ulnar excision or radioulnar fusion with the creation of a more proximal ulnar pseudarthrosis to restore pronation and supination.

Palmar synovium may be reached through the dorsal approach by applying distal traction to the hand and using a pair of fine tipped rongeurs, unless a decision was made preoperatively to use an additional palmar approach. A synovectomy of the

(*Text continues on page 372.*)

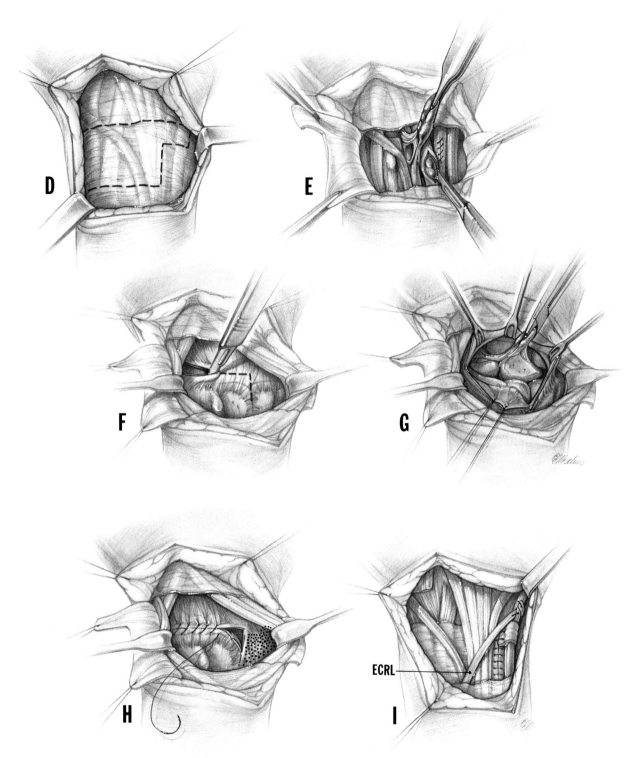

Fig. 18-1. (cont.) (*D*) A step-cut retinacular incision is used. (*E*) Both retinacular flaps are elevated. Tendon synovectomy, excision of intratendinous nodules, and tendon repair may now be performed. (*F*) Tendons are retracted medially and laterally and the dorsal radioulnocarpal capsule is divided using an L-shaped incision. (*G*) The articular stage of the procedure is completed. (*H*) Capsular closure. (*I*) The supratendinous retinaculum is placed under the extensor tendons. The long slip of retinaculum, from the initial step-cut incision, is looped around the extensor carpi ulnaris. The drawing depicts a transfer of the extensor carpi radialis longus tendon to the extensor carpi ulnaris, just proximal to its insertion.

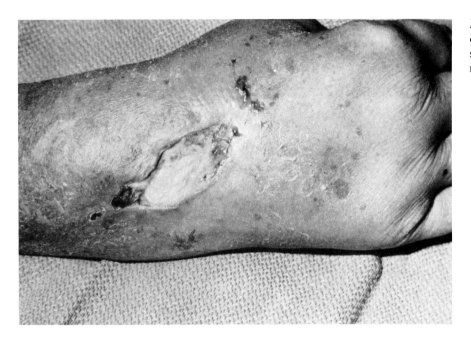

Fig. 18-2. Necrosis of skin edges following dorsal tenosynovectomy in patient with rheumatoid arthritis.

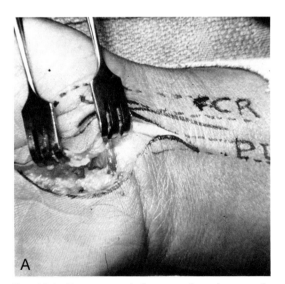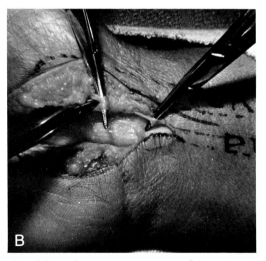

Fig. 18-3. Recommended approach to the carpal tunnel and the palmar compartments of the wrist. *A:* Incision (see text). The flexor carpi radialis (FCR) and palmaris longus (PL) tendons are projected on the skin. Between them (solid line) is the palmar cutaneous branch of the median nerve. *B:* The carpal tunnel is exposed. The median nerve can be seen in the depth of the wound. The composite flap of skin, subcutaneous tissue, and transverse carpal ligament carries with it the intact palmar cutaneous nerve and its divisions. (From Taleisnik J: The palmar cutaneous branch of the median nerve and the approach to the carpal tunnel. An anatomical study. J Bone Joint Surg [Am] 55:1212, 1973.)

Fig. 18-4. Synovitis of palmar compartment of the wrist joint. *A*: Synovial proliferation between fibers of radiocarpal ligaments. *B*: Synovium being removed (arrow). *C*: Appearance after synovectomy. The patient's hand is to the left. Tendons retracted ulnarward. (From Taleisnik J: Rheumatoid synovitis of the volar compartment of the wrist joint: It's radiological signs and its contribution to wrist and hand deformity. J Hand Surg 4:526, 1979.)

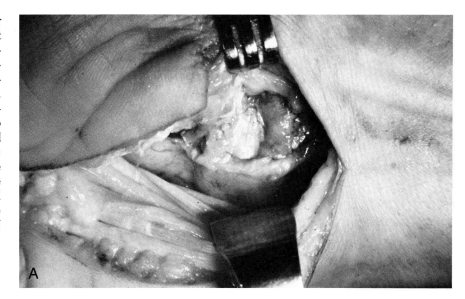

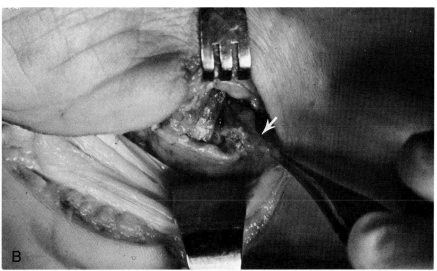

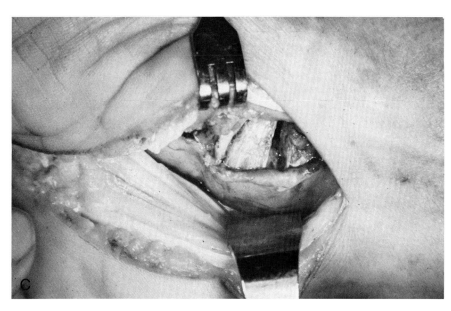

palmar joint and tendon compartments may be done at the same time of a dorsal synovectomy or as an independent procedure. The palmar approach starts distally and proceeds proximally, initially along the interthenar crease, reaching the wrist crease on the ulnar side of the axis of the ring finger ray (Fig. 18-3A). At the level of the transverse wrist creases, it curves radially to just the medial margin of the flexor carpi radialis tendon. It then curves back proximally and in an ulnar direction. In this fashion, the palmar cutaneous branch of the median nerve remains protected under the flexor carpi radialis tendon, and its terminal branches remain intact within the radial palmar skin flap (Fig. 18-3B).[44] A flexor tenosynovectomy and a decompression of the median nerve are done when needed. The floor of the carpal canal may also be exposed and evaluated by inspection and palpation. Inspection may show synovium protruding through the weak capsular areas between the fibers of the palmar radiocarpal ligaments (Figs. 18-4A, 10C). Palpation may disclose sharp bony spicules protruding through the floor of the carpal canal (Fig. 16-8). Using very fine-tipped rongeurs a palmar synovectomy can be done. The radiocarpal and radioulnar ligaments are usually intact (Fig.

18-4C); through a gap between their fibers the scaphoid may be seen in a palmarflexed position, its waist detached from the undersurface of the radiocapitate ligament. When a scapholunate dissociation is present, the proximal pole of the scaphoid is subluxated dorsally and appears to be deep when visualized from the palmar side. With the dorsal joint still exposed, a ligament reconstruction (Fig. 18-5), or else a modified dorsal capsulodesis[4] may then be performed to stabilize the scaphoid (Fig. 11-24). The weak areas between the fibers of the palmar ligaments are repaired. Sharp bony spicules should be removed and bare bone covered by local soft tissue. A flexor tenosynovectomy is completed. It is important at this point to assess the freedom of excursion of the individual tendons. If full range of finger motion is not restored, further exploration of the tendons within the palm or within the fingers is indicated.[27] The tourniquet may be released and hemostasis completed at this stage. If there is persistent "surface bleeding" the tourniquet is reinflated, the operation completed, and a suction drain is used for 24 to 48 hours. Closure of the dorsal incision is performed in layers. When a tenosynovectomy is performed the dorsal retinaculum is placed under the extensor tendons, both to pro-

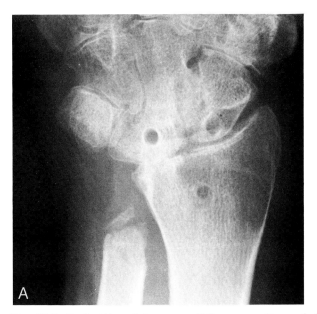 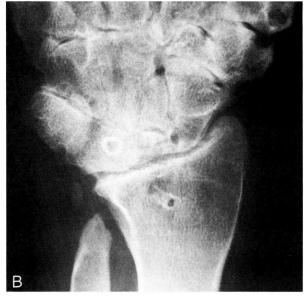

Fig. 18-5. Early (A) and three-year follow-up radiograph (B) of wrist with scapholunate dissociation in patient with rheumatoid arthritis, treated by ligamentous reconstruction (see Fig. 11-19).

vide support to the underlying joint and to place the tendons in an environment where recurrent synovitis will not be a problem.[1,37] The step-cut opening of the pretendinous retinaculum provides a radially based flap which is then used to loop around the extensor carpi ulnaris to retain it in a more dorsal position (Figs. 18-1I, 20-6H). When an extensor tendon synovectomy was not performed, and the dorsal retinaculum was incised over the extensor pollicis longus, the retinaculum is repaired but placed under the extensor pollicis longus, leaving only this tendon superficial to the retinacular plane. Subcutaneous and subcuticular skin closure is preferred. When a palmar synovectomy was performed, and after the capsular rents or openings are repaired, the transverse carpal ligament is left unsutured and only the skin is closed. A bulky dressing with plaster reinforcement is usually applied. When suction drainage is used, it is passed through intact skin and is left accessible through the dressings, to be removed 24 to 48 hours following surgery without disturbing the postoperative dressings. Full finger motion is encouraged immediately after surgery. The bulky dressing is replaced with a short arm circular plaster or splint 3 to 5 days postoperatively. This immobilization is continued for no longer than 7 to 10 days for synovectomies alone, or for 3 to 4 weeks when tendon repair or transfer or a dorsal capsulodesis of the scaphoid were performed. It is not unusual to incorporate dorsal extensor assist devices to preserve full finger extension. Following synovectomies, a program of gradual wrist exercises with intermittent support provided by removable splints is allowed after the surgical incision is healed and the postoperative reaction has subsided. The length of postoperative immobilization may vary if additional procedures (i.e., Lauenstein's or Darrach's) were performed.

CAPSULAR AND LIGAMENT
REPAIR AND RECONSTRUCTION

Capsular and ligament deficiencies maybe suspected preoperatively, but are more frequently found and treated during synovectomies. Placement of the dorsal retinaculum deep to the extensor tendons is the most common type of capsular

reinforcement. The indication for a ligamentous reconstruction to correct a scapholunate dissociation in rheumatoid arthritis is exceptional (Fig. 18-5). One of several techniques may be used.[16,35] It is important to differentiate a true scapholunate dissociation from a type II ulnar translocation (see Chapter 13). The distinction is important, for in true scapholunate dissociation the scaphoid is the only *abnormal* carpal bone, while in a type II ulnar translocation, the scaphoid is the only *normal* carpal bone, left behind by the ulnarly displaced carpus (Fig. 13-4). Any attempts to join the scaphoid to the displaced lunate will succeed only in adding the scaphoid to the abnormally subluxated carpus (Fig. 18-6). For true scapholunate dissociations, most patients with rheumatoid disease will do well if the scaphoid is just reduced and pinned to the lunate and capitate for 6 to 8 weeks. An alternative to this is to anchor the distal pole of the scaphoid in a dorsal position by a modification of the dorsal capsulodesis procedure described by Blatt.[4] The distal pole of the scaphoid is brought dorsally, and sutured to the dorsal capsule using nonabsorbable material that is passed through the capsule and through drill-holes in the scaphoid distal to its axis of rotation (Fig. 11-24).

Capsular repair is also indicated for areas of weakness that are found during palmar synovectomies (spaces of Poirier; see Chapter 2). The treatment of the unstable distal ulna and the restoration of ulnocarpal relationship are discussed later.

TENDON TRANSFERS,
RELOCATIONS, AND REPAIRS

Relocation of the extensor carpi ulnaris dorsal to the distal ulna has already been discussed. For those patients exhibiting excessive radial metacarpal shift, correction of alignment may be achieved by detaching the extensor carpi radialis longus from the base of the second metacarpal and transfering its insertion to the ulnar side of the carpus (Fig. 18-1I).[9,12] This removes its radially deviating influence on the metacarpals. By attaching it under tension to the insertion of the extensor carpi ulnaris *distal* to the ulnar head, additional benefits are derived. The transferred tendon provides a pulleylike effect on the underlying finger extensors assisting

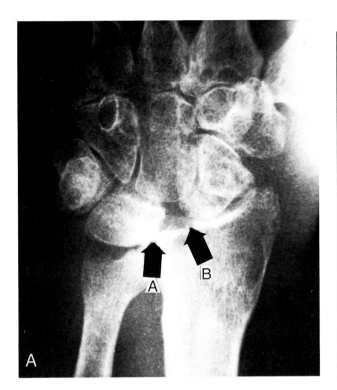

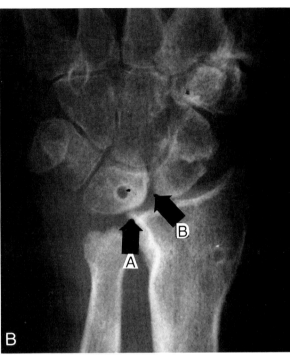

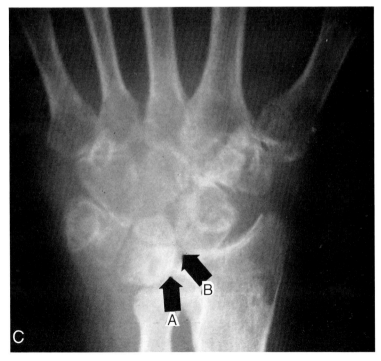

Fig. 18-6. True scapholunate dissociation should be differentiated from a type II ulnar translocation. *A:* Ulnar translocation type II shows scapholunate gap A-B, erroneously diagnosed as a simple scapholunate dissociation. *B:* Ligamentous reconstruction results in closure of scapholunate gap A-B. *C:* The ulnar translocation continues uncorrected. Scapholunate tenodesis succeeded only in changing a type II ulnar translocation into a type I.

in preventing bowstringing after the dorsal retinaculum is rerouted deep to the extensor compartment. This transfer also assists in keeping the extensor carpi ulnaris in its more dorsal position. Finally, it tends to elevate the ulnar carpus from its subluxated position, therefore correcting carpal malrotation and decreasing metacarpal descent. In laboratory studies in cadaver models Boyce and collaborators[5] confirmed the rebalancing potential of this transfer for those patients who have lost the stabilizing influence of dorsoulnar ligaments and fibrocartilaginous structures. The potential effect of the extensor carpi radialis longus transfer on the ulnar drift of the fingers at the metacarpophalangeal joints is not as clear.[5] However, persistence of the uncorrected radial metacarpal shift may be a factor in the recurrence of ulnar drift of the fingers after metacarpophalangeal procedures with or

Fig. 18-7. Clinical (*A*) and intraoperative (*B*) appearance of distal ulna in patient with multiple extensor tendon ruptures. Rough bone spicule from ulnar head is seen through dorsal capsule.

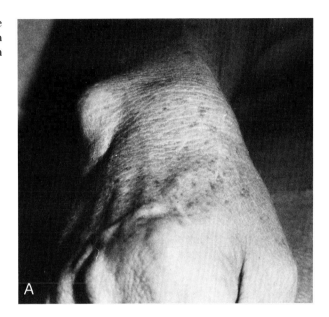

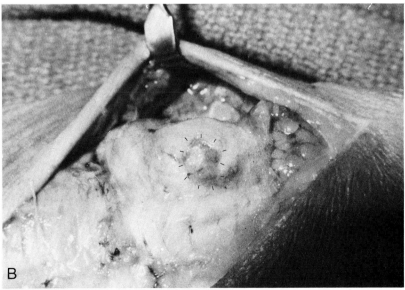

without arthroplasties. Transfer of the extensor carpi radialis longus to the lunate has also been proposed for the correction of VISI deformities.[23]

Tendon ruptures in the presence of rheumatoid disease were described in 1956 by Straub and Wilson.[43] These tears are due to mechanical or chemical causes and are secondary to invasion of the tendon substance by rheumatoid tissue, to constriction of tendons under the dorsal retinaculum, and to attrition against rough bony surfaces (Figs. 16-8, 18-7).[46,47] Other ruptures may follow repeated local steroid injections,[29] local tendon infarcts produced by the occlusion of vincular vessels by rheumatoid tissue[24,36] fibrinoid degeneration of collagen fibers in the tendons[21,36] interference by the thickened synovium with normal fluid exchange[7] and ischemic changes within the tendon due to compression.[13] In all likelihood most ruptures are secondary to a combination of factors.[13] Prevention of ruptures is preferable to their surgical correction.[39] Persistent tenosynovitis, the "scallop sign" (Fig. 18-8),[14] a dorsal displacement of the ulna in relation to the carpus (Fig. 18-7), and wrist pain during finger motions, all suggest the need for truly prophylactic treatment by tenosynovectomy and by correction of the distal radioulnar joint relationship.[8,13,19,49] Tendon ruptures in patients with rheumatoid disease are seldom amenable to direct repair. At times gaps left by tendon retraction and attrition can be bridged by using interposed tendon grafts, particularly in the case of a relatively recent rupture of the extensor pollicis longus. In my experience, however, loss of extensor tendons to the digits is best treated by tendon transfers. As soon as one extensor tendon is ruptured, the wrist should be splinted and, in many cases, active dynamic assist provided to all fingers to delay or prevent further ruptures until tendon repair is performed. The choice of procedure depends on the number of torn tendons, and the availability of suitable transfers. In my opinion, the isolated loss of extension to the little finger is satisfactorily corrected by end-to-side tenodesis of the distal stump of the extensor digiti quinti to the extensor tendon to the ring finger (Fig. 18-9A). This procedure requires meticulous postoperative supervision, for improper tension at the junction and postoperative adhesions may compromise mo-

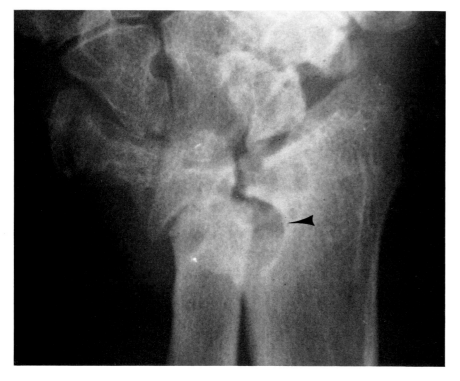

Fig. 18-8. "Scallop sign" (cavitation of distal radius opposite ulnar head: arrow) is a frequent radiographic sign in patients with rheumatoid arthritis and rupture of extensor tendons.

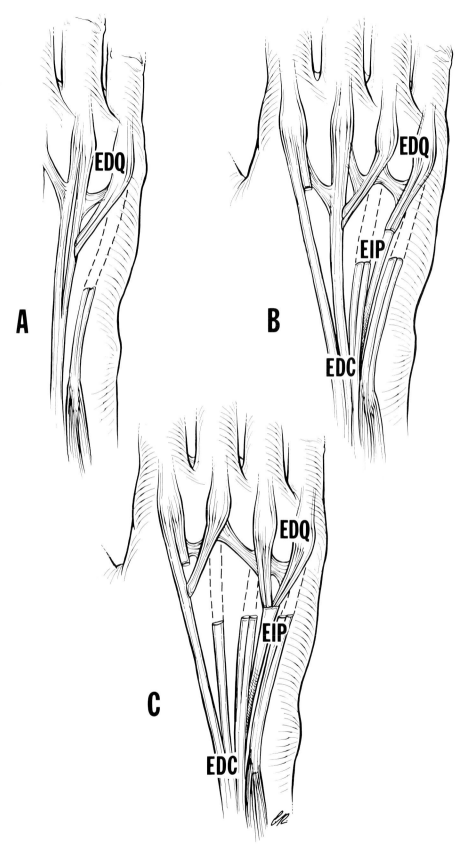

Fig. 18-9. Diagrammatic representation of common techniques recommended for the treatment of extensor and flexor tendons rupture or tear.
(Fig. continues on next page.)

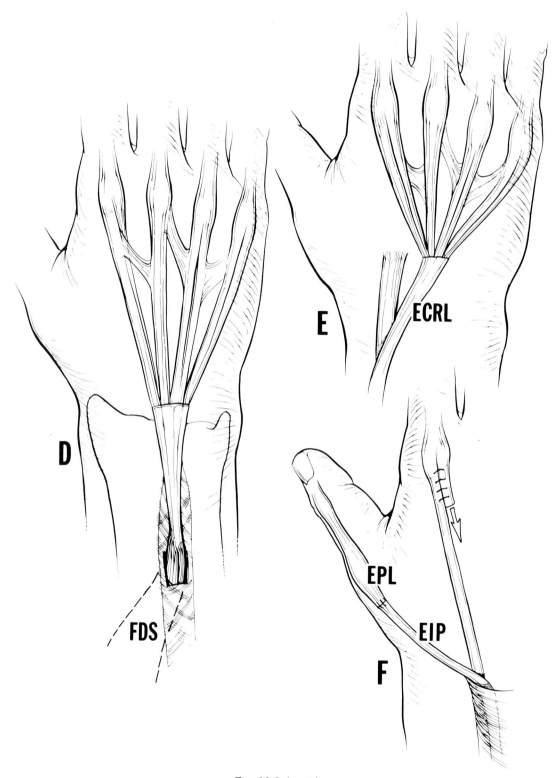

D

FDS

E

ECRL

EPL

EIP

F

Fig. 18-9 (cont.)

Fig. 18-9 (cont.)

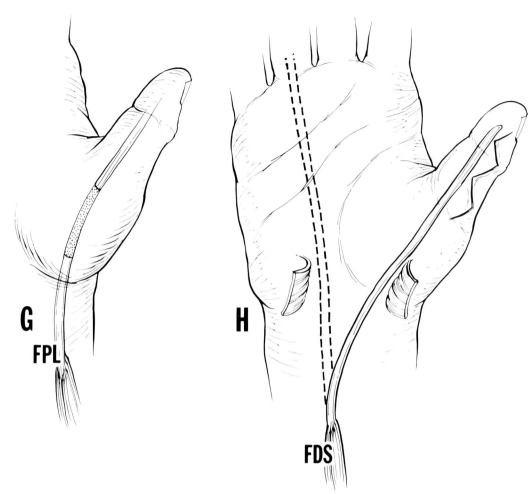

tion of both the recipient little finger and the donor ring finger. These difficulties have prompted some surgeons to abandon this technique in favor of tendon grafting, using the palmaris longus, the plantaris, or both, or one half of the extensor carpi radialis longus as donors. The anatomic characteristics of the extensor mechanism to the little finger should be kept in mind. The incidence of a relatively large extensor digitorum communis to this digit is only 23 percent.[34] In most cases, this tendon is just a junctura tendinii from the communis tendon to the ring finger. Therefore, in most cases, a double tendon going to the little finger does not represent independent extensor digitorum communis and extensor digiti quinti tendons, but rather a large, split, double extensor digiti quinti.

The loss of extensors to both ring and little

fingers may be treated by a transfer of the extensor indicis proprius to the extensor digiti quinti and an end-to-side tenodesis of the ring finger extensor to that of the long finger (Fig. 18-9B). If the latter is also torn, then the transferred extensor indicis proprius is used to activate both the ring and little finger extensors, while the long finger extensor is tenodesed to that of the index finger (Fig. 18-9C). An alternate plan calls for the transfer of a flexor digitorum superficialis to the long and ring fingers, and of the extensor indicis proprius to the extensor digiti quinti.[31] In general, however, Clayton's suggestion that "the simplest procedure is probably the best" is most valid in these cases.[8] If the extensor indicis proprius is needed to activate a torn extensor pollicis longus, then a more distant transfer utilizing a wrist motor, particularly the extensor carpi radialis longus,[39] or one of the flexor digitorum superficialis may be used.[27] When all finger extensors have ruptured, Backhouse and co-workers[3] recommend the use of the intact extensor pollicis longus as a common motor for the fingers, with restoration of extension to the thumb by activation with the extensor pollicis brevis or the abductor pollicis longus. My preference for rupture of all extensors is the use of the flexor digitorum superficialis, as proposed by Nalebuff,[31] when the proximal interphalangeal (PIP) joints of the fingers are stable (Fig. 18-9D). In the presence of swan neck deformities, it is preferable to leave the superficialis tendons intact, and to use a wrist extensor as the motor (Fig. 18-9E).

Rupture of the extensor pollicis longus can rarely be repaired directly. Infrequently, continuity may be restored using an intervening tendon graft. In

most patients tendon transfers are needed, usually using the extensor indicis proprius (Figs. 16-5 and 18-9F), although other tendons (extensor pollicis brevis, a slip of the abductor pollicis longus, the palmaris longus)[3,18] have also been proposed. The choice of donor depends on the surgeon's experience, on the number of transfers required and on the availability of intact motors. The most frequent rupture of flexor tendons involve the flexor pollicis longus and the flexors to the index. It may be treated by a transfer of a flexor digitorum superficialis to the flexor pollicis longus (Fig. 18-9H), and an end-to-side tenodesis of the profundus flexor to the index to that of the long finger. The isolated loss of a profundus tendon to a single digit with a satisfactory flexor digitorum superficials may not require treatment or may be treated by stabilization of the involved distal joint by tenodesis or by fu-

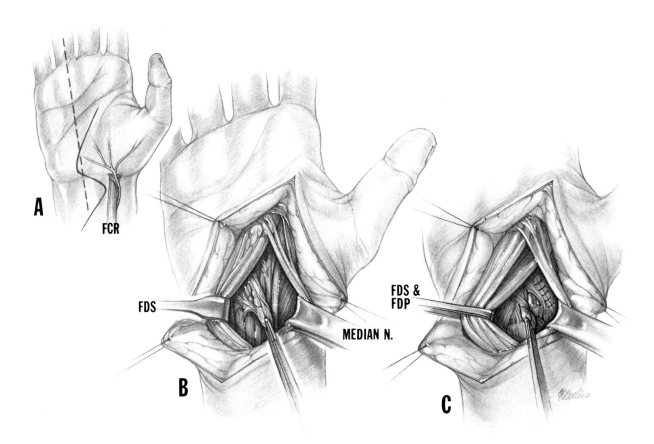

Fig. 18-10. Surgical approach recommended for palmar synovectomy of the wrist. *A*: Surgical incision. *B*: Tendon stage of the procedure. *C*: Joint exposure, palmar synovectomy, and repair of capsule.

sion, when the distal joint itself is destroyed by the disease or unstable. In general, attempts at restoration of profundus function are reserved for those patients with loss of *both* flexors to any single digit (Fig. 18-11), or of multiple flexors, or when the repair is simply done by suture to an adjacent digit's tendon. The condition of the middle and distal digital joints should be good enough to warrant the operative treatment and the prolonged postoperative care. In all cases, the cause of the tendon rupture should be found and corrected. When both flexor tendons to a finger are ruptured, and the digital joints are less than satisfactory, a fusion of both middle and distal joints may be performed, particularly for the index finger, where it will provide a stable pillar for pinching against the thumb.

TECHNIQUE OF TENDON TRANSFER

Single or Multiple Ruptures of Extensor Tendons to the Fingers

The repair of torn extensor tendons is usually performed after a dorsal tenosynovectomy, and any additional procedures have been completed (i.e., joint synovectomies, arthrodeses or arthroplasties, excision of the distal ulna) (Fig. 18-9). A smooth gliding bed must be provided by placing the extensor retinaculum deep to the repair.[8,9] In the case of a single loss, frequently to the little finger, the extensor digiti quinti tendon is sutured to the extensor tendon to the ring finger. Usually, the distal stump of the extensor digiti quinti is too short to allow weaving it to the donor tendon, a more secure fixation. The tension applied to the the suture should be such that full extension of the digit is obtained with the wrist in palmarflexion, and satisfactory flexion is produced with the wrist in full dorsiflexion. Full passive digital flexion should be possible without tearing the sutured junction when the wrist is held in neutral or slight dorsiflexion. The stump of the ruptured tendon is sutured to the neighboring intact extensor using # 4-0 nonabsorbable material. When the extensor indicis proprius is to be used as a donor, it should be divided distally enough to provide sufficient length. The extensor indicis proprius tendon is

always ulnar and deep to the extensor digitorum communis to the index finger. Prior to its division, it is my preference to suture the distal portion of the extensor indicis proprius to the communis tendon while slight proximal traction is placed on the extensor indicis proprius tendon. This should prevent excessive extension lag of the index during the immediate and early postoperative period.[8] The tendon is then divided just proximal to this suture line and transferred to activate either the extensor digiti quinti alone, or the extensors to both ring and little fingers. Either a side-to-side or a weave-through technique is used. Sutures are always fine and nonabsorbable. The tension applied to the transfer is similar to that described for the repair of the isolated rupture of the extensor digiti quinti. This procedure may be performed under regional intravenous anesthesia, in which case, once the sutures are completed, the tourniquet may be released and the patient requested to actively extend the fingers. The tension can then be adjusted and the skin closed under local anesthesia.[15,25,27] When all finger extensors are torn, a different transfer is required. This must be strong enough to activate all four fingers, and must have a similar excursion to allow for satisfactory extension without loss of flexion. Nalebuff and Patel[32] have advocated the use of flexor digitorum superficialis transfers, a procedure first proposed by Boyes[6] for patients with radial nerve palsy. Instead of bringing the superficialis tendon to the dorsum through a window in the interosseous membrane, Nalebuff and Patel proposed that the transfer be passed subcutaneously around the radial border of the forearm. Two incisions are needed in addition to the one used to expose the dorsum of the wrist: one in the distal palmar crease to explore the tendons and divide them proximal to their decussation, and a second on the anterior aspect of the forearm, longitudinal, and ulnar to the midline, to retrieve the tendons. These are then routed subcutaneously around the ulnar border of the forearm, brought into the dorsal wrist incision, and sutured into the distal stumps of the finger extensors. Usually, one superficialis tendon, that of the ring finger, suffices to activate all four finger extensors. Transfer through the interosseous membrane, as originally suggested by Boyes,[6] provides a more direct line of pull. The type of distal suture and the tension to be applied to the transfer follow principles already mentioned. A special circumstance is present in patients where tendon ruptures will require arthroplasties of dislocated metacarpophalangeal joints.[27] Although it is my general preference to complete the wrist stage prior to initiating reconstructive procedures for the hand, in these cases the approach is reversed. Otherwise, the tendon transfers will be inactive or poorly active until the metacarpophalangeal arthroplasties are performed, increasing the potential for adhesions. Unless both procedures (arthroplasties and tendon repairs) are done simultaneously, which requires a more sophisticated and complex postoperative management, it is preferable to do the arthroplasties first, keep these movable through passive exercises and dynamic exten-

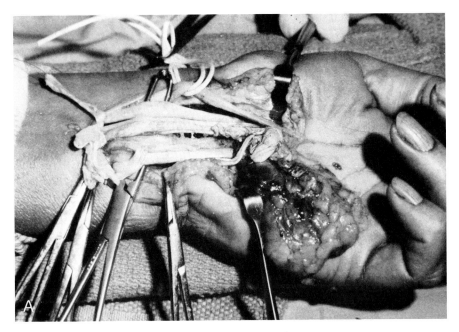

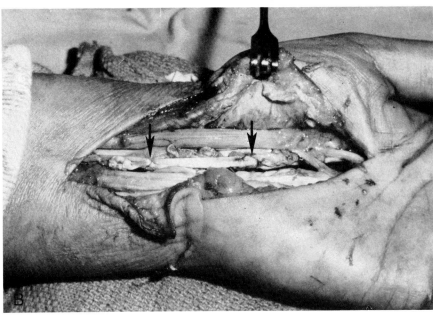

Fig. 18-11. A: Patient with rheumatoid arthritis shows multiple superficial flexor tendon ruptures. Flexor profundi are preserved except for the index finger. B: Appearance after insertion of a tendon graft to bridge gap between ends of flexor profundus to index finger (arrows).

sor splints, completing the repair of the extensor tendons during a second stage.[27] Postoperatively the wrist and hand are placed in a well-padded compression dressing, reinforced with plaster splints supporting the proximal phalanges of the donor (index) and recipient fingers, with the proximal joints 10 to 20 degrees short of full extension. The wrist is maintained in neutral from dorsal or palmar flexion, particularly from dorsiflexion, since this would allow the tendons to bowstring against the dorsal surgical incision.[8] Both interphalangeal joints are left free. Motion of these joints is encouraged as soon as the patient is comfortable. This exercise program will not interfere with the tendon suture, and will help to prevent excessive postoperative edema, and to preserve gliding of the extensor structures. Three to four days later, the bulky dressings are removed. If immobilization of the wrist is required (i.e., following excision of the distal ulna, wrist arthroplasties or fusions), a short or long arm circular plaster dressing is applied; otherwise, a removable splint may be used. In either case, dorsal dynamic assistance is provided to the proximal phalanges of each finger. The middle and distal joints remain free to move. Carefully supervised, gentle active flexion against dorsal rubber-band traction is permitted. At three to four weeks after the operation, the patient is allowed to remove all splints several times a day and the fingers and wrist are freely exercised. All immobilization is discontinued at six weeks postoperatively, although night splinting may be necessary for a longer time, particularly if an extension lag of the fingers is present. Limitation of passive flexion of the little finger may develop quite rapidly. The surgeon should be well aware of this potential and treat it by appropriate splinting as soon as it becomes apparent. Gliding of the repaired extensor mechanism should be secured while fixed unyielding adhesions are avoided throughout the postoperative period (Fig. 16-4).

Extensor Indicis Proprius Transfer for Rupture of the Extensor Pollicis Longus

A curvilinear incision is used along the ulnar border of the first metacarpal, starting proximally at the level of Lister's tubercle, and prolonged distally to allow a comfortable exposure of the distal stump of the extensor pollicis longus. The extensor

indicis proprius tendon is exposed through a short longitudinal incision ulnar and proximal to the second metacarpophalangeal joint. It is divided using the same technique and precautions discussed for its use as a transfer for multiple extensor tendon ruptures. The tendon is then withdrawn through the first incision and is then woven through the distal stump of the extensor pollicis longus. The tension of the transferred tendon should be enough to produce full firm extension of the thumb with the wrist in palmar flexion, and to allow full thumb adduction and flexion with the wrist in dorsiflexion (Fig. 16-5). Fine nonabsorbable sutures are used. A synovectomy must be done at the same time and any areas of roughness that could have contributed to the tendon tear are excised and covered with soft tissue. The postoperative management is identical to that recommended for the extensor tendons of the fingers.

Rupture of Flexor Digitorum Profundus and Superficialis at the Wrist

The flexor tendon compartment is exposed using a universal carpal tunnel incision (Fig. 18-10) that is prolonged proximally and distally to provide for a satisfactory exposure of the involved synovium and of the tendon rupture or ruptures. A synovectomy is performed; any rough bony ridges or spicules that are palpable in the floor of the carpal canal are excised and raw areas covered with adjacent soft tissues. Isolated profundus ruptures are easily treated by side-to-side suture to an adjacent intact profundus tendon. When the proximal tendon excursion is satisfactory, continuity may be restored by a tendon graft to the distal tendon stump (Fig. 18-11B). The postoperative care is similar in principle to that used for extensor tendon repairs and transfers. Dynamic substitutes for finger flexion are provided by rubber bands passed through hooks cemented to the nails of the involved digits, and through a safety pin or band on the anterior aspect of the wrist.

Rupture of the Flexor Pollicis Longus

Exposure is similar to that for palmar tenosynovectomies. Rupture of the flexor pollicis longus is frequently caused by attenuation and attrition against a bony roughness arising from either the distal pole of the scaphoid or the tubercle of the trapezium (Fig. 16-8) poking through the palmar ligaments and capsule. A synovectomy is performed, and the rough bony prominence is excised; the remaining raw area of bone is covered with adjacent soft tissues. If the distal tendon stump is easily accessible, and excursion of the muscle-tendon unit is satisfactory, a bridge graft is a good solution to the problem (Fig. 18-9G). The donor tendon may be the palmaris longus, a slip from the flexor carpi radialis or from the abductor pollicis longus.[27] A slip of a flexor digitorum superficialis may also be used. When the distal tendon cannot be retrieved into the wrist incision, a transfer is preferable. The flexor digitorum superficialis of the ring finger is a suitable donor, provided its excision does not result in increased instability of the proximal interphalangeal (PIP) joint (Fig. 18-9H). The thumb is exposed using a midlateral incision or a zigzag approach that does not cross the entire width of the digit, but just one half. The flexor digitorum superficialis is then threaded along the flexor pollicis longus tunnel and is retrieved distally. A routine pull-out wire technique is used to attach the tendon to the insertion site of the flexor pollicis longus on the distal phalanx. The tension of the transferred tendon is such that in full wrist dorsiflexion, with the digit's incision closed, full flexion of the thumb is obtained. Conversely, in palmarflexion of the wrist, full extension of the thumb should be possible without disruption of the repair. After skin closure, a well-padded compression dressing is applied, incorporating a dorsal plaster splint with the wrist in 30 degrees of palmarflexion, the thumb metacarpal palmar to the second metacarpal, and the proximal and distal joints of the thumb in slight semiflexion. At three to five days postoperatively, this dressing is removed, a metal hook is cemented to the nail (usually distal to the button used for the pull-out wire suture), and a short arm thumb spica is applied, maintaining the wrist and thumb in the position described. The palmar half of the cast opposite the thumb is removed to allow rubber band-assisted flexion, and active extension to the dorsal plaster stop. At three weeks postoperatively continuous immobilization is discontinued and a splint is applied, which the patient removes several times a day for active exercises. At six weeks postoperatively all immobilization and protection are discarded.

REFERENCES

1. Abernethy PJ, Dennyson WG: Decompression of the extensor tendons at the wrist in rheumatoid arthritis. J Bone Joint Surg [Br] 61:64, 1979
2. Arden GP: The results of synovectomy in rheumatoid arthritis. In Chapchal G: Synovectomy and Arthroplasty in Rheumatoid Arthritis. Georg Thieme, Stuttgart, 1967
3. Backhouse KM, Harrison SH, Hutchings RT: Color Atlas of Rheumatoid Hand Surgery. Yearbook Medical Publications, Chicago, 1981
4. Blatt G: Personal communication, 1981
5. Boyce T, Youm Y, Sprague BL, Flatt AE: Clinical and experimental studies on the effect of extensor carpi radialis longus transfer in the rheumatoid hand. J Hand Surg 3:390, 1978
6. Boyes JH: Bunnell's Surgery of the Hand. 5th Ed. Lippincott, Philadelphia, 1970
7. Campbell RD Jr, Straub LR: Surgical consideration for rheumatoid disease in the forearm and wrist. Am J Surg 109:361, 1965
8. Clayton ML: Surgical treatment at the wrist in rheumatoid arthritis. A review of thirty-seven patients. J Bone Joint Surg [Am] 47:741, 1965
9. Clayton ML, Ferlic DC: The wrist in rheumatoid arthritis. Clin Orthop 106:192, 1975
10. Clayton ML: The caput ulnae syndrome: Update. In Strickland JW, Steichen JB (eds): Difficult Problems in Hand Surgery. p 199. Mosby, St. Louis, 1982
11. Eiken O: Assessment of surgery of the rheumatoid wrist. Scand J Plast Reconstr Surg 9:207, 1975
12. Ferlic DC, Clayton ML: Tendon transfer for radial rotation in the rheumatoid wrist. J Bone Joint Surg [Am] 55:880, 1973
13. Flatt AE: Care of the Arthritic Hand. 4th Ed. Mosby, St. Louis, 1983
14. Freiberg RA, Weinstein A: The scallop sign and spontaneous rupture of finger extensor tendons in rheumatoid arthritis. Clin Orthop 83:128, 1972
15. Goldner JL: Tendon transfers in rheumatoid arthritis. Orthop Clin North Am 5:425, 1974
16. Green CP: Carpal dislocation. In Green DP (ed): Operative Hand Surgery. Vol. I. p 703. Churchill Livingstone, New York, 1982
17. Helweg JL: Snapping finger. Ugeskr Laeger 86:546, 1924
18. Henderson ED, Lipscomb PR: Surgical treatment of rheumatoid hand. JAMA 175:431, 1961
19. Jackson IT, Milward TM, Lee P, Webb J: Ulnar head resection in rheumatoid arthritis. Hand 6:172, 1974
20. Kahlmeter G: Rheumatic affections of tendons and muscle attachments (tendinitis). Lancet 1:1338, 1933

21. Kellgren JH, Ball J: Tendon lesions in rheumatoid arthritis. A clinico-pathological study. Ann Rheum Dis 9:48, 1950
22. Kleinert HE, Frykman G: The wrist and thumb in rheumatoid arthritis. Orthop Clin North Am 4:1085, 1973
23. Linscheid RL, Dobyns JH: Rheumatoid arthritis of the wrist. Orthop Clin North Am 2:649, 1971
24. Mannerfelt L, Norman O: Attrition ruptures of flexor tendons in rheumatoid arthritis caused by bony spurs in the carpal tunnel. J Bone Joint Surg [Br] 51:270, 1969
25. Millender LH, Nalebuff EA, Albin R, et al: Dorsal tenosynovectomy and tendon transfer in the rheumatoid hand. J Bone Joint Surg [Am] 56:601, 1974
26. Millender LH, Nalebuff EA: Preventive surgery. Tenosynovectomy and synovectomy. Orthop Clin North Am 6:765, 1975
27. Millender LH, Nalebuff EA, Feldon PG: Rheumatoid arthritis. In Green DP (ed): Operative Hand Surgery. Churchill Livingstone, New York, 1982
28. Mitchell NS, Shepard N: The effect of synovectomy on synovium and cartilage in early rheumatoid arthritis. Orthop Clin North Am 4:1057, 1973
29. Moberg E: Tendon grafting and tendon suture in rheumatoid arthritis. Am J Surg 109:375, 1965
30. Mongan ES, Boger WM, Gilliland BC, Meyerowitz S: Synovectomy in rheumatoid arthritis. A retrospective study. Arthritis Rheum 13:761, 1970
31. Nalebuff EA: Surgical treatment of tendon rupture in the rheumatoid hand. Surg Clin North Am 49:811, 1969
32. Nalebuff EA, Patel MR: Flexor digitorum sublimis transfer for multiple extensor tendon ruptures in rheumatoid arthritis. Plast Reconstr Surg 52:530, 1973
33. Namba H: Clinical result of synovectomy for rheumatoid wrist compared with the opposite side. Nippon Seikeigeka Gakkai Zasshi 55:527, 1981
34. Nicolle FV, Dickson RA: Surgery of the Rheumatoid Hand. A Practical Manual. Yearbook Medical Publishers, Chicago, 1979
35. Palmer AK, Dobyns JH, Linscheid RL: Management of post-traumatic instability of the wrist secondary to ligament rupture. J Hand Surg 3:507, 1978
36. Potter TA, Kuhns JG: Rheumatoid tenosynovitis. Diagnosis and treatment. J Bone Joint Surg [Am] 40:1230, 1958
37. Savill DL: Combined management of rheumatoid arthritis. Manitoba Med Rev 46:527, 1966
38. Scudamore C: A Treatise on the Nature and Cure of Rheumatism; With Observations on Rheumatic Neuralgia, and on Spasmodic Neuralgia, or Tic Douloureaux. Longman, Rees, Orme, Brown and Green, London, 1827
39. Shannon FT, Barton NJ: Surgery for rupture of extensor tendons in rheumatoid arthritis. Hand 8:279, 1976
40. Souter WA: Planning treatment of the rheumatoid hand. Hand 11:3, 1979
41. Spinner M, Kaplan EB: Extensor carpi ulnaris: Its relationship to the stability of the distal radioulnar joint. Clin Orthop 68:124, 1970
42. Steiger U, Morscher E: Indications for synovectomy in rheumatoid arthritis. In Chapchal G (ed): Synovectomy and Arthroplasty in Rheumatoid Arthritis. Georg Thieme, Stuttgart, 1967
43. Straub LR, Wilson EH: Spontaneous rupture of the extensor tendons in the hand associated with rheumatoid arthritis. J Bone Joint Surg [Am] 38:1208, 1956
44. Taleisnik J: The palmar cutaneous branch of the median nerve and the approach to the carpal tunnel: An anatomical study. J Bone Joint Surg [Am] 55:1212, 1973
45. Taleisnik J: Rheumatoid synovitis of the volar compartment of the wrist joint: Its radiological signs and its contribution to wrist and hand deformity. J Hand Surg 4:526, 1979
46. Vaughan-Jackson OJ: Rupture of the extensor tendon by attrition at the inferior radioulnar joint. Report of two cases. J Bone Joint Surg [Br] 30:528, 1948
47. Vaughan-Jackson OJ: Attrition ruptures of tendons in the rheumatoid hand. (Abstract). J Bone Joint Surg [Am] 40:1431, 1958
48. Vaughan-Jackson OJ: Rheumatoid hand deformities considered in the light of tendon imbalance. J Bone Joint Surg [Br] 44:764, 1962
49. Vaughan-Jackson OJ: Personal impressions of synovectomy in rheumatoid arthritis after 6 years. In Chapchal G (ed): Synovectomy and Arthroplasty in Rheumatoid Arthritis. Georg Thieme, Stuttgart, 1967
50. Zancolli E: Structural and Dynamic Bases of Hand Surgery 2nd Ed. Lippincott, Philadelphia, 1979

19 Treatment: Bone and Joint Procedures

TOTAL ARTHRODESIS

Although total arthrodesis of the wrist is an excellent procedure,[13–15,17,19–21,25,26,37,39,45,48,57,58,62,64,77] it is performed rather infrequently, particularly for rheumatoid arthritis. There are three main reasons for this. First, many patients with rheumatoid arthritis of the wrists will retain relatively good function and remain largely pain-free after synovectomies and stabilization,[35,49,50,77] even in the presence of a degree of joint destruction that would be incompatible with a pain-free function in a nonrheumatoid patient (Fig. 18-5B). Second, maintenance of wrist motion is helpful to increase tendon excursion in patients who require tendon transfers or repairs, or who have severe disease of the digital joints requiring arthroplasties. In these patients wrist motion assists to obtain greater tendon excursion at the finger level. Third, the involvement of ipsilateral joints in the upper extremities, particularly elbow and shoulder, or the contralateral wrist, greatly hamper the functional capacity of these patients and their ability to place one or both hands in space for the activities of daily living. Furthermore, although arthrodeses may be done at a time when other joints of the same or of the opposite upper extremity are highly functional, the likelihood of these joints becoming involved later on is serious enough that a severe handicap may eventually be expected in most of these patients. Total wrist arthrodeses are usually reserved for the completely destroyed painful wrist in the younger, more vigorous patients, particularly when the ipsilateral elbow, shoulder, and hand are fairly functional and largely uninvolved, or when these joints, although involved, may be made functional through arthroplasties (Fig. 19-1). Arthrodeses are also indicated when wrist extensors are destroyed.[19] This is the procedure of choice as a salvage operation for failed arthroplasties in frail or very unstable wrists (Fig. 19-2). It may free tendons for transfers in very special circumstances. Arthrodesis is not difficult to obtain in the rheumatoid wrist, in spite of osteoporosis. The selection of the surgical technique will be influenced by the nature of the disease, and the radiographic and surgical findings, particularly the bone stock available, and the degree of preexisting stability. Thus, the surgeon should be prepared to use local bone from the distal radius, or from an excised distal ulna, or cortical, cancellous, or corticocancellous bone grafts from the iliac crest, with or without internal fixation with Kirschner wires or Steinmann or Rush pins.[17,19,20,51,58–60,73] Failure to obtain a solid fusion may still result in a painless wrist, a stable pseudoarthrosis (Fig. 19-3).[59]

The position of wrist fusion has been the subject of some controversy. Haddad and Riordan[33] recommended 10 degrees of dorsiflexion, while Boyes[12] suggests 20 to 30 degrees of dorsiflexion as measured on the radiograph. Clayton[19] favors a neutral position from palmar and dorsiflexion, and about 10 degrees of ulnar deviation,[20] even for bilateral fusions. In some patients, particularly fe-

387

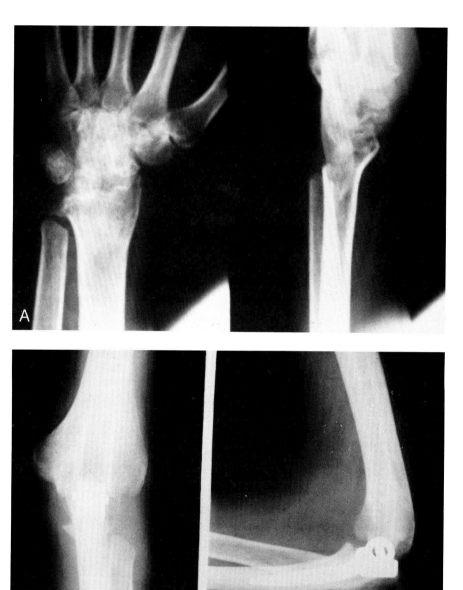

Fig. 19-1. Total wrist arthrodesis (*A*) in patient who later required a total elbow arthroplasty (*B*).

males, the preoperative position of the wrist is not symmetrical, with one of the two joints in considerably more palmarflexion than the other. In these cases, when a bilateral fusion is indicated, it is my preference to fuse the palmar flexed wrist in approximately 20 to 30 degrees of palmar flexion, and the opposite wrist in neutral. This seems to facili-

tate some activities, particularly personal hygiene for women. Clayton[20] pointed out the advantage derived from a fusion in neutral, over one in dorsiflexion, for placement of the hand at table-top level (Fig. 19-4). With the wrist dorsiflexed 30 degrees, the point of contact of the thumb pinching against the fingertips is essentially along the axis of forearm

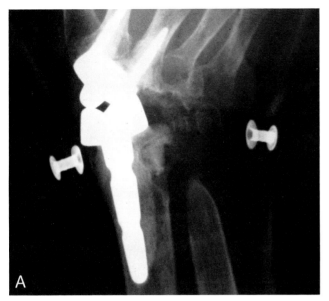 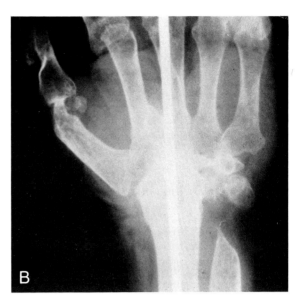

Fig. 19-2. *A*: Failed total wrist arthroplasty. *B*: The implant has been removed, and a total wrist arthrodesis performed.

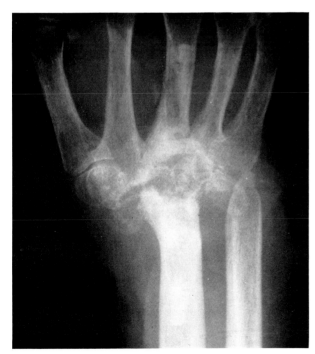

Fig. 19-3. Painless, stable pseudarthrosis of the wrist of patient with rheumatoid arthritis. The arthrodesis was an attempt to stabilize the wrist following a failed total wrist implant.

rotation. Therefore, during pronation and supination, this point of contact moves very little, and along a restricted arc of no more than 5 cm. With the wrist in neutral, the point of thumb-to-fingertip contact is approximately 7.5 cm palmar to the axis of rotation of the forearm and can, in consequence, traverse a much greater arc from full pronation to supination and vice versa allowing a less awkward placement of the hand in space.

TECHNIQUE OF TOTAL WRIST ARTHRODESIS

The universal longitudinal approach to the wrist is used similar to that described for dorsal synovectomies (Fig. 18-1). If a tenosynovectomy is not required, and whenever possible, the dorsal tendon compartments are not entered. This will preserve an intact envelope around the extensor tendons, and facilitate postoperative tendon gliding over the fused wrist. The exception is the extensor pollicis longus, which is lifted to enter the joint through the floor of its tunnel (Fig. 18-1B,C). The capsule is incised longitudinally between the extensor carpi radialis brevis and the extensor indicis proprius. An

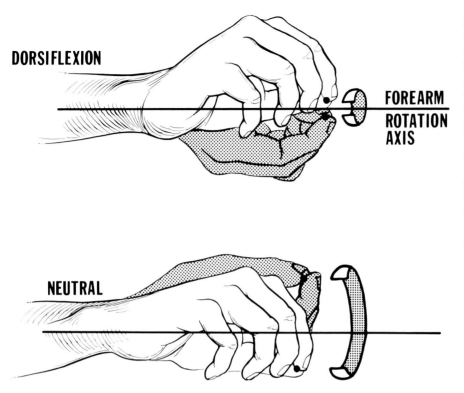

DORSIFLEXION

FOREARM ROTATION AXIS

NEUTRAL

Fig. 19-4. In wrist fusions with the joint dorsiflexed (top), the contact point between thumb and fingertips is along the axis of rotation of the forearm. The resulting arc of motion during pronation and supination is restricted. With the wrist in neutral (bottom) the contact point between thumb and fingertips is approximatly 7.5 cm removed from the axis of forearm rotation. Consequently, this contact point traverses a much greater arc during pronation and supination.

extensive subperiosteal and subcapsular dissection will result in a satisfactory exposure of the entire joint, including the distal ulna, which may need to be excised. When a tenosynovectomy is required, or tendons need to be repaired or transferred, it is better to incise the dorsal retinaculum between the extensor digiti quinti and the extensor carpi ulnaris (Fig. 18-1D). This allows elevation of a retinacular flap based radially, in a single piece, and avoids the placement of a suture line directly beneath repaired or synovectomized tendons. The capsule in these cases is incised transversely, just distal to the dorsal rim of the radius, elevating a large capsular flap based distally to expose the radiocarpal joint and the carpus (Fig. 18-1F). Exposure of the ulnar head is completed with a vertical incision at the radioulnar level. In either case, elevation of the lateral half of the capsule from the radius must be done close to bone, to avoid injury to the adductor pollicis longus and extensor policis brevis tendons, which are in very close proximity to the surface of the radius. Radiocarpal and intercarpal joints are denuded of cartilage, down to subcortical, cancellous bone. The amount of bone excised must be

enough to realign the radius and carpus. Longitudinal traction will help to relocate the carpus at the end of the radius, providing at the same time some biologic compression after the traction is released. In some patients, local bone from the excised ulna, and from the distal radius, may be enough to pack all denuded interstices. In some, an iliac bone graft is needed. The iliac crest from the same side is utilized as the donor site. This will allow the patient to ambulate postoperatively, using a cane held in the contralateral hand for support. In some cases a walker or bilateral crutches with forearm platforms are required. Carroll and Dick[17] advise the routine use of a radiometacarpal inlay cortical cancellous bone graft usually obtained from the iliac crest. In my experience this is not always necessary in the rheumatoid patient. Internal fixation is required in most cases, for the quality of the rheumatoid bone, and the support that may be afforded with a bone graft alone, may result in insufficient stability unless internal skeletal support is added. This may be provided by the use of crisscross Steinmann pins or large Kirschner wires,[49,77] or with longitudinally inserted Steinmann pins or Rush rods with additional rotatory stabilization provided by staples or Kirschner wires.[19,51,58,59] Clayton proposed in 1965[19] to use an axial fixation with a buried Steinmann pin, inserted retrograde along the third metacarpal and into the radius. Later[20] a ⅛-inch Rush pin was used, introduced at the distal end of the third metacarpal from the radial side, and into the radius for about 15 to 20 cm. After this is in place, manual compression is applied, and a staple (or buried Kirschner wires) is used for rotational stability and to maintain satisfactory bony contact. This is similar to the technique described by Mannerfelt and Malmsten[51] in 1971, using a Rush pin introduced through the ulnar side of the third metacarpal and a staple on each side of the Rush pin, at the radiocarpal level. The second metacarpal may be used instead of the third[58] or the space between either the second and third or the third and fourth metacarpals.[59] Millender and Nale-

buff[59] described a modification of Mannerfelt's technique of wrist arthrodesis using a simple Steinmann pin for fixation (Fig. 19-5). The medullary canal of the radius is perforated with a pointed awl. The largest Steinmann pin that will fit into the canal is chosen and drilled distally through the carpus to emerge between the second and third or between the third and fourth metacarpal, according to the patient's wrist and hand alignment. If the metacarpophalangeal joint is destroyed, needing a replacement arthroplasty, the pin may be introduced along the third metacarpal and through the metacarpal head. It is then tapped retrograde and countersunk approximately 2 cm proximal to the metacarpophalangeal joint to allow for the insertion of a metacarpophalangeal joint implant. If additional fixation of the radiocarpal joint is needed, staples or Kirschner wires may be utilized. By necessity, the position of the arthrodesed wrist using this

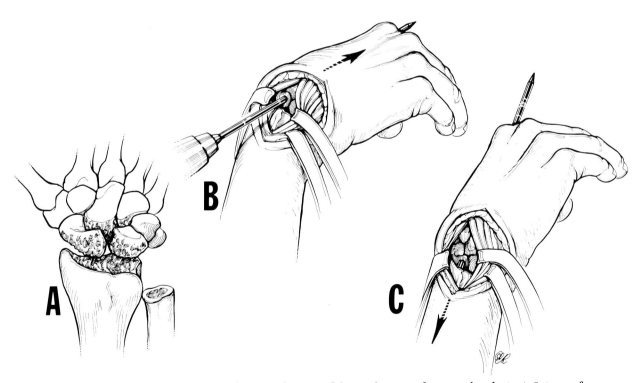

Fig. 19-5. Millender and Nalebuff's modification of Mannerfelt's technique of wrist arthrodesis. *A:* Joint surfaces are excised exposing healthy cancellous bone. The head of the ulna is excised. The medullary canal of the radius is perforated with a pointed awl, and the largest Steinmann pin that will fit the canal is selected. *B:* The pin is driven distally through the carpus, to emerge between the second and third, or between the third and fourth metacarpals. *C:* The pin is then tapped retrograde into the radius. If additional fixation is required, staples or Kirschner wires may be used.

technique will be very close to neutral. A few degrees of palmarflexion may be obtained by directing the Steinmann pin toward the dorsal cortex of the radius[60] or simply by bending it manually after insertion.[20] Because of the large surface of cancellous bone that is exposed, it is my preference in these patients to use postoperative suction drainage. Closure is performed in layers with or without placement of the dorsal retinaculum deep to the extensor tendons according to the approach that had been used. A well-padded compression dressing is applied and incorporated into a long arm circular plaster dressing to be worn at least for the immediate postoperative period, particularly if the distal ulna had been excised and appeared unstable, in which case the forearm needs to be kept in supination. An alternative is to fix the distal radioulnar joint with a distal radioulnar pin utilizing a short arm immobilization for the postoperative care. The suction tubing is left sticking through the dressings and cast in a straight line, to be pulled out 24 to 48 hours later without disturbing the postoperative dressings. The fingers are left free and should be exercised as soon as possible during the immediate postoperative period. At five to seven days, the dressings are removed, radiographs obtained, and a routine plaster dressing is applied to replace the bulky compression immobilization used after operation. If extensor tendons were repaired, or if the extensor effort is poor, dynamic traction may be incorporated. At two to three weeks postoperatively, the elbow may be freed and pronation-supination encouraged. A short arm circular plaster or splint is then worn, usually for no more than an additional three to five weeks period. When the internal fixation is stable and bone stock satisfactory external immobilization may be discontinued much earlier, depending on the patient's comfort and cooperation.

LIMITED ARTHRODESIS

These are excellent procedures in the wrist of patients with rheumatoid arthritis, whether performed alone or in association with partial arthroplasties. The type and location of a partial fusion is determined by the preoperative radiographic eval-

(Text continues on page 396.)

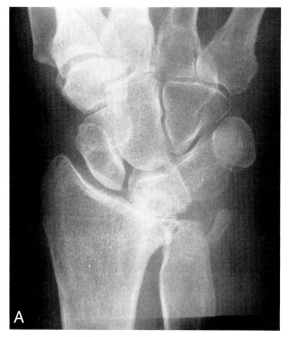 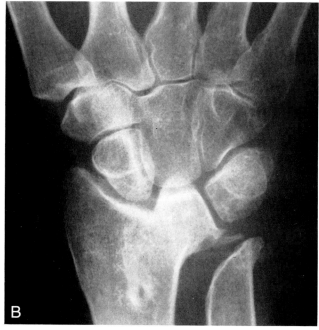

Fig. 19-6. Stabilization of the wrist by radiolunate arthrodesis. *A:* Arthritic joint changes localized to radiolunate and distal radioulnar joints and to ulnar head. There is an early type **I** ulnar translocation of the carpus. *B:* radiograph obtained four years after radiolunate fusion, synovectomy, and excision of the distal ulna.

Fig. 19-7. Radioscapholunate arthrodesis in patient with minimal or absent residual synovitis. *A:* Preoperative radiograph. *B:* Radiograph obtained two years postoperatively.

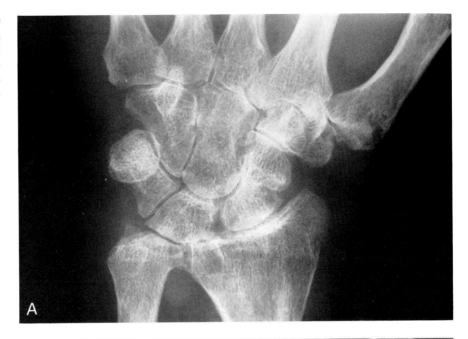

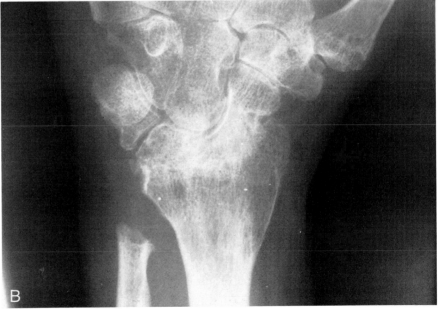

uation, by the findings at the time of operation and by the needs of the patient, which vary considerably according to sex, occupation, hand dominance, and the involvement of joints other than the wrist. In my opinion, whenever possible, a subtotal arthrodesis with or without the use of a small carpal implant is preferable to complete fusions, total joint replacement or to proximal row carpectomies or attempts at stabilization without fusion. There are several combinations that may be utilized. Campbell and Straub[15] point out that in the presence of a very active synovitis, with advanced carpal destruction, an excessive excision of the distal ulna may lead to ulnar drift of the carpus. They recommended that the excised ulna be used as a graft "from the radius to the capitate" to secure

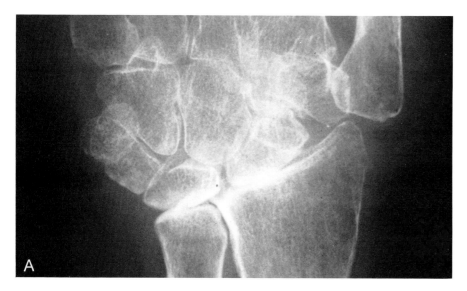

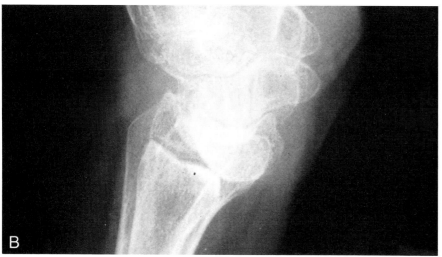

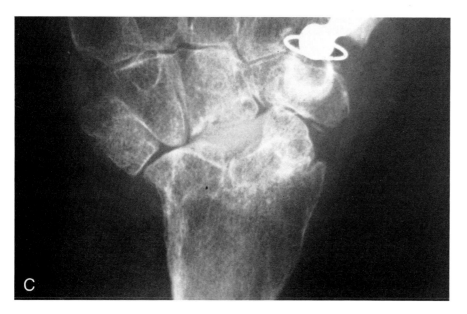

Fig. 19-8. Type I ulnar translocation of the wrist with palmar radiocarpal subluxation. The surfaces of the scapholunocapitate joint were found denuded of articular cartilage at operation. A: Preoperative AP radiograph. B: Preoperative lateral radiograph. C: Postoperative radiograph two years later. There is a solid radioscapholunate fusion. The head of the capitate was excised and replaced with a condylar silicone implant. Also seen is a total trapeziometacarpal joint for realignment of a dislocated first metacarpal (see A). The distal ulna was excised.

Fig. 19-8 (continued) *D*: Lateral radiograph. *E*: Postoperative range of dorsiflexion. *F*: Postoperative range of palmar flexion.

(Figure continues on next page.)

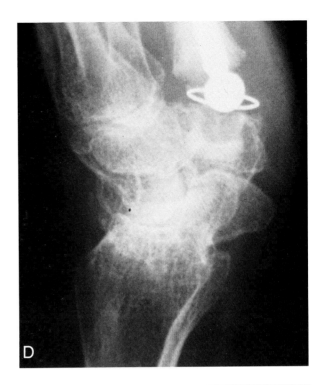

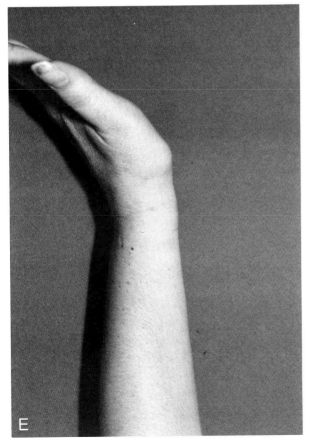

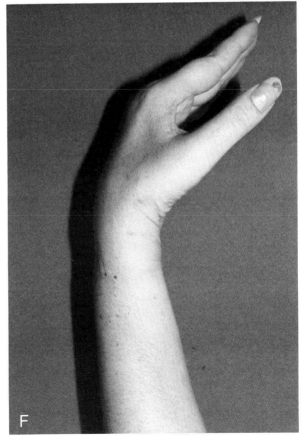

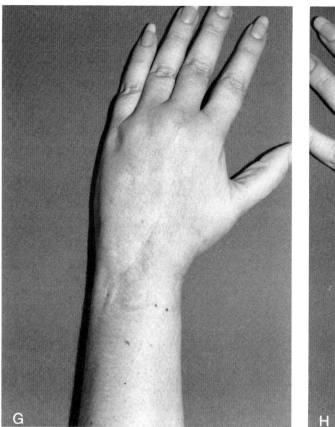 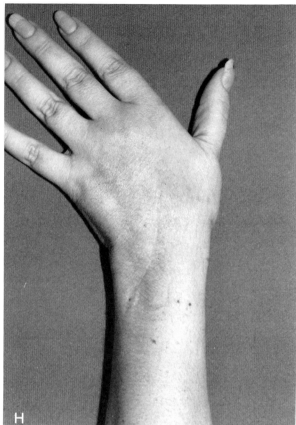

Fig. 19-8 (cont.) G: Radial deviation. *H*: Ulnar deviation.

radiocarpal alignment. When joint architecture is preserved, carpal stablization by radiolunate fusion is preferable to radiocapitate fusion (Fig. 19-6) and is the procedure of choice to anchor a reduced ulnar translocation of the carpus (Fig. 13-6).[18,83,84] The postoperative range of motion that may be expected still falls well within functional requirements. In many patients, the head of the capitate appears well preserved in preoperative radiographs, at a stage when the radioscapholunate interface is completely destroyed, unstable or dislocated. A radioscapholunate arthrodesis is a satisfactory procedure for these patients when active synovitis is either controlled or no longer present (Fig. 19-7). This situation is more likely to be found in patients with psoriatic arthritis than in those with rheumatoid arthritis. When the head of the capitate is not satisfactory initially, or when it

deteriorates due to persistent synovitis after the radiocarpal stabilization is completed, it may be excised and replaced with a silicone condylar implant or an "anchovy" type of soft-tissue filler, allowing wrist motion to continue on a stable midcarpal arthroplasty (Fig. 19-8). In some patients, the scaphoid alone may be excised and replaced with an implant, while at the same time a load-bearing column is restored by a limited arthrodesis performed either at the midcarpal joint level or between radius and lunate (Fig. 19-9).[90]

ARTHROPLASTIES

These procedures are indicated in patients for whom arthrodesis would be performed, were it not for the need to preserve motion. Their wrists are

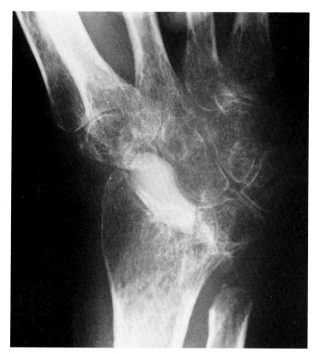

Fig. 19-9. Severe ulnar translocation with a poor radial styloid-scaphoid joint, treated by carpal relocation, stabilization by radiolunate fusion, excision of the head of the ulna, and insertion of a scaphoid silicone implant.

painful, with destruction or dislocation of both radiocarpal and intercarpal joints, and with severe functional limitations. In addition, these patients present similar destructive changes in other joints of the same extremity or in the opposite wrist. The goal of a successful arthroplasty is to relieve pain, correct deformity, and preserve some motion without loss of stability.[31] Augmentation of the effective range of finger motion is also enhanced by the tenodesis effect that is present when wrist motion is preserved to any degree. For the patient with isolated unilateral wrist disease with similar findings, partial and total arthrodesis with or without the use of partial carpal implants should be performed instead. Meuli[55] attributes to Beyer, a German military surgeon, the first wrist joint resection arthroplasty, performed during wartime in 1762. In 1967 Doebeli[24] presented a 28-year follow-up of what may be the first successful arthroplasty in a patient with rheumatoid arthritis performed in 1939 by a Swiss surgeon, Hans Budliger. Joint resections alone, or proximal row carpecto-

mies without the use of some type of interposition arthroplasty, are rarely indicated for rheumatoid arthritis.

ARTHROPLASTIES WITHOUT
ENDOPROSTHESIS

Dorsal wrist stabilizations[15,41,42,48,49,77] or pseudofusions[35] are procedures resembling arthrodeses, except that no attempt is made to achieve a solid fusion. Rather, a synovectomy is performed and, even if articular crtilage is destroyed, radiocarpal alignment is restored and temporarily maintained with internal fixation. The goal of these procedures is the creation of a fibrous ankylosis (Fig. 19-10). Of all the joints of the upper extremity, the wrist is most amenable to this type of reconstruction. Internal fixation must, therefore, be removed early, usually at six weeks postoperatively, before ankylosis occurs.[35,41,42,45,49,77] Upon removal of the internal fixation, a true fibrous ankylosis will be present, allowing a limited range of motion, which is usually free of pain. Albright and Chase[2] described a variation of this technique. These authors observed an abnormal profile of the distal radius in lateral radiographs consisting of an excessive palmar slant and palmar marginal spurs that interfere with reduction when the carpus is dislocated volar to the radius. They suggested that the use of interposition materials is actually not necessary to produce a movable space, provided cancellous bone is not allowed to come in contact with cancellous bone. They proposed a modification of stabilization procedures whereby the carpus is replaced opposite the radius, and prevented from further palmar dislocation by a short palmar shelf, constructed from the volar cortical rim of the radius. In general, however, these are unpredictable procedures, because of the potential for recurrent deformity, and for gradual wrist collapse and destruction, even though some long-term resections have shown some maintenance of comfortable, stable, limited motion.[42] More consistent results and a smoother postoperative course are achieved by the insertion of interposition materials, or by combinations of limited arthrodeses and arthroplasties.

A surgically created radiocarpal space may be maintained by the insertion of the patient's own

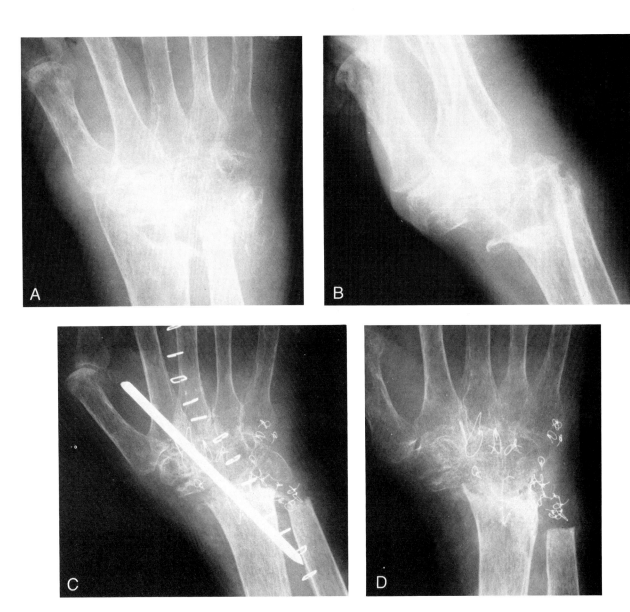

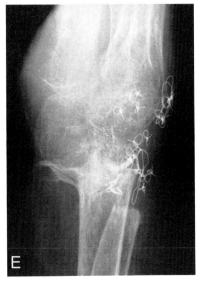

Fig. 19-10. Wrist stabilization or pseudofusion for an infection of the wrist in a patient with severe rheumatoid arthritis. *A*: Preoperative AP radiograph. *B*: Preoperative lateral view. *C*: Early postoperative appearance following synovectomy, joint debridement, delayed closure, and stabilization. *D* and *E*: Late (one year) postoperative appearance.

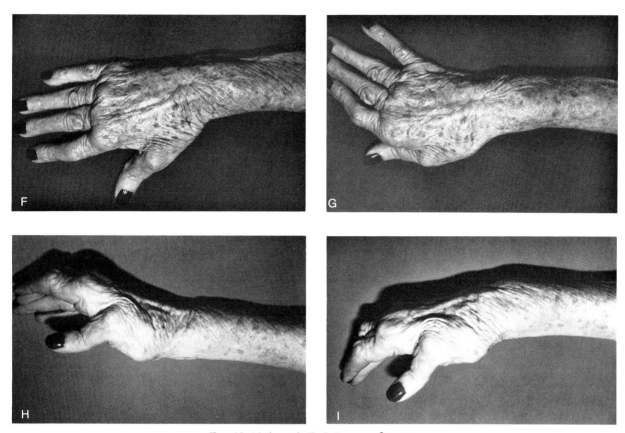

Fig. 19-10 (cont.) F–I: Range of motion.

tissues (perichondrum,[27,63,65,66,74,75] dorsal retinaculum,[85] palmar capsule[85]) by the interposition of silastic sheeting[37] or by the introduction of flexible[78] or mechanical articulated implants.[53,86] Skoog[74,75] was the first to investigate the potential of free perichondral grafts in the regeneration of articular cartilage. This potential was further researched by Engkvist and collaborators[27] and by Ohlsen.[63] In 1979 Pastacaldi and Engkvist[65] presented their clinical experience with the use of perichondral arthroplasties for the wrist. In one case a biopsy obtained four months later showed newly formed cartilaginous tissue in the reconstructed joints. A follow-up study in 1982[66] reinforced earlier expectations demonstrating longlasting relief of pain and persistence of satisfactory function. I believe that this procedure has exciting but limited applications; it is particularly indicated in the young patient with adult onset rheumatoid disease, in whom larger sheets of perichondrum

can be harvested, and who presents destructive changes at both radiocarpal and midcarpal joint levels, with preserved radiocarpal longitudinal alignment (Fig. 19-11A–D). Bone stock is not sacrificed with this technique (Fig. 19-11E), motion (although limited) is maintained, and relief of pain is effective and durable (Fig. 19-11F–I). Recurrence of synovitis in the newly created joint has not been a problem. The patient's rheumatoid process, however, must be maintained under satisfactory medical control. This is a technique that will require extensive evaluation before its indications can be properly determined. Similarly, Tillman and Thabe[85] presented resection arthroplasties with resurfacing using either the palmar capsule or the dorsal retinaculum.

Instead of the patient's own tissues, Jackson and Simpson[37] advocate interposition arthroplasties using a silastic sheet. These authors classify the diseased wrists into three groups. In the first, the least

(Text continues on page 403.)

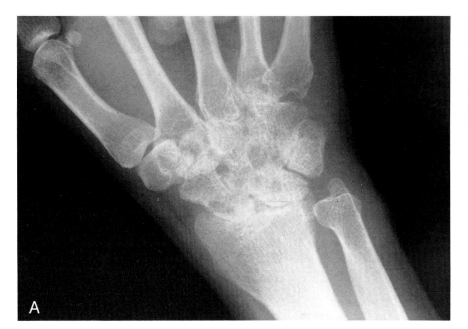

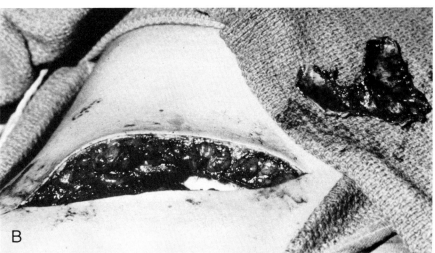

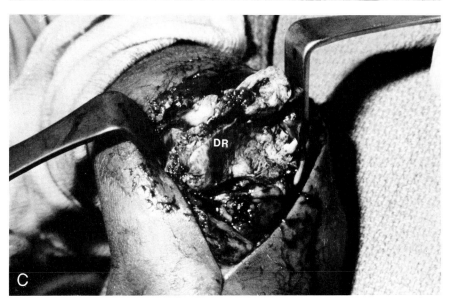

Fig. 19-11. Perichondral arthroplasty for young patient with adult onset of rheumatoid arthritis. *A:* Preoperative radiograph. All joint levels are destroyed. *B:* Perichondral grafts are obtained. *C:* Resurfacing of distal radius (DR).

Fig. 19-11 (cont.) D: Resurfacing of newly fashioned proximal carpal condyle. This required a midcarpal fusion (DR: distal radius; PC: proximal carpus). *E*: Postoperative radiograph. In addition to the midcarpal fusion and the creation of a congruent proximal carpal condylar surface, the distal ulnar head was fused to the radius, and forearm rotation was restored by the creation of a pseudarthrosis of the ulna.

(Fig. continues on next page.)

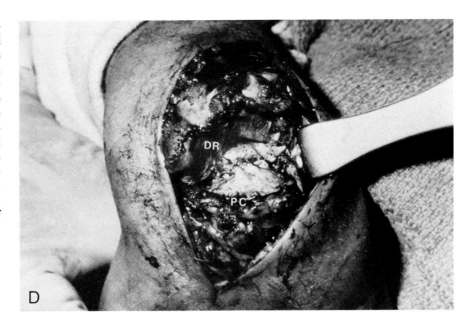

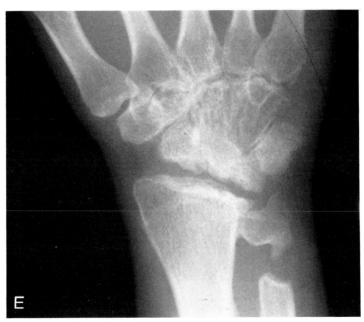

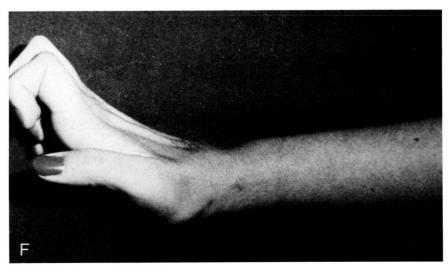

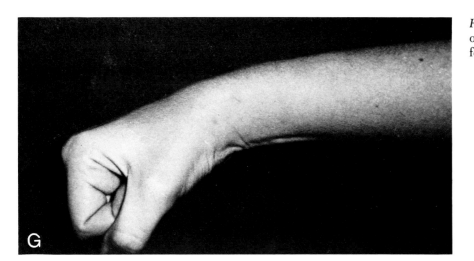

Fig. 19-11 (cont.) F–I: Post-operative range of motion four years following surgery.

G

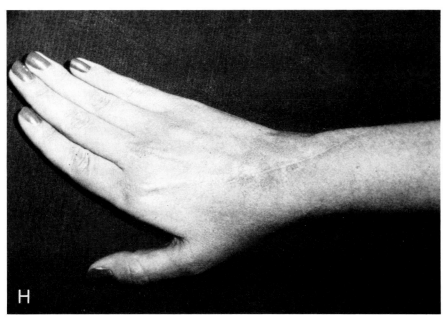

H

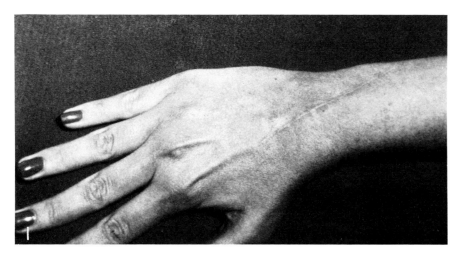

I

involved group, synovitis without joint changes can be managed by nonoperative measures, or by synovectomies if nonsurgical treatment fails. The most involved third group includes the destroyed, ankylosed, or dislocated wrists that are beyond salvage and are treated by arthrodeses or by the insertion of endoprostheses. In their opinion, it is the second, the intermediate group, which represents a problem in the selection of a surgical treatment. These are patients with painful but relatively stable joints, with synovitis and with joint changes which preclude synovectomy alone as the treatment of choice. For these cases they recommend the insertion of medical grade silastic sheeting, 3 mm thick, as an interposition material. Fragmentation is a problem, although the authors stress that if the silicone breaks and the wrist becomes symptomatic, replacement can be done easily and rapidly. Since bone stock is preserved a fusion or a formal implant arthroplasty may also be performed later.

SILICONE IMPLANT ARTHROPLASTY AND ENDOPROSTHESES

Swanson[79,81] postulated that the insertion of a flexible implant as an adjunct to resection arthroplasties would improve the predictability of the procedure and its results. Shortly thereafter, other investigators[53,86] developed mechanical or articulated prostheses for the wrist. This followed the successful use of the total joint replacement concept for the hips and knees and applied to orthopaedic surgery the technique of molding of monomer-polymer dough, a technique first introduced in 1938 in the fabrication of dentures.[16] Both types of implants are indicated for painful, destroyed wrists, when other joints of the same limb or the contralateral wrist are involved and in addition, when deformity is severe and interferes with hand function. All implants are successful in relieving pain and in preserving some motion,[3,5-8,23,31,53-56,72,78-82,86-89,92] although in general there seems to be a direct relationship between the range of preoperative motion and that obtained after insertion of the implant. Patients exhibiting greater preoperative mobility will most likely develop a better postoperative motion.[3] The implant allows the arc of motion to be positioned within a more

functional range. In general, especially for the flexible implants, it is not wise to push for greater motion for this may result in increased instability and in a greater potential for breakage or failure. Improvement should be expected for all activities that are facilitated by a better arc of motion with increased dorsiflexion capability, although stressful loading of these implants should be avoided. Fine digital dexterity, of course, should not be expected to change,[22] since this depends on the condition of the finger joints and is independent from that of the wrist. Contraindications include a recent history of infection, loss of wrist extensors,[43] young patients with open epiphyses, and, for the most part, the heavy manual workers.[22,82] The use of implants should be discouraged for the nonrheumatoid patients with single joint involvement. Rheumatoid patients should be cautioned against unrestricted loading of the arthroplasty, and permanent restrictions must be placed for their use in heavy activities, or for lifting of more than 10 lb, or for pounding and sports involving repetitive impact to the hand and wrist.[7,22] In the arthritic patients, the demands on the wrist may be even greater, for many of them will require to bear weight on the hands for support of involved lower extremities. This may result in unnatural loads upon the wrist implants,

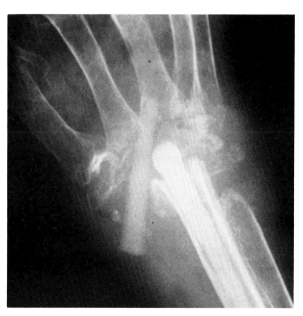

Fig. 19-12. Fracture of flexible wrist implant.

that cannot be met by present materials and designs. Modification of support devices used for ambulation, such as the addition of forearm platforms to crutches or walkers, will fulfill the patient's needs better than any attempts at designing more complex wrist prostheses.

Complications may include fracture of the flexible implant (Fig. 19-12), dislocation of the total joint replacement (Fig. 19-13), recurrence of deformity, infection, bone resorption, bony erosions, and settling of the implants (Fig. 19-14).

Flexible Implant Arthroplasty

Flexible implant arthroplasty involves the use of a double-stemmed flexible hinge, with a barrel-

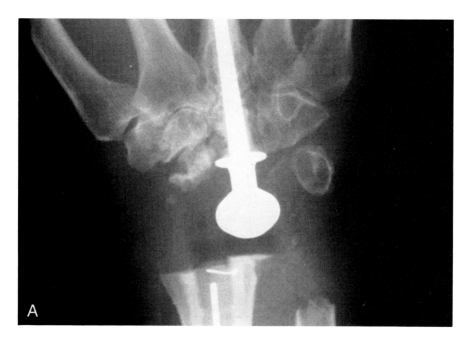

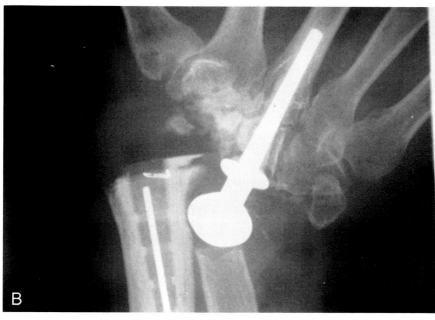

Fig. 19-13. Dislocation of a total wrist implant. *A:* Early postoperative alignment is satisfactory. *B:* Appearance at six months following operation.

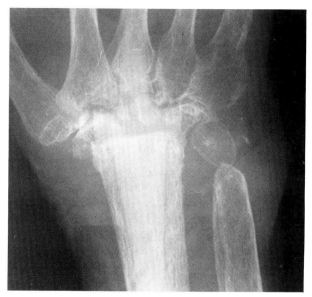

Fig. 19-14. Settling of a flexible wrist implant. This wrist was asymptomatic at the time the radiograph was obtained.

shaped midsection, slightly flattened on the dorsal and palmar surfaces, and with a Dacron reinforcement core, for increased axial stability and resistance to rotatory torque (Fig. 19-15).[82] Since 1974, the implant has been made of high performance silicone elastomer, improving its mechanical properties, reliability, and durability.[82] A newer wider design is now available. The purpose of the implant is to facilitate management following resection arthroplasties, to relieve pain and maintain a joint space, preserve alignment, and provide a mold for the development of a capsular support system. It must be remembered that the use of an implant is only a step in the reconstruction of the destroyed, unstable, painful wrist, and to be successful, the implant must be surrounded by a satisfactory, balanced, soft tissue envelope. The concept of implant encapsulation is most important.[80] Capsule formation and implant stability can be manipulated to a considerable extent by the amount of bone resected, and by the use of tendon slips to reinforce soft tissue closure over the implant, and postoperatively by the length of immobilization. A great advantage of this type of arthroplasty is its salvageability. It can be easily converted into a resection arthroplasty or revised by the insertion of a new implant, or changed into an arthrodesis with the

insertion of a suitable bone graft. Marked deformity or instability and excessive loss of bone stock are specific contraindications for the use of flexible arthroplasties,[31] in addition to the contraindications common to all types of implants.

Technique of Flexible Implant Arthroplasty (Swanson). A routine longitudinal dorsal incision is preferred. Superficial sensory branches of radial and ulnar nerves are identified and preserved. The extensor retinaculum is incised close to its ulnar attachment; a step-cut incision is preferred (Fig. 18-1D). Both retinacular flaps are then reflected, successively exposing the second through sixth dorsal extensor compartments. A dorsal tenosynovectomy is now completed. The dorsal wrist capsule and ligaments are sharply and carefully separated from the distal radius, and elevated from the carpus beneath, as a single, distally based flap (Fig. 19-16A).

As dissection of the distal radius proceeds toward the base of the styloid process, care should be taken to avoid injury to the tendons of the abductor pollicis longus and extensor pollicis brevis, which are in very close proximity to the bony surface. The palmar rim should be freed also, attempting to preserve intact the attachments of the very strong palmar radiocarpal ligaments and capsule. If these are detached, they should be sutured to bone just prior to the insertion of the implant (Fig. 19-16B,C). Scaphoid and lunate, usually destroyed, fragmented, and dislocated, are resected (Fig. 19-16D). In many cases it is preferable to excise just the proximal half of the scaphoid leaving the distal half in place to provide additional support to the thumb ray. Likewise, the medial half of the triquetrum may be preserved.[31] The head of the capitate is excised and the end of the radius is squared off, in a plane grossly parallel to the carpal cut. If additional bone excision is needed, because of severe soft tissue contractures, it is performed at the end of the radius, rather than from the carpal bones. Just enough space is created for the proper sized implant. The body of the capitate is reamed first and through it the medullary canal of the third metacarpal is identified by passing a fine Kirschner wire until it exits through the third metacarpal head; a fine curet may also be used to "feel" the walls of the canal. If in doubt, intraoperative radiographs may be obtained to secure placement of the distal stem of the implant through the body of the

(Text continues on page 408.)

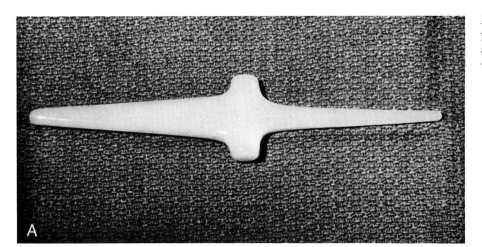

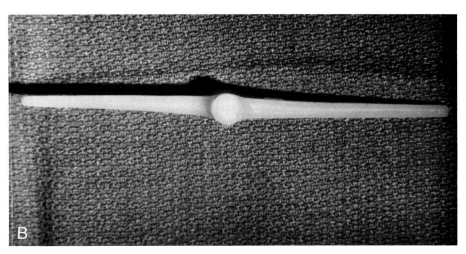

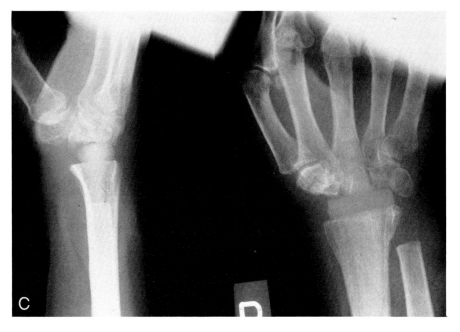

Fig. 19-15. Flexible wrist implant (Swanson's design). *A* and *B*: Frontal and side view. *C*: Postoperative radiographs.

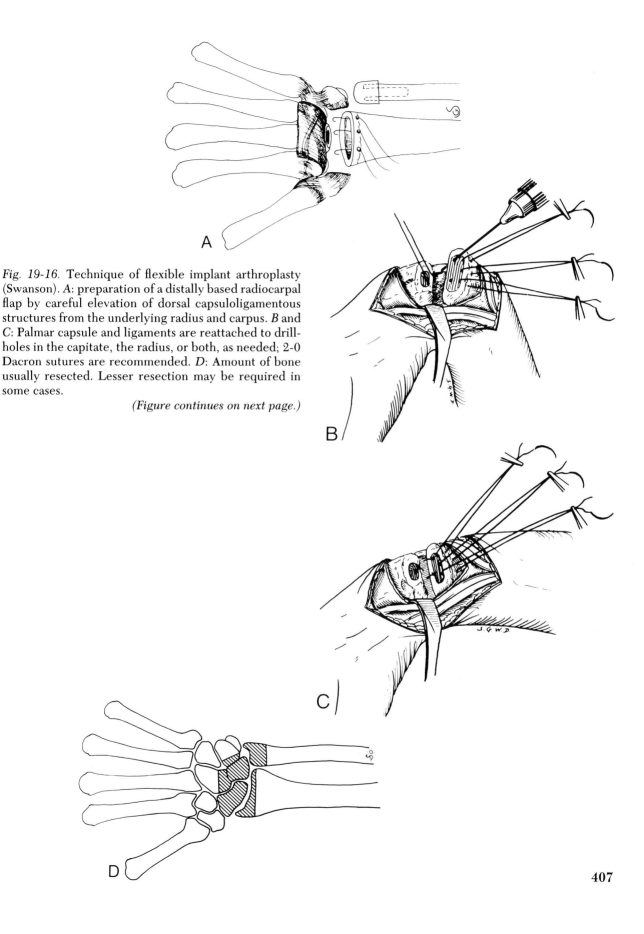

A

Fig. 19-16. Technique of flexible implant arthroplasty (Swanson). *A:* preparation of a distally based radiocarpal flap by careful elevation of dorsal capsuloligamentous structures from the underlying radius and carpus. *B* and *C:* Palmar capsule and ligaments are reattached to drill-holes in the capitate, the radius, or both, as needed; 2-0 Dacron sutures are recommended. *D:* Amount of bone usually resected. Lesser resection may be required in some cases.

(Figure continues on next page.)

B

C

D

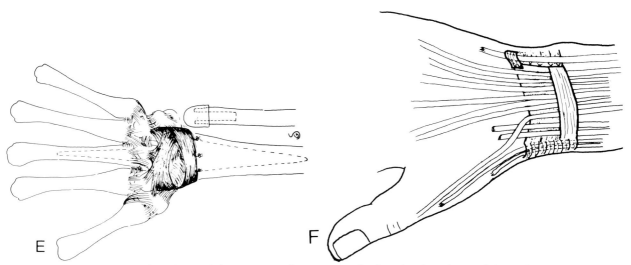

E

F

Fig. 19-16 (cont.) **E:** The dorsal capsuloligamentous flap is reattached to the dorsal rim of the radius. Sutures (3-0 Dacron) are passed through small drill holes and tied using an inverted knot technique. **F:** Technique recommended for replacement of the extensor (supratendinous) retinaculum. (*A* and *E* from Swanson AB, de Groot Swanson G: Flexible implant resection arthroplasty: A method for reconstruction of small joints in the extremities. Am Acad Orthop Surgeons Instruct Course Lect 27:27, 1978. *B* and *C* from Swanson AB, Herndon, JH, de Groot Swanson G: Complications of arthroplasty and joint replacement of the wrist. In Epps CH (ed): Complications in Orthopaedic Surgery. Lippincott, Philadelphia, 1978. *D, E,* and *F* from Swanson AB: Flexible Implant Resection Arthroplasty in the Hand and Upper Extremity. Mosby, St. Louis, 1973.)

capitate and along the axis of the third metacarpal. Placement of the distal stem of the implant outside the medullary canal of the metacarpal is not, however, a reason for failure. The largest implant is selected, provided it seats flush against the carpus. The medullary canal of the radius is next widened to accept the proximal stem. The head of the ulna is excised. When indicated, the palmar radiocarpal capsule is reattached to the radius through drill-holes, using nonabsorbable sutures (Fig. 19-16B,C). The proximal stem of the implant is inserted first into the radius, then the distal stem. The wrist is passively moved; buckling of the implant should be corrected by additional bone resection or reaming, or by switching to a smaller size implant. The dorsal capsule and ligaments are firmly sutured through drill-holes in the dorsal cortex of the radius (Fig. 19-16E). The distal ulna is stabilized next, including a palmar capsulodesis if needed (Fig. 20-6F).[11] Rowland[69] believes that a tenodesis of the distal-ulnar half of the extensor carpi ulnaris through the distal ulna after the insertion of a radiocarpal implant is helpful to maintain alignment of the prosthesis and to prevent popping, snapping or subluxation of the distal ulna. Swanson advises testing the capsular repair surrounding the implant to ensure approximately 45 degrees of extension and flexion range, and 10 degrees of radial and ulnar deviation on passive manipulation. The retinaculum is replaced under the extensors, and sutured to itself and to the underlying capsule. The extensor carpi ulnaris is secured over the dorsum of the ulna in the usual manner using the radially based retinacular flap created by the step-cut division of the dorsal retinaculum (Fig. 19-16F). Whatever tendon repair or reconstruction is required should be completed at this time, including rebalancing of wrist extensors to secure satisfactory dorsiflexion without deviation. Closure is completed and a bulky dressing is applied and incorporated into a plaster splint with the wrist in neutral position. Because ulnar stabilization is usually performed, plaster immobilization frequently includes the elbow with the forearm in supination, or sugar tong splints are applied. At three to five days this immobilization is removed and replaced with a circular plaster that is worn for at least three weeks. If extensor tendons were repaired, outriggers are provided with rubber-band slings to support the fingers. Long arm immobilization is then discontinued. A removable below elbow splint is then worn for three additional weeks, or until enough stability is present without external support. This splint is removed daily and wrist motion and pronation-supination exercises are allowed during this stage. A frequent mistake is to place the patient on an agressive early exercise program toward increased range of motion. A more stable but less movable arthroplasty with a range of 50 to 60 degrees of total flexion-extension is preferable.

Total Wrist Prostheses

Meuli[53] and Volz[86] designed the first commercially available prostheses for clinical use in the United States. These are articulated implants designed to reproduce the normal biomechanical characteristics of the wrist. Total wrist arthroplasties are potentially more stable than the flexible implants, and may be utilized to distract the collapsed radiocarpal joint,[8] thereby increasing the effective lever arm for the extrinsic muscles crossing the wrist. There are two formal contraindications among those that have previously been mentioned for all implants, namely, previous sepsis and absence of appropriate motors to control the wrist, particularly the extensor carpi radialis brevis.[43] These total joint implants are usually constructed of high molecular weight polyethylene and metal and are cemented to bone.

Meuli's prosthesis is a three-part trunnion design that allows triaxial motion.[53-56] It consists of a metallic stem that is introduced into the radius, and a metallic cup mounted on stems usually placed into the second and third metacarpals. Between these, a polyethylene ball is interposed. Both metal parts are made of protasul and are anchored to bone using cement, although isolated reports suggest that the prosthesis may be used without cement.[52] The stems can be bent to allow easier fit and a better centering of the prosthesis (Fig. 19-17).

In 1976 Volz[86,87] reported his experience with the use of a new total wrist prosthesis, a semiconstrained unit with radial and metacarpal compo-

nents. The intersurface represents a toroid sector, which is a sphere with two different radii. The prosthesis has a carpal height of 2 cm. The initial design of the distal component presented two prongs, for insertion into the second and third metacarpals (Fig. 19-18). The prosthetic axis of rotation was radial and dorsal to that of the normal wrist, in line with the center axis of the radius. The prosthetic design allowed 50 degrees of radioulnar deviation and 90 degrees of palmar-dorsal motion. This unit has been modified since, first with the introduction of a single central distal prong, and more recently by moving the prosthetic axis of rotation to coincide with the instant axis of joint motion. A recent improvement has been the addition to the prosthetic stems of a porous coating for a cementless fixation to bone. Experience with the use of both these total wrist prostheses has shown that the most predictable result observed postoperatively was relief of pain and the second most predictable result was the preservation or restoration of a useful, stable arc of motion.[7,28,43,56,89] Volz points out that many patients with rheumatoid arthritis undergoing this type of reconstruction exhibit sufficient metacarpophalangeal and interphalangeal joint disease that significant grip strengths are not attainable.[89] This may actually be an argument in favor of the use of flexible implants for most of these joints, since the pain relief and the motion obtained differ very little from those following total joint arthroplasties, and the demands that these patients may place on the implants are usually very limited. The most difficult problem associated with these total wrist replacements has been the attainment of a well-balanced wrist joint.[8,9,28,43,55,56,88] This has been attributed in part to loss of volitional control of wrist extension, and in part to a faulty placement of the prosthetic axis of rotation. Volz has called attention to an abnormal shortening-reflex of the flexor carpi ulnaris, requiring tenotomy or lengthening through a separate incision if found after the prosthesis is inserted.[88] The functional integrity of the extensor carpi radialis brevis and the degree of palmar and ulnar contracture have been found to be the most important factors influencing the ultimate results.[43]

Linscheid and coworkers[47] reviewed 135 cemented wrist arthroplasties performed at the Mayo

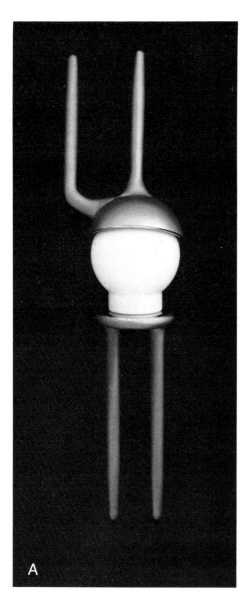

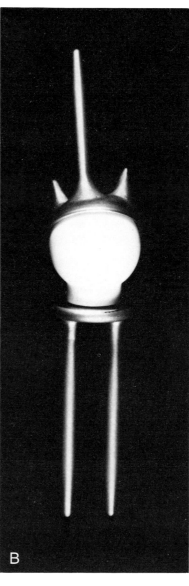

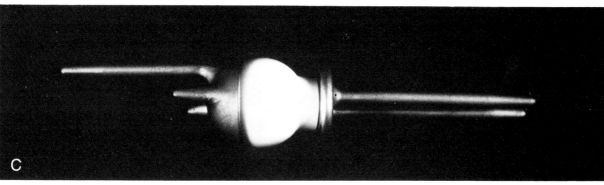

Fig. 19-17. A: The Meuli prosthesis with an offset two-prong distal component. *B:* Mayo's modification of the Meuli prosthesis. There is a single-stemmed component, offset dorsal to the radial component *(C).* (From Beckenbaugh RD, Linscheid RL: Arthroplasty in the hand and wrist. In Green DP (ed): Operative Hand Surgery. Vol. 1. Churchill Livingstone, New York 1982.)

Fig. 19-18. A: Double-pronged AMC total wrist prosthesis, designed in 1973. B: Single-pronged AMC total wrist prosthesis, designed in 1977, in an attempt to correct the problem of postoperative radioulnar imbalance. (Photographs courtesy of Robert G. Volz, M.D., The University of Arizona College of Medicine, Tucson, AZ.)

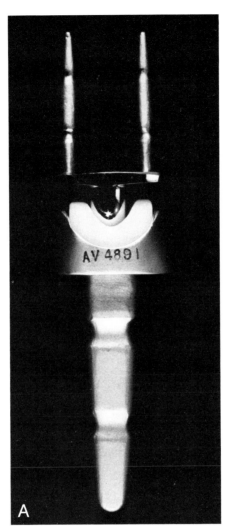

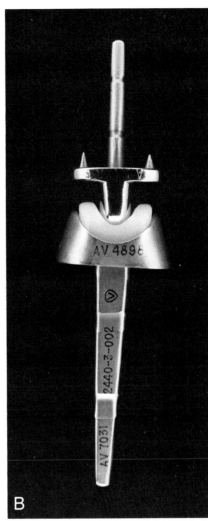

Clinic during a five-year period; 36 percent of these required reoperations, in most cases for a revision of the arthroplasty. They report, however, an improved later record, attributed to better cement techniques, and modifications in the design of the prosthesis, particularly because of a more accurate centering of the device in relation to the biologic center of rotation of the wrist. A review of the modified Meuli prosthesis shows, however, the center of rotation still in line with the longitudinal axis of the radius, rather than ulnar to it. An accurate placement of the prosthetic axis of rotation has, therefore, been a frequent problem, leading to gradual ulnar deviation of the hand.[5-8,9,28,43,55,56,87-89] The axis of prosthetic motion of Meuli and Volz' original designs, as well as some of the modified later units, was dorsal and radial to the actual biologic axis of wrist motion.[34] This has resulted in longer lever arms for the motor units that determine ulnar deviation and palmar flexion, producing a gradual ulnar deviation and palmar flexion of the hand on the forearm. Initially, correction for this problem was attempted through soft tissue rebalancing (i.e., flexor carpi ulnaris tenotomy[6,43,56,87] or transfer,[6,56] and palmaris longus tenotomy[43]) and postoperative splinting to induce restricted encapsulation[6] or by preservation of the triquetrum as a block to ulnar drift.[6] Intraoperative

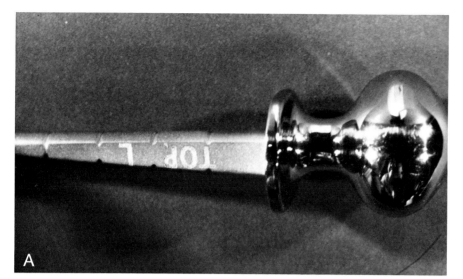

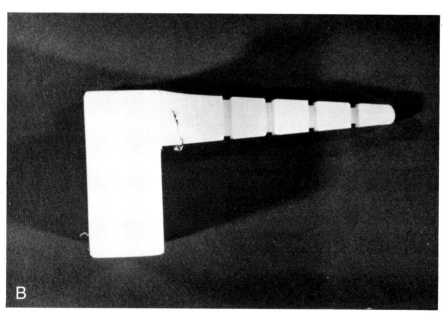

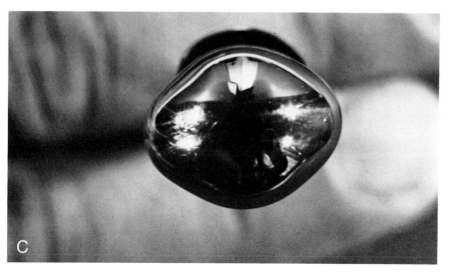

Fig. 19-19. Distal (A) and proximal (B) components of a self-centering articulated total wrist implant designed by the author. C: Distal component presents an ovoid element designed to reproduce and favor the normal functional range of the wrist (see Fig. 3-3A,B).

Fig. 19-19 (cont.) D, E: Both
components articulated.

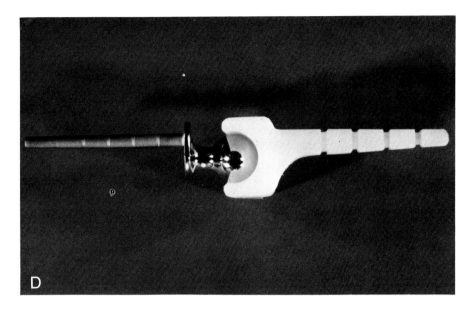

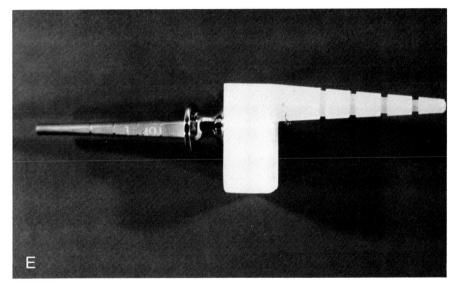

modification of the prosthesis, usually by changing
metacarpal components,[5,43] has also been proposed. This is a highly unreliable technique.
Hamas[34] presented a quantitative method to determine the location of the prosthetic center of motion, eventually evolving into a precentered modified Meuli-type design in which the axes of motion
are placed within 1.5 mm of the optimal location
for almost any size wrist.

Ranawat and collaborators,[67] in an attempt to improve stability and to simulate a more normal wrist
motion, introduced a spherical-triaxial wrist prosthesis (STW). It consists of metacarpal and radial
components, a plastic bearing, and an axle mechanism. Its center of rotation is preset in a palmar and
ulnar direction to place it within the instant center
of motion of the wrist, and allows 85 degrees of
flexion-extension, 10 degrees of radioulnar deviation, and greater than 10 degrees of axial rotation.
Similar to all other wrist implants, the main benefit
derived from the use of this particular design was
relief of pain. Range of motion was improved in

most patients, or placed within a more functional arc. Grip strength improved "modestly," because of the associated polyarthropathy of the hand itself.

Because of the intricacy of wrist function, a satisfactory replacement capable of reproducing radiocarpal function is extremely difficult to design. In my opinion, requisites for a total wrist implant are as follows:

1. Placement of the prosthetic center of rotation ulnar and palmar to the central axis of the radius, corresponding to the instant center of rotation within the head of the capitate, but allowed to find its own balance through self-centering.

2. Reproduction of the normal ballistic motion of the wrist, from dorsiflexion and radial deviation to palmarflexion and ulnar deviation, with built-in stops against excessive rotation, to allow stable loading in ulnar deviation and transmission of pronation and supination from the forearm to the hand.[38,46]

2. Reduction of loads and stresses at the cement-bone interface, particularly of the shear type.[44] A semiconstrained fit secures stable fixation during the surgical procedure, yet it allows stresses to dissipate without concentrating at the prosthesis-cement, cement-bone, or prosthesis-bone interfaces, thereby reducing the potential for loosening. The device should preserve the stability

of the carpometacarpal joints of the thumb, fourth and fifth digits.[46]

4. A range of motion that is less than 50 percent of normal; it is desirable to sacrifice high mobility for the sake of durable, stable, pain-free motion.

5. Salvageability. The amount of bone excised for the insertion of the implant should be minimal enough, to allow for either a conversion into an implant arthroplasty, or a fusion.

With these requisites in mind, an articulated, self-centering unit was designed, with an ovoid distal component eccentrically placed to reproduce the normal functional motion, from dorsiflexion and radial deviation to palmar flexion and ulnar deviation (Fig. 19-19). The implant allows a limited *prosthetic* range of motion of 40 degrees of palmar flexion, 40 degrees of dorsiflexion, 20 degrees of ulnar deviation, and 10 degrees of radial deviation. This translates into a more limited *clinical* range, usually associated with greater dorsiflexion than volarflexion (Figs. 19-20, 19-21). With rare exceptions, experience with this design has failed to show a clear advantage over other, more conservative techniques (i.e., limited arthrodesis combined with arthroplasties) or over the use of Swanson's flexible implant.

In spite of their more sophisticated designs, total wrist prostheses share a number of problems, some

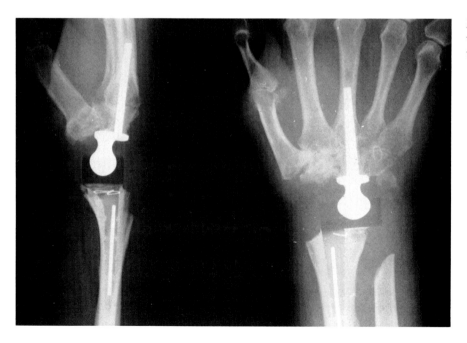

Fig. 19-20. Radiographs of wrist following insertion of total joint implant.

Fig. 19-21. A–D: Postoperative range of motion.

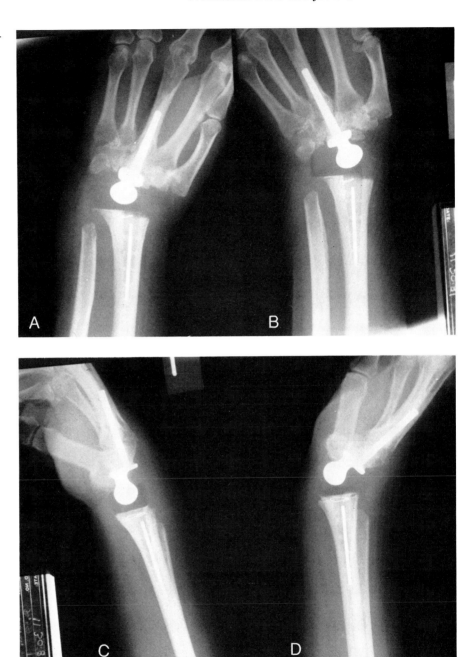

of which may still arise from faulty design, while others are secondary to the unresolved biological response that leads to bone absorption and implant loosening. Deep wound sepsis and hypersensitivity to the implanted foreign materials are the primary causes of biological failure.[29] Revisions or salvage procedures are more difficult, although possible (Figs. 19-2B, 19-22). Complications are less forgiv-

ing; those peculiar to the total wrist implant include loosening, dislocation, progressive deformity, and protrusion of the implant into the carpal canal, with subsequent median nerve compression and tendon fraying and rupture. The insertion of these implants is also technically more demanding. Placement must be exact. The introduction of cement itself must follow precise guidelines to

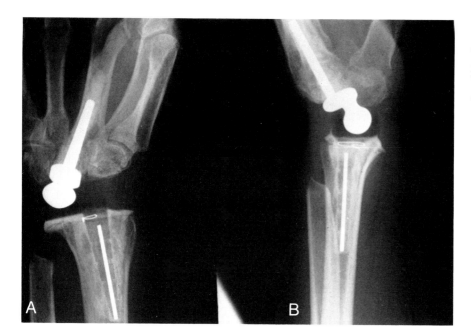

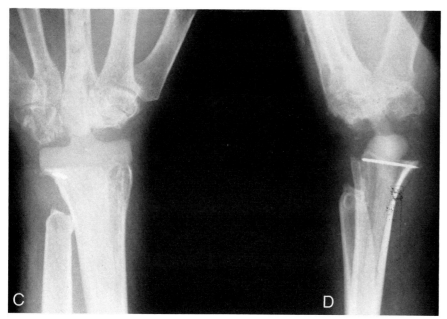

Fig. 19-22. A,B: Failed unstable total joint implant. *C,D:* The total joint implant was removed and a silicone rubber arthroplasty (Swanson's design) was inserted.

achieve a satisfactory mechanical interlocking with bone, and with the prosthetic components.[44] After all, acrylic cement has no adhesive properties of its own.

Overall, the results from all different types of articulated prostheses are not significantly better than those obtained with the use of the more forgiving flexible implants, and do not justify, in my opinion, the increase in operative complexity and in potential complications. For the future, more reliable total joint replacements may result from improvements in design and technique,[38] from investigations into new materials, and from cement-free implant fixation,[1,4,10,23,30,32,36,40,68,70,71,91] obtained through the use of porous coating, allowing bone ingrowth for fixation, with a modulous of elasticity close to that of bone. This would also allow a more effective load transfer and minimize stress shielding and stress concentration.[23,76] While this modulous should be low enough to permit transmission of stress to ingrowing bone, it must be high enough to prevent deformity during implantation.[23] Other considerations are the pore size, an intimate press-fit between the surfaces of the porous implant and the bone surface, and rigid postoperative immobilization to secure satisfactory ingrowth.[61] Although fixation through bone ingrowth is likely to improve results, it may create a set of problems all of its own, not the least important of which will be the challenge faced by a surgeon about to remove a biologically incorporated prosthesis.[29] Many problems remain, however, and until these are solved, and the efficacy of articulated prostheses clearly surpasses that of implantless arthoplastics, combined arthroplasty–partial arthrodesis, and flexible implant arthroplasty, clinical trials may best be limited to medical centers with vast experience in this type of surgery.

REFERENCES

1. Albrektsson T, Branemark P-T, Hansson H-A, Lindström J: Oseointegrated titanium implants. Requirements for ensuring a long-lasting, direct bone-to-implant anchorage in man. Acta Orthop Scand 52:155, 1981

2. Albright JA, Chase RA: Palmar-shelf arthroplasty of the wrist in rheumatoid arthritis. J Bone Joint Surg [Am] 52:896, 1970

3. Allieu Y, Asencio G, Brahin B, et al: First results of arthroplasty of the wrist by Swanson's implant. Twenty-five cases. Ann Chir Main 1:307, 1982

4. Anderson R, Cook SD, Weinstein AM: The interface mechanics of LTI pyrolytic carbon, porous titanium, and carbon-coated porous titanium implants. Trans Orthop Res Soc 7:178, 1982

5. Beckenbaugh RD: New concepts in arthroplasty of the hand and wrist. Arch Surg 112:1094, 1977

6. Beckenbaugh RD, Linscheid RL: Total wrist arthroplasty: A preliminary report. J Hand Surg 2:336, 1977

7. Beckenbaugh RD: Total joint arthroplasty. The wrist. Mayo Clin Proc 54:513, 1979

8. Beckenbaugh RD, Linscheid RL: Arthroplasty in the hand and wrist. In Green DP (ed): Operative Hand Surgery. Vol. I. Churchill Livingstone, New York, 1982

9. Bedeschi P, Luppino T, Fiocchi R, Balli A: Complications and technical errors on endo- and arthroprostheses of the wrist and hand. Ital J Orthop Traumatol 6:343, 1980

10. Blaha JD, Insler HP, Freeman MAR, et al: The fixation of a proximal tibial polyethylene prosthesis without cement. J Bone Joint Surg [Br] 64:326, 1982

11. Blatt G, Ashworth CR: Volar capsule transfer for stabilization following resection of the distal end of the ulna. Orthop Trans 3:13, 1979

12. Boyes JH: Bunnell's Surgery of the Hand. 5th Ed. Lippincott, Philadelphia, 1970

13. Bracey DJ, McMurtry RY, Walton D: Arthrodesis in the rheumatoid hand using the AO technique. Orthop Rev 9:65, 1980

14. Bunnell S: Surgery of the rheumatoid hand. J Bone Joint Surg [Am] 37:759, 1955

15. Campbell RD Jr, Straub LR: Surgical considerations for rheumatoid disease in the forearm and wrist. Am J Surg 109:361, 1965

16. Cannon SL: The role of bone cements in total joint replacement. Preliminary report of effort to toughen acrylic. Orthop Rev 7:63, 1978

17. Carroll RE, Dick HM: Arthrodesis of the wrist for rheumatoid arthritis. J Bone Joint Surg [Am] 53:1365, 1971

18. Chamay A, Della Santa D, Vilaseca A: Radiolunate arthrodesis. Factor of stability for the rheumatoid wrist. Ann Chir Main 2:5, 1983

19. Clayton ML: Surgical treatment at the wrist in rheumatoid arthritis. A review of thirty-seven patients. J Bone Joint Surg [Am] 47:741, 1965

20. Clayton ML: Arthrodesis of the wrist (position and technique). In Strickland JW, Steichen JB (eds): Difficult Problems in Hand Surgery. Mosby, St. Louis, 1982

21. Cregan JCF: Indications for surgical intervention in rheumatoid arthritis of the wrist and hand. Ann Rheum Dis 18:29, 1959

22. Davis PR: Some significant aspects of normal upper limb functions. In Joint Replacement in the Upper Limb. Mechanical Engineering Conference Publications, New York, 1977

23. Davis RJ, Spector M, Harmon SL, Irvin MP: The role of porous plastics in total joint arthroplasty. Orthop Rev 8:81, 1979

24. Doebeli H: Total resection of the wrist joint in rheumatoid arthritis. In Chapchal G (ed): Synovectomy and Arthroplasty in Rheumatoid Arthritis. Georg Thieme, Stuttgart, 1967

25. Dupont M, Vainio K: Arthrodesis of the wrist in rheumatoid arthritis. A study of 140 cases. Ann Chir Gynaecol Fenn 57:513, 1968

26. Eiken O: Assessment of surgery of the rheumatoid wrist. Scand J Plast Reconstr Surg 9:207, 1975

27. Engkvist O, Johansson SH, Ohlsén L, Skoog T: Reconstruction of articular cartilage using autologous perichondrial grafts. A preliminary report. Scand J Plast Reconstr Surg 9:203, 1975

28. Ferlic DC, Clayton ML: Total joint arthroplasty of the large joints of the upper extremities, as relief for degeneration and rheumatoid arthritis. Colorado Med 78:262, 1981

29. Fitzgerald RH, Kelly PJ: Total joint arthroplasty. Biologic causes of failure. Mayo Clin Proc. 54:590, 1979

30. Galante J, Rostoker W, Leuk R, Ray RD: Sintered fiber metal composites as a basis for attachment of implants to bone. J Bone Joint Surg [Am] 53:101, 1971

31. Goodman MJ, Millender LH, Nalebuff EA, Philips CA: Arthroplasty of the rheumatoid wrist with silicone rubber: An early evaluation. J Hand Surg 5:114, 1980

32. Griss P, Heimke G, Andrian-Werburg A von, et al: Morphological and biochemical aspects of Al_2O_3 ceramic joint replacement. Experimental results and design considerations for human endoprosthesis. J Biomed Mater Res Symp 6:177, 1975

33. Haddad RJ, Riordan DC: Arthrodesis of the wrist. A surgical technique. J Bone Joint Surg [Am] 49:950, 1967

34. Hamas RS: A quantitative approach to total wrist arthroplasty: Development of a "precentered" total wrist prosthesis. Orthopedics 2:245, 1979

35. Hooper J: The surgery of the wrist in rheumatoid arthritis. Aust NZ J Surg 42:135, 1972

36. Hulbert SF, Cooke FW, Klawitter JJ, et al: Attachment of prostheses to the musculoskeletal system by tissue ingrowth and mechanical interlocking. J Biomed Mater Res Symp 4:1, 1973

37. Jackson IT, Simpson RG: Interpositional arthroplasty of the wrist in rheumatoid arthritis. Hand 11:169, 1979

38. Kapandji JA: Principles and experimentation of wrist prostheses of the universal joint type. Ann Chir Main 1:155, 1982

39. Kessler I, Vainio K: Posterior (dorsal) synovectomy for rheumatoid involvement of the hand and wrist. J Bone Joint Surg 48:1085, 1966

40. Klawitter JJ, Hulbert SF: Application of porous ceramics for the attachment of load bearing internal orthopaedic appliances. J Biomed Mater Res Symp 2:161, 1971

41. Kleinert HE, Frykman G: The wrist and thumb in rheumatoid arthritis. Orthop Clin North Am 4:1085, 1973

42. Kulick RG, DeFiore JC, Staub LR, Ranawat CS: Long-term results of dorsal stabilization in the rheumatoid wrist. J Hand Surg 6:272, 1981

43. Lamberta FJ, Ferlic DC, Clayton ML: Volz total wrist arthroplasty in rheumatoid arthritis: A preliminary report. J Hand Surg 5:245, 1980

44. Lee AJC, Ling RSM: The optimised use of PMMA bone cement and some limitations of its use in the fixation of upper limb prostheses. In Joint Replacement in the Upper limb. p 41. Mechanical Engineering Conference Publications, New York, 1977

45. Linscheid RL: Surgery for rheumatoid arthritis. Timing and techniques: The upper extremity. J Bone Joint Surg [Am] 50:605, 1968

46. Linscheid RL, Beckenbaugh RD: Total arthroplasty of the wrist to relieve pain and increase motion. Geriatrics 31:48, 1976

47. Linscheid RL, Beckenbaugh RD, Dobyns JH: Total wrist arthroplasty. In Inglis AE (ed): American Academy of Orthopaedic Surgeons. Symposium on Total Joint Replacement of the Upper Extremity. Mosby, St. Louis, 1982

48. Lipscomb PR: Synovectomy of the wrist for rheumatoid arthritis. JAMA 194:655, 1965

49. Lipscomb PR: Surgery of the arthritic hand: Sterling Bunnell Memorial Lecture. Mayo Clin Proc 40:132, 1965

50. Lipscomb PR: Surgery for rheumatoid arthritis. Timing and techniques: Summary. J Bone Joint Surg [Am] 50:614, 1968

51. Mannerfelt L, Malmsten M: Arthrodesis of the wrist in rheumatoid arthritis. A technique without external fixation. Scand J Plast Reconstr Surg 5:124, 1971

52. Mantero R, Bertolotti P, Ferrari GL: Meuli's total prosthesis in severe rheumatoid osteoarthrosis of the wrist. Ital J Orthop Traumatol 3:47, 1977

53. Meuli HCh: Arthroplastie du poignet. Ann Chir 27:527, 1973

54. Meuli HCh: Alloarthroplastik des Handgelenks. Z Orthop 113:476, 1975

55. Meuli HCh: Total wrist joint replacement. In Joint Replacement in the Upper Limb. p 117. Mechanical Engineering Conference Publications, New York, 1977

56. Meuli HCh: Arthroplasty of the wrist. Clin Orthop 149:118, 1980

57. Mikíc ZDJ, Helal B: The value of the Darrach procedure in the surgical treatment of rheumatoid arthritis. Clin Orthop 127:175, 1977

58. Mikkelsen OA: Arthrodesis of the wrist joint in rheumatoid arthritis. Hand 12:149, 1980

59. Millender LH, Nalebuff EA: Arthrodesis of the rheumatoid wrist. An evaluation of sixty patients

and a description of a different surgical technique. J Bone Joint Surg [Am] 55:1026, 1973

60. Millender LH, Nalebuff EA, Feldon PG: Rheumatoid arthritis. In Green DP (ed): Operative hand surgery. Churchill Livingstone, New York, 1982

61. Miller JE: Biologic fixation of implants. Symposium. Contemp Orthop 6:123, 1983

62. Nicolle FV, Dickson RA: Surgery of the Rheumatoid Hand. A Practical Manual. Yearbook Medical Publishers, Chicago, 1979

63. Ohlsén L: Cartilage formation from free perichondrial grafts: An experimental study in rabbits. Br J Plast Surg 29:262, 1976

64. Papaioannou T, Dickson RA: Arthrodesis of the wrist in rheumatoid disease. Hand 14:12, 1982

65. Pastacaldi P, Engkvist O: Perichondrial wrist arthroplasty in rheumatoid patients. Hand 11:184, 1979

66. Pastacaldi P: Perichondrial wrist arthroplasty. Ann Plast Surg 9:146, 1982

67. Ranawat CS, Green NA, Inglis AE, Straub LR: Spherical-tri-axial total wrist replacement. In Inglis AE (ed): American Academy of Orthopaedic Surgeons Symposium on Total Joint Replacement of the Upper Extremity. Mosby, St. Louis, 1982

68. Ranawat CS, Weinstein AM, Homsy CA, Hedley AK: Alternatives to bone cement. Symposium. Contemp Orthop 4:230, 1982

69. Rowland SA: Stabilization of the ulnar side of the rheumatoid wrist following radio-carpal arthroplasty and resection of the distal ulna. Orthop Trans 6:474, 1982

70. Salzer M, Locke H, Engelhardt H, Zweymüller K: Keramische Endoprothesen der oberen Extremität. Z Orthop 113:458, 1975

71. Salzer M, Knahr K, Locke H, et al: A bioceramic endoprosthesis for the replacement of the proximal humerus. Arch Orthop Traumatol, Surg 93:169, 1979

72. Schernberg F, Gerard Y, Collin JP, Teinturier P: Arthroplasty of the rheumatoid wrist by silicone implants. Experience with forty cases. Ann Chir Main 2:18, 1983

73. Skak SV: Arthrodesis of the wrist by the method of Mannerfelt. Acta Orthop Scand 53:557, 1982

74. Skoog T, Ohlsén L, Sohn SA: Perichondrial potential for cartilaginous regeneration. Scand J Plast Reconstr. Surg 6:123, 1972

75. Skoog T, Johannsson SH: The formation of articular cartilage from free perichondrial grafts. Plast Reconstr Surg 57:1, 1976

76. Spector M, Michno MJ, Smarook WH, Kwiatkowski GT: A high-modulus polymer for porous orthopaedic implants: Biomechanical compatibility of porous implants. J Biomed Mater Res 12:665, 1978

77. Straub LR, Ranawat CS: The wrist in rheumatoid arthritis. Surgical treatment and results. J Bone Joint Surg [Am] 51:1, 1969

78. Swanson AB: Flexible Implant Resection Arthroplasty in the Hand and Extremities. Mosby, St. Louis, 1973

79. Swanson AB: Flexible implant arthroplasty for arthritic disabilities of the radiocarpal joint. A silicone rubber intramedullary stemmed flexible hinge implant for the wrist joint. Orthop Clin North Am 4:383, 1973

80. Swanson AB: Implant arthroplasty in the hand and upper extremity and its future. Surg Clin North Am 61:369, 1981

81. Swanson AB: Arthroplasty in the rheumatoid hand. In Lamb DW, Kuczynski K (ed): The Practice of Hand Surgery. Blackwell Scientific Publications, Boston, 1981

82. Swanson AB, deGroot Swanson G: Flexible implant arthroplasty of the radiocarpal joint: Surgical technique and long-term results. In Inglis AE (ed): American Academy of Orthopaedic Surgeons Symposium on Total Joint Replacement of the Upper Extremity. Mosby, St. Louis, 1982

83. Taleisnik J: Post-traumatic carpal instability. Clin Orthop 149:73, 1980

84. Taleisnik J: Rheumatoid arthritis of the wrist. In Strickland JW, Steichen JB (ed): Difficult Problems in Hand Surgery. Mosby, St. Louis, 1982

85. Tillman K, Thabe H: Technique and results of resection and interposition arthroplasty of the wrist in rheumatoid arthritis. Reconstr Surg Traumatol 18:84, 1981

86. Volz RG: Clinical experiences with a new total wrist prosthesis. Arch Orthop Unfallchir 85:205, 1976

87. Volz RG: The development of a total wrist arthroplasty. Clin Orthop 116:209, 1976

88. Volz RG: Total wrist arthroplasty. A new approach to wrist disability. Clin Orthop 128:180, 1977

89. Volz RG: Total wrist arthroplasty: A clinical and biomechanical analysis. In Inglis AE (ed): American Academy of Orthopaedic Surgeons Symposium on Total Joint Replacement of the Upper Extremity. Mosby, St. Louis, 1982

90. Watson HK, Goodman ML, Johnson TR: Limited arthrodesis. Part II. Intercarpal and radiocarpal considerations. J Hand Surg 6:223, 1981

91. Welsh RP, Pilliar RM, McNab A: Surgical implants: the role of surface porosity in fixation to bone and acrylic. J Bone Joint Surg [Am] 53:963, 1971

92. Zolczer L, Somogyvári K, Nyári T, et al: A Kéztőcsontok pótlása szilikon protézissel. Magy Traumatol 24:282, 1981

20 The Distal Ulna in the Wrist with Rheumatoid Arthritis

CLINICAL EVALUATION

In the wrist with rheumatoid arthritis, a complete dislocation of the distal radioulnar joint, with total loss of contact between radius and ulna, may be pain-free, without limitation of pronation and supination, but with a sensation of instability and attending loss of power and strength. Conversely, maintenance of distal radioulnar contact, but with rheumatoid involvement of the joint surfaces, may be painful and may be accompanied by limited forearm rotation and by a palpable, and at times audible, crepitation at the distal radioulnar joint level. Synovitis may not only involve the radioulnar joint, but also the ulnocarpal space, with or without synovitis of the extensor carpi ulnaris. The clinical complex involving the ulnar head in the patient with rheumatoid arthritis, was described by Bäckdahl,[2] who named it the "caput ulnae syndrome". It includes the following:

1. Wrist weakness and pain on pronation and supination
2. Dorsal prominence of the ulnar head
3. Limitation of pronation and supination
4. Swelling over the distal radioulnar area
5. Secondary tendon changes, including possible ruptures of the long extensors of the fingers

The dorsal dislocation of the ulna (or rather the palmar dislocation of the carpus) is a deformity accentuated by forearm pronation. The "piano key-board" sign[2,32] is produced when the ulnar head is manually depressed and it springs back up dorsally after the pressure is released, a finding not present in the stable radioulnar joints. The extensor carpi ulnaris is subluxated palmarward (Fig. 16-10), contributing to changes of carpal alignment secondary to the loss of this tendon's support. The examiner must carefully evaluate the entire radioulnocarpal relationship, because what appears as a simple dorsal dislocation of the ulna, may in effect be a palmar dislocation of the carpus (Fig. 16-10B), placing the emphasis of repair at a different location during the process of reconstructive surgery.

RADIOGRAPHIC EVALUATION

Radiographs should be carefully studied, not only for the relationship between radius, ulna, and carpus, and for the degree of destruction of the radioulnar joint, but also for changes in the contour and integrity of the ulnar carpus and of the distal-ulnar corner of the radius. Destruction of the ulnar corner of the radius,[6] or remodeling of its distal articular aspect into a surface that is sharply slanted in a proximal and ulnar direction, strongly suggests that an excision of the ulnar head may further destabilize this potentially unstable wrist, permitting progressive ulnar translocation of the carpus. Preexistent carpal ulnar translocation must also be noted, for this deformity is a formal contraindication to ulnar head excision, unless radioulnar

421

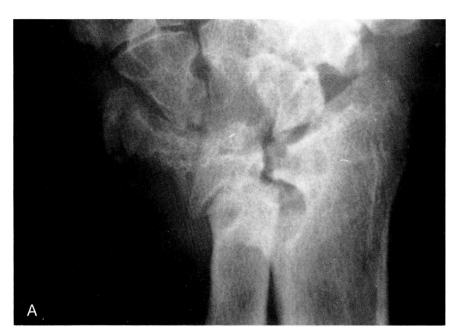

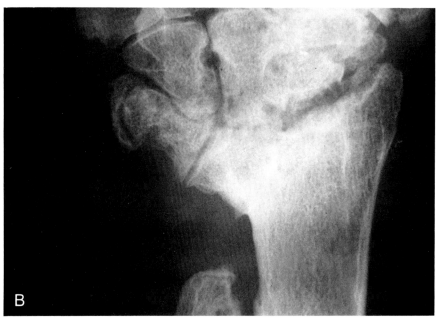

Fig. 20-1. A: Severe ulnar translocation. Also visible is the "scallop" sign opposite the head of the ulna. Excision of the ulnar head is contraindicated in this wrist, unless radiocarpal stability is restored. *B:* Same wrist after radiolunate fusion, soft tissue interposition arthroplasty between scaphoid and radius, and excision of ulnar head.

alignment and stability are restored first (Fig. 20-1).[10,60,62,63] The "scallop" sign, a semicircular loss of contour of the radius opposite the head of the ulna, is a radiographic finding described in 1972 by Freiberg and Weinstein.[24] It is frequently associated with spontaneous rupture of digital extensor tendons (Fig. 20-2).

TREATMENT OF THE DISTAL RADIOULNAR JOINT IN THE RHEUMATOID PATIENT

RESTORATION OF ULNOCARPAL ALIGNMENT

In the presence of a distal radioulnar dislocation, the head of the ulna may still show a well-preserved cartilaginous cover and may still be reducible with relative ease by supination of the forearm. Unlike chronic traumatic dislocations, which require a much stronger and more sophisticated distal radioulnar and ulnocarpal reconstruction,[8,31,38] the dislocated ulnar head in rheumatoid arthritis may be effectively reduced in supination, and stabilized by imbrication of the dorsal capsule, reinforced with a strip of dorsal retinaculum passed deep to the extensor carpi ulnaris. It is further supported by relocating the extensor carpi ulnaris dorsal to the ulnar head, holding it in position by a retinacular flap based radially, looped around the tendon, and sutured to itself. Since this is, in effect, a palmar dislocation of the carpus with ulna dorsal, the ulnocarpal relationship may be restored by a transfer of the extensor carpi radialis longus to the insertion of the extensor carpi ulnaris.[13,22] This provides additional dorsal support to the ulnar carpus. Should this fail to secure radioulnar congruency, the ulnocarpal relationship may be further stabilized by using one half of the flexor carpi ulnaris tendon left attached distally, passed obliquely proximally, dorsally, and radially through the ulnar head, looped over the head, and sutured to itself (Fig. 20-3).[31] Postoperative immobilization in supination for three weeks is sufficient, followed by a gradual exercise program to restore pronation.

RESECTION OF THE DISTAL ULNA

Resection of the distal ulna was first mentioned by Desault.[19] In 1880 Moore[45] described a resec-

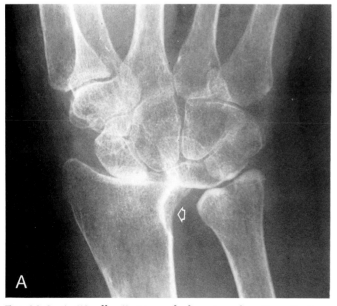
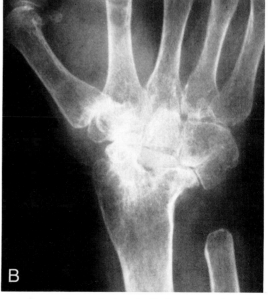

Fig. 20-2. A: "Scallop" sign and ulnar translocation. *B:* Appearance after radioscapholunate fusion, insertion of a condylar implant for the excised head of the capitate, and excision of the ulnar head.

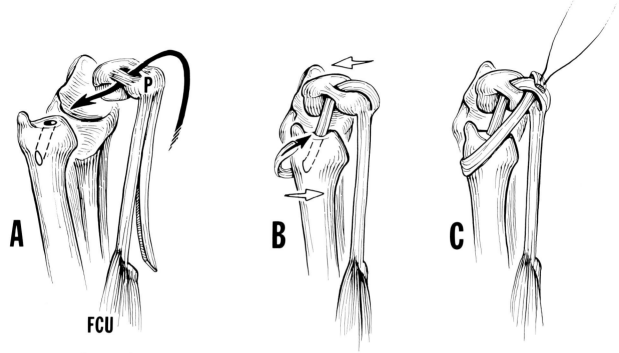

Fig. 20-3. Technique of augmentation tenodesis for the distal radioulnar joint. *A*: The ulnar head is exposed using a longitudinal dorsal skin incision, longitudinal division of the supratendinous retinaculum and of the infratendinous retinaculum radial to the fibrous tunnel for the extensor carpi ulnaris tendon. A tunnel is drilled through the ulnar head, from near the base of the ulnar styloid, proximally and dorsally, to emerge at the synovial reflection of the radioulnar joint. A slip of flexor carpi ulnaris (FCU) tendon is created from the medial half of the tendon, is left attached distally and passed through the pisotriquetral capsule with a tendon passer (P, pisiform). *B*: The tendon slip is then passed through the tunnel in the head of the ulna, and is looped over and around the medial aspect of the head. The forearm is supinated, the radioulnar joint reduced and reduction maintained with a 0.062 Kirschner wire passed from ulna to radius, *proximal* to the radioulnar joint. *C*: The tendon slip is pulled taut, superficial to the radioulnar capsule, and is sutured to the pisotriquetral ligament. (Modified from Hui FC, Linscheid RL: Ulnotriquetral augmentation tenodesis: A reconstructive procedure for dorsal subluxation of the distal radioulnar joint. J Hand Surg 7:230, 1982.)

tion of the distal end of the ulna in connection with a distal radioulnar fracture dislocation, with protrusion of the ulna through the skin. The ulnar head was sawed off to allow reduction. In 1887 Lauenstein[37] described a more formal surgical excision of the distal ulna for a healed Colles-type fracture with radioulnar dysfunction, and in 1908 Angus[1] described the same procedure for a 15-year-old patient who presented a chronic dislocation of the ulnar head. This technique was later popularized by Darrach,[16–18] and now carries his name. In 1943 it was reported in patients with rheumatoid arthritis by Smith-Peterson and collaborators[54] and has since become an accepted part of the surgical ar-

mamentarium for the treatment of rheumatoid arthritis.[2,3,12,15,28,29,32,34,35,41,44,58] There are two main indications for ulnar head excision: disabling pain during pronation and supination, arising from distal radioulnar joint changes, and rupture of extensor tendons by attrition against an abnormal ulnar head, even in the presence of a pain-free radioulnar function. A third reason for excision of the ulnar head in rheumatoid disease is to allow exposure for a complete synovectomy of the distal radioulnar and ulnocarpal joint spaces.[34,35] Actually, isolated excision of the head of the ulna is rarely performed for rheumatoid arthritis; it is usually part of a more extensive procedure that includes dorsal synovectomies of tendons or joints, wrist arthroplasties, or fusions.

Several authors have warned against excessive excision of the distal ulna.[9,41,47,48] The two most frequent complications from this procedure are ulnar instability and rupture of the digital extensors; both can be prevented by excising only enough to correct the radioulnar dysfunction, and by a careful reconstruction of soft tissue support dorsal to the ulna, including the creation of a palmar capular restraint.[7] Even with such an economical excision, however, the carpus may migrate toward the recessed ulna[9,11,15,21,23,27,30,32,36,39,43, 50,54,60,61] or progressive ulnar deviation may occur.[21,46] It should be stressed that ulnar translocation, and eventual dislocation of the carpus, may occur in the presence of an intact ulna as the outcome of significant radiocarpal disease, unrelated to excision of the ulnar head.[43] The carpus simply slides palmar to or over the ulnar head to migrate medially (Figs. 13-2, 20-4).

Excision of the head of the ulna without simultaneous radiocarpal stabilization is contraindicated when the radiographic features suggest an impending dislocation or translocation (Fig. 20-2A). For these patients, either the ulnar head is preserved as a supportive block,[4] or is fused to the distal radius (Lauenstein),[26,52,55-57] or else the radiocarpal joint is stabilized (Fig. 20-2B). After radioulnar fusion, forearm rotation is restored by the creation of a surgical pseudarthrosis of the ulna proximal to the fixation site (Fig. 20-5).

Technique of Excision of the Distal Ulna

This procedure is usually performed in the course of tendon or wrist joint synovectomies, arthroplasties, or fusions. The ulnar head is exposed by retraction of the medial skin flap and through a longitudinal incision at the level of the radioulnar joint capsule, deep to the extensor tendon layer (Figs. 18-1F,G). When the surgical procedure is strictly limited to an excision of the ulnar head, and is performed independently, a longitudinal skin incision is used along the palpable subcutaneous border of the ulna, from 2 to 3 cm proximal to the prominence of the ulnar head to just distal to it (Fig. 20-6A). In this fashion, the dorsal branch of the ulnar nerve will remain distal to the operative field, as it traverses in a dorsal and distal direction bisecting the space between the ulnar styloid and the pisiform. The pretendinous retinaculum is exposed. It may be incised directly over the extensor carpi ulnaris. Frequently, however, the extensor

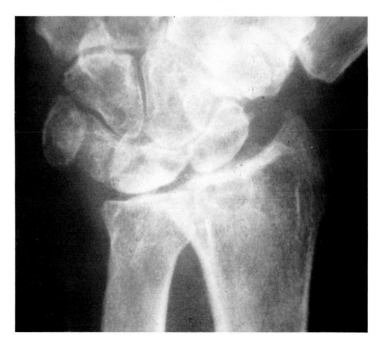

Fig. 20-4. Severe type I ulnar translocation. The carpus subluxes palmar to the intact ulnar head.

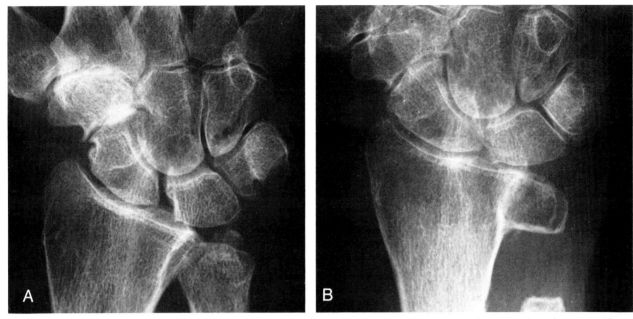

Fig. 20-5. Wrist with mild rheumatoid synovitis and painful radioulnar rotation, treated by radioulnar fusion and by creation of surgical pseudarthrosis proximal to the fusion. *A:* Preoperative radiograph. *B:* Postoperative appearance.

carpi ulnaris is displaced in a palmar direction, and the exposure is best performed along the space between the fifth and sixth dorsal extensor tendon tunnels. Since the pretendinous retinaculum is not adherent to the underlying capsule, it can be lifted with ease, creating a larger medial and a smaller lateral retinacular flap, which remains attached to the dorso-ulnar corner of the radius. If relocation of the extensor carpi ulnaris dorsal to the ulna and its retention by a retinacular loop is anticipated, the distal portion of the retinacular incision should be planned accordingly, leaving a "tongue" of tissue based radially, to be wrapped or looped later on around the extensor carpi ulnaris (Fig. 20-6B). The dorsoulnar capsule is now exposed and can be incised longitudinally (Fig. 20-6C). This capsule also has a strong attachment on the dorsal rim of the sigmoid cavity of the distal radius. This attachment must be preserved for a satisfactory dorsoulnar reconstruction. Frequently, a large synovial sac will then come into view. A synovectomy is performed. The neck of the ulna is exposed subperiosteally and sharply divided along a plane that is slanted somewhat distally and medially (Fig. 20-6D). There is no need to measure the length of ulna to be resected:

the osteotomy must be placed just proximal to the proximal rim of the sigmoid cavity of the radius.[20] The detached head is now grasped with a metal clip and, through traction and rotation, it is sharply freed up from all surrounding tissues and removed together with its styloid process. Although Darrach[16] had recommended that the excision be performed subperiosteally and with preservation of the styloid process, this has not been required in my experience. Dingman[20] compared the results of extra- and subperiosteal resections, with or without the ulnar styloid, and found no significant difference. Through the space created by this resection a synovectomy of the distal radioulnar and ulnocarpal spaces, and at times of the radiocarpal joint as well, can be completed. Also the palmar capsular-periosteal layer comes into view. A flap can be then raised from this palmar capsule and left hinged distally, to be brought over the cut end of the ulna.[7] The edges of the ulnar stump are carefully rounded off until no sharp areas can be felt by palpation (Fig. 20-6E). While the assistant holds the ulna depressed palmarward, this capsular flap is brought over the dorsal rim of the cut end of the ulna and is attached to periosteum or through drill-

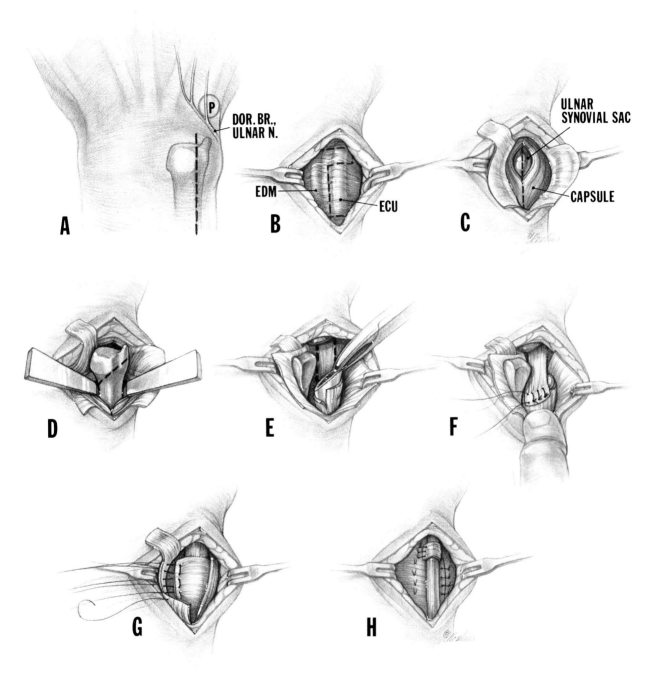

Fig. 20-6. Technique of excision of the head of the ulna. *A*: Incision along the subcutaneous border of the ulna, proximal to the projection of the dorsal branch of the ulnar nerve. *B*: The supratendinous retinaculum is exposed and divided along the interrupted line (ECU, extensor carpi ulnaris; EDM, extensor digit minimi). *C*: The retinacular flaps are elevated. Underlying capsule and synovial sac are divided longitudinally. *D*: The neck of the ulna is exposed subperiosteally and is divided along an oblique plane (interrupted line). *E*: The sharp margins of the cut end of the ulna are rounded off. A palmar capsular flap can be seen, delineated between two interrupted lines. *F*: This flap is freed-up, divided proximally, left attached distally, and brought over the dorsum of the ulna, to which is sutured while an assistant keeps the ulna depressed in a palmar direction. *G*: Dorsal capsule, and *H*: Dorsal retinaculum, are imbricated and sutured. A loop of retinaculum is passed around the ECU tendon, and is sutured to itself.

holes to bone, using nonabsorbable sutures (Fig. 20-6F). If, upon release of the pressure on the ulna and during hyperpronation, the fixation remains firm, no additional support is used. If there are any questions as to the quality of this repair, the forearm is supinated and is kept supinated throughout the remainder of the procedure and early postoperative period. An alternative is to drive a large Kirschner wire across the ulna and radius to maintain supination until stability is achieved at approximately three weeks postoperatively. The rest of the soft tissue repair is completed with the forearm in supination. In some author's experience, stabilization of the ulnar stump may also be achieved by the use of one half of the extensor carpi ulnaris tendon, left attached distally and threaded through the end of the ulna.[25,51] This would accomplish three major objectives: to elevate the ulnar carpus, to depress the ulna palmarward, and to maintain the extensor carpi ulnaris in a corrected dorsal position. Clayton[14] recommended suture of the ulnopalmar capsule to the dorsum of the distal radius to elevate and derotate the ulnar carpus. This capsuloplasty reproduces the direction and function of the ulnocarpal complex (see Chapter 2), which is usually destroyed or detached by rheumatoid disease. The capsule dorsal to the ulna can usually be imbricated over the ulnar stump. The extensor retinaculum is also imbricated, deep to the extensor

carpi ulnaris (Fig. 20-6G), and the extensor carpi ulnaris is brought over dorsally and secured in this position using the retinacular loop previously mentioned (Fig. 20-6H). In some patients, when a transfer of the extensor carpi radialis longus to the insertion of the extensor carpi ulnaris is also contemplated as part of the surgical plan,[13,22] the extensor carpi radialis longus is detached at this point through a small transverse incision on the radial aspect of the base of the second metacarpal. It is withdrawn at the musculotendinous junction and then rerouted subcutaneously into the first ulnar exposure for its attachment to the extensor carpi ulnaris. This transfer, which overlies the cut end of the ulna, helps to further reinforce this dorsal reconstruction. The extensor carpi radialis longus is then sutured to the tendon of the extensor carpi ulnaris, close to its insertion. The skin is closed in layers, and a well-padded dressing is applied. Drains are rarely required. The postoperative care depends on the stability of the distal ulnar stabilization. When this appears strong, postoperative immobilization in supination is recommended for the first seven to ten days, followed by a program of gradual exercises from this resting position in supination toward full pronation. At three weeks postoperatively a short arm splint is used for support and discontinued at six weeks following surgery. If there is any question as to the stability of the ulnar

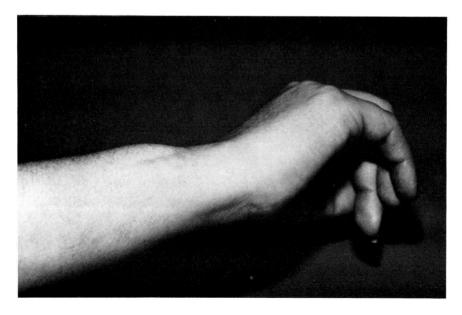

Fig. 20-7. Unstable distal ulna and carpus, following excessive excision of the ulna.

Fig. 20-8. The appearance of the wrist is satisfactory, following distal radioulnar fusion and surgical pseudarthrosis of the ulna (Lauenstein procedure).

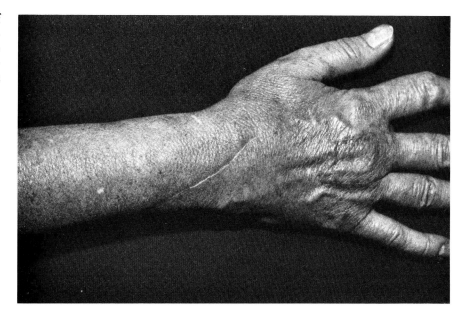

stump, immobilization in supination should be continued for a minimum of three weeks, or else the radioulnar pin introduced during the operative procedure should be maintained for a similar length of time. At three weeks the long arm immobilization is discontinued or the radioulnar pin is removed and an exercise program is begun, using intermittent short arm splinting for comfort and support. At the end of six weeks, all immobilization is discontinued.

TREATMENT OF THE UNSTABLE DISTAL ULNA AFTER EXCISION OF THE ULNAR HEAD

Excessive excision of the ulnar head carries a potential for instability of the ulnar stump. This complication is easier to prevent than to treat.[49] Instability is manifested as an unsightly prominence of the cut end of the ulna against the dorsal skin (Fig. 20-7) and is accompanied by pain, weakness of grip, and clicking during pronation and supination. The clicking may disappear on its own after weeks, (or, rarely, months) of exercises. More frequently, however, it persists and remains disabling, and may occasionally produce bony changes of the radius opposite the end of the ulna. Several techniques have been proposed for the correction of this prob-

lem, all having in common the creation of a palmar restraint to the ulnar stump. If a palmar capsulodesis was not performed at the time of the original excision of the ulnar head, it may be used at this time.[7] The palmaris longus may be detached distally, passed through a drill-hole in the radius, looped around the ulna and sutured to itself,[49] or else used as free graft looped around the flexor carpi ulnaris tendon, to provide a dynamic restraint to the ulna during power gripping.[8] A strip of extensor carpi ulnaris tendon left attached distally and threaded through a drill-hole in the cut end of the ulna has also been proposed as an effective technique for ulnar stabilization.[25]

THE LAUENSTEIN AND BALDWIN PROCEDURES

In 1940, 1946, and 1947, Steindler[55–57] described a procedure which he attributed to Lauenstein, consisting of a fusion across the distal radioulnar joint and an osteotomy proximal to the fusion for restoration of pronation and supination. A search of Lauenstein's contributions to the treatment of wrist problems failed to produce such an article. This operation was actually described by Sauvé and Kapandji in 1936.[52] Lauenstein's name, however, has remained associated with this procedure, largely because of Steindler and also following Gonçalves' report on correction of distal radioulnar joint disorders by what he called "artificial pseudoarthrosis of the ulna."[26] In 1921 Baldwin[4] described an operation consisting of the extracapsular excision of a 1-cm segment of ulna proximal to the ulnar head for the restoration of pronation and supination following radioulnar ankylosis, malunited Colles fractures, or fractures of the shaft of the radius. Baldwin's operation was mentioned by McMurray in his textbook, *A Practice of Orthopaedic Surgery*,[42] and was resurrected by Kersley in a presentation to the autumn meeting of the British Orthopaedic Association in 1977[33] and by Thomas and Matthewson in 1982.[64] According to Gonçalves, both these operations, Lauenstein's and Baldwin's, share all the advantages of the Darrach procedure, but avoid its potential complications, particularly progressive ulnocarpal translocation, ulnar deviation with accompanying instability, pain, and weakness of grip.[26] Gonçalves recommends the Baldwin operation for blocked forearm rotation secondary to malunion of radial fractures with an intact radioulnar joint, and the Lauenstein procedure when the distal radioulnar joint is abnormal due to either subluxation, dislocation, or arthritis. I believe that distal radioulnar fusion with ulnar osteotomy is an excellent operation for the younger patients with painful radioulnar dysfunction: it preserves intact all ulnocarpal support, provides a stable fixation to the ulnar head with restoration of pronation and supination and results in a more pleasing appearance of the wrist, when compared with simple excision of the ulnar head (Fig. 20-8). The second important indication for the Lauenstein operation is the patient in whom the architecture of the distal radius is modified by rheumatoid arthritis, creating the condition for a gradual ulnar translocation of the carpus (Fig. 20-5). The third indication is found in those patients requiring a stable proximal radioulnar surface, either for the support of a proximal carpal row implant or arthroplasty (Fig. 19-11E), or else for patients requiring radiolunate fusions in whom the bony surface opposite the lunate can be augmented by the addition of the ulnar head to the radiolunate fusion mass (Fig. 20-9).

Technique of the Lauenstein Procedure

The distal ulna is approached in a manner similar to that described for simple excision of the ulnar head. After the ulna is exposed supperiosteally, a Kirschner wire is driven through the ulnar head to be used as a handle to manipulate it. The insertion of the Kirschner wire also assures that no artificial rotations will be placed on the ulnar head as it is fused to the distal radius. A small towel clip may be used instead (Fig. 20-10A). An osteotomy is performed tangential to the proximal margin of the flare of the ulnar head, no more than 1 or 2 mm proximal to the border of its articular cartilage. When radioulnar length discrepancy is present and needs correction, usually because of the ulna being too long, the ulnar head must be recessed proximally until it faces the sigmoid cavity of the radius. In all cases, after this ulnar relationship is restored, a segment of ulna is excised, measuring 12 to 14 mm (Fig. 20-10A). Care should be taken to protect the extensor carpi ulnaris while these osteotomies are completed. Using the Kirschner wire or the

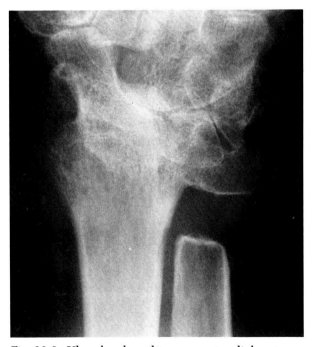

Fig. 20-9. Ulnar head used to augment radiolunate surface area for a radioscapholunate fusion.

Fig. 20-10. The Lauenstein procedure: The distal ulna and the distal radioulnar joint are exposed (see Fig. 20-6A,B,C). *A*: A segment of ulna (12–14 mm in width) is excised (arrow) immediately proximal to the articular surface of the ulnar head (UH). The end of the proximal ulna (PU) can be seen. A towel clip (A) is used to manipulate the ulnar head, and to secure that it is properly oriented for the radioulnar fusion. *B*: The ulnar head is hinged away from the radius. This allows visualization of the ulnocarpal complex (UCC). Excision of the articular surface of the radius is carried out using a power gauge (B). *C*: After both articular surfaces have been excised (arrows), the ulnar head is brought against the radius, to which it is fixed with Kirschner wires or a single screw.

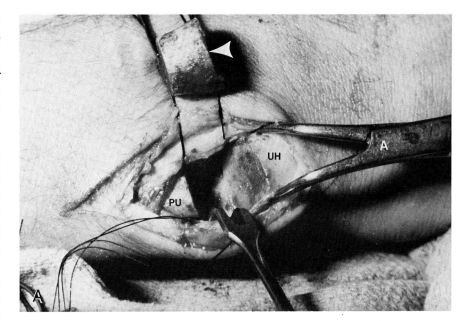

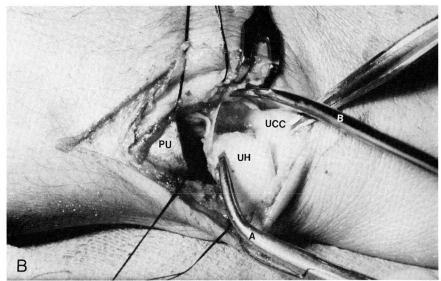

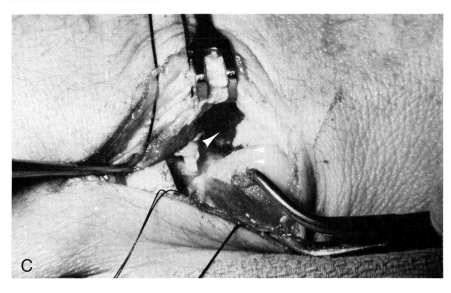

towel clip to handle the head of the ulna, this is hinged away from the radius (Fig. 20-10B), thus exposing both opposing radioulnar articular surfaces; these are excised down to cancellous bone (Fig. 20-10C). The ulnar head is then brought against the radius and is pinned to it using two crisscross 0.054 Kirschner wires (Fig. 20-11). The wires are driven through the radius until their tips are palpable under the skin on the radial aspect of the wrist, from which they will be removed after the fusion becomes solid. On the medial side, they are cut flush with the ulnar surface. Bone grafts obtained from the portion of the ulna that was excised can be inserted into the fusion site to enhance healing. The treatment of the ulnar stump is then completed in a manner similar to that described for a simple excision of the distal ulna, including a palmar capsuloplasty, and dorsoulnar soft tissue reconstruction. The postoperative care is also similar to that described for simple excision of the ulnar head. Controlled motion with intermittent protective splinting may begin a few days after operation, and progress according to the patient's comfort. Splinting should continue for at least four weeks to secure an uneventful fusion of the radioular joint. At this point, one of the two Kirschner-wires is removed. The second Kirschner-wire is maintained until the fusion appears radiologically solid.

RESECTION OF ULNAR HEAD AND ULNAR CAPPING (SWANSON)

In 1972, Swanson introduced the use of a silicone rubber implant, first developed in 1966, for the capping of the ulna following excision of the ulnar head.[59,61] The success of bone capping had been demonstrated in amputation stumps in animals and in the control of overgrowth of long bones in juvenile amputees. Design requisites included a cuff no longer than 1 cm, which was not excessively constrictive of the bony end. The periosteum over the cut end of the ulna was left intact. According to Swanson,[60] this procedure allows a more economical bone resection, maintains the physiologic ulnar length, and consequently helps to prevent ulnocarpal shift. It also provides a smooth surface for articulation with the radius and the carpus, and for the gliding of overlying extensor tendons, and decreases potential bony overgrowth.[5,60,61] The main advantage of this procedure may be a smoother, less painful recovery of function following surgery. Several authors[14,48,53] either consider this an unnecessary addition to the more simple excision of the distal ulna or have abandoned the procedure altogether. The prevention of ulnar translocation is better accomplished with other techniques (Lauenstein's radiolunate fusions). A good indica-

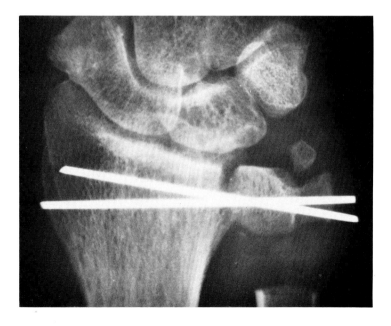

Fig. 20-11. Radiographic appearance immediately following completion of a Lauenstein procedure.

Fig. 20-12. Technique presently recommended by Swanson for fixation of a silicone rubber implant to cap the distal ulna (Modified from Swanson AB: Ulnar head implant resection arthroplasty for disabilities of distal radioulnar joint. In Swanson AB (ed): Flexible Implant Resection Arthroplasty in the Hand and Extremities. Mosby, St. Louis, 1973.)

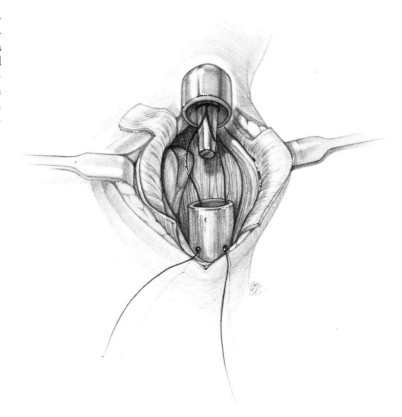

tion for ulnar capping may be the revision of Darrach procedures, when tendon ruptures, or scissoring and snapping of the cut end of the ulna against the radius, have developed postoperatively. Ulnar capping itself is not, unfortunately, free of complications. These include subluxation or dislocation of the implant, which may be minimized by fixation with different suture techniques, and excessive bone resorption under the implant, attributed by Swanson to early design problems producing a too-tight fit of bone between the central stem of the prosthesis and the peripheral cuff. Linscheid[40] described an ulnocarpal implant carved at the time of operation from a block of medical grade silicone, to fill the ulnocarpal space after the ulnar head is removed.

Technique of Implant Resection Arthroplasty of the Distal Ulna (Swanson)

The implant resection arthroplasty of the distal ulna may be performed independently, or as part of more extensive procedures (i.e., radiocarpal arthroplasty). The details of surgical exposure and of excision of the ulnar head have already been presented. After the ulna is sectioned at the neck, and the head excised, the periosteum is not stripped off, but muscle attachments on the anterior surface of the ulnar stump are released over the distal 2 cm. A synovectomy is performed when indicated. The cut end of the ulna is smoothed, and the medullary canal is appropriately reamed to accept a snugly fitting stem. The cuff of the implant should seat loosely over the end of the bone. The implant presents a nonabsorbable polyester retention cord which is passed through two small drill-holes in the distal ulna (Fig. 20-12). Once the implant is well seated, the ends of the cord are tied together. The passage of the cord is facilitated by the use of a looped wire. The usual dorsal soft tissue reconstruction is performed over the implant. The postoperative care is similar to that following a simple excision of the head of the ulna.

REFERENCES

1. Angus: Dislocation of head of ulna, caused by a "back-fire" in starting a motorcar. Northumberland Durham Med J 18:23, 1908–1909

2. Bäckdahl M: The caput ulnae syndrome in rheumatoid arthritis: A study of the morphology, abnormal anatomy and clinical picture. Acta Rheum Scand Suppl 5:1–75, 1963

3. Backhouse KM, Harrison SH, Hutchings RT: Color Atlas of Rheumatoid Hand Surgery. Yearbook Medical Publishers, Chicago, 1981

4. Baldwin WI: In Jones Sir Robert (ed): Orthopedic Surgery of Injuries. Henry Frowde and Hodder and Stoughton, London, 1921

5. Berg E: Indications for and results with the Swanson distal ulnar prosthesis. South Med J 69:858, 1976

6. Black RM, Boswick JA Jr, Wiedel J: Dislocation of the wrist in rheumatoid arthritis. The relationship to distal ulnar resection. Clin Orthop 124:184, 1977

7. Blatt G, Ashworth CR: Volar capsule transfer for stabilization following resection of the distal end of the ulna. Orthop Trans 3:13, 1979

8. Boyes JH: Bunnell's Surgery of the Hand. 5th Ed. Lippincott, Philadelphia, 1970

9. Campbell RD Jr, Straub LR: Surgical considerations for rheumatoid disease in the forearm and wrist. Am J Surg 109:361, 1965

10. Chamay A, Della Santa D: Cinématique du poignet rhumatoïde après résection de la tête du cubitus. Ann Chir 34:711, 1980

11. Chamay A, Della Santa D, Vilaseca A: Radiolunate arthrodesis. Factor of stability for the rheumatoid wrist. Ann Chir Main 2:5, 1983

12. Clayton ML: Surgical treatment at the wrist in rheumatoid arthritis. A review of thirty-seven patients. J Bone Joint Surg [Am] 47:741, 1965

13. Clayton ML, Ferlic DC: Tendon transfer for radial rotation of the wrist in rheumatoid arthritis. Clin Orthop 100:176, 1974

14. Clayton ML: The caput ulnae syndrome: Update. In Strickland JW, Steichen JB: Difficult Problems in Hand Surgery. Mosby, St. Louis, 1982

15. Cracchiolo A, Marmor L: Resection of the distal ulna in rheumatoid arthritis. Arthritis Rheum 12:415, 1969

16. Darrach W: Anterior dislocation of the head of the ulna. Ann Surg 56:802, 1912

17. Darrach W, Dwight K: Derangements of the inferior radioulnar articulation. Med Rec 87:708, 1915

18. Darrach W: Fractures of the lower extremity of the radius. Diagnosis and treatment. JAMA 89:1683, 1927

19. Desault M: Extrait d'un mémoire de M. Desault sur la luxation de l'extrêmité inferieure du radius. J Chir 1:78, 1791

20. Dingman PVC: Resection of the distal end of the ulna (Darrach operation). An end result study of twenty-four cases. J Bone Joint Surg [Am] 34:393, 1952

21. Eiken O: Assessment of surgery of the rheumatoid wrist. Scand J Plast Reconstr Surg 9:207, 1975

22. Ferlic DC, Clayton ML: Tendon transfer for radial rotation in the rheumatoid wrist. J Bone Joint Surg [Am] 55:880, 1973

23. Flatt AE: Care of the Arthritic Hand 4th Ed. Mosby, St. Louis, 1983

24. Freiberg RA, Weinstein A: The scallop sign and spontaneous rupture of finger extensor tendons in rheumatoid arthritis. Clin Orthop 83:128, 1972

25. Goldner JL, Hayes MG: Stabilization of the remaining ulna using one-half of the extensor carpi ulnaris tendon after resection of the distal ulna. Orthop Trans 3:330, 1979

26. Gonçalves D: Correction of disorders of the distal radio-ulnar joint by artificial pseudoarthrosis of the ulna. J Bone Joint Surg [Br] 56:462, 1974

27. Hastings DE, Evans JA: Rheumatoid wrist deformaties and their relation to ulnar drift. J Bone Joint Surg [Am] 57:930, 1975

28. Henderson ED, Lipscomb PR: Surgical treatment of the rheumatoid hand. JAMA. 175:431, 1961

29. Henderson ED, Lipscomb PR: Rehabilitation of the rheumatoid hand by surgical means. Arch Phys Med Rehabil 42:58, 1961

30. Hooper J: The surgery of the wrist in rheumatoid arthritis. Aust NZ J Surg 42:135, 1972

31. Hui FC, Linscheid RL: Ulnotriquetral augmentation tenodesis: A reconstructive procedure for dorsal subluxation of the distal radioulnar joint. J Hand Surg 9:230, 1982

32. Jackson IT, Milward TM, Lee P, Webb J: Ulnar head resection in rheumatoid arthritis. Hand 6:172, 1974

33. Kersley JB: Baldwin's operation for malunited Colles' fracture. J Bone Joint Surg [Br] 60:136, 1978

34. Kessler I, Vainio K: Posterior (dorsal) synovectomy for rheumatoid involvement of the hand and wrist. J Bone Joint Surg 48:1085, 1966

35. Kessler I, Hecht O: Present application of the Darrach procedure. Clin Orthop 72:254, 1970

36. Kulick RG, DeFiore JC, Straub LR, Ranawat CS: Long-term results of dorsal stabilization in the rheumatoid wrist. J Hand Surg 6:272, 1981

37. Lauenstein C: Zur Behandlung der nach karpaler Vorderarmfraktur zurückbleibenden Störung der Pro- und supinations-Bewegung. Zentralbl Chir 23:433, 1887

38. Liebolt FL: A new method for repair of the distal radioulnar ligaments. NY State J Med 50:2817, 1950

39. Linscheid RL: Mechanical forces affecting the deformity of the rheumatoid wrist. Presented at the meeting of the American Society for Surgery of the Hand, New York, 1969

40. Linscheid RL, Dobyns JH: Rheumatoid arthritis of the wrist. Orthop Clin North Am 2:649, 1971

41. Lipscomb PR: Surgery of the arthritic hand: Sterling Bunnell Memorial Lecture. Mayo Clin Proc 40:132, 1965

42. McMurray TP: A Practice of Orthopaedic Surgery. 3rd Ed. Williams & Wilkins, Baltimore, 1949

43. Mikíc ZDJ, Helal B: The value of the Darrach procedure in the surgical treatment of rheumatoid arthritis. Clin Orthop 127:175, 1977

44. Moller M: Forty-eight cases of caput ulnae syndrome treated by synovectomy and resection of the distal end of the ulna. Acta Orthop Scand 44:278, 1973

45. Moore EM: Three cases illustrating luxation of the ulna in connection with Colles' fracture. Med Rec 17:305, 1880

46. Nalebuff EA, Potter TA: Rheumatoid involvement of tendons and tendon sheaths in the hand. Clin Orthop 59:147, 1968

47. Newmeyer WL, Green DP: Rupture of digital extensor tendons following distal ulnar resection. J Bone Joint Surg [Am] 64:178, 1982

48. Nicolle FV, Dickson RA: Surgery of the Rheumatoid Hand. A Practical Manual. Yearbook Medical Publishers, Chicago, 1979

49. Noble J, Arafa M: Stabilization of distal ulna after excessive Darrach's procedure. Hand 15:70, 1983

50. Rana NA, Taylor AR: Excision of the distal end of the ulna in rheumatoid arthritis. J Bone Joint Surg [Br] 55:96. 1973

51. Rowland SA: Stabilization of the ulnar side of the rheumatoid wrist following radio-carpal arthroplasty and resection of the distal ulna. Orthop Trans 6:474, 1982

52. Sauvé, Kapandji: Nouvelle technique de traitement chirurgical des luxations récidivantes isolées de l'extrémité inferieure du cubitus. J. Chir 47:589, 1936

53. Schernberg F, Gerard Y, Collin JP, Teinturier P: Arthroplasty of the rheumatoid wrist by silicone implants. Experience with forty cases. Ann Chir Main 2:18, 1983

54. Smith-Peterson MN, Aufranc OE, Larson CB: Useful surgical procedures for rheumatoid arthritis involving joints of the upper extremity. Arch Surg 46:764, 1943

55. Steindler A: Orthopedic Operations: Indications, Technique and Results. Charles C Thomas, Springfield, IL, 1940

56. Steindler A, Marker JL: The Traumatic Deformities and Disabilities of the Upper Extremity. Charles C Thomas, Springfield, IL, 1946

57. Steindler A: Orthopedic Operations: Indications, Technique and Results. 4th prtg. Charles C Thomas, Springfield, IL, 1947

58. Straub LR, Wilson EH: Spontaneous rupture of the extensor tendons in the hand associated with rheumatoid arthritis. J Bone Joint Surg [Am] 38:1208, 1956

59. Swanson AB: The ulnar head syndrome and its treatment by implant resection arthroplasty. (Abstract). J Bone Joint Surg [Am] 54:906, 1972

60. Swanson AB: Flexible implant resection arthroplasty in the hand and extremities. Mosby, St. Louis, 1973

61. Swanson AB: Implant arthroplasty for disabilities of the distal radioulnar joint. Use of a silicone rubber capping implant following resection of the ulnar head. Orthop Clin North Am 4:373, 1973

62. Taleisnik J: Post-traumatic carpal instability. Clin Orthop 149:73, 1980

63. Taleisnik J: Rheumatoid arthritis of the wrist. In Strickland JW, Steichen JB: Difficult Problems in Hand Surgery. Mosby, St. Louis, 1982

64. Thomas TL, Matthewson MH: Habitual anterior subluxation of the head of the ulna treated by Baldwin's operation. A case report. Hand 14:67, 1982

Index

Page numbers in italic represent illustrations.

A

Anterior interosseous artery
  anatomic location of, 51–54
  recent studies of, 61–62, *64*
Arthrodesis, limited or partial, 135–
  138, *137*
Arthrography, 95–97, *99*

B

Baldwin procedure, 429
Basal metacarpal arch, recent
  studies of, *58*, 59
Bentzon's procedure, in scaphoid
  fracture, 139–140
Bone graft, in scaphoid fracture,
  118–119, *125–129*
Bone scintigraphy, 102
Bones of wrist, 1–12. *See also*
  individual bones.

C

Capitate, 9–10
  intraosseous arterial circulation
    of, *75*, 76–77
  ligament attachment to, 25
Capitate fracture, *159–161*, 160–
  163
  diagnosis of, *161*, 162
  historical, 160

mechanism of injury in, 160–162
  in multiple injuries, *159*, 160, *161*
  treatment of, 162–163
Carpal arcs, radiographic, 81–82, *81*
Carpal bones, 1–12. *See also*
  individual bones.
  dorsal blood supply to, 55,
    64–65, *64*
  palmar, 64–65, *64*
    blood supply to, 55–56, *57*
  vulnerable zone of, 149, *150*
Carpal bridge radiograph, 92–94, *94*
Carpal dislocation and fracture-dis-
    location, 195–228
  classification in, 196, *196*, *197*
  diagnosis of, *200–208*, *202–205*
    radiographic features in,
      202–208, 203–205
    unrecognized, *200–201*,
      202–203
  dorsal transscaphoid perilunate
    dislocation in, *214–217*,
    216–218
  historical, 195
  mechanisms of injury in, 196–
    202, *199*
  in palmar perilunate dislocation
    in, 200–202
  progressive perilunar instability
    in, 198–199, *199*
  terminology in, 195
  transradial-styloid perilunate
    transtriquetral fracture-dislo-
    cation in, 221, 223

transscaphoid perilunate fracture-
    dislocation in, 199–200
  treatment of, 205–225
    dorsal perilunate dislocation,
      206–211, *208–212*
    greater arc injuries, 216–223
    lesser arc injuries, 206–216
    open reduction in, 206
    volar lunate dislocation in,
      211–213
    volar perilunate dislocation/dorsal
      lunate dislocation in, 214–
      216
    volar transscaphoid perilunate
      fracture-dislocation in,
      218–223
Carpal height, 82, *83*
Carpal instability, 229–238
  anatomic basis for classification
    of, 233
  classification of, 233–237
  historical, 229–231
  lateral, 233–235. *See also* Lateral
    carpal instability.
    scaphocapitate diastasis in,
      234–235
    scapholunate dissociation in,
      233–234
    scaphotrapezium-trapezoid
      instability in, *233–234*, 235
  major types of, *230–231*, 231
  medial, 235–237, 281–303. *See
    also* Medial carpal instability
  proximal, *236*, 237, 305–326.

437

Carpal instability *(Continued)*
    See also Proximal carpal
        instability.
    static and dynamic, *230–232,*
        231–233
Carpal kinematics, 39–49
    columnar carpus in, 39–47. *See*
        also Columnar carpus.
    unstable wrist in, *46–47, 47–48*
Carpal translocation
    dorsal, 307–317. *See also* Dorsal
        carpal translocation.
    palmar, *317–321, 320–322. See*
        also Palmar carpal transloca-
        tion.
Carpal tunnel, 1, *2*
Carpal tunnel view, 87–90, *90*
Cineradiography, 95
Clenched-fist radiograph, 94
Columnar carpus, 39–47
    central flexion extension column:
        radiolunocapitate link in,
        40–41
    historical, 39–40, *40–41*
    lateral mobile column: scaphoid
        in, 41–44, *43*
    medial rotation column: trique-
        trum in, *43,* 44–47
Common interosseous artery,
    anatomic location of, 51–54
Computed tomography, 97, *102*

D

Darrach procedure, 423–429, *427*
Deep radioscapholunate ligament.
    See Radioscapholunate
    ligament.
Deep radiolunotriquetral ligament.
    See Radiolunotriquetral
    ligament.
Deltoid ligament, *24,* 25
Digital fluorography, *100–101*
DISI deformity, 291–303
Dorsal carpal arch
    anatomic location of, 54
    in extraosseous circulation, 63
    recent studies of, 58–59, *58*
Dorsal carpal translocation, 307–
    317
    diagnosis of, 308, *316*
    in distal radial fracture, 307–308,
        314–315

dorsal open wedge osteotomy of
    distal radius in, 310–311,
    317, *317–319*
    treatment of, 308, 310–311,
        317, *317–319*
Dorsal intercarpal arch, recent
    studies of, *58,* 59
Dorsal intercarpal ligament, *23,* 25
Dorsal interosseous artery. *See*
    Posterior interosseous artery.
Dorsal radiocarpal arch, recent
    studies of, *58,* 59
Dorsal radiocarpal ligament,
    22–23, *23*
Dorsal radiotriquetral fascicle, 22
Dorsal retinaculum, 29–37, *30–37.*
    See also Extensor retinaculum.

E

Extensor compartments, 31–37,
    33–37
Extensor retinaculum
    infratendinous, 30–31, *30*
    supratendinous, 30, *30–34*
Extraosseous arterial circulation,
    62–66, *65*
Extrinsic ligaments, 13–23, *14. See*
    also individual ligaments.

F

Fluorography, digital, *100–101*
Frondiform ligament, 7
Fusions, limited or partial, 135–
    138, *137*

H

Hamate, 9, *11*
    intraosseous arterial circulation
        of, 77, *77*
Hamate fracture, *162–164, 163–*
    166
    of body, *162,* 164
    diagnosis and treatment in,
        165–166
    of hook, *163–164,* 164
    mechanism of injury in, 164–165
Hereditary multiple exostis, ulnar
    translocation in, 305, *308*

I

Intraosseous arterial circulation,
    66–77
    anterior, 51–54, 61–62, *64*
    capitate, *75,* 76–77
    common, 51–54
    hamate, 77, *77*
    lunate, 68–72, *70–71*
    pisiform, 72, *73*
    posterior, 52–55
    scaphoid, 66–68, *66–69*
    trapezium, 72–76, *76*
    trapezoid, *74,* 76
    triquetrum, 72, *73*
Intrinsic ligaments, *14,* 23–25. *See*
    also individual ligaments.
    intermediate, 24–25, *24*
    long, *24,* 25
    short, 23, *23*

K

Kienböck's disease, 169–194
    avascular necrosis in, 169–170
    capitate-hamate fusion technique
        in, 189
    classification of, 189–190, *190*
    diagnosis of, 174–176, *174–177*
    etiology of, 169–174
    fractures in, 170, *171*
    intercarpal arthrodesis in,
        185–189, *186–189*
    joint leveling operations in,
        181–183, *183*
    lunate excision in, 177–178
        prosthetic replacement with,
            178–180, *179*
    lunate implant in, 180–181,
        181–182
    lunate load stresses in, 173, *173*
    lunate position in, 171, *173*
    lunate types in, 171, *172*
    minus variant theory in, 170
    nonoperative treatment in, 178
    progressive stages of, 189, *190*
    radial shortening technique in,
        183, 184–185
    radiography in, 174–176,
        174–177
    scaphotrapezium-trapezoid
        arthrodesis in, 189. *See also*

Scaphotrapezium-trapezoid fusion, technique. subperiosteal wedge resection of distal radius in, 185, *185* treatment in, 176–190 ulnar minus variant, theory in, 170 ulnar lengthening technique in, 183–184, *184* Kuenz and Testut, ligament of, 15, *18–19*

L

Lateral carpal instability, 233–235
Laterovolar vessels to the scaphoid, *66,* 67
Lauenstein procedure, 429–432, *431–432*
Ligament of Kuenz and Testut, 15, *18–19*
Ligaments of wrist, 13–38. *See also individual ligaments.*
    classification of, *14*
    extrinsic, 13–23
    intrinsic, 23–25
    recapitulation of, 25–29
Linea jugata, 22, *22,* 36, *37*
Lunate, 3–5, *6–7. See also* Kien- böck's disease.
    angle of inclination of, 3, *6*
    dislocation of, volar, 211–213
    intraosseous arterial circulation of, 68–72, *70–71*
    lesion of, radiographic, 82, *82*
    ligament attachment to, 25
Lunatomalacia. *See* Kienböck's disease.
Lunotriquetral ligament, 24
Lunotriquetral instability, 235–236, 281–291

M

Medial carpal instability, 281–303
    triquetrohamate, 236–237, *236,* 291–303
    triquetrolunate, 235–236, *235,* 281–291
Meniscus. *See* Ulnocarpal meniscus homologue.
Meuli wrist prosthesis, 409, *410*
Midcarpal instability, in malunited distal radial fracture, 321– 325, *323–325*

Moneim's tangential posteroanterior radiograph, 91, *93*

N

Navicular fat stripe, in scaphoid fracture, 107–108, *108*

O

Os centrale, 2, *3*

P

Palmar artery, deep, variations of, 54–55
Palmar carpal arch
    anatomic location of, 54
    superficial, 54
    variations of, 55, *56*
Palmar carpal translocation, 317–321, *320–322*
    in Barton's fracture, 317, *320*
    diagnosis of, 319
    rare volar subluxation in, 319, *320*
    treatment of, 319–321, *322*
Palmar radiocarpal ligaments. *See* Volar radiocarpal ligaments.
Palmar radiocarpal ligaments, in radial, neutral, and ulnar de- viation, 26, *26*
Palmar tilt of radius, 80, *81*
Partial arthrodeses (fusions), 135–138, *137*
Pericarpal arterial network, 51–62, *52–64*
    common interosseous artery in, 51–54
    dorsal, *52*
    dorsal carpal arch in, 54
    main artery branches in, 54
    palmar, *53*
    palmar carpal or transverse arch in, 54
    radial artery in, 51
    recent studies on, 56–62
        anterior interosseous artery in, 61–62, *64*
        dorsal arches in, 58–59, *58*
        radial artery in, 60, *60–61*
        recurrent arteries in, 62

techniques for, 56–58
        ulnar artery in, 60–61, *63*
        volar arches in, 59–60, *59*
    superficial and deep palmar arches in, 54
    ulnar artery in, 51
    variations in, 54–56, *56*
Perilunate dislocation, 198–199, *199*
    dorsal, treatment of, 206–211, *208–212*
    dorsal transscaphoid, *214–217,* 216–218
    palmar, 200–202
    volar, dorsal lunate dislocation and, 214–216
Perilunate fracture-dislocation transscaphoid, 199–200, 218– 223
    transtriquetral transradial-styloid, *221,* 223
Pisiform, 7, *8–10*
    intraosseous arterial circulation of, 72, *73*
Pisiform fracture, 152–155, *155–156*
    diagnosis in, 153, *155*
    excision, technique, 153
    mechanism of injury in, 152–153
    treatment in, 153–155, *156*
Poirier, space of, 25
Posterior interosseous artery
    anatomic location of, 52–54
    variations of, 55
Prosthesis, total wrist, 409–417, *410–416*
Proximal carpal instability, 305–326
    dorsal carpal translocation in, 307–317
    malunited distal radius fracture in, 321–325
    palmar carpal translocation in, 317–321
    ulnar translocation in, 305–307
Psoriatic arthritis, ulnar transloca- tion in, 305, *307*

R

Radial artery
    anatomic location of, 51
    recent studies of, 60, *60–62*
    variations of, 54–55

Radial collateral ligament, 13–15, *14–17*
Radial inclination or angulation, *80,* 81
Radial length, *80,* 81–82
Radial recurrent artery, recent studies of, 62
Radiate ligament, 25
Radiocapitate ligament, 15, 27, *27*
Radiocarpal dislocation, *223–224,* 224
Radiographic examination, 79–104
  carpal bridge view, 92–94, *94*
  carpal tunnel view, 87–90, *90*
  clenched-fist, 94
  dynamic view, 90–91, *91–92*
  routine projections in, 79–86
    anteroposterior, 82–83, *84*
    carpal height, 82, *83*
    lateral, 83–85, *85–87*
    oblique, 85–86, *88*
    palmar tilt, *80,* 81
    posteroanterior, lateral, oblique, 79–81, *80*
    radial inclination or angulation, *80,* 81
    radial length, *80,* 81–82
  scaphoid view, 86–87, *89*
  special procedures in, 95–102
  tangential posteroanterior, 91, *93*
  trapezium view, 95, *96*
Radiolunate fusion, 307
Radiolunate ligament, 15
Radiolunocapitate system, in central flexion extension column, 40–41
Radiolunotriquetral ligament, 23, *23*
Radioscaphocapitate ligament, 15, 27, *27*
Radioscapholunate fusion, 307, *313*
Radioscapholunate ligament, 15, *18–19*
Radius, distal, anatomy of, 11
  palmar and dorsal aspects of, 1, *2*
Retinacular septa, 31–37, *33–37*
Rheumatoid arthritis
  arthroplasty in, 396–417
    without endoprosthesis, 397–403, *398–402*
    with endoprosthesis, 409–417, *403–416*
    with flexible implant, 403–409, *406–408*

    indications in, 396–397
    with total wrist prosthesis, 409–417, *410–416*
  basic patterns of, *331,* 332–333
  capsular and ligament repair and reconstruction in, *372,* 373, *374*
  clinical evaluation in, 335–345
    abnormal metacarpal descent in, 345, *346*
    deformity in, 344–345, *345–350*
    extensor tendon rupture in, 341, *344*
    flexor tendon rupture in, 339, *342*
    flexor tenosynovitis in, 339, *342*
    palmar carpal subluxation in, 345, *348*
    palmar subluxation of radius and carpus in, 344–345, *345*
    sublimis test in, 339, *341*
    synovitis in, 335, *336–338*
    tendon ruptures in, 335–344, *339–344*
    tenosynovitis in, 338
  distal ulna in, 412–435
    clinical evaluation of, 421
    implant resection arthroplasty of, 433, *433*
    Lauenstein and Baldwin procedures for, 429–432, *429–432*
    radiographic evaluation of, 421–423, *422–423*
    resection of, 423–429, *425–427*
    restoration of ulnocarpal alignment in, 423, *424*
    treatment of, 423–433
    ulnar head resection and capping in, 432–433
    unstable, ulnar head excision and, *428,* 429
  historical, 327–328
  juvenile, surgery in, 329–332, *330*
  limited arthrodesis in, 392–396, *392–397*
  necrotizing vasculitis and gangrene in, *330*
  radiocarpal dislocation in, *331,* 333

    radiographic evaluation in, 345–355
    distal radioulnar joint in, 351–353
    erosion of ulnar corner of radius and triquetrum in, 351, *354–355*
    pseudocyst of radius and scapholunate dissociation in, 348, *352*
    scaphoid grooving in, 348, *351*
    ulnar styloid and prestyloid recess in, 351, *355*
    ulnar translocation in, 348–351, *353*
    VISI deformity in, 353–355
  stages of, *332–333,* 333–334
  surgery in, 329–334
    indications for, 329
    selection of, 329
  synovectomy in, 365–373
    dorsal, 366
    historical, 365
    indications for, 366
    pain relief in, 366
    surgical technique in, 367–373, *368–372*
  tendon transfers, relocations, repairs in, 373–384
    extensor carpi ulnaris, 373–376
    extensor indicis proprius transfer in, 383
    extensor pollicis longus rupture in, 380–381
    extensor tendon ruptures, 376–383, *377, 378*
    flexor digitorum profundus and superficialis rupture in, *380–382,* 383
    flexor pollicis longus rupture in, 383–384
    flexor tendon rupture in, 380–381, *382*
    loss of little finger extension and, 376, *377–379,* 379
    loss of ring and little finger extension in, *377–379,* 379–380
    scallop sign and, 376, *376*
    single or multiple ruptures of extensor tendons in, 381–383
    surgical technique in, 381–384
    tendon rupture and, *375,* 376

total arthrodesis in, 387–392
  indications for, 387, *388–389*
  Millender and Nalebuff's
    technique in, 391, *391*
  position of wrist fusion in, 387–
    389, *390*
  technique for, 389–392, *391*
treatment of, 365–419. *See also
  individual treatments.*
  bone and joint procedures,
    387–419
  soft tissue procedures, 365–385
ulnar translocation in, 305, *306*
wrist deformity in, 357–363
  coordinates for metacarpal and
    finger deviation in, 357, *359*
  extensor carpi ulnaris in, 359
  intrinsic and extrinsic musculo-
    tendinous units in, 359, *360*
  intrinsic ulnar wing contracture
    in, 357, *358*
  stages of, 357
Rotary subluxation of the scaphoid,
  233–234, 239–279. *See
  Scapholunate dissociation.*
Russe bone graft, in scaphoid
  fracture, 119, *125*

S

Sauvé and Kapandji procedure, 429
Scaphocapitate diastasis, 234–235
Scaphocapitate fracture syndrome,
  159, 160, 161
Scaphocapitate space, 2, *4*
Scaphoid, 3, *5*
  bipartite, 108–110, *110*
  intraosseous arterial circulation
    of, 66–68, *66–69*
  in lateral mobile column, 41–44,
    43
  ligament attachment to, 27, *27*
Scaphoid fat stripe, in scaphoid
  fracture, 107–108, *108*
Scaphoid fracture, 105–148
  bipartition vs, 108–110, *110*
  diagnosis of, 105–111, *106–110*
  of distal third, *141–142*, 142
  fat stripe sign, 107–108, *108*
  history in, 105
  incidence of, 105

laminogram and isotopic scanning
  in, 108, *109*
mechanism of injury in, 111, *112*
of middle third, 112–140
  arthroplasty in, 122–133,
    131–136
  asymptomatic nonunion in,
    117, *124*
  Bentzon's procedure in,
    139–140
  bone graft in, 118–119,
    125–129
  classification of, 114, *114*
  DISI pattern in, *108*, 112
  displaced, 116, *123*
  horizontal fracture, 114, *116*
  immobilization in, 114–115,
    118–122
  nonoperative treatment in,
    114–115, *114, 116–122*
  operative treatment of, 116–
    140
  osteosynthesis in, 120–122,
    129–130
  partial arthrodesis in, 133–
    138, *137*
  prosthetic replacements in,
    124–125, 130, *131–135*
  proximal row carpectomy in,
    130–133, *136*
  pulsing electromagnetic field
    treatment in, 115, *120–122*
  radial styloidectomy in,
    138–139, *138–139*
  scaphoid excision in, 122–123
  screw fixation in, 121–122,
    129–130
  transverse fracture, 114, *116*
  vertical oblique fracture, 114,
    117
  VISI pattern in, 112, *113*
  navicular fat stripe in, 107–108,
    108
  of proximal third, *139–140*,
    141–142
  radiography in, 105–107,
    106–107
  treatment of, 111–142
Scaphoid view, 86–87, *89*
Scaphoid-trapezium ligaments, 24,
  24
Scapholunate dissociation, *230*,
  233–234, 239–279

diagnosis in, 242–254
  arthrography in, 254
  associated dissociation in, 243,
    243–245
  bone scan in, *251*, 254
  cineradiograph in, 248–249,
    251, 254
  cortical ring sign in, 245,
    248–250
  dynamic subluxation of scaph-
    oid in, 243, *246*
  frontal radiograph in, 245–
    248, *248–250*
  lateral radiograph in, 248, *250*
  primary dissociations, *241*, 242
  scaphoid foreshortening in,
    245, *248–250*
  scaphoid ring proximal pole
    distance in, 245, *250*
  scapholunate gap in, 245,
    248–249
  scapholunotriquetral correla-
    tion in, 245, *248–250*
  secondary dissociations, 242–
    243, *242*
mechanism of injury in, 239–
  242, *240*
treatment in, 254–277
  chronic dissociation in, *256–
    261*, 258
  dorsal capsuloligamentodesis
    in, 258, 262, *262*
  fusion in, *276*, 277
  osteoarthritis in, 270–277,
    272–276
  primary dissociation, *252–254*,
    255
  scaphoid-trapezium-trapezoid
    arthrodesis in, 262–270,
    264–271
  scaphotrapezium trapezoid
    fusion in, 264–270, *264–271*
  secondary dissociation, *254–
    255*, 255–258
Scapholunate ligament, 25
Scaphotrapezium-trapezoid fusion
  (technique), 267–270, 271
Scaphotrapezium-trapezoid
  instability, 233–234
Scintigraphy, bone, 102
Space of Poirier, 25
Swanson wrist implants
  lunate, 180

Swanson wrist implants (*Continued*)
  scaphoid, 130
  ulnar lead, 432
  wrist, 403–409

T

Tomography, 95, *98*
  computed, 97, *102*
Transverse arch, anatomic location
    of, 54
Trapezium, 11
  intraosseous arterial circulation
    of, 72–76, *76*
Trapezium fracture, 155–158
  diagnosis in , 156–157
  dislocation in, 156, *157*
  isolated, 155, *156*
  mechanism of injury in, 156
  treatment in, 157–158
Trapezium view, 95, *96*
Trapezoid, 11
  fracture of, 158–160, *158*
  intraosseous arterial circulation
    of, *74*, 76
Triangular fibrocartilage, 17–20,
    20–21
Triquetrohamate dissociation. *See*
    Triquetrohamate instability.
Triquetrohamate instability,
    236–237, *236*, 291–303
  diagnosis of, *294–297*, 297–298
  historical, 291–294
  lunate stabilization, tenodesis,
    capsulodesis in, *298–301*,
    299–301
  mechanism of, *291–293*, 294–297
  midcarpal stabilization in,
    301–303, *302*
  treatment of, 298–303, *298–302*
Triquetrolunate dissociation. *See*
    Triquetrolunate instability.
Triquetrolunate instability, 235–
    236, *235*, 281–291

diagnosis of, 284–288, *287–288*
  historical, 281
  mechanism of, 281–284, *282–
    286*
  treatment of, 288–291, *289–291*
Triquetropisiform system, 7
Triquetrum, 5–7, *7–8*
  fracture of, 149–152, *150–155*
  intraosseous arterial circulation
    of, *72, 73*
  ligament attachment on, 27–29,
    28–29
  in medial rotation column, *43*,
    44–47
Triquetrum fracture, 149–152,
    150–155
  avulsion, 150, *151*
  diagnosis of, 150–151, *152*
  dislocation in, *154–155*
  dorsal cortical, 150, *152*
  lunate aspect in, 149, *151*
  mechanism of injury in, 149–
    150, *150–151*
  transverse, 149, *150*
  treatment of, 152, *154*

U

Ulna, distal, palmar and dorsal
    aspects of, 1, *2*
Ulna, variants, 170
Ulnar artery
  anatomic location of, 51
  recent studies of, 60–61, *63*
  variations of, 54–55
Ulnar collateral ligament, 20
Ulnar recurrent artery, recent
    studies of, 62
Ulnar styloid, varying lengths in,
    17, *19*
Ulnar translocation, 305–307
  diagnosis of, 305–306, *309–310*
  in hereditary multiple exostosis,
    305, *308*

in psoriatic arthritis, 305, *307*
  radiolunate and radioscapholun-
    ate fusion in, 307, *313*
  in rheumatoid arthritis, 305, *306*
  treatment of, 306–307, *311–313*
Ulnocarpal complex, 17–22, *19–22*
Ulnocarpal meniscus homologue,
    17–20, *20–21*
Ulnolunate ligament, 20
Unstable wrist, *46–47, 47–48*

V

V ligament, *24*, 25
Vascular anatomy of wrist, 51–78.
    See also individual vessels.
  extraosseous arterial circulation,
    62–66
  intraosseous arterial circulation,
    66–77
  pericarpal arterial network,
    51–62
VISI, dynamic, 291–303
VISI, static, 281–291
Volar carpal arch
  in extraosseous circulation, 63
  recent studies of, 59–60, *59*
Volar carpal translocation. *See* Pal-
    mar carpal translocation.
Volar intercarpal ligament, long, *24*,
    25
Volar radiocarpal arch, 59
  recent studies of, 59, *59*
Volar radiocarpal ligaments, 15,
    17–19, 24
Volz wrist prosthesis, 409, *411*

W

Watson's test, 244–245, 247
Wrist, unstable, *46–47, 47–48*